CANCER SYMPTOM MANAGEMENT

Jones and Bartlett Series in Oncology

CANCER SYMPTOM MANAGEMENT

Second Edition

EDITED BY

Connie Henke Yarbro, RN, MS, FAAN

Clinical Associate Professor
Division of Hematology/Oncology
Adjunct Clinical Assistant Professor
Sinclair School of Nursing
Editor, *Seminars in Oncology Nursing*
University of Missouri–Columbia
Columbia, Missouri

Margaret Hansen Frogge, RN, MS

Vice President, Strategic Development
and System Integration

Riverside Health Care
Kankakee, Illinois

Assistant Professor, Associate Faculty
Rush University College of Nursing

Rush-Presbyterian-St.Luke's Medical Center
Chicago, Illinois

Michelle Goodman, RN, MS

Oncology Clinical Nurse Specialist
Rush Cancer Institute
Assistant Professor of Nursing
Rush University College of Nursing

Rush-Presbyterian–St. Luke's Medical Center
Chicago, Illinois.

JONES AND BARTLETT PUBLISHERS
Sudbury, Massachusetts
BOSTON   TORONTO   LONDON   SINGAPORE

World Headquarters
Jones and Bartlett Publishers
40 Tall Pine Drive
Sudbury, MA 01776
978-443-5000

Jones and Bartlett Publishers Canada
2100 Bloor Street West
Suite 6-272
Toronto, ON M6S 5A5
CANADA

Jones and Bartlett Publishers International
Barb House, Barb Mews
London W6 7PA
UK

Copyright © 1999 by Jones and Bartlett Publishers, Inc.

Library of Congress Cataloging-in-Publication Data

Cancer symptom management / edited by Connie Henke Yarbro . . . [et al.].
—2nd ed.
    p.   cm. — (Jones and Bartlett series in oncology)
    Includes bibliographical references and index.
    ISBN 0-7637-0864-X
    1. Cancer—Nursing.   2. Cancer—Palliative treatment.
I. Groenwald, Susan L.   II. Series: The Jones and Bartlett series
in oncology
    [DNLM 1. Oncologic Nursing—methods.   2. Neoplasms—nursing.
3. Neoplasms—complications.   WY 156 C2205 1999]
RC266.C35644   1999
616.99′406—dc21
DNLM/DLC
for Library of Congress   98-43134
                                                                                 CIP

Acquisitions Editor: Greg Vis
Production Editor: Linda DeBruyn
Manufacturing Buyer: Therese Brauer
Design/Editorial Production Service/Typesetting: Modern Graphics
Cover Design: Dick Hannus
Printing and Binding: Courier Westford

Printed in the United States of America
02 01 00 99   10 9 8 7 6 5 4 3 2 1

Contents

v

Contributors

Laurel A. Barbour, RN, MSN, AOCN
Department of Surgical Oncology
University of Illinois at Chicago
Chicago, IL

Andrea M. Barsevick, RN, DNSC, AOCN
Psychosocial Support Nurse
Director of Nursing Research and Education
Fox Chase Cancer Center
Philadelphia, PA

Susan L. Beck, PhD, AOCN, APRN
Research Associate Professor
Nurse Researcher
University of Utah, College of Nursing
Salt Lake City, UT

Donna L. Berry, RN, PhD, AOCN
Research Assistant Professor
Behavioral Nursing and Health Systems
University of Washington
Seattle, WA

Virginia Bourne, RN, MSN
Clinical Nurse Specialist, Thanatology/Oncology
St. Luke's Medical Center
Milwaukee, WI

Deborah Watkins Bruner, RN, MSN
Clinical Nurse Specialist
Director, Prostate Cancer Risk Assessment Program
Department of Radiation Oncology
Fox Chase Cancer Center
Philadelphia, PA
Doctoral student
University of Pennsylvania

Carol P. Curtiss, RN, MSN, OCN®
Clinical Nurse Specialist Consultant
Consultant, Cancer Care
Greenfield, MA

Marylin J. Dodd, RN, PhD, FAAN
Professor and Associate Dean
Department of Physiological Nursing
University of California
San Francisco, CA

Jane V. Dyonzak, PhD
Assistant Professor, Psychology and Social Sciences
Laboratory Director, Sleep Disorders Service and
    Research Center
Rush-Presbyterian–St. Luke's Medical Center
Chicago, IL

Margaret Hansen Frogge, RN, MS
Vice President, Strategic Development and System
    Integration
Riverside Health Care
Kankakee, IL
Assistant Professor, Assistant Faculty
Ruch University College of Nursing
Rush-Presbyterian-St. Luke's Medical Center
Chicago, IL

Michelle Goodman, RN, MS
Oncology Clinical Nurse Specialist
Rush Cancer Institute
Assistant Professor of Nursing
Rush University College of Nursing
Rush-Presbyterian–St. Luke's Medical Center
Chicago, IL

Barbara Holmes Gobel, RN, MS
Oncology Clinical Nurse Specialist
Gottlieb Memorial Hospital
Melrose Park, IL
Instructor, Complemental
Rush University College of Nursing
Chicago, IL
Adjunct Faculty
Northern Illinois University
Dekalb, IL

Mel Haberman, PhD, RN, FAAN
Associate Dean for Research and Professor
Washington State University College of Nursing
Spokane, WA

Kerry V. Harwood, RN, MSN
Clinical Nurse Specialist
Director, Cancer Patient Education Program
Duke University Medical Center
Durham, NC

Carol S. Heckman, RN, BSN
Director, Healing Partners
Annapolis, MD

Ryan R. Iwamoto, MN, ARNP, AOCN
Clinical Nurse Specialist
Section of Radiation Oncology
Virginia Mason Clinic
Seattle, WA
Clinical Instructor
Department of Physiological Nursing
School of Nursing
University of Washington
Seattle, WA

Lucinda A. (Cindy) Jones, RN, MS, AOCN
Oncology Clinical Nurse Specialist
San Diego Veterans Healthcare System
San Diego, CA

Barbara Hansen Kalinowski, RN, MSN, AOCN
Oncology Clinical Nurse Specialist
Clinical Research Nurse
Joint Center for Radiation Therapy
Boston, MA

Patricia E. Lawler, RN, MS
Educator/Private Practice
Glenview, IL

Virginia R. Martin, MSN, RN, AOCN
Clinical Director, Ambulatory Care
Fox Chase Cancer Center
Philadelphia, PA

Carole Hennessy Martz, RN, MS, OCN®
Clinical Coordinator
Breast Health and Mammography Center
Evanston Hospital
Evanston, IL

Roxanne W. McDaniel, RN, PhD
Associate Professor
Sinclair School of Nursing
University of Missouri–Columbia
Columbia, MO

Ann E. McDonald, RN, MN
Oncology Nurse Manager
Group Health Plan
Brentwood, MO

Judith Kehs Much, RN, MSN, AOCN
Oncology Clinical Nurse Specialist
Psychosocial Support Nurse
Fox Chase Cancer Center
Philadelphia, PA

Judith A. Paice, RN, PhD, FAAN
Clinical Nurse Specialist, Pain Management
Department of Neurosurgery
Rush-Presbyterian–St. Luke's Medical Center
Chicago, IL
Associate Professor, College of Nursing
Rush University
Chicago, IL

Julie Pruett, RN, MS
Clinical Nurse Specialist
Bone Marrow Transplant
Rush Cancer Institute
Rush-Presbyterian–St. Luke's Medical Center
Chicago, IL

Dianne M. Reeves, RN, OCN®
Head, Protocol Office
Medicine Branch, COP, DCT
National Cancer Institute
Bethesda, MD

Verna A. Rhodes, RN, EdS, FAAN
Associate Professor
Sinclair School of Nursing
University of Missouri–Columbia
Columbia, MO

Alison M. Seiz, RN, MSN, AOCN
Breast Case Nurse Specialist
Cancer Institute of St. John's Hospital
Springfield, IL

Brenda K. Shelton, RN, MS, CCRN, AOCN
Critical Care Clinical Nurse Specialist
The Johns Hopkins Oncology Center
Baltimore, MD

Nancy S. Tait, RN, BSN, OCN®
Research Nurse
Greenbaum Cancer Center
Baltimore, MD

Lisa Turnbough, RN, AA
Nurse Clinician II
The Johns Hopkins Oncology Center
Baltimore, MD

Janet Ruth Walczak, RN, MSN, CRNP
Nurse Practicioner
Breast Cancer Program
The Johns Hopkins Oncology Center
Baltimore, MD

Rita Wickham, RN, PhD, AOCN
Assistant Professor
Rush College of Nursing
Practitioner-Teacher
Rush-Presbyterian–St. Luke's Medical Center
Chicago, IL

Gail M. Wilkes, RNC, MSN, ANP, AOCN
Oncology Nurse Practioner
Boston Medical Center
Cancer Care Center
Boston, MA

Maryl L. Winningham, MSN, APRN, PhD, FACSM
Executive Director
Institute for the Advancement of Health
   Care Engineering
Salt Lake City, UT

Debra Wujcik, RN, MSN, AOCN
Clinical Director
VCC Affiliate Network Office
The Vanderbilt Cancer Center
Adjunct Faculty
Vanderbilt University School of Nursing
Nashville, TN

Connie Henke Yarbro, RN, MS, FAAN
Clinical Associate Professor
Division of Hematology/Oncology
Adjunct Clinical Assistant Professor
Sinclair School of Nursing
Editor, *Seminars in Oncology Nursing*
University of Missouri–Columbia
Columbia, MO

Suzanne B. Yellen, PhD
Assistant Professor, Psychology and Social Sciences
Clinical Director, Division of Psychosocial Oncology
Rush Cancer Institute
Rush-Presbyterian–St. Luke's Medical Center
Chicago, IL

Preface

When patients with cancer and their families are asked what bothers them most about their treatment or disease, they respond with examples of how the problems resulting from cancer or its treatment affect their daily activities. Although these problems may seem minor to health professionals, they often make life difficult and frustrating for the individual experiencing the problem. The nurse who is trying to help the patient and family needs information about the problems that occur, identification of available options for management of the problem, and information about how to teach the patient and family to provide care at home.

Cancer Symptom Management continues to provide such information to the clinical oncology nurse. The most common problems experienced by individuals with cancer are addressed. All problems are identified as "symptoms" in this text. We recognize that some of the problems identified are not symptoms but *signs* or *syndromes*; however, rather than concern ourselves with the semantic distinctions among these terms we have focused on the important task of identifying the most common problems that individuals with cancer experience, describing how the problem affects the quality of the individual's life and identifying what the nurse can do to help relieve or diminish the patient's and family's suffering.

The health care environment for the majority of individuals with cancer has shifted from the hospital to the ambulatory care setting and the home. The challenge to health professionals is to provide quality care and to meet the educational and care needs of patients within the fluid environment of the ambulatory care setting and the home. Early hospital discharge and the performance of procedures on an outpatient basis have resulted in inadequate opportunity for patient teaching, and often patients and families are ill-prepared for the problems that may occur once they are home. Nurses are therefore challenged as to how to provide patients and their families with the information they need in the short time allotted.

Cancer Symptom Management is written by nurses and allied professionals who are recognized for their expertise as practitioners and who understand the frustrations of the changes in the health care arena and the impact these changes have had on quality of patient care. In Chapter 1, Rhodes and McDaniel define terms and differentiate between symptom occurrence and experience. In Chapter 2, Haberman identifies the ways in which symptoms are measured so that nurses can evaluate the impact of their interventions. In Chapter 3, Dodd describes the importance of self-care and how nurses can assist patients and families to prepare to care for the patient at home. The contributors of the remaining chapters provide updated creative approaches to management of the most common problems experienced by cancer patients. These include symptoms of disturbances of comfort, alterations in nutrition, disturbances of protective mechanisms, alterations in fluid and electrolyte balance, disturbances in elimination, and alterations in coping.

Two new chapters have been added to this second edition. Because new chemotherapy drugs and biologic response modifiers have caused an increased incidence of arthralgias and myalgias in many patients, a chapter has been devoted to this problem. The other new chapter to this edition is entitled "Saying Good-Bye". Based on clinical experience, reader input and comments from patients and families, it was apparent that too often discussions regarding end-of-life issues do not occur. This chapter describes ways in which the nurse can help patients to begin thinking more about end-of-life issues, how they want to be remembered, and how they want to say good-bye to their loved ones.

Unique to this text are the patient self-care guides. For each problem discussed, at least one self-care tool is provided at the end of the chapter to assist in teaching the patient and family how to provide care at home. Feedback from our readers, patients, and family members have been incorporated in these updated self-care guides. They are written in a form that patients can understand and use. The reader is encouraged to adapt these self-care guidelines to their practice.

We acknowledge the challenges and opportunities faced by our readers and their patients who provide our purpose for this endeavor. We hope that this text will be helpful to both nurses and their patients, whatever the clinical setting.

Connie Henke Yarbro
Margaret Hansen Frogge
Michelle Goodman

PART I

THE PROBLEMS OF SYMPTOM DISTRESS

CHAPTER 1

The Symptom Experience and Its Impact on Quality of Life

Verna A. Rhodes, RN, EdS, FAAN
Roxanne W. McDaniel, RN, PhD

The Symptom Experience

Each patient's journey with cancer is unique. While different individuals may develop the same symptoms, the cause of and the person's response to those symptoms may vary. In most instances, the distress a person experiences from a symptom becomes greater as the symptom persists, even if the symptom does not intensify.

Management of the symptom experience merits high priority for both the patient with cancer and the nurse caring for the patient. Appropriate management of symptoms promotes higher quality of life, preventing needless suffering and distress. Teaching the patient and family about the symptom experience enhances coping and self-care behaviors and eases the journey.

Definitions

Symptom

A *symptom* is a patient's subjective evidence of disease or of physical disturbance. As differentiated from *signs*, which are objective and observable, symptoms are not observable. They can be perceived and verified only by the person experiencing them; they cannot be observed, perceived, or verified by others. Symptoms may or may not be related specifically to a medical problem and may have a strong psychosocial element. They may be either continuous or intermittent. The distress caused by a symptom may escalate over time. Therefore, the symptom experience affects patients' self-care and coping abilities and their quality of life.[1]

Symptom experience

The concepts of symptom occurrence and symptom distress were first linked with the term "symptom experience" when Rhodes et al.[2] discussed nausea and vomiting in terms of patterns of symptom experiences. *Symptom experience* was defined as the patient's perception and response to symptom occurrence and distress.[2]

Symptom occurrence

Symptom occurrence comprises the *frequency* (the number of times the event occurs within a given time frame), the *duration* (the persistence or continuance of the prevailing subjective happening), and *severity* (the amount and degree of discomfort) with which the symptom occurs.[3] The severity or harshness of symptoms can be perceived, verified, and rated by the individual according to the amount or degree of discomfort: i.e., mild, moderate, or severe.

Symptom distress

Symptom distress is an entity different from symptom occurrence. It is the degree or amount of physical or mental upset, anguish, or suffering experienced from the specific symptom.[3] The ability of the individual to be aware of or to perceive the degree of physical or mental anguish caused by the symptom experience is affected by various factors, e.g., age, socioeconomic levels, culture, family role, education, health knowledge, values, and past experiences. Distress can best be measured with self-report tools. Each symptom can be assessed separately for occurrence and for the distress.

Conceptual Framework

Although symptoms have been referred to frequently in the nursing literature and nursing texts since Nightingale, most nursing authors and theorists have failed to provide a framework for the appropriate application of knowledge about symptom experience to nursing practice. The theory of self-regulation is used to explain the mechanisms underlying the behavioral component of coping in response to a stressful event.[4] The depth and research base of their self-regulation theory make it useful to the practitioner. Of particular importance is the description of parallel responses to stressful stimuli; i.e., a single stressful event evokes both a cognitive (objective) response and an emotional (subjective) response. Symptoms are described as concrete representations of disease that are components of cognitive processing by the individual experiencing the symptom. Emotional responses to the stress of symptoms of disease and to the disease itself are separate responses. This differentiation of the occurrence of a symptom (a concrete, objective event) from the emotional response to the event is critical to the further understanding and treatment of the individual experiencing symptoms.

Individuals exert control over their life situations by caring for themselves. Orem's Self-Care Deficit Theory of Nursing provides a framework in which to assess the ability of the individual experiencing symptoms from cancer to care for himself or herself, and helps define appropriate nursing actions.[5] An individual is assessed for (1) the capacity or potential for action, (2) the demand or need for action, and (3) the ability to meet the demand. Human and environmental factors ("basic conditioning factors") are used to examine a patient's needs for self-care and his or her ability to cope based on past, present, and future conditions. Table 1-1 provides an example of an assessment of basic conditioning factors.[6] Once an individual's ability to care for self is assessed, Orem's theory provides a framework for identifying the method or measure most appropriate to meet the required action.

Larson et al.[7] developed a model for symptom management applicable to symptoms and patient populations in a variety of settings. The model has three dimensions—symptom experience, management strategies, and symptom outcomes—and was derived from research and practice. The premise of the theory is that to manage a symptom effectively, all three dimensions must be considered. The model is in early stages of development and will require further research for refinement.

Assessment

Because the symptom experience is not outwardly observable, it can be measured only through the report of the person being assessed. Accurate assessment techniques and reliable and valid measurement tools that measure symptom occurrence separately from symptom distress and thus adequately assess a patient's symptom experiences are required.

Several researchers have developed instruments to measure symptom distress and symptom occurrence. Instruments are available to measure a single symptom, such as the Piper Fatigue Scale[8] and the Rhodes Index of Nausea and Vomiting.[9] Other instruments measure the occurrence and distress of a variety of symptoms. For example, Rhodes, Watson, and Johnson developed the Adapted Symptom Distress Scale Form 1 (ASDS-1) in 1984.[10] Further revision and differentiation between the occurrence of the symptom and the emotional response to the symptom resulted in Form 2 of the ASDS.[11] The ASDS-2 established separate scales for distress and occurrence of fourteen symptoms, thereby producing a measurement of symptom experience. Appearance, lacrimation, changes in body temperature, nausea, vomiting, breathing, sleeping, pain, concentration, restlessness, coughing, bowel elimination, eating, and fatigue are the symptoms measured by the ASDS-2. The ASDS-2 has been used extensively to study the components and dimensions of nausea, vomiting, and concomitant symptoms, and to aid in the development of effective nursing interventions.[12] It has also been used to examine the symptom experience of women receiving chemotherapy for breast cancer,[13] and to measure the effect of antiemetic regimens in the control of postchemotherapy symptoms.[14]

In the 1990s, research began to expand the focus to understanding symptoms from the perspective of caregivers and patients. One study correlated patient and caregiver rating of cancer pain[15] and discovered that caregivers often seriously underestimate the amount of pain the patient experiences. Another study documented that patients with late-stage cancer reported a higher prevalence of dyspnea than nurses reported.[16] In a study of bone marrow transplant patients, it was reported that nurses' overall perceptions of symptom distress were less than those of their patients.[17] Kurtz et al.[18] found that family caregivers accurately reported patients' symptom occurrence approximately 71% of the time. Fatigue was the symptom most often accurately reported by family caregivers. Rhodes, McDaniel, and Matthews[19] found that

TABLE 1-1   An Example of an Assessment of the Basic Conditioning Factors

Personal and sociocultural	
Age	30 years
Sex	Male
Family	Married (2nd marriage) with a son, 2, and a daughter, 8 (daughter from first marriage); mother and father divorced, 1 stepbrother.
Education level	Two years junior college
Occupation	Cook at pizza parlor; works 60 hours per week.
Religion	Baptist; not currently attending.
Sociocultural orientation	White, lower middle class, raised by mother, stepfather on West Coast.
Relevant life experience	Grandmother had lung cancer and received chemotherapy: "She had a horrible death." Believes cancer is one of the worst things that can happen to a person.
Social roles	Husband, father, breadwinner
Patterns of living	
Living environment and family system	Lives with wife and children in ground-level duplex with one bathroom, 40 miles from hospital; wife doesn't drive.
Health habits (self-care practices)	Considers himself to have good body and oral hygiene, although his teeth are in poor repair; doesn't eat well-balanced meals; prefers food high in fat. Sees a physician or dentist only when he has a problem—no routine checkups.
	Takes Tylenol for pain; uses over-the-counter cold medications when needed.
Support systems	Main source of support is his wife; describes himself as not having many friends: "I've moved around a lot"; communicates very little with extended family.
Preferred learning style	Likes to read; does not feel comfortable in groups; prefers one-to-one demonstration.
Health state and healthcare systems	
Present health concerns	Recently diagnosed with lymphoma. Patient sought medical help for neck pain following a mishap at work, and feeling tired. Neck pain presently controlled by pain medications. Hospitalized for diagnostic workup and treatment.
Previous health concerns and self-care actions	Previous problem with drug abuse. Quit "cold turkey"; neck pain due to work injury; took prescribed medications and used local comfort measures that were effective. No other hospitalizations.
Perception of healthcare	Generally views system as helpful, but somewhat distrustful due to experience with grandmother with cancer.
Developmental state	Early adult transitions—does not consider himself to have yet found a career; interested in becoming a chef.
Self-management system for care—physical, emotional, spiritual	Seeks medical advice/help only when he has a problem. Usually waits to see if it will get better before seeking help due to financial concerns. Copes by being by himself and talking to his wife; smokes more when upset. Requested to see chaplain.

Johnson MH, Rhodes VA: Patient education, in Perry MC (ed): *The Chemotherapy Source Book* (ed 2). Baltimore: Williams & Wilkins, 1997, p. 1009.[6] Reprinted by permission.

nurses caring for hospice patients tended to rate symptom experience higher than patients themselves.

Chapter 2 of this book, The Measurement of Symptom Distress, provides a thorough discussion of various measurement instruments and how they are used.

Relationship of the Cancer Experience to Quality of Life

Definitions of Quality of Life

The term "quality of life" entered the American vocabulary in the middle of the twentieth century. Although the term is used in many different contexts, there is a lack of agreement about its definition and proper use in nurs-ing and healthcare. To further complicate matters, "quality of life" is often used interchangeably with the term "quality life," giving the impression that quality of life is always positive. "Quality of life" is often used in legislation and development of public policy, and the aim of improving quality of life is frequently used as a research goal. It has become a common outcome variable in evaluating cancer treatment and nursing care for these patients. However, the literature fails to reveal a consistent definition for the term.

Several dimensions of quality of life have been identified in the literature. The most commonly listed are socioeconomic status, physical health, relationships with friends and family, and satisfaction with self.[20–22] According to Grant et al.,[23] quality of life is "a personal statement of the positivity or negativity of attributes that characterize life" (p. 108). Bland[20] maintains that quality of life is determined by the patient's perception of the physical, psychosocial, and emotional outcomes of healthcare treatment. The terms "well-being" and "satisfaction" are often used interchangeably for quality of life.[24,25] Ferrell[26] defines quality of life as a personal sense of well-being, encompassing physical, psychological, social, and spiritual dimensions. Others include well-being as a dimension of quality of life.[27,28]

"Life satisfaction" is frequently used as a synonym for quality of life. Many authors view life satisfaction as an indication of an individual's well-being.[21,27] Salamon[29] maintained that "the concept of life satisfaction is a construct universally accepted as a valid measurement of qualify of life" (p. 45).

McDaniel and Bach[30] contend that quality of life is a more inclusive concept than life satisfaction. Life satisfaction or dissatisfaction may be one expression used to describe quality of life, but the terms are not synonymous. Based on a concept analysis, McDaniel and Bach defined quality of life as a unique, individual, dynamic concept that is influenced by the various dimensions of an individual's life. Quality of life is relative to the situation of each individual. The experience of cancer and the symptom occurrence and symptom distress associated with cancer may change an individual's criteria and evaluation of quality of life.

Impact of the Cancer Symptom Experience on Quality of Life

The meanings people assign to physical sensations may have profound implications for their physical and psychological health and, therefore, their quality of life. Somatic perception incorporates the attributions, goals, coping strategies, and prior hypotheses of the perceiver.[31–33] In fact, symptoms initiate the decision-making process and play a continuing role throughout the patient's experience of cancer. During the acute illness episode, symptoms serve as targets for coping and as points of reference for appraising coping outcomes. Although actual physical functioning and occurrence of symptoms may influence a person's quality of life, what may be more important is the extent to which the deficits and symptoms cause distress to the patient. This is exemplified in a study by Rathmell et al.,[34] which compared the quality of life of patients with head and neck cancer who received radiation therapy alone to the quality of life of those who received both radiation and surgical therapy. Similar quality of life in areas of pain severity, mouth dryness, and taste and appetite impairment was reported for both groups. However, qualitative data from these two patient groups indicated that self-reported quality of life was diminished when patients were unable to eat normally, had a reduced capacity to carry out self-care and domestic tasks, and had uncertainty regarding the outcome of their disease and the future.

The cancer symptom experience (symptom occurrence and symptom distress) may affect all components of quality of life: socioeconomic, physical health, relationships with friends and family, and satisfaction with self. The concern about quality of life during and after cancer treatment has increased dramatically because of the heightened awareness of the effect of cancer treatment on all dimensions of quality of life. Living with cancer requires adaptation to the experience and the changes over time. Included in these changes are symptom occurrence and symptom distress.

The relationship of symptom experience to quality of life has become increasingly important in oncology nursing care and research. The existing literature in oncology nursing raises a number of issues for further study:

- a more complex description of factors influencing symptom distress
- the interrelationship of individual symptoms on total symptom experience
- more information about the threshold for symptom distress
- actual descriptions of patients' symptom experiences
- knowledge of the influence of nutritional status, multiple stressors, personal control, family functioning, and social support on symptom distress
- coping types and coping strategies to deal with symptom experience

A full explanation of the relationship between symptom distress and quality of life necessitates identification of intervening variables. Symptom distress as an independent variable has been shown to partially explain social dependency, mood disturbance, and individual concerns. Symptom distress may be an important variable in predicting the quality, as well as the quantity, of survival for patients with cancer. For example, women diagnosed with breast cancer continued to experience symptoms that adversely affected their quality of life many years later.[35] Sarna[36] found that symptom distress was strongly related to quality of life in women with lung cancer and that symptom distress predicted 53% of the variance in quality of life.[37]

Symptom distress may alter the cancer experience and the individual's quality of life; consequently, symptom distress as an indicator of the effectiveness of nursing interventions on patient quality of life should be examined. Further research is needed in the nursing management of symptom distress, taking into account the individual's perception of both symptom distress and quality of life. Ethical, contractual, and situational issues require systematic examination in planning and testing management strategies. Among the numerous questions that still need to be answered are the following:

- How is quality of life affected over time by changes in symptom experience, symptom occurrence, and symptom distress?
- What nursing interventions are useful to reduce symptom distress, as opposed to symptom occurrence?

- Is symptom distress paired to the occurrence of single symptoms, or is it a generalized response to the occurrence of multiple symptoms?
- Are anxiety, depression, worry, and fear symptoms or expressions of symptom distress?
- How should information about symptom experience—symptom occurrence and symptom distress—be used in the formulation of nursing diagnoses?

Symptom occurrence and distress have been discussed since medieval times, yet inadequate attention has been given to why and how they are important to individual patients and specific healthcare providers. Nurses have assumed that knowledge of symptoms and symptom distress was essential to practice but have failed to focus on how to use this knowledge and how to reduce symptom distress.

Assessment of Quality of Life

The overall goal of assessing quality of life is to obtain information that will improve the care and treatment of patients. Evaluation of quality of life of individuals with cancer can be used to measure the effectiveness of treatments, nursing interventions, and self-care activities.

Quality of life may be determined by subjective or objective report; as with instruments to measure symptom experience, self-report measures are considered the best sources of information. Quality-of-life instruments may assess overall quality of life or several dimensions. Instruments that measure multiple dimensions often include symptoms and functioning. Quality-of-life instruments may yield quantitative data such as Ferrans's and Powers's Quality of Life Index Cancer Version,[21] or qualitative data such as Frank-Stromborg and Wright's[38] Health Survey.

To measure quality of life, an instrument must be appropriately conceptualized. An adequately conceptualized instrument will contain items from all the domains of quality of life and include a range of responses to reflect aspects of quality of life. It must have acceptable reliability and validity, be responsive to changes in quality of life, be based on patient-generated data, and be acceptable to patients and healthcare providers. Several quality-of-life instruments are reviewed by Haberman in Chapter 2.

Teaching the Patient and Family Self-Care

Inherent in nursing is the responsibility to provide sufficient educational instruction, information, and materials to enable patients to perform adequate self-care. Shortened hospital stays, the increasing use of antineoplastic therapies in the outpatient and home settings, and the increasing older population in the United States all provide a challenge for, and emphasize the importance of, patient preparation, education, and guidance.

The extended span (from 55 to over 100 years of age) for the single developmental stage of older adults now approximates in extent that of all other developmental stages combined (infancy through mid-adulthood). Because of the increased incidence of cancer in the older adult group, attention must be paid to the multiple familial demands borne by these adults.[39] Persons aged 55 years and over may still have children at home. This same household may have one or more parents or grandparents in or outside the home who are also dependent. Individuals 85 years and older are the fastest growing segment of the older population. Care for this group is a major concern because of their vulnerability. The complex care requirements of this large group underscore the need for a thorough patient and family assessment.

Nursing practice often involves caring for patients with signs and symptoms—e.g., fatigue, fever, confusion, nausea, and vomiting—that may or may not be specifically related to a medical problem. The clinical interpretation and management of these signs and symptoms are often the primary responsibility of the nurse. Nurses frequently provide information to patients about an impending event in order to prepare them for unpleasant medical procedures and treatments. Such preparatory information helps reduce patient distress and fear of the unknown by enhancing the patient's perceived control and understanding of the procedure.

Gammon and Mulholland[40] found that providing patients with preparatory information prior to elective total hip replacement surgery significantly reduced anxiety and depression. They concluded that these psychological benefits enhance patients' ability to cope and may be associated with earlier discharge. McDaniel and Rhodes[41] found that providing preparatory sensory information helped women receiving chemotherapy for breast cancer to develop anticipatory coping and self-care behaviors. Johnson et al.[42] examined the effects of self-regulation theory–based nursing care for patients who were receiving radiation therapy. Patients in the theory-based care group had significantly less disruption in activities of daily living during and after radiation therapy. Self-regulation theory provided the basis for nursing care. Tishelman, Taube, and Sachs[43] examined 46 hospitalized cancer patients, aged 29 to 88 years, to determine what they experienced and how they coped with their sickness. Although few age-related differences in symptom distress were found, some differences were seen in patients' perception of the response of the professional healthcare system. Older patients explained that they perceived less sense of engagement and concern from the professional healthcare sector. The findings suggest that age may be used by patients to explain a variety of situations, functioning as a means to "make sense" of sickness experiences.

Haberman[44] supported the need for preparatory information in a group of bone marrow transplant patients. He suggested that patients need preparatory information regarding treatment and effective coping to decrease symptom distress.

Conclusion

Nurses assist patients to cope with symptom experience, while physicians are primarily concerned with symptom occurrence in the diagnosis or treatment of disease. Patients' perceptions of their abilities to cope with symptom experience vary. Without effective interventions to alter (restrain or produce) their own actions to cope with symptoms, patients may withdraw from potentially curative treatments.

Symptom distress hampers self-care and threatens independence. Consequently, social dependency, the need to ask others to assist with activities that are ordinarily accomplished by oneself, may produce additional distress. How individuals monitor and react to symptoms changes over the course of an illness, and how this affects behavior, self-care activity, and response to therapy require assessment. Without adequate assessment of the symptom experience and appropriate intervention, symptom occurrence and symptom distress may increase, and additional problems may develop for the patient with cancer.

At times, the diverse perceptions, evaluations, and responses to illness greatly affect the degree to which symptoms interfere with usual life routines, chronicity, attainment of proper care, and participation in self-care practices. Successful coping and self-care behaviors reduce symptom distress, thus improving quality of life.

References

1. Watson PM, Rhodes VA, Germino BB: Symptom distress: Future perspectives for practice, education, and research. *Semin Oncol Nurs* 3:313–315, 1987
2. Rhodes VA, Watson PM, Johnson MH, et al: Patterns of nausea, vomiting, and distress in patients receiving antineoplastic drug protocols. *Oncol Nurs Forum* 14:35–44, 1987
3. Rhodes VA, Watson PM: Symptom distress—the concept: Past and present. *Semin Oncol Nurs* 3:242–247, 1987
4. Johnson JE, Fieler VK, Jones LS, et al: *Self-Regulation Theory: Applying Theory to Your Practice*. Pittsburgh: Oncology Nursing Press, 1997
5. Orem DE: *Nursing Concepts of Practice* (ed 4). St. Louis: Mosby-Year Book, 1991
6. Johnson MH, Rhodes VA: Patient education, in Perry MC (ed): *The Chemotherapy Source Book* (ed 2). Baltimore: Williams & Wilkins, 1997, pp. 1007–1020
7. Larson PJ, Carrieri V, Dodd MJ, et al: Proceedings from the First International Symposium for Symptom Management. *Image* 26:272, 1994
8. Piper BF, Lindsey A, Dodd MJ, et al: The development of an instrument to measure the subjective dimension of fatigue, in Funk SG, Tornquist EM, Champagen MT, et al. (eds): *Key Aspects of Comfort: Management of Pain, Fatigue, and Nausea*. New York: Springer, 1989, pp. 199–208
9. Rhodes VA, McDaniel RW: Measuring nausea, vomiting, and retching, in Frank-Stromborg M, Olsen SJ (eds): *Instruments for Clinical Research in Healthcare* (ed 2). Norwalk, CT: Appleton & Lange, 1997, pp. 509–518
10. Rhodes VA, Watson PM, Johnson MH: Development of reliable and valid measures of nausea and vomiting. *Cancer Nurs* 7:33–41, 1984
11. Rhodes VA, McDaniel RW, Hanson B, et al: A reliable and valid measurement of symptom experience: Symptom occurrence and symptom distress. Columbia, MO: University of Missouri, 1995
12. Rhodes VA: Nausea, vomiting, and retching. *Nurs Clin North Am* 25:885–900, 1990
13. Berman AJ: Sailing a course through chemotherapy: The experience of women with breast cancer. *Dissertation Abstracts International*. 55-02B:363, 1993
14. Simms SG, Rhodes VA, Madsen RW: Comparison of prochlorperazine and lorazepam antiemetic regimens in the control of postchemotherapy symptoms. *Nurs Res* 42:234–239, 1993
15. Grossman SA, Sheidler VR, Swedeen K, et al: Correlation of patient and caregiver ratings of cancer pain. *J Pain Symptom Manage* 6:53–57, 1991
16. Roberts DK, Thorne SE, Pearson C: The experience of dyspnea in late-stage cancer. *Cancer Nurs* 16:310–320, 1993
17. Larson PJ, Viele CS, Coleman S, et al: Comparison of perceived symptoms of patients undergoing bone marrow transplant and the nurses caring for them. *Oncol Nurs Forum* 20:81–88, 1993
18. Kurtz ME, Kurtz JC, Given CC, Given B: Concordance of cancer patient and caregiver symptom reports. *Cancer Pract* 4:185–196, 1996
19. Rhodes VA, McDaniel RW, Matthews CA: Hospice patients' and nurses' perceptions of self-care deficits based on symptom experience. *Cancer Nurs* 21:143–148, 1998
20. Bland KI: Quality of life management for cancer patients. *CA Cancer J Clin* 47:207–217, 1997
21. Ferrans C: Development of a quality of life index for patients with cancer. *Oncol Nurs Forum* 7:15–21, 1990
22. Ferrell BR, Grant M, Funk B, et al: Quality of life in breast cancer Part II: Psychological and spiritual well-being. *Cancer Nurs* 21:1–9, 1998
23. Grant MM, Ferrell BR, Padilla GV, et al: Assessment of quality of life with a single instrument. *Semin Oncol Nurs* 6:260–270, 1990
24. Stenstrup EZ: Graduate student scholarship. Review of quality of life instrumentation in the oncology population. *Clin Nurs Spec* 10:164–169, 1996
25. Cella DF: Methods and problems in measuring quality of life. *Supp Care Cancer* 3:11–22, 1995
26. Ferrell BR: The quality of lives: 1,525 voices of cancer. *Oncol Nurs Forum* 23:907–916, 1996
27. Cella DR, Tulsky DS: Measuring quality of life today: Methodological aspects. *Oncology* 4:29–38, 1990
28. Taylor EJ, Jones P, Burns M: Quality of life, in Lubkin

IM(ed): *Chronic Illness: Impact and Intervention* (ed 3). Sudbury: Jones & Bartlett, 1995, p. 195

29. Salamon M: Clinical use of the life satisfaction in the elderly scale. *Clin Gerontol* 8:45–54, 1988

30. McDaniel RW, Bach CA: Quality of life: A concept analysis. *Rehab Nurs Res* 3:18–24, 1994

31. Rhodes VA, McDaniel RW, Hanson B, et al: Sensory perceptions of patients on selected antineoplastic protocols. *Cancer Nurs* 17:45–51, 1994

32. Ciossi D: Beyond attentional strategies: A cognitive-perceptual model of somatic interpretation. *Psychol Bull* 109:25–41, 1991

33. McDaniel RW, Rhodes VA, Nelson RA, Hanson B: Sensory perceptions of women receiving Tamoxifen for breast cancer. *Cancer Nurs* 18:215–221, 1995

34. Rathmell A, Ash D, Howes M, et al: Assessing quality of life in patients treated for advanced head and neck cancer. *Clin Oncol* 3:10–16, 1991

35. Ferrell BR, Grant M, Funk B, et al: Quality of life in breast cancer Part I: Physical and social well-being. *Cancer Nurs* 20:398–404, 1997

36. Sarna L: Correlates of symptom distress in women with lung cancer. *Cancer Pract* 1:21–28, 1993

37. Sarna L: Women with lung cancer: Impact on quality of life. *Qual Life Res* 2:13–22, 1993

38. Frank-Stromborg M, Wright P: Ambulatory cancer patients' perceptions of the physical and psychosocial changes in their lives since the diagnosis of cancer. *Cancer Nurs* 7:117–130, 1984

39. Wells NL, Lodovico B: Geriatric oncology: Medical and psychosocial perspectives. *Cancer Pract* 5:87–91, 1997

40. Gammon J, Mulholland CW: Effect of preparatory information prior to elective total hip replacement on psychological coping. *J Adv Nurs* 24:303–308, 1996

41. McDaniel RW, Rhodes VA: Development of a preparatory sensory information videotape for women receiving chemotherapy for breast cancer. *Cancer Nurs* 21:312–319, 1998

42. Johnson JE, Fieler VK, Wlasowicz GS, et al: The effect of nursing care guided by self-regulation theory on coping with radiation. *Oncol Nurs Forum* 24:1041–1050, 1997

43. Tishelman C, Taube A, Sachs L: Self-reported symptom distress in cancer patients: Reflections of disease, illness or sickness? *Soc Sci Med* 33:1229–1240, 1991

44. Haberman M: The meaning of cancer therapy: Bone marrow transplantation as an exemplar of therapy. *Semin Oncol Nurs* 11:23–31, 1995

CHAPTER 2

The Measurement of Symptom Distress

Mel Haberman, PhD, RN, FAAN

Today, more than at any time in its history, nursing is being challenged to demonstrate the effectiveness of its therapeutics through research that examines the link between specific nursing interventions and patient outcomes. Moreover, healthcare reform has shifted many aspects of cancer care away from the clinical arena and into the home and community setting. Nurses are responsible for teaching persons with cancer and family caregivers how to monitor symptoms and implement self-care measures for the relief of symptom distress. However, the private and subjective nature of cancer symptoms poses many problems for nursing assessment and the objective measurement of symptom occurrence and perceived distress.[1] In light of the demands for outcome research, the changing healthcare delivery system, and the complexity of developing reliable and valid instruments to measure symptom distress, a critical need remains for nurse clinicians and researchers to work together to establish a research base for practice. New nursing interventions that are aimed at improving the management of disease and treatment-related symptoms must be devised and tested.

The purpose of this chapter is to provide an overview of some of the key issues influencing the selection of research instruments for measuring symptom occurrence and distress. Knowing the methodologic issues that influence the choice of a research instrument offers a basis for critiquing published studies. Moreover, nurses can structure their patient assessments and teaching based on their understanding of the way researchers measure symptoms. Understanding the issues that underlie the measurement of symptoms can make nurses better clinicians, reviewers of research, and patient advocates.

Theoretical Definitions and Conceptual Issues

Theoretical definitions that lack clarity continue to be a major problem in nursing outcome research.[2] The theoretical definition of a clinical phenomenon is important because it directs how the investigator will ultimately operationalize or measure the concept. Rhodes and Watson[1] make a distinction between the terms "symptom distress" and "symptoms of distress." *Symptom distress* refers to the "degree or amount of physical or mental upset, anguish, or suffering experienced from a specific symptom, e.g., nausea, fatigue, insomnia" (p. 243). *Symptoms of distress* is a more global concept that refers to the psychological, social, mental, neurophysiologic, and immunologic responses to illness and stress.[1] These global aspects of illness may be covariates with symptom distress. From a research viewpoint, McCorkle[3] defined measurement of symptom distress as the "systematic attempt to measure the person's level of distress from a specific symptom being experienced" (p. 248).

It is quite common for researchers to assess symptoms by using questionnaires that measure both the occurrence as well as the perceived intensity of symptoms. However, as McClement et al.[4] note, the perceived intensity of a symptom may not equate with the degree of suffering or distress the symptom causes. Consequently, researchers and clinicians are encouraged to take a meaning-centered approach to assess the nature of patients' total symptom experience, including independent assessment of personal meaning, occurrence, intensity, and distress.[4,5] Symptom experience is a multidimensional, dynamic process of deriving meaning from a subjective, out-of-the-ordinary sensation—a synthesis of symptom occurrence and perceptions of intensity and distress.[4,5] A discussion of the research-design issues that influence the measurement of symptom distress, and in some cases the measurement of symptoms of distress, follows.

Measurement Issues in Conducting Research on Symptom Distress

In this chapter, the terms "questionnaire," "measure," "instrument," and "tool" are used interchangeably for the measurement technique. Table 2-1 provides a summary of the methodologic issues that guide the selection of a symptom-distress instrument.

Measurement Framework

How does one know which symptom-distress variable is the most important outcome to measure in a given clinical situation? To answer this question, Strickland[2] points out that the investigator needs to understand (1) the health problems that are the focus of specific nursing interventions, (2) the various components of these nursing interventions and their anticipated therapeutic effects, (3) the conceptual and clinical links between the health problems and interventions, and (4) the sensitivity of specific measures to quantify desired outcomes. Additionally, understanding the nature and temporality of nursing interventions is critical to the selection of specific symptom-distress variables and to identifying the proper time to measure the anticipated outcomes.[2]

There is probably no symptom-occurrence and distress tool that is designed to assess patient outcomes in every situation. The purpose and specific aims of the research study will determine which symptom-distress variables or end points are of primary and secondary

TABLE 2-1   Guidelines for Evaluating Symptom Distress Instruments

Theoretical foundation	Are the symptom occurrence and/or distress-related concepts theoretically defined?
Measurement framework	What symptoms are measured?
	In what populations and settings has the instrument been developed, and has it been used in your population/setting?
	Is the instrument capable of detecting the changes in symptoms that occur at different times in the disease and treatment trajectory?
Data collection methods	Will the data-gathering methods provide the appropriate data to answer the specific aims of the study?
	What data-gathering approaches will be used: self-report, symptom checklists, observer ratings, symptom diaries, open-ended questions?
Measurement standardization	Are the data collection and scoring procedures standardized across different interviewers, populations, settings, and intervention/control groups?
Single or repeated measurement	What is the rationale for choosing a single measurement occasion or multiple occasions?
	Are the measurement occasions properly timed to reflect the clinical course of the disease and of treatment?
Measurement error	Have potential sources of random and systematic error been identified and minimized?
Reliability and validity	Is there empirical evidence to support the instrument's reliability and validity?
	What types of reliability and validity testing are reported?
Scaling, aggregation, and scoring	Are similar items grouped into scales, and if so, are the items highly interrelated?
	Will the scaling method result in a response bias or set?
	Is it appropriate to aggregate or sum the individual items and scales to obtain a total score?
	Are all items and scales weighted equally?
Staff and responder burden	How long does it take to complete the questionnaire and/or interview?
	Are there sufficient staff resources to handle data collection?
	Will the data collection procedures result in lower accrual and higher attrition rates?
Pilot study	Is a trial run needed to evaluate the data-gathering procedures?
	Is a pretest of the instrument needed to assess clarity, comprehensiveness, and responder burden?
Ethical implications	Has permission been obtained from the tool's developer to use the instrument?
	Will the tool need modification?
	Is the tool copyrighted and/or in the public domain?
	Is there a fee involved for using the tool?

interest. If symptom distress is the primary end point, then the researcher may choose to measure any number of clinical phenomena, e.g., the regimen-related toxicities and perceptions of symptom distress that accompany a particular chemotherapy regimen. The more global concept of symptoms of distress may provide secondary end points of lower priority, e.g., the effect of therapy on mood changes, social support, and activities of daily living. After determining which end points to measure, potential questionnaires need to be examined item by item to determine the relevancy of the items for measuring the selected end points. The population that the tool was originally designed to assess and the setting in which it was originally developed should also be evaluated.[2]

The operational definition will specify how symptom occurrence and distress will be measured and the activities necessary to quantify or manipulate the variable.[6] There are any number of operational definitions for a given concept, as evidenced by the vast array of instruments that are now available to measure different aspects of symptoms. It may be necessary to use more than one instrument to achieve conceptual and operational congruency.[2] One option is to use an assortment of standardized questionnaires, each one tailored to provide a comprehensive measurement of one specific symptom, e.g., anxiety, depression, fatigue, cognitive impairment. A second method is to use a multidimensional instrument that is designed to measure a wide range of different symptoms, e.g., sleep and eating disturbances, social roles, mood states, changes in activities of daily living, and regimen-related toxicities. A more recent trend, popular in the quality-of-life literature, is the use of a modular approach to measurement. The modular approach combines a core questionnaire that measures symptoms common to a wide variety of cancers with a disease- or treatment-specific symptom module. Symptom modules have been developed for the late complications of bone marrow transplant,[7] lung cancer,[8,9] and breast, bladder, colorectal, ovarian, head/neck, prostate, pancreatic, brain, and cervical cancer.[9]

Data Collection Methods

The choice of data collection strategies is determined by the specific aims and design of the study.[10] Quantitative research designs incorporate a conceptual framework that identifies the salient concepts to measure and a set of strict operational definitions that specify exactly how the concepts will be measured. Alternatively, qualitative designs follow a more flexible process of concept discovery and evolution. Consequently, the investigator tries to avoid writing a rigid theoretical framework and relies on the empirical findings to guide concept definition. It is becoming increasingly common for nurse researchers to triangulate methods of data collection and research designs, i.e., to use multiple methods of data collection and

to combine aspects of both quantitative and qualitative designs.

Self-report questionnaires usually are regarded as the best source of patient information because they obtain the unique perspective of the person with cancer. Self-assessment tools, in the form of fixed-item or alternative-choice scales, obtain the same "standardized" data from all participants. The advantages of self-administered questionnaires are that they do not require extensive interviewer training and that they negate the potential problems that often occur with observer or interviewer bias.[3] The investigator may want to enhance objectivity by obtaining ratings from various family members, such as the designated caregiver, from other nurses and physicians, or from a trained interviewer. Lobchuk et al.[11] administered the McCorkle and Young Symptom Distress Scale (SDS) to 37 patient and family caregiver dyads and found moderate correlations between the two sets of scores for 10 of the 13 symptoms on the SDS. However, the comparison of different perceptions of symptom distress may be problematic due to the subjective and private nature of symptoms.[12] An outside observer or rater can never directly experience the patient's symptoms but must make a supposition about the occurrence or intensity of the symptoms. McCorkle[3] notes that it is quite common to obtain discrepant results when the symptom reports of patients and observers are compared and that a failure to achieve congruence does not mean the symptom distress measure is invalid. For instance, Kurtz et al.[13] investigated whether 216 family caregivers agreed with the symptom reports of patients with cancer. The caregivers were accurate for only 71% of the symptoms, with the highest accuracy for fatigue and lowest for insomnia. The disadvantage of self-assessment questionnaires is that they assume the respondents can read and comprehend the items. Moreover, self-assessments can be biased by the effects of medications, cognitive impairment, cultural differences, age, and educational level.[2] Because of the limitations of self-report questionnaires, the investigator may want to choose a combination of quantitative and qualitative data collection methods.

Qualitative methods allow people to describe in rich detail the personal meaning of their symptoms. Several popular qualitative methods of measurement include the use of open-ended interviews and questionnaires, symptom diaries, telephone interviews, and participant observation. McDaniel et al.,[5] for example, used an open-ended questionnaire to collect data from 20 women about the sensory effects of receiving tamoxifen for breast cancer. A combination of data collection methods is often preferable, as it provides different vantage points from which to examine the same clinical phenomenon. A fixed-item scale that measures fatigue, for instance, may indicate that the respondent's daily average distress level is high, a rating of 4 on a 5-point scale. To supplement this single numerical rating, participants can be interviewed and asked to describe the broader impact of their fatigue and the time of day when episodes of fatigue usually occur.

From these qualitative data, the investigator may be able to identify patterns of fatigue, link episodes of fatigue with certain activities of daily living, and describe the more global consequences of fatigue, e.g., the loss of mobility, social isolation, mood swings, and weight loss from not having enough energy to prepare meals.

Measurement Standardization

Standardizing all data collection and scoring procedures is necessary to ensure reliable measurement. For example, it is essential to determine the extent to which one or more raters can generate similar symptom distress scores for different persons experiencing similar levels of distress.[3] Standardizing the timing of data collection is both a conceptual and an operational issue. Conceptually, the symptom occurrence and distress variables selected for measurement must clearly reflect the outcomes of nursing care that are expected to occur at specific points in treatment, and the administration of instruments must be properly timed to capture the desired changes in symptoms.[2] Operationally, the timing of data collection also must be standardized across treatment or intervention groups, often referred to as *study arms*. When a research protocol has two or more study arms—such as standard therapy versus experimental treatment—symptom occurrence or distress should be measured at the same point in treatment in each arm. Moreover, the same tools should be used at all measurement occasions, unless the length of the instrument overburdens the respondent. If the instrument or packet of several tools is large, a full complement of questionnaires can be given at baseline and at some point in the future, such as at the end of therapy. A smaller subset of instruments or single items from one instrument can be administered at strategic points falling between the initial baseline and last measurement occasion. Of course, if single items are used from a larger questionnaire, the scores on these items can be compared only with themselves and not with the scores on the instrument as a whole (obtained at other time points). Standardizing the timing of measurements and using the same instruments and single items allows the investigator to examine changes in symptoms over time and to make meaningful comparisons across study arms.

Single or Repeated Measurements

Cross-sectional designs obtain a single measure of a symptom at one point in time. A repeated-measures design allows for the examination of the dynamic nature of symptoms and the changes in symptom occurrence, duration, and intensity that occur across time. The *sensitivity* of an instrument refers to its ability to detect small changes in the outcome variable (symptom distress and occurrence) from one testing occasion to the next. Sensitivity is a serious issue, especially in those situations in which the investigator is trying to distinguish between patients who show symptom improvement and those who do not, and in those cases in which the desired patient outcome is probably present but the instrument may lack the sensitivity to detect it.[2]

The number of measurement occasions will be determined by such factors as the specific aims of the study, the amount of funding and time frame available for completing the study, the burden that repeated measurement places on the staff and respondent, and the nature of the disease and clinical trajectory. In the field of quality-of-life measurement, a minimum of three measurement occasions is recommended: (1) at baseline before the initiation of therapy, (2) sometime during therapy when symptoms are at their maximum intensity and frequency, (3) and at the end of treatment.[14] It should always be remembered that repeated-measures designs are extremely sensitive to issues of measurement error, especially the reliability of measurement. If an instrument has measurement-error problems during the first testing occasion, these problems will be repeated and compounded at subsequent measurement occasions.

Measurement Error, Reliability, and Validity

Measurement error

The observed score on a symptom-distress measure is a combination of a true score (what the participant's symptom score would be if the tool were perfect) and random and systematic error.[15] *Random error* occurs from unpredictable fluctuations or chance variations in either the tool, procedures for data collection, or participants. Sources of random error include questionnaire directions that are confusing, poorly worded items, fatigue, guessing, lapses in memory, nausea or vomiting during data collection, a noisy laminar air flow room, and so on. Random error can also be caused by the interviewer's asking questions in different ways at different times or by a lack of consistency among several interviewers.[3] The larger the random error, the lower the reliability coefficient of the tool and the less likely the tool will be useful for describing symptom distress or testing relationships.[15] Random error can be minimized by the careful control of the measurement conditions (standardization, randomization, large sample sizes), by increasing the reliability of the measures themselves, and by doing a pilot test of the questionnaires to detect poorly worded or confusing items.[3,16]

Systematic error occurs when some extraneous factor affects every measurement in the same way,[15] systematic error is usually associated with individual differences among participants and interviewers. For example, in a randomized clinical trial, people in the experimental and control group may vary systematically by some unmeasured or uncontrolled characteristic. People in the experimental group, for instance, may be less motivated to adhere to the research protocol than those individuals in the control group. Other sources of systematic error include such factors as differences in intelligence, pain tolerance, chronic fatigue, and tolerance for ambiguity.[17] Interviewers can introduce systematic error into the measurement procedures, for instance, by interviewing all participants before they undergo the initial regimen of chemotherapy, when individuals tend to be anxious, distracted, and mentally focused on the upcoming therapy. The aim of all reliability and validity estimates is to minimize the portion of the participant's score that is due to error and to maximize the portion that is true.[15]

Types of reliability

Every effort should be made to select research questionnaires with known reliability and validity. The investigator should determine how well an instrument has performed previously in samples having age, gender, cultural background, diseases, and treatments similar to those for which it will be used in the current study.[2] Most of the popular tools that measure symptom occurrence and distress, symptoms of distress, and quality of life have published empirical estimates of reliability and validity.[18–20] In general, *reliability* refers to the stability or dependability of measurement, i.e., the ability to consistently repeat the same findings time after time. A *reliability coefficient* indicates whether the obtained score is likely to be a stable indication of the person's performance on a given symptom questionnaire or due to some type of measurement error.[17]

Internal consistency reliability This form of reliability measures the degree to which all items on a scale or questionnaire measure the same thing.[21] In general, the higher the intercorrelation of items (1.0 is the maximum), the more confident the investigator is that all of the items are internally consistent and measuring the same concept, attribute, trait, characteristic, or symptom. Common correlation coefficients for estimating internal consistency reliability include Kuder-Richardson formulas (KR20, KR21), Cronbach's alpha, and split-half reliability.[6,22] *Split-half reliability* is determined by correlating the scores on half of the items on a questionnaire against scores on the other half, as an indication of both the internal consistency and the stability of the entire questionnaire.[17]

Test-retest reliability *Test-retest reliability* refers to the repeatability of measurements from one testing occasion to the next.[21] For example, if a symptom-distress questionnaire is given on two occasions at 2-week intervals, the closer the correlation of the two scores is to 1.0 (known as the coefficient of stability), the more stable the instrument is presumed to be. An instrument must demonstrate stability over short periods of time before it can be used by clinicians to document changes in symptoms.[3]

Many phenomena of interest to nurse researchers and clinicians are dynamic and tend to fluctuate over time; therefore, one would anticipate a low coefficient of stability. For example, pain intensity ratings and perceptions of nausea may vary extensively from moment to moment or within a short period of time. Conceptually, a fluctuation in pain and nausea scores would not be interpreted as measurement error but as an indication of the clinical nature of these symptoms. Statistically, however, such variations in an unstable symptom act like measurement error in that they tend to attenuate correlations with other variables.[22] A great deal of research is still needed to determine how well various symptom-distress tools are able to detect, with high reliability, changes in symptoms from one time period to another.[3]

Parallel/alternative forms reliability Another type of reliability applicable to the measurement of symptom distress is *parallel* or *alternative forms reliability*. When the same questionnaire is given to a person repeatedly, as in the case of a repeated-measures or longitudinal research design, the respondent may memorize the questions and answer them in a set pattern from memory (*response set*) rather than according to present circumstances.[21] When response set becomes a problem, a parallel or alternative version of the questionnaire should be administered such that both forms measure exactly the same symptoms with slightly different questions. The investigator must statistically examine the equivalency of the two versions. The correlation between the alternative versions is a measure of the equivalency (a criterion of .80 or higher is considered good).

Types of validity

Measurement reliability is necessary for validity, although neither measurement issue alone guarantees the other. Validity provides some assurance that the instrument is measuring what it claims to be measuring, e.g., nausea, insomnia, pain, fatigue, anxiety.

Face and content validity The terms "face validity" and "content validity" are often used interchangeably. *Face validity* is the extent to which an instrument appears to measure what it claims to measure. For instance, every item on a scale that measures the side effects of chemotherapy and radiation therapy should "look like" it measures a relevant symptom. Similarly, *content validity* involves a nonempirical, common-sense examination of the items and subscales of an instrument to see if they are representative of the entire universe of items that could, theoretically, be designated to measure the concept.[3,10] Content and face validity are usually determined by a panel of individuals who are regarded as exerts in the area under study.

Criterion-related validity   This form of validity refers to the degree to which scores on one scale correlate with a *criterion measure,* i.e., an instrument previously shown to validly measure the variable under consideration.[21] Criterion validity has two forms—concurrent and predictive. The difference between the two forms of validity is essentially a difference in the time at which the scores of the criterion measure (often called the "gold standard") are available. *Concurrent validity* can be tested when both the symptom-distress scale and criterion measure of symptom distress are administered at the same moment in time. Alternatively, *predictive validity* refers to the degree to which scores on a scale, available at the present time, correlate with a criterion measure that is not immediately available but can be obtained only in the future.[23] For instance, the scores on a scale that measures acute regimen-related toxicities could be correlated with the scores obtained six months later on a symptom checklist that has previously been shown to validly measure the toxicities of marrow transplantation. The magnitude of the correlation coefficient gives an indication in that case of how well the acute toxicity scale predicts the scores obtained on the symptom checklist (the higher the correlation, the better the predictive validity).

Construct validity   *Construct validity* is the validation of theory. Establishing construct validity is a multistep process. First, the investigator proposes a set of hypotheses about the theoretical relationships that exist among the concepts, and then these relationships are tested. The investigator attempts to demonstrate that a given measure correlates with other instruments that the theory specifies should correlate with the measure.[23]

Construct validity can be examined in several ways. In the *contrasted groups approach,* an instrument is administered to at least two groups—one group known to be high and another known to be low in the characteristic under study, e.g., symptom distress.[24] If the group's symptom distress scores differ significantly, then construct validity is supported based on the finding that the tool is capable of discriminating group differences in the hypothesized directions (high or low).

The *multitrait-multimethod approach* to construct validity is based on the principles of convergent and discriminant validity.[6,15] In a multitrait-multimethod analysis, more than one variable and more than one data collection method are used to establish construct validity. The simplest form of such an analysis is the intercorrelation of two variables (e.g., symptom distress and self-care) and two methods of measuring each variable (e.g., self-report and observer rating). Convergence occurs when the same variables measured differently intercorrelate highly with each other. Discriminant validity is supported when different variables intercorrelate poorly with each other.

Instrument Scaling, Aggregation, and Scoring Issues

Scaling issues

Another aspect to examine when choosing an instrument to measure symptom distress is the scaling method chosen by the tool's developer. It is necessary to distinguish between the terms "scales" and "dimensions." *Scale* refers to the technique that is employed when one or more individual items are grouped together in order to form a single score.[25] *Dimension* represents an underlying characteristic, measured by the scale, that describes the responses at a conceptual level.[25] For example, a scale comprising three symptoms (headache, nausea, pain) may represent the conceptual dimension of physical symptoms, while a scale composed of three other items (anxiety, depression, uncertainty) may represent a psychosocial dimension. The extent to which individual items can be placed on a single scale without losing descriptive or explanatory information is governed by the criterion of dimensionality.[25] The individual items or variables on a scale should be highly intercorrelated if, in fact, they are measuring the same underlying dimension or concept. However, if the inter-item correlations are low, the investigator needs to consider the possibility that several dimensions exist.

Scales are constructed for several reasons. In general, they reduce the complexity of the data by aggregating a set of individual items into a single score, so that analysis can be simplified.[25] Moreover, investigators may want to test the hypothesis that a scale composed of several items actually does, in fact, measure a single underlying conceptual dimension.[25] For example, an investigator may want to intercorrelate several pain items (joint/muscle pain, bone pain, skin pain, tooth pain) to determine if the items represent a single conceptual dimension and, therefore, can be summed into a single score. Last, scales are used to reduce measurement error and thereby improve the reliability of the data that are used in analysis.[25]

Individual items may be scaled on a categorical level ("yes/no") or on a numerical system. Likert-type scales are the most typically used form of summated or aggregated scales. A typical Likert-type scale has five degrees of response intensity: (0) not at all, (1) a little bit, (2) moderately, (3) quite a bit, and (4) extremely. Within limits, the reliability of a scale increases as the number of possible alternative responses increases.[25] For this reason, some investigators prefer to use seven-point Likert-type scales or 100-mm visual analogue scales to obtain more precise information about the individual's degree of symptom distress. Questionnaires containing items in identical scale or response formats, such as a Likert-type scale, are highly prone to bias from response sets. A response set in this case occurs when participants respond to the items in a set pattern regardless of the item content.[15]

Another scaling format is the visual analogue scale (VAS) in which respondents quantify their symptoms by making a mark on a 100-mm line. The phrases chosen to anchor each end of a VAS scale are largely determined by the symptom being measured. For example, in rating the degree of perceived nausea, the 0-mm end of the scale may be labeled "no nausea at all" and the 100-mm end of the scale may be labeled "the worst nausea imaginable." Despite the popularity of VAS scales, many respondents find them conceptually confusing and difficult to fill out. Moreover, the hand scoring of VAS scales is highly labor-intensive because the investigator needs to measure each response on a 100-mm ruler. Electronic scanners can be used to measure the lines with high precision and reliability. The scanners enter the score directly into a computer for subsequent analysis.

Aggregation issues

Not all symptom-occurrence and distress scales group similar items into composite scales. However, if a symptom-distress scale is used that claims to be composed of one or more scales, the scales should always be examined to determine whether their dimensionality remains intact in a new population or setting. The existence or nonexistence of a scale's unidimensionality should be tested as a research hypothesis just like any other hypothesis.[25] Methods for testing the dimensionality of a scale were previously discussed in the sections on internal consistency reliability and scaling issues.

The dimensionality of a scale influences how the individual items or scales can be aggregated for analysis. Generally speaking, the individual items on a questionnaire are each given a numerical score and these scores are summed to obtain a total score of symptom occurrence and distress. However, depending on the underlying conceptual foundation and dimensionality of a questionnaire, some scales cannot easily be aggregated into a single total score.

Scoring issues

When scoring a symptom-occurrence and distress questionnaire, a related concern is whether all items or scales can be weighted equally. The aggregation of items into total scores and the assigning of different weights to items or scales remains an issue of some controversy.[23] Some psychometricians[23] argue that total scores are conceptually and statistically meaningless when they are based on the summation of different types of items or scales; e.g., when items or scales that measure physical symptoms, psychosocial symptoms, social functioning, and spirituality are summed into a total score. If items are given some preferred weight (preference-weighting), then weights are usually assigned by different rules and statistical procedures, such as paired comparisons, magnitude estimation, and category scaling.[2] Most importantly,

these statistical approaches allow the respondent's own preferences to be given more weight in the scoring procedure. In nonpreference weighting, the researcher assigns weights to each item, often using a Likert-type scale that is summated.

Regardless of the type of weighting given to the items by the instrument's developer, care should be taken to examine all items and scales within a tool. As is often the case, the score on a single item or scale may provide valuable information about a patient outcome.[2] When scores are aggregated to provide some type of summary or total score, information about a specific symptom may be hidden or lost in this process.[3]

Responder Burden

Two basic rules of thumb must be remembered when selecting an instrument to measure symptom occurrence and/or distress. As the responder burden increases, respondents are more likely to refuse participation in the study, and higher attrition rates can be expected once the study is under way. Attrition is often a serious problem in studies that use a repeated-measures design. Common sources of responder burden include fatigue, emotional distress, and the time needed to complete a long questionnaire or packet of questionnaires. Instruments that are long and comprehensive may be reliable and valid, but they are of little use when an acutely ill person becomes too fatigued to finish completing the questionnaire.

Pretests and Pilot Studies

One way to determine the degree of responder burden is to conduct a pretest or pilot study. A *pretest* involves trying out the symptom distress questionnaire on a few volunteers for the purpose of evaluating the clarity of instructions, wording and interpretation of items, social sensitivity or desirability of items, and the time needed to complete the questionnaire. A *pilot study* involves a small-scale trial run of the procedures for accruing participants, collecting data, managing a new data set, and standardizing the consistency of scoring by the interviewers.[3,15] A sample size of 10 to 20 participants is suitable for a pilot study, and the participants should be as similar as possible to those eligible for accrual in the eventual study.[15] A pilot study should always include the debriefing session so participants and staff can express their reactions to the entire research process and offer their suggestions for improving the questionnaire or study procedures.

Ethical Implications

The responsible researcher always obtains written permission from the author of a questionnaire before using the tool for research or clinical purposes. The user also requests the developer's permission to modify the tool in any way, such as the addition or deletion of items or the rewording of items. Similarly, at the end of the study, the user sends the developer a copy of the findings, a description of the sample, a copy of the modified tool, and a report of any reliability and validity testing conducted on the original or modified tool. The use of some tools that are trademarked or copyrighted by the developer may involve the payment of a fee by the user. If an entire instrument is published in a journal, then it is considered a part of the public domain and may be used without formal permission from the developer, unless the author retains the copyright on the tool as indicated in the publication.[15] However, even if a tool is obtained from the public domain, it is a common courtesy to inform the developer of your intent to use the tool. A copyrighted tool should be properly cited and the published source of a tool should always be referenced.

Symptom Distress Scales

Although studies on symptom distress have proliferated in the last few years, there remains a need for investigators to precisely define the difference between the measurement of symptom occurrence, symptom intensity, and symptom distress.[4] Many of the tools still in use, such as the Sickness Impact Profile and Sickness Checklist 90, were not originally designated for use with populations of cancer survivors.[4] Though only a few tools focus solely on the measurement of symptom distress, a wide variety of questionnaires are now available to measure symptom occurrence and intensity. This new generation of multidimensional tools is largely the result of the recent boom in quality-of-life research.[26] Many quality-of-life tools include either generic symptom inventories that are applicable to many types of cancer, or specific symptom checklists that apply only to one type of cancer.[26] Quality-of-life tools are often designed to measure the occurrence of social, psychological, physical, and spiritual symptoms of distress. These tools also may obtain ratings of symptom intensity; however, most quality-of-life questionnaires do not measure the suffering, mental anguish, or distress a symptom causes. Further understanding of the relationship between the concepts of quality of life and symptom distress is clearly needed.[4]

McCorkle[3] noted that there are three primary methods for measuring symptom distress, including a clinical assessment of the patient's symptoms, the patient's self-report of symptoms and his or her perceived level of distress, and symptom ratings performed by a trained observer. Table 2-2 lists many of the most common tools that are designed to measure symptom occurrence and symptom distress and symptoms of distress. Quality-of-life

TABLE 2-2   Instruments to Measure Symptom Occurrence and Distress, Symptoms of Distress, and Quality of Life

---

Symptom Occurrence and Distress and Symptoms of Distress

- Brief Symptom Inventory (BSI)[28]
- Demands of Illness Inventory (DOII)[29]
- Demands of Bone Marrow Transplant Recovery[7]
- Illness Distress Scale[30]
- Medical Outcomes Study (MOS) Short Form General Health Survey[31]
- Nottingham Health Profile[32]
- Profile of Mood States (POMS)[33]
- Psychosocial Adjustment to Illness Scale—Self-Report (PAIS-SR)[34]
- Rand Health Insurance Study Scales[35]
- Rotterdam Symptom Checklist[36]
- Symptom Checklist 90 (SCL-90)[37]
- Symptom Distress Scale—Original 10-Item Scale[38]
- Symptom Distress Scale—Revised 13-Item Scale[39]
- Symptom Experience Scale[40]
- Sickness Impact Profile (SIP)[41]
- Symptom Profile Instrument (SPI)[42]

Quality of Life

- Late Complications of Bone Marrow Transplant Symptom Checklist[7]
- Breast Cancer Chemotherapy Questionnaire[43]
- Cancer Rehabilitation Evaluation System (CARES)[44]
- City of Hope Quality of Life: Bone Marrow Transplantation[45]
- European Organization for Research and Treatment of Cancer (QLQ-C30)[8]
- Functional Assessment of Cancer Therapy (FACT)[46]
- Functional Living Index—Cancer (FLIC)[47]
- Karnofsky Performance Status[48]
- Linear Analogue Self-Assessment (LASA)[49]
- Spitzer Quality-of-Life Index (QL-Index)[50]
- Ferrans and Powers Quality-of-Life Index (QLI)[51]
- Padilla et al. Quality-of-Life Scale for Cancer (QOL-CA)[52]
- Southwest Oncology Group Quality-of-Life Questionnaire[14]
- Memorial Symptom Assessment Scale—Cancer Specific[53]
- Quality Adjusted Life-Year (QALY)[54]
- Quality Adjusted Time Without Symptoms of Toxicity (Q-TWiST)[55]

---

tools are included because many of these instruments contain symptom occurrence and distress scales. Additional instruments can be found in several resources that provide a compilation of research instruments for nursing.[3,18–20,27]

Conclusion

Several theoretical issues need further elaboration. Although self-report ratings of symptom distress have been shown to predict survival in persons with cancer, there remains a need to examine other variables that mediate perceptions of symptom distress, such as the type of therapy, types of cancer, gender, and age.[4] Moreover, it cannot be assumed that the mere occurrence of a symptom is stressful to the person with cancer. Factors such as the symptom's frequency, duration, periodicity, predictability, and intensity will all influence the saliency attributed to the symptom.[1,3,29] In addition, little is known about what in fact constitutes a problematic level of symptom distress, especially in situations in which survivors of cancer report a high incidence of symptoms but a low level of symptom distress and a high overall quality of life and health.[7] A high incidence of the lingering toxicity effects of chemotherapy and radiation therapy may not be as important as the resiliency of individuals. Cancer survivors are adept at "getting on with their lives" and finding ways to compensate for the deleterious effects of unresolved symptoms.[7] Moreover, the presence of a single or a few repeated symptoms that have a compelling significance and eventually exhaust the individual's or family's efforts to cope may be more detrimental to health than a high number of trivial, minor symptoms.[7,29]

In conclusion, an extensive variety of instruments now exists to measure symptom occurrence and intensity. Many of the newest generation of tools that measure the quality of life of survivors of cancer include scales that measure symptom occurrence and intensity. Measures of symptom occurrence and distress can be used to quantify the effectiveness of nursing interventions that are designed either to provide symptom relief or to enhance self-care ability. Symptom inventories can also be used for making clinical assessments and for helping persons with cancer and their families identify the symptoms that are most likely to be problematic at different points in therapy. Moreover, nurses can provide accurate information about the symptoms that are expected to persist indefinitely after aggressive cancer therapy, in an effort to help cancer survivors better anticipate the future.

References

1. Rhodes VA, Watson PM: Symptom distress—The concept: Past and present. *Semin Oncol Nurs* 3:242–247, 1987
2. Strickland OL: Measures and instruments, in *Patient Outcomes Research: Examining the Effectiveness of Nursing Practice.* U.S. Dept. of Health and Human Services, NIH Publication No. 93-3411, U.S. Government Printing Office, Washington, DC, October 1992, pp. 145–153
3. McCorkle R: The measurement of symptom distress. *Semin Oncol Nurs* 3:248–256, 1987
4. McClement SE, Woodgate RL, Degner L: Symptom distress in adult patients with cancer. *Cancer Nurs* 20:236–243, 1997
5. McDaniel RW, Rhodes VA, Nelson RA, et al: Sensory perceptions of women receiving tamoxifen for breast cancer. *Cancer Nurs* 18:215–221, 1995
6. Kerlinger FN: *Foundations of Behavioral Research* (ed 2.) New York: Holt, Rinehart and Winston, 1973
7. Bush NE, Haberman MR, Donaldson G, et al: Quality of life of 125 adults surviving 6–18 years after bone marrow transplantation. *Soc Sci Med* 40:479–490, 1995
8. Aaronson NK, Ahmedzai S, Bergman B, et al: The European organization for research and treatment of cancer QLQ-C30: A quality of life instrument for use in international clinical trials in oncology. *J Natl Cancer Inst* 85:356–376, 1993
9. Cella DF, Tulsky DS: Measuring quality of life today: Methodological aspects. *Oncology* 4:29–39, 1990
10. Haberman M: Advancing cancer nursing through nursing research, in Groenwald SL, Frogge MH, Goodman M, Yarbro CH (eds): *Cancer Nursing: Principles and Practice* (ed 4). Sudbury: Jones & Bartlett, 1997, pp. 1678–1690
11. Lobchuk MM, Kristjanson L, Degner L, et al: Perception of symptom distress in lung cancer patients: I. Congruence between patients and primary family caregivers. *J Pain Symptom Manage* 14:136–146, 1997
12. McDaniel RW, Rhodes VA: Symptom experience. *Semin Oncol Nurs* 11:232–234, 1995
13. Kurtz ME, Kurtz JC, Given CC, et al: Concordance of cancer patient and caregiver symptom reports. *Cancer Pract* 4:185–190, 1996
14. Moinpour CM, Hayden KA, Thompson LM, et al: Quality of life assessment in Southwest Oncology Group trials. *Oncology* 4:79–89, 1990
15. Jacobson SF: Evaluating instruments for use in clinical nursing research, in Frank-Stromborg M, Olsen SJ (eds): *Instruments for Clinical Healthcare Research* (ed 2). Sudbury: Jones & Bartlett, 1997, pp. 3–19
16. Isaac S, Michael WB: *Handbook in Research and Evaluation: For Education and the Behavioral Sciences* (ed 2). San Diego: EdITS, 1971
17. Haberman M: Research in ambulatory care settings: The need for and how to do research, in Buchsel PA, Yarbro CH (eds): *Oncology Nursing in Ambulatory Settings: Issues and Models of Care.* Sudbury: Jones & Bartlett, 1993, pp. 307–340
18. Frank-Stromborg M, Olsen SJ (eds): *Instruments for Clinical Healthcare Research* (ed 2). Sudbury: Jones & Bartlett, 1997
19. Waltz CF, Strickland OL (eds): *Measurement of Nursing Outcomes: Measuring Client Outcomes,* vol 1. New York: Springer, 1988
20. Strickland OL, Waltz CF (eds): *Measurement of Nursing Outcomes: Measuring Client Self-Care and Coping Skills,* vol 4. New York: Springer, 1991
21. Atwood J: Definition of the research variables, in Grant MM, Padilla GV (eds): *Cancer Nursing Research: A Practical Approach.* Norwalk, CT: Appleton & Lange, 1990, pp. 101–116
22. Nunnally JC: *Psychometric Theory* (ed 2). New York: McGraw-Hill, 1978
23. Edwards AL: *The Measurement of Personality Traits by Scales and Inventories.* New York: Holt, Rinehart and Winston, 1970
24. Waltz C, Bausell RB: *Nursing Research: Design, Statistics and Computer Analysis.* Philadelphia: F.A. Davis, 1981

25. Selltiz C, Wrightsman LS, Cook ST: *Research Methods in Social Relations* (ed 3). New York: Holt, Rinehart and Winston, 1976

26. King CR, Haberman M, Berry DL, et al: Quality of life and the cancer experience: The state-of-the-knowledge. *Oncol Nurs Forum* 24:27–41, 1997

27. Quality of Life in Current Oncology Practice and Research. *Oncology* 4: Whole Issue, 1990

28. Derogatis LR, Melisaratos N: The brief symptom inventory: An introductory report. *Psychol Med* 13:595–605, 1983

29. Haberman MR, Woods NF, Packard NJ: Demands of chronic illness: Reliability and validity assessment of a demands-of-illness inventory. *Holist Nurs Pract* 5:25–35, 1990

30. Noyes R, Kathol RG, Debelius-Enemark P, et al: Distress associated with cancer as measured by the illness distress scale. *Psychosomatics* 31:321–330, 1990

31. Ware JE, Sherbourne CD: A 36-item short form health survey (SF-36): A conceptual framework and item selection. *Med Care* 30:473–483, 1992

32. Hunt SM, McKenna SP, McEwen J, et al: The Nottingham Health Profile: Subjective health status and medical consultations. *Soc Sci Med* 15A:221–229, 1981

33. McNair DN, Lorr M, Droppleman LF: *Profile of Mood States.* San Diego: EdITS, 1981

34. Derogatis LR, Lopez MC: *PAIS & PAIS-SR: Administration, Scoring and Procedures Manual—I.* Baltimore: Clinical Psychometric Research, 1983

35. Brook RH, Ware JE, Davies-Avery A, et al: Overview of adult health status measures fielded in Rand's health insurance study. *Med Care* 17 (suppl):1–131, 1979

36. deHaes JCJM, Welvaart K: Quality of life after breast cancer surgery. *J Surg Oncol* 28:123–125, 1985

37. Derogatis LR, Rickels K, Rock A: The SCL-90 and the MMPI: A step in the validation of a self-report scale. *Br J Psychiatry* 128:280–289, 1976

38. McCorkle R, Young K: Development of a symptom distress scale. *Cancer Nurs* 1:373–378, 1978

39. McCorkle R, Quint-Benoliel J: Symptom distress, current concerns and mood disturbance after diagnosis of life-threatening disease. *Soc Sci Med* 17:431–438, 1983

40. Samarel N, Leddy SK, Greco K, et al: Development and testing of the symptom experience scale. *J Pain Symptom Manage* 12:221–228, 1996

41. Bergner M, Bobbitt RA, Carter WB, et al: The sickness impact profile: Development and final revision of a health status measure. *Med Care* 19:787–806, 1981

42. King KB, Nail LM, Kreamer K, et al: Patients' descriptions of the experience of receiving radiation therapy. *Oncol Nurs Forum* 4:55–61, 1985

43. Levine MN, Guyatt GH, Gent M, et al: Quality of life in stage II breast cancer: An instrument for clinical trials. *J Clin Oncol* 6:1798–1810, 1988

44. Schag CA, Ganz A, Heinrich RL: Cancer Rehabilitation Evaluation System—Short Form (CARES-SF). *Cancer* 68:1406–1413, 1991

45. Ferrell B, Schmidt GM, Rhiner M, et al: The meaning of quality of life for bone marrow transplant survivors: 1. The impact of bone marrow transplant on quality of life. *Cancer Nurs* 15:153–160, 1992

46. Cella DF, Tulsky DJ, Gray G, et al: The Functional Assessment of Cancer Therapy Scale: Development and validation of the general measure. *J Clin Oncol* 11:570–579, 1993

47. Schipper H, Clinch J, McMurray A, et al: Measuring the quality of life of cancer patients—The functional living index-cancer: Development and validation. *J Clin Oncol* 2:472–483, 1984

48. Karnofsky DA, Burchenal JH: The clinical evaluation of chemotherapeutic agents in cancer, in McCleod CM (ed): *Evaluation of Chemotherapeutic Agents.* New York: Columbia University Press, 1949

49. Priestman TJ, Baum M: Evaluation of quality of life in patients receiving treatment for advanced breast cancer. *Lancet* 1:899–901, 1976

50. Spitzer WO, Dobson AJ, Hall J, et al: Measuring the quality of life of cancer patients: A concise QL-index for use by physicians. *J Chronic Dis* 34:585–597, 1981

51. Ferrans CE, Powers MJ: Quality of life index: Development of psychometric properties. *Adv Nurs Sci* 8:15–24, 1985

52. Padilla GV, Grant MM, Lipsett J, et al: Health quality of life and colorectal cancer. *Cancer* 70 (5 suppl):1450–1456, 1992

53. Portenoy RK, Thaler HT, Kornblith AB, et al: The memorial symptom assessment scale: An instrument for the evaluation of symptom prevalence, characteristics and distress. *Eur J Cancer* 30A:1326–1336, 1994

54. Kaplan RM: Quality of life assessment for cost/utility studies in cancer. *Cancer Treat Rev* 19 (suppl A):85–96, 1993

55. Gelber RD, Goldhirsch A, Cole BF: Evaluation of effectiveness: Q-TWiST. The international breast cancer study group. *Cancer Treat Rev* 19 (suppl A):73–84, 1993

Chapter 3

Self-Care and Patient/Family Teaching

Marylin J. Dodd, RN, PhD, FAAN

The Problem of Self-Care

Since the 1960s, healthcare professionals have incorporated a self-care component into their practices. However, in this era of dwindling community health resources and shortened inpatient lengths of stay, the concept of self-care has taken on central importance in the attainment of quality health promotion and illness-related care. Now, individuals simply must manage more by themselves. The mandate for nurses to provide needed information, skills, and support is clear.

The concept of self-care varies based on the degree to which the patient relies on the healthcare system and its professional practitioners. Among healthcare professionals, perspectives range from a conservative ideology,[1-3] with emphasis on minimal dependence on the healthcare system, to a less conservative view,[4] in which the healthcare professional plays a significant role, not only in assisting the patient and family in the acquisition of self-care skills but in managing the patient's self-care. In Orem's self-care deficit theory,[4] the concept of self-care is defined as "the practice of activities that individuals initiate and perform on their own behalf in maintaining life, health, and well-being" (p. 117). She clearly emphasizes the significant role of the nurse in assisting patients to meet their self-care demands when actual or potential deficits exist.

Self-care theorists view the individual as knowledgeable, skillful, and autonomous. Presumably, before a diagnosis of cancer, individuals and family members managed quite well on their own. With a diagnosis of cancer, however, the nurse must augment the knowledge and skills of patients and family members, and provide support—areas that will be discussed in turn in this chapter. The role of the nurse is critically important, because over the years cancer treatment has become more aggressive and complex. For example, unless patients are adequately prepared to manage the side effects of chemotherapy, the resulting morbidity may require reduced chemotherapy dosages, treatment delays, and changes in the chemotherapy agents used—all of which adversely affect an individual's chances for cure or prolonged survival,[5] not to mention diminishing quality of life.

Without specific instruction, patients have only limited knowledge of their cancer treatment, and this knowledge erodes quickly without reinforcement. While treatment knowledge does not guarantee that self-care activities will be performed, participation in care (or self-care) cannot occur without treatment knowledge. The assessment of patients' treatment knowledge and timely reinforcement of information are carried out periodically during the course of treatment, preferably at intervals coinciding with predictable toxicity.

If left on their own, patients undertake modest levels of self-care activities to manage the side effects of treatment, but virtually no self-care to prevent side effects from occurring in the first place. Patients typically wait until the side effects are severe and persistent before initiating self-care, and the range of their self-care activities is limited. The assessment of patients' treatment related self-care and the nurse's role in augmenting patients' self-care is discussed throughout this text, with special emphasis on the management of the symptoms of cancer and its treatment through the use of self-care guides.

Support by the nurse may take on many forms. For example, for patients and their families, the diagnosis of cancer evokes strong emotions, including fear of dying. Careful listening and correction of misconceptions about cancer treatment greatly increase the likelihood of optimal self-care behavior during this difficult period. Support may also come in the form of physical care for patients during times of exacerbation of acute illness and complications from aggressive treatment protocols. Supportive nursing practice and mobilization of community resources are even more crucial when no family members are able to assist patients in their care.

Self-care studies provide compelling data indicating that the whole family is affected by the cancer experience. The American Cancer Society[6] estimates that three out of four families in the United States will have at least one family member diagnosed with cancer. In families that had experienced difficulties prior to the patient's diagnosis with cancer, preexisting problems such as alcohol or drug use were exacerbated. Often, family members commented that it seemed more difficult to stand by and try to help than to be the patient. As such, some family members need self-care interventions for themselves, to help promote healthy coping behaviors.

Some patients do not have available and capable family members to assist them with the more common needs of cancer treatment (e.g., transportation to treatment) or with more complex care demands (e.g., catheter care, parenteral feedings). Their family members may be older or have disabling medical conditions themselves. In such circumstances, the nurse's role is to assess the personal resources of the family and to work with family members to determine how they will manage the family-care needs. Assessment and coordination of additional healthcare services for the family are often required and are facilitated jointly by members of the healthcare team.

What emerges from a review of the literature on self-care are several concepts: the individual's readiness to learn about a health- or disease-related situation,[7,8] knowledge of what to do,[8–12] beliefs in ability,[9,11,13,14] and possession of the functional abilities to perform self-care activities.[8,11,15–17] These concepts coincide with Orem's model of self-care deficit[4] through her proposed power components of self-care agency (one's ability to care for self). Table 3-1 details the power components. The power components are needed to engage in self-care operations.

Assessment

Readiness to Learn

Assessment of patients' and family members' readiness to learn is based on the clinical assessment of these individuals. A positive assessment may be rendered if the individuals appear to be listening, maintaining their attention, and exercising the requisite vigilance with respect to self and the situation. Patients and family members who are fully engaged in the interaction will ask relevant questions, demonstrating their readiness to learn. Clinical realities dictate, however, that whether or not the patient or family members are ready, they must be taught the

TABLE 3-1 Self-Care Concepts and Self-Care Agency Power Components and Operations

Concept	Power Component Operations
Readiness to learn about health or disease-related condition • ability to maintain attention and to exercise requisite vigilance with respect to self and external conditions (power component)	*Estimative operations* of inquiry that seek both empirical and technical knowledge about what is, what can, and what should be brought about with respect to self-care
Knowledge about what to do • ability to reason within a self-care framework • ability to acquire technical knowledge **Beliefs in ability**	*Transitional operations* of reflecting, judging, and deciding with respect to self-care requisites (needs) and measures for meeting them
Functional abilities • controlled use of available physical energy • ability to control the position of the body, e.g., psychomotor skills • possessing cognitive, perceptual, communication, and interpersonal skills • ability to make decisions about self-care requisites	*Productive operations* of performance of self-care activities, monitoring performance, and evaluation of effectiveness of self-care

Orem, D: *Nursing Concepts of Practice* (ed 5). St. Louis: Mosby, 1995.[4] Reprinted with permission.

potentially life-threatening signs and symptoms of disease and treatment-related complications. When patients are reluctant, nurses shift their focus and attempt to teach the "most ready" family member. Such an approach is not ideal, because the patient is the focus of self-care. Addressing the patient at subsequent sessions or visits is recommended, as the lack of readiness may resolve with time.

Difficulties in readiness derive from several potential sources. For example, cognitive impairment, profound psychological and emotional responses to the cancer experience, and lack of motivation for self-care all adversely affect individuals' readiness to learn about their conditions. To participate in self-care, certain higher-order cognitive abilities are required: (1) ability to order discrete self-care actions into relationships with prior and subsequent actions; (2) ability to learn the technical aspects of care; and (3) ability to reason within the self-care frame of reference.[4] For individuals who are moderately to severely cognitively impaired, self-care beyond basic hygiene is not realistic. In such an instance, the nurse works with a family member, or other designated caregiver, who has provided care to the individual before the diagnosis of cancer.

High anxiety's negative effect on an individual's readiness to take in information is well documented, and its occurrence compels the nurse to include less anxious family members in the discussion. It is recommended that the highly anxious patient or family member not be excluded during self-care teaching sessions; instead, the nurse works with the highly anxious individual in concert with the less anxious patient or family member. Giving individuals who are moderately anxious discrete, sequential tasks to perform may lessen their anxiety.

Finally, a lack of motivation to understand the situation and the required self-care measures has a negative impact on the ultimate success of self-care activities. For people who are not sufficiently motivated, despite the nurse's efforts to provide information, self-care may not be a realistic goal. However, today, unlike in the past, choosing not to participate in self-care is not a viable option; it is an expectation. Orem suggests that when working with less motivated individuals, the nurse should encourage them to think about their self-care role, their ability to care for themselves, and the benefits derived from practicing self-care.[4] Components of assessment and strategies for teaching self-care, for this and following sections, are summarized in Table 3-2.

Patients' and Family Members' Knowledge

Assessing patients' and family members' knowledge of the situation and what needs to be done, such as potential side effects that may occur and the self-care that is needed, lends itself to both clinical evaluation by the nurse and the use of instruments such as the Chemotherapy Knowledge Questionnaire.[18] (Patient feedback on the self-care guides that are presented throughout this text may also aid in knowledge assessment.) Individuals who possess a repertoire of skills that can be adapted to the performance of self-care are at an advantage. Knowledge about the specific situation is a necessary precursor to preventive self-care, as it may help the patient to avoid the side effect or to minimize its occurrence. Knowledge is also necessary for the timely initiation of self-care if the side effect is experienced.

Nail et al.[19] have developed the Self-Care Diary, in which the common side effects of chemotherapy are presented, along with a list of self-care activities. The patients are asked if they experienced these side effects and to indicate which self-care activities they performed. An instrument that consists of a pre-existing list of possible responses is less challenging to individuals than one having an open-ended format (in which they write their responses with no prompting). When developing a knowledge questionnaire, it is helpful to break down the content to be tested into specific items. This strategy permits more discrete indications of where the patients and families are lacking knowledge. For example, if the content to be tested is preventive self-care activities for the potential side effects of doxorubicin, the patient's knowledge of those potential side effects must be established before any preventive activities can be realized.

Beliefs in Ability and Effectiveness of Self-Care

Assessing individuals' beliefs in their ability and their confidence that their self-care activities will positively affect their health outcomes is a newer area of assessment. This dimension of clinical assessment stems from Bandura's work with the theory of "self-efficacy."[20] There are two sequential components to the theory: (1) the individuals' belief that they can perform the needed self-care, and (2) their confidence that their self-care will positively affect the desired outcome. Motivation to do self-care is directly linked to these beliefs—if people do not believe they can perform the required self-care or that it will make a difference, it is unlikely that self-care will be tried. This issue may be most relevant for some of the more demanding self-care tasks, such as intravenous line care or the injection of medications.

Talking to individuals about their self-care is probably the most likely way to detect difficulties with either dimension of self-efficacy. A method of assessing belief in ability consists of asking individuals to demonstrate the skill (*return demonstration*). Lack of confidence that self-care activities will make a difference in outcomes is more difficult to detect. In the example of the return demonstration, the individuals may be fully capable of doing the task, but because of lack of confidence in the worth of

TABLE 3-2 Clinical Nursing Guide: Teaching Self-Care

Areas for Assessment	Methods/Strategies
1. Readiness to learn Observe patient/family for: • appearance of listening and attention behaviors • asking relevant questions • cognitive impairments • high emotional distress • motivation	Clinical assessment including: • asking patients and family members if they are ready to learn • working with the persons who are ready • asking patients and family members what it would take for them to feel more ready • asking them what they want to know first
2. Treatment knowledge of patients and family members	Ask patients and family members questions about their treatment. • provide needed information, and correct misinformation • provide potentially life-threatening information first; repeat this information at return clinic visits
Self-care behaviors to be performed to prevent side effects and to manage them once they have occurred	• assess what the patients/family members know and do for the side effects of treatment • augment their knowledge with additional self-care behaviors to be performed
3. Assessing beliefs in ability and effectiveness of self-care behaviors	• ask how confident patients/family members feel to perform self-care behaviors • provide practice sessions and return demonstrations • ask how effective they believe the self-care behaviors will be in obtaining better results, i.e., does it work? does it help? • relate past clinical experiences in which self-care behaviors resulted in better outcomes • cite studies' findings in which self-care behaviors assisted patients/family members in realizing better outcomes
4. Functional abilities/constitutional status, e.g., fatigue	Using Karnofsky Performance Scale or other cooperative groups' functional status instruments:
Fine-motor abilities	• observe return demonstration of self-care skills and provide more practice as needed • if patients and family members are unable to perform the needed care activities, give referral to an agency that can provide this care
5. Evaluation of self-care activities	• have patient/family members keep a Self-Care Log (Appendix 3A) of side effects experienced and self-care behaviors performed to manage these side effects • review their recordings with them for severity of side effects and effectiveness of the self-care behaviors • augment what they are already doing by suggesting other self-care behaviors to be tried
Symptom and side effect status	• Clinical assessment of specific symptoms and side effects; if a symptom or side effect persists or is particularly severe, consult members of the multidisciplinary team for their recommendations

doing it, sustained self-care activity—particularly when not directly supervised—becomes less likely. Simply asking individuals if they believe that the self-care will make a difference in the outcome may prompt a socially desirable, rather than an honest, response: "Yes, of course it will make a difference!"

Different strategies are used by the nurse when bolstering patients' confidence in their ability to perform the required self-care and when encouraging their confidence in its value. In the first instance, the nurse can

guide, coach, and support patients. Supervised practice sessions enhance patients' confidence that they can do the activities on their own. The strategies used to enhance patients' perceptions of the value of performing self-care are more challenging. The nurse may draw on personal experience with other patients who experienced better outcomes by using the suggested self-care activities or may cite research studies (where available) that have demonstrated the benefit of specific self-care activities. Examples include the benefit of taking antiemetic medications on a prescribed schedule, not as needed, and the benefit of performing systematic mouth care when at risk for chemotherapy-induced mucositis.

Functional Abilities to Perform Self-Care

Assessment of functional abilities of the person with cancer includes not only the consequences of pre-existing comorbid conditions (e.g., arthritis, diabetes) but also the current loss or projected loss of functioning due to the disease and its treatment. There are general instruments to determine physical capabilities of activities of daily living—for example, the Functional Assessment Inventory.[21] There are also instruments to measure the functional abilities of people with specific conditions, such as arthritis, vision loss, or motor deficits. In cancer practice, an example of a general measure of functional ability is the Karnofsky Performance Scale[22] or the Oncology Cooperative Group's scale for functional status. These instruments are useful in determining the overall constitutional abilities of individuals and can measure the disease and treatment sequelae of fatigue and weakness. Functional abilities are important to the repeated performance of needed self-care activities. Assessment of functional abilities also includes the discrete fine-motor movements needed for specific self-care activities. Observation of fine-motor performance in practice is essential because instruments have not been developed and tested for skill-specific self-care activities. The return demonstration of the fine-motor skills needed to perform self-care activities would be helpful to evaluate performance. A one-time repeat demonstration does not assess performance repeatedly over time, that is, the ability to perform consistently over time.

A few agencies and hospitals have developed "learning labs" for patients and their families to gain knowledge and skills in selected self-care activities. These labs are often adjacent to the agency or hospital and provide a quiet, unhurried environment in which to learn, by simulation and other methods, for example, to give injections, change dressings, and provide catheter care. Learning labs are more cost-effective than hospitalization of patients and, because they are available to patients until skills are mastered, they are more likely than hospitalization to enhance quality of care.

Early in the cancer experience, family members may assist patients with care, such as driving them to clinic visits and to radiation therapy treatments, and preparing favorite foods to counteract the patients' diminished appetite or when the patients are too fatigued to carry out self-care activities. With the eventual onset of the patients' diminished physical capabilities, the family members' roles change. If family members are included in teaching sessions from the outset, the change in activities can be less overwhelming. The suggested techniques for evaluating the patients' performance of self-care apply to family members as well.

Self-Care Management

Preventive Self-Care

Prevention through self-care of a symptom or complication of cancer and the side effects of treatment is an important goal. To fulfill this goal, patients and family members must know two things: (1) what the risks are for developing symptoms and (2) the self-care that is appropriate. When the nurse has provided the information needed for patients to monitor adequately for the development of potential side effects, major benefits are realized. First, patients are sufficiently educated to assess for the initial phases of the side effect and are less likely not to notice subtle manifestations or to falsely attribute bodily sensations to the treatment. Secondly, patients can initiate timely self-care activities, which may include alerting their healthcare provider of problems, if they have been instructed to do so. The nurse, by fulfilling the role of educator, provides patients with information about what to watch for, the meaning of the side effect, and recommended activities to be performed to manage the side effect.

Empirically tested self-care that can prevent or diminish the occurrence of disease symptoms and side effects of treatment is limited. For example, we know that alopecia occurs with some chemotherapy drugs, and while it is advised that patients not color hair or get a permanent because these activities potentially exacerbate hair loss, at the same time we cannot prescribe self-care activities that will totally prevent the hair loss from occurring. Similarly, we prescribe a systematic oral care protocol for patients who are receiving oral mucositis-inducing chemotherapy agents; though this protocol may not prevent oral mucositis from developing in all patients, it is helpful for many patients.[23]

Early Stage Self-Care

What to teach patients and family members first is in part a function of what is essential for them to know immediately. For example, self-care knowledge and skills for potentially, life-threatening events, such as fever and infection in immunosuppressed individuals, are critically important. The early self-care needed in this situation would consist of having patients and family members monitor something that might seem innocuous to them, such as a low-grade fever, and then to contact the healthcare provider in a timely manner. The timing of the content in other teaching sessions might be driven by the knowledge of what symptoms and side effects are likely to occur. For example, oral mucositis can occur within the first several days of the first cycle of chemotherapy; whereas, treatment-related fatigue is likely to occur in subsequent cycles of chemotherapy. Knowing this, one would individualize the teaching to present the information and self-care skills to assess for, prevent, and then treat oral mucositis, before presenting similar information about fatigue. Early self-care includes teaching patients and family members about necessary self-care *before* the need presents itself.[24] For example, it is a practice in one bone marrow transplant unit to have the patients learn about and practice systematic oral care and to exercise on stationary bicycles with intravenous pumps and other apparatus prior to receiving the transplant, so that when they are feeling much more ill during the early stages of the transplant, they already know and have had some practice at the necessary self-care that must be performed.

Later Stage Self-Care

Later stage self-care is as important as early stage self-care. Its components include the sustained performance of activities by the patients, the breadth of their self-care repertoire, and an active role for nursing. Many of the symptoms of the disease and side effects of treatment are not exclusively acute events (e.g., pain and fatigue) and therefore carry with them an added challenge to patients: They need to be consistent and persistent in their self-care activities. This is especially true when individuals' stamina and energy stores are at low levels. Every self-care activity must be effective, and because of the more chronic nature of some symptoms, individuals have to be more creative, as self-care activities that worked previously may lose their effectiveness over time. Having a large repertoire of self-care activities on which to draw helps enormously. However, from experience, it is clear that most individuals do not possess a large repertoire, but rather a modest list of things to do that have worked for ailments in the past. When patients come to the end of their limited repertoires, they either decrease their self-care activities or they persist in familiar self-care activities, even though they know that they are being minimally effective. At this critically important juncture, it is the nurse's job to assess individuals' self-care activities or the lack thereof; to evaluate the effectiveness of the self-care; and to augment individuals' self-care repertoire through clinical experiences of what has been effective and knowledge of current literature.

Enhancing patients' self-care creativity and expanding their self-care repertoire clearly is an important role for nursing. The art of managing these situations comes in the nurse's ability to match the appropriateness of the suggested new self-care activity with the individual patient. For example, guided imagery and hypnosis have been demonstrated to be very effective in managing several symptoms and side effects. However, some patients may find the thought of these activities aversive. Trying new self-care activities when the patient is feeling ill and discouraged due to the lack of effectiveness of earlier self-care activities requires much encouragement and creative

intervention on the part of the nurse. Most importantly, the nurse must communicate the belief that with some effort a successful alternative approach to managing the problem will be found.

Evaluation of Management Strategies

There are two aspects to the evaluation of management strategies: (1) the evaluation of individuals' self-care activities, and (2) the evaluation of the effectiveness of these activities through the assessment of the symptom or side effect status.

Several established instruments are available for use by individuals to report symptoms or side effects, rate their intensity and severity, report what they have done or are doing for each symptom or side effect, rate the effectiveness of each of their self-care activities, and finally to give the source of their idea for each self-care activity. Instruments on which the individuals write in their responses to questions, such as the symptom or side effect that they experienced and what they have done or are doing,[25–26] are appropriate for use for a variety of symptoms and side effects and across treatment modalities. An example of one of these instruments is the self-care log (Appendix 3A).[26] Individuals who are beginning their cancer treatment are given a log. They record the side effects of treatment as they occur and rate the side effects' levels of intensity and distress. Next, the individuals record what they did to manage the side effect. The individuals then rate the effectiveness of their self-care activities and report the source of the ideas for the self-care activities. The individuals bring in their logs at the next treatment and show them to their nurse or physician, who studies what the individuals have experienced and what they have done to manage. The individuals take their logs home and continue reporting in them as side effects are experienced. Other instruments have the format of a preexisting list of symptoms, side effects, and self-care activities. By design, therefore, these instruments are used with specific cancer treatment modalities—for example, for radiation therapy patients or chemotherapy patients.[8,19,26]

The goal of self-care is not to have individuals overly active in their self-care but, rather, to encourage individuals to practice informed, effective self-care activities. The effectiveness of self-care is based on symptom or side effect status. As mentioned, there are instruments available that ask individuals to rate the effectiveness of each of their self-care activities in alleviating a symptom or side effect. The format of this evaluation is usually on a Likert scale of 0 (i.e., activity did not help at all) to 5 (i.e., completely alleviated the symptom or side effect). However, a numerical scale may not provide sufficient detail for more precise evaluations of exactly what self-care activities are working for what aspects of the symptom or side effect experience.

There are some general principles to follow when

choosing a clinical instrument. First and most important, the patients and families must understand the instructions and what is being asked. The instrument must be easy to complete and brief, asking only what is needed. Ideally, the instrument should be able to be completed by patients and families on their own with a minimum of guidance by the nurse. From the nurses' perspective, the instrument must be easy to interpret or score in clinical settings. The instrument should lend itself to being included in the patients' medical records, so that the patients' and families' learning needs are clearly documented, as is the teaching provided by the nurse to meet those needs. Finally, the instrument should be understandable to other healthcare providers, who will thereby have access to the patients' and families' data to guide their own practice.

A recently developed tool (Figure 3-1) for documenting the patient's learning needs, instruction/information provided to the patient, and planned reinforcement of the information is completed by the patient's nurses on an ongoing basis. The level of the patient's skills are assessed by return demonstrations. The patient initials entries on the tool. This documentation tool is designed to be used with a comprehensive patient education packet and is a permanent part of the patient's medical record.

The Future of Self-Care in the Changing Healthcare Environment

Currently, most oncology nurses practice in specific healthcare settings such as diagnostic/procedure and day-surgery settings, radiation therapy departments, and chemotherapy outpatient clinics. The fragmentation of patient care resulting from this current model is well documented. The rare exception is the joint-practice model, in which the advanced nurse practitioner (i.e., clinical nurse specialist and nurse practitioner) follows a caseload of oncology patients along with the oncologist through the treatment phases of the cancer experience, from the diagnosis of cancer, through surgery, radiation therapy, and chemotherapy. This practice model requires the nurse to have expertise in a variety of diagnostic and treatment regimens, but it has greater likelihood of achieving continuity of care. Another proposed model is that of nurse-run clinics. Central questions to be answered concerning this model of care include where and how patients and families access the nurse, and how these programs can become financially self-sufficient. The problem of reimbursement for independent nursing services hinders the progress that could be made in establishing more free-standing nurse-run clinics.

The concept of managed care has gained attention from all healthcare providers. For nurses, managed care will likely contract for nursing services through large health maintenance organizations (HMOs) and other healthcare–providing agencies/insurers. This will most likely occur for outpatient services (in the community and patients' homes), as the need for these services will continue to increase. Ensuring a role for nursing in contracted managed care will be most appropriate and cost effective for insurers. By providing information, skills, and support, nurses prepare patients and families to manage the care needed for the patient/family member, thereby decreasing care delivery in more expensive settings.

The provider expectation is that when patients have diminished capabilities to care for themselves, family members will become the primary caregivers in the home. This expectation exists despite reports that many families feel unprepared to provide care.[27–28] Yet, in the face of having few or no other options, patients and family members generally take pride in their abilities.[29] Still, when problems occur for which neither the patient nor the family are prepared, they feel terribly responsible and guilty for not having the knowledge. The implications for nursing are clear—if patients and family members are expected to carry increased responsibility, then they need to be educated proactively, *not* reactively when difficulties have already occurred. The need for self-care will continue to escalate as more care is provided on an outpatient basis, as patients are discharged from hospitals "sicker and quicker," and as healthcare technologies continue to become more complex.

Conclusion

In self-care studies, it has been documented that with treatment-related information, patients' knowledge and self-care activities have been significantly improved.[18,25,30,31] These findings have not consistently translated into statistically significant improvement in side effect status, but patients and families report liking the self-care interventions and feeling more empowered and in control of the situation by being participants in their care.[32] For these patients and families, the nursing intervention positively influenced their quality of life.

Research findings are lagging behind clinical practice observations that self-care information, skills, and support do make a difference in patients' treatment-related morbidity. Similarly, the cost-effectiveness of self-care interventions is currently observed in clinical practice; i.e., patients who have been prepared for self-care have prevented or managed treatment-related complications adequately rather than requiring additional care and perhaps hospitalization. Ongoing and future studies must continue to investigate the effectiveness of self-care interventions in affecting side effect and symptom status; the cost of these interventions, including the human costs to patients and family members; and the costs that result from not preparing patients and families adequately to manage their care.

STANFORD HEALTH SERVICES
STANFORD, CALIFORNIA 94305

HEMATOLOGY / ONCOLOGY
TEACHING DOCUMENTATION - Page 1 of 2

ADDRESSOGRAPH - PATIENT NAME, MEDICAL RECORD NUMBER

Hematology/Oncology Documentation	Written Instruction	Video	First Review	Second Review	Patient Initials	Caregiver Present	Comments
Date and Initial Each Encounter							
Type of Cancer_____							
Primary Caregiver							
Definitions: Neutropenia / Nadir / ANC							
Anemia							
Thrombocytopenia							
Bone Marrow Biopsy							
Chemotherapy							
Radiation Therapy							
Growth Factor:_____							
SQ Administration of Growth Factor							Return Demonstration:_____
Side Effects:							Type:_____
Central Line Catheter							Return Demonstration:_____
Dressing Changes							Return Demonstration:_____
Line Flushing / Cap Changes							
Neutropenia Precautions							
Thrombocytopenia Precautions							
Anemia / Fatigue							
Treatment: Chemotherapy							
1.							
2.							
3.							
4.							
Radiation Therapy							
Symptom Management: Nausea							
Vomiting							
Diarrhea							
Mouth Sores							
Hemorrhagic Cystitis							
Peripheral Neuropathy							
Skin Rash / Changes							
Alopecia							
Fevers							

INITIALS	SIGNATURE					
1		4			8	
2		5			9	
3		6			10	
		7			11	

15-1276 (8/97)

FIGURE 3-1   Hematology/Oncology Teaching Documentation

STANFORD HEALTH SERVICES
STANFORD, CALIFORNIA 94305

HEMATOLOGY / ONCOLOGY
TEACHING DOCUMENTATION - Page 2 of 2

ADDRESSOGRAPH - PATIENT NAME, MEDICAL RECORD NUMBER

Hematology/Oncology Documentation	Written Instruction	Video	First Review	Second Review	Patient Initials	Caregiver Present	Comments
Symptom Management: Xerostomia							
Esophagitis							
Constipation							
Insomnia							
Other: 1.							
2.							
3.					•		
Transfusion of RBC / Platelets							
Daily Hygiene: Mouth Care							Return Demonstration:
Hepafilter Mask / Proper Fitting							Return Demonstration:
Coach							Return Demonstration:
Perirectal Care							
Skin Care							
Gonadal Suppression							
Sexual Activity							
Preparing the Home							
D/C Medications							
Reportable Signs & Symptoms							
Dietary: Low Microbial Diet							
Special Diet Needs							
Other:							
Physical Therapy							
Social Work: Housing							
Durable Power of Attorney							
Disability / Return to Work							
Community Resources							
Psychosocial Issues							
Case Management: Home Care Agency							
Pharmacy							
Equipment							
Home Care Management:							
Pump Teaching							Return Demonstration:
Self Administration of Medications							Return Demonstration:

INITIALS	SIGNATURE	4		8	
1		5		9	
2		6		10	
3		7		11	

15-1276 (8/97)

FIGURE 3-1   (continued) Source: Olsen, M. Stanford Health Services. Used with permission.

References

1. Levin L, Katz A, Holst E: *Self-Care: Lay Initiatives in Health.* New York: Prodist, 1976

2. Levin L: Self-care: An international perspective. *Soc Policy* 7:70, 1976

3. Levin L: Patient education and self-care: How do they differ? *Nurs Outlook* 26:170–175, 1978

4. Orem D: *Nursing: Concepts of Practice* (ed 5). St. Louis: Mosby, 1995

5. Peters L, Ang K: Altered fractionation schemes, in Mauch PM, Loeffler JS (eds), *Radiation Oncology: Technology and Biology.* Philadelphia: W.B. Saunders, 1994, pp. 545–565

6. Landis SH, Murray T, Bolden S, Wingo PA: Cancer statistics, 1998. *CA Cancer J Clin* 48:6–9, 1998

7. Dodd MJ, Dibble SL: Predictors of self-care: A test of Orem's model. *Oncol Nurs Forum* 20:895–901, 1993

8. Hagopian G: The effects of informational audiotapes on knowledge and self-care behaviors of patients undergoing radiation therapy. *Oncol Nurs Forum* 23:697–700, 1996

9. Lev EL: Triangulation reveals theoretical linkages and outcomes in a nursing intervention study. *Clin Nurse Specialist* 9:300–305, 1995

10. Fujita LY, Dungan JD: High risk for ineffective management of therapeutic regimen: A protocol study. *Rehabilitation Nurs* 19:75–79, 1994

11. Williams-Utz S, Shuster G, Merwin E, Williams B: A community-based smoking-cessation program: Self-care behaviors and success. *Public Health Nurs* 11:291–299, 1994

12. Robinson KD, Posner JD: Patterns of self-care needs and interventions related to biologic response modifier therapy: Fatigue as a model. *Semin Oncol Nurs* 8:17–22, 1992

13. Hurley AC: Measuring self-care ability in patients with diabetes: The Insulin Management Diabetes Self-Efficacy Scale, in Strickland OL, Watz CF (eds): *Measurement of Nursing Outcomes: Measuring Client Self-Care and Coping Skills,* vol 4. New York: Springer, 1990, pp. 28–44

14. Gortner S, Jenkins L: Self-efficacy and activity level following cardiac surgery. *J Adv Nurs* 15:1132–1138, 1990

15. Hart MA: Orem's self-care deficit theory: Research with pregnant women. *Nurs Sci Q* 8:120–126, 1995

16. Vesely C: Pediatric patient—Controlled analgesia: Enhancing the self-care construct. *Pediatric Nursing* 21:124–128, 1995

17. Dennis CM: *Self-Care Deficit Theory of Nursing.* St. Louis: Mosby, 1997

18. Dodd MJ: Chemotherapy knowledge in patients with cancer: Assessment and informational interventions. *Oncol Nurs Forum* 9:39–44, 1982

19. Nail L, Jones LS, Greene D, et al: Use and perceived efficacy of self-care activities in patients receiving chemotherapy. *Oncol Nurs Forum* 18:887–983, 1991

20. Bandura A: Self-efficacy mechanisms in human agency. *Am Psychol* 37:122–147, 1982

21. Pfeiffer E: *Functional Assessment Inventory.* Tampa: University of South Florida College of Medicine, 1980

22. Karnofsky DA, Burchenal JH: The clinical evaluation of chemotherapeutic agents in cancer, in MacLeod CM (ed): *Evaluation of Chemotherapy Agents.* New York: Columbia University Press, 1949, pp. 45–49

23. Dodd MJ, Larson P, Dibble SL, Miaskowski C, et al: Randomized clinical trial of chlorhexidine versus placebo control for prevention of oral mucositis in patients receiving chemotherapy. *Oncol Nurs Forum* 23:921–927, 1996

24. Dodd MJ. *Suggestions for Managing the Side Effects of Chemotherapy and Radiation Therapy: A Handbook for Patients and Families* (ed 3). San Francisco: UCSF School of Nursing Press, 1996

25. Dodd MJ: Assessing patient self-care for side-effects of cancer chemotherapy. *Cancer Nurs* 5:447–451, 1982

26. Dodd MJ: Measuring self-care activities, in Frank-Stromborg M, Olsen S (eds): *Instruments for Clinical Healthcare Research* (ed 2). Sudbury, MA: Jones & Bartlett, 1997, pp. 378–388

27. Stetz K: Caregiving demands during advanced cancer. *Cancer Nurs* 10:260–268, 1987

28. Dodd MJ: Self-care: Ready or not! *Oncol Nurs Forum* 24:981–990, 1996

29. Weiner C, Dodd MJ: Coping amid uncertainty: An illness trajectory perspective. *Sch Inq Nurs Pract* 7:17–31, 1993

30. Dodd MJ: Efficacy of proactive information on self-care in radiation therapy patients. *Heart Lung* 16:538–544, 1987

31. Dodd MJ: Efficacy of proactive information on self-care in chemotherapy patients. *Patient Educ Couns* 11:215–225, 1988

32. Dodd MJ, Lovejoy N, Larson P, et al: *Self-Care Intervention to Decrease Chemotherapy Morbidity.* Final Report of National Cancer Institute Research Grant ROI CA48312, 1992

Self-Care Log

Problem or Major Complaint	Severity/Distress	Actions Taken	Effectiveness of Actions		Sources of Suggestions for Actions
			not relieved at all	completely relieved	
	a) Severity, i.e., how intense is it?	a.	0 1 2 3 4 5		a.
	barely most noticeable severe 1 2 3 4 5	b.	0 1 2 3 4 5		b.
	b) Distress, i.e., how much does it bother you?	a.	0 1 2 3 4 5		a.
	minor extremely annoyance distressing 1 2 3 4 5	b.	0 1 2 3 4 5		b.
	a) Severity, i.e., how intense is it?	a.	0 1 2 3 4 5		a.
	barely most noticeable severe 1 2 3 4 5	b.	0 1 2 3 4 5		b.
	b) Distress, i.e., how much does it bother you?	a.	0 1 2 3 4 5		a.
	minor extremely annoyance distressing 1 2 3 4 5	b.	0 1 2 3 4 5		b.

(continued)

Source: Dodd MJ: Measuring self-care activities, in Frank-Stromborg M, Olsen S (eds): *Instruments for Clinical Research in Healthcare* (ed 2). Sudbury: Jones & Bartlett.[26] Used with permission. © 1997 Jones & Bartlett Publishers.

Questions to ask the nurse and physician

1. Question: _____
_____ Date: _____

1a. Answer: _____
_____ Date: _____

2. Question: _____
_____ Date: _____

2a. Answer: _____
_____ Date: _____

3. Question: _____
_____ Date: _____

3a. Answer: _____
_____ Date: _____

4. Question: _____
_____ Date: _____

4a. Answer: _____
_____ Date: _____

5. Question: _____
_____ Date: _____

5a. Answer: _____
_____ Date: _____

6. Question: _____
_____ Date: _____

6a. Answer: _____
_____ Date: _____

7. Question: _____
_____ Date: _____

7a. Answer: _____
_____ Date: _____

8. Question: _____
_____ Date: _____

8a. Answer: _____
_____ Date: _____

PART II

SYMPTOMS OF DISTURBANCES OF COMFORT

CHAPTER 4

Arthralgias and Myalgias

Virginia R. Martin, MSN, RN, AOCN

The Problem of Arthralgias and Myalgias in Cancer

New chemotherapy drugs and biologic response modifiers have caused an increased incidence of arthralgias and myalgias in patients with cancer. *Arthralgia* is joint pain. *Myalgia* is diffuse muscle pain, usually accompanied by malaise. Both are often listed as neurotoxicities for an individual drug, though the neuromuscular toxicity is a more precise description. Table 4-1 provides a list of chemotherapy drugs and biologic response modifiers that may cause arthralgias and myalgias.

Incidence

Arthralgias and myalgias have long been associated with chronic illness such as rheumatoid arthritis or fibromyalgia. The taxane drugs cause arthralgias and myalgias in as many as 96% of patients.[1] The intensity of these symptoms is related to the dose of paclitaxel given; however, it is not a dose-limiting toxicity. The reported incidence of severe arthralgias and myalgias is 8%, which was noted at doses of more than 200 mg/m^2.[2] Another drug in the taxane category, docetaxel, also produces arthralgias and myalgias. The vinca alkaloid drugs and the colony-stimulating factors are also associated with arthralgias and myalgias, but the incidence is less frequent and accompanied by other flulike symptoms that have been reported more regularly. Vinblastine, when used at high doses in the treatment of testicular cancer, caused severe myalgias—a clear dose-related phenomena.[3] The colony-stimulating factors produce flulike symptoms that include, but are not limited to, arthralgias and myalgias. The new approach to mobilization of peripheral blood stem cells with granulocyte colony-stimulating factor (G-CSF), with or without interleukin-3, has produced up to 83% incidence of arthralgias and myalgias.[4,5]

Impact on Quality of Life

The impact of arthralgia and myalgia on the patient's quality of life can be significant. If the severity of the symptoms is great enough, patients' ability to perform their normal activities of daily living may be impaired. Most chemotherapy drugs have overlapping side effects. Fatigue, malaise, decreased appetite, and lack of energy are common complaints. The addition of joint and muscle aches can substantially reduce the patient's quality of life.

Etiology

How chemotherapeutic agents cause joint and muscle pain is uncertain. It is interesting to note, however, that the agents associated with significant joint and muscle pains are agents that inhibit microtubular function (i.e., the vinca alkaloids, particularly vinblastine and vindesine, and the taxanes, paclitaxel and docetaxel). The antimi-

TABLE 4-1   Chemotherapy/Biologic Response Modifiers That May Cause Arthralgias and Myalgias

Classification/Drugs	Comments
Taxanes	
Paclitaxel	Dose-related: mild discomfort at doses <170 mg/m²; more frequent and severe with doses >200 mg/m².
	Schedule related: mild symptoms with 24-hour infusion; severity increases with 1-hour infusion
	Arthralgias and myalgias increase when G-CSF added.
	Transient pain in muscles and joints, especially large axial, shoulder, and paraspinal muscles
Docetaxel	Transient myalgias and arthralgias
Vinca alkaloids	
Vincristine	Myalgias
Vinblastine	Myalgias; dose-related: severe muscle pain with high doses
Vindesine	Muscle weakness
Biologic response modifiers	
Filgrastim	Flulike syndrome that includes arthralgias and myalgias
Sargramostim	Skeletal pain
Interferon	Arthralgias and myalgias of transient duration; involves proximal muscles of lower extremities
Interleukin-2	Arthralgias and myalgias; more significant at high doses
Rituximab	Arthralgias and myalgias

crotubule agents are among the most important anticancer drugs and have contributed significantly to the therapy of most curable neoplasms, such as Hodgkin's and non-Hodgkin's lymphomas, germ cell tumors, and childhood leukemias.[6,7] At a subcellular level, these agents are very potent; a few molecules can disrupt the microtubular structure.[8]

Vinca Alkaloids

With the vinca alkaloids and taxanes, there is a clear dose-response relationship with arthralgias and myalgias. This is most striking with vinblastine. The cure of advanced testicular cancer was heralded by the report by Einhorn and Donahue[9] in the late 1970s and later in subsequent studies.[10–12] The original Einhorn regimen employed vinblastine at a dose of 0.4 mg/kg administered in two equally divided doses (0.2 mg/kg) on the first and second day of therapy. This high-dose program was associated with

intense myelosuppression, as was to be expected, but there were also two nonhematologic toxicities that were profound. One was neurotoxicity, which was generally seen at lower doses, and the second was severe muscle pain. This symptom developed a few days after drug administration and lasted for several days. It manifested as severe back and abdominal pain, and in its worse form required opiate analgesics. Sometimes dose adjustments were required to convince patients to continue treatment. Einhorn et al.[3] studied maintenance therapy with vinblastine after the success of primary therapy. Eighteen of 58 patients (31%) randomized to take maintenance therapy with vinblastine refused to take the drug; others who took the drug refused to complete therapy due to toxicity. Clinical trials investigating lower doses of vinblastine (0.1 to 0.2 mg/kg) revealed that the associated muscle pain was much milder, thus toxicity was dose-related. The introduction of etoposide into the primary regimen for testicular cancer abolished this toxicity as a major therapeutic problem.[13] Now used at much lower doses, the vinca alkaloids are still associated with occasional muscle pain, but rarely, if ever, is the pain as severe as that which was seen with high-dose vinblastine.

Taxanes

Paclitaxel

From the initial clinical trials, it was quickly shown that paclitaxel was associated with joint and muscle pain. It is described as a paroxysmal pain that involves muscles and bones, mainly in the lower extremities, with or without painful dysesthesia.[14] It is described by patients as aching in the hips, thighs, and upper legs, and can also include the shoulders. This reaction is often now referred to as arthralgia or myalgia and is considered an expression of neurotoxicity.[1,15] Overall, 24% of paclitaxel courses administered in one study required opiate analgesics due to the severity of the symptom.[16]

Transient arthralgias and/or myalgias are commonly observed after treatment with moderate to high doses of paclitaxel administered over a variety of infusion times, from 1 to 24 hours.[1,2,15–22] As with vinblastine, this toxicity appears to be dose-related, but in contrast to the vinblastine experience, rarely does it require dose adjustment. The administration schedule influences the incidence of arthralgias and myalgias. Langer et al.[21] reported mild symptoms in a 24-hour schedule; whereas, the incidence climbed to 54% when the paclitaxel was given over 1 hour. In contrast to the pain associated with high-dose vinblastine, with paclitaxel there is less truncal pain and more pain in the distal muscles and joints. Large axial muscles, particularly shoulder and paraspinal muscles, are frequently involved.[17]

In neither vinblastine nor paclitaxel has there been any evidence suggesting that this toxicity was associated with inflammation. Elevations of muscle enzymes such as creatinine phosphokinase have not been observed in patients treated with paclitaxel.[2,7] The dose-related nature of the toxicity suggests that the drug affects the muscle directly and, although it is speculation, this suggests an effect on the microtubular system, which is so critical to maintaining normal muscle function and physiology. While these symptoms are usually mild at doses of paclitaxel less than 170 mg/m², they become more frequent and severe at doses greater than 200 mg/m².[17,23] Severe muscular complaints usually occur more often at paclitaxel doses greater than 250 mg/m².[17,24,25] In a study of escalating doses of paclitaxel plus cisplatin, 27 of 28 patients (96%) reported arthralgias and myalgias. All were reported as grade 1 or 2, except for four patients who reported grade 3. Those four patients were at higher dose levels (260–300 mg/m²). It was also noted that arthralgias and myalgias increased when G-CSF was used.[26] The use of cisplatin in combination with paclitaxel does not appear to affect the severity of myalgias relative to single-agent paclitaxel at comparable doses.[17,24,27]

A myopathy has been documented in patients treated with high doses of paclitaxel (250–350 mg/m²) in combination with cisplatin (75–100 mg/m²) and G-CSF.[28,29] Another investigator reported a patient who developed progressive muscle weakness, involving both the upper and lower extremities while receiving 19 courses of paclitaxel, with doses ranging from 120–250 mg/m².[29] In both cases, electromyogram (EMG) studies revealed myopathic findings. Distal muscle weakness was also reported in other patients, two of whom had diabetes mellitus while receiving single-agent paclitaxel at a dose of 250 mg/m².[24]

Docetaxel

Phase I studies revealed the incidence of arthralgias and myalgias in docetaxel therapy.[30] Reversible grade 3 and grade 4 arthralgias and myalgias have been noted in clinical trials of docetaxel.[31] Frances et al.,[32] in a phase II trial of docetaxel given to patients with platinum-refractory ovarian cancer, reported that 40% of patients experienced myalgias during the week after drug administration. After phase II trials of docetaxel revealed significant fluid retention toxicity and dermatologic toxicity, it was recommended that, to ameliorate toxicities, patients be given dexamethasone 8 mg PO bid starting 24 hours before treatment and continuing for up to 5 days after administration.[33] It is likely that this premedication regimen also influenced the incidence of myalgias, because recent clinical trials mention this problem less frequently. Although comparison trials have not been fully reported, it is believed that docetaxel is associated with less neuropathy and fewer myalgias, and arrhythmias than paclitaxel.[34]

Biologic Response Modifiers

Toxicities associated with interferon include an acute syndrome characterized by arthralgias and myalgias.[35] Most symptoms in the musculoskeletal system are related to the flulike syndrome caused by interferon. Symptoms consist of self-limited arthralgias and myalgias of transient duration. Severe myalgias were reported in 4 of 27 patients (15%) whose chronic myelogenous leukemia was treated with interferon.[35] The myalgias involved the proximal muscles of the lower extremities and were associated with limited movement. Treatment consisted of bed rest and therapy with steroids and opiate analgesics. Testing revealed a negative EMG and no elevated muscle enzymes. G-CSF and granulocyte-macrophage colony-stimulating factor (GM-CSF) are well known to produce flulike syndrome side effects that include the joint pain and muscle aches of arthralgias and myalgias. New approaches to mobilization of peripheral blood stem cells include administration of G-CSF sequentially or simultaneously with interleukin-3 (IL-3) or with G-CSF alone; these methods produced up to an 83% incidence of arthralgias and myalgias.[4,5]

Arthralgias and myalgias occur at high doses of interleukin-2 (IL-2) due to an accumulation of cytokine deposits in the joint spaces. Potential toxicities of rituxan, a monoclonal antibody, include alteration in comfort, and more specifically arthralgias and myalgias usually 2 to 8 hours after the dose is given.

There is a report on a postchemotherapy rheumatism syndrome in eight patients treated with adjuvant therapy for breast cancer. Symptoms appeared within a few months of completing combination chemotherapy and were collectively described as a musculoskeletal syndrome.[36] Serologic tests for autoimmune markers, and bone and joint scans were not remarkable, but there was noted mild periarticular swelling.[36] Symptoms abated over several months for these patients. Nonsteroidal analgesics were ineffective in relieving pain, but one patient was treated effectively with low-dose steroids.[36] Loprinzi et al.[36] concluded that the etiology was unclear for this syndrome.

Pathophysiology

The pathophysiologic mechanism of arthralgia and myalgia remains unclear, and a specific treatment is not available. *Microtubules* are polymers of tubulin believed to function as the major constituent of the mitotic spindle apparatus. The microtubules are also critical for maintenance of cell shape, motility, anchorage, mediation of signals between cell surface receptors and the nucleus, and for intracellular transport.[37] Microtubules are important in axonal transport and other vital neuron functions, and it is known that neurotoxicity is a major toxicity of antimicrotubule drugs.

Microtubule assembly and disassembly are in dynamic equilibrium. The vinca alkaloids induce microtubule disassembly, whereas the taxanes promote microtubule assembly and stabilization. The vinca alkaloids interact with the tubulin and disrupt the microtubules, inducing metaphase arrest in dividing cells.[38] The stabilization of the microtubules by paclitaxel inhibits mitosis in the G2 and M phases of the cell cycle, inhibits fibroblast cell migration, and causes cell death.[8] The microtubules formed in the presence of paclitaxel are extraordinarily stable and dysfunctional, causing the death of the cell by disrupting the reorganization of the microtubule network.[7]

Assessment

Myalgia is sometimes associated with muscle tenderness and sometimes not. Arthralgia and myalgia following chemotherapy are not associated with physical findings. Arthralgia and myalgia secondary to chemotherapy should be distinguished from fibromyalgia, viral infections, an overuse syndrome, neuropathies, and hypothyroidism.[39] Joint symptoms may be due to trauma, infection, crystal-induced inflammation (gout), or primary inflammatory arthritis.[39] Myalgias may be secondary to a localized problem (trauma or overuse), a systemic disorder (acute or chronic infection, toxic or metabolic disorders), or less commonly it may reflect a primary muscle disease.[39] Differential diagnosis is based on the physical examination and history.[40]

Muscle pain differs from cutaneous pain in several ways: (1) it is usually described as aching or cramping rather than stabbing or sharp; (2) it is poorly localized, whereas cutaneous pain is localized with great accuracy; (3) it is generally referred to other deep somatic structures (muscles, fascia, tendons, ligaments, and joints), whereas cutaneous pain is not referred.[40]

Typical pain from arthralgias and myalgias develops in the large joints of the arms and legs 48 to 72 hours after treatment and disappears within 4 to 7 days. Patients report that the discomfort is constant—it does not wax and wane during those days but ends predictably within this time frame. It can be described by patients as varying from a mild ache to a severe pain. It is similar to arthritic pain, as it is worse or more pronounced on movement and more relieved at rest. Many patients state they do not feel the discomfort until they attempt to get out of bed in the morning. Others describe a feeling that comes over them, similar to a flulike ache, that begins the manifestation of the symptom. Myalgias generally involve shoulder muscles, the arms, and the leg joints.[41] The weakness is greater in the lower extremities than in the upper extremities.[28] Arthralgias and myalgias are dose-related and generally recur with repeated paclitaxel treatment but are not predictable. The discomfort also varies from cycle to cycle; thus, it is not predictable. The unpredictability and the fluctuation in severity of the symptoms contribute to anxiety in the patient. In addition, the joint

and muscle aches can influence the patient's ability to function normally.

The muscle and bone pain experienced by patients receiving paclitaxel can be compared to that experienced with a bout of influenza or following administration of high doses of vinblastine or etoposide.[42] Shoulder and paraspinal muscles are usually involved, and arthralgias in the large joints of the arms and legs are most frequently reported by patients.[28,41]

Impaired physical mobility related to limitation of joint function and pain can have a deleterious effect on a patient's work, home, and leisure activities. Assessment of sociological and psychological factors is important in judging the strengths and resources the patient brings to coping with the condition. Functional changes can lead to depression, anxiety, and loss of confidence.

Risk Factors

The most important risk factor for developing arthralgias and myalgias is the dose of the chemotherapy. Risk factors for arthralgias and myalgias include:[23]

- antecedent peripheral neuropathy
- history of diabetes
- alcohol use
- high individual doses of paclitaxel at >250 mg/m^2
- high-dose vinblastine
- concurrent administration of paclitaxel with cisplatin
- administration of biologic response modifiers
- age
- prior neurotoxic chemotherapy
- history of arthritis

Patients with prior peripheral neuropathies related to ethanol were more likely than patients without an alcohol history to develop neurotoxicities that were severe.[25]

Physical Assessment

The first component of an assessment includes a thorough history and physical examination with a focus on pain assessment. Detail concerning the character of the pain, such as the location and quality of the discomfort or pain, its time of onset, and factors that make it worse or better are important clues to cause. Ask the patient to describe the severity of the pain using a numerical scale from 0 to 10 (0 = no pain, 10 = worst pain). Ask if the pain is present at rest or not, if it is present on movement or not, and the time of day the pain occurs. Differentiation must be made from neurologic pain, which is described as a numbness, "falling asleep," burning, shooting, or a pins-and-needles pain, which is often a neurologic rather than a neuromuscular toxicity. Important in the differentiation process is ascertaining whether the pain is described as an ache, which is often the case with arthralgias, versus a burning pain in an extremity, which may indicate neuropathy. Many of the chemotherapy drugs also cause neurologic toxicity, including peripheral neuropathy affecting both sensory (pain and temperature) and motor pathways, and/or autonomic pathways. Rowinsky et al.[17] suggest research aimed at identifying patients who are likely to develop complications, perhaps by using nerve conduction studies, quantitative sensory testing, or limited selective examinations. Patients also should be asked about accompanying stiffness or swelling in joints and any complaints of limited motion. Weakness and fatigue are common general complaints.[9]

Careful listening during the assessment is essential. Encouraging the patient to call or come to the office when the symptom is present may be helpful. Trying to assess patients' limitations with the activities of daily living and trying to sort out the primary cause are important. Often neuromuscular pain is managed over the phone, so paying careful attention to what the patient is describing is most important. Confounding factors include patients receiving multiple drugs at one time with overlapping side effects; giving premedications to ameliorate the hypersensitivity reactions (i.e., decadron 20 mg IV) complicate the symptom as well. Corticosteroids can cause myopathy, and their withdrawal may result in a rheumatologic syndrome that includes arthralgias and myalgias. Patients experience a "high" feeling from the steroid, which wears off in about 48 hours, precisely the time when the rheumatologic syndrome often may start. The authors that documented a postchemotherapy rheumatism in breast cancer patients considered the intermittent boluses of steroids as a possible cause of the syndrome.[36] They concluded that the pulse administration of corticosteroids with chemotherapy did not seem to contribute to the postchemotherapy rheumatism syndrome.[36] This is a phenomena that should be studied more in the new population of patients getting paclitaxel weekly with steroid boluses. This group may be better able to document whether the side effects are more prevalent with steroid boluses and whether they are caused by the steroids.

Patients with cancer who have arthritis and a long history of aches and pains and a long history of medication use to manage their pain are a complicated group to assess. It is important to be aware of the signs and symptoms of arthritis. The symptoms include: stiffness, pain, weakness, fatigue, and emotional depression or lability. The signs include: tenderness localized over an afflicted joint, swelling, heat and erythema, crepitus, and bony spurs. Careful documentation of medication history and baseline data of functional status and pain are critical in the successful management of this group of patients. It is important to remember that the underlying cancer can cause additional symptoms or problems at any time,

and those need to be ruled out as well. Usually the finite time that this symptom manifests itself makes it easy to rule out a new metastasis, because the pain associated with that does not dissipate. Concomitant use of colony-stimulating factors may exacerbate the arthralgias and myalgias or may be the root cause of the symptoms, and differentiation is important.

Diagnostic Tests

Concurrent signs of inflammation and elevations of muscle enzymes have not been noted.[42] Whereas proximal muscle weakness and elevated creatinine phosphatase enzyme levels suggest inflammatory myopathy,[39] the discomfort is not associated with fever or joint swelling. No specific diagnostic tests are recommended for making the diagnosis; it is made instead from a careful history and physical examination.

Degree of Toxicity

Arthralgias and myalgias should be graded using the common toxicity criteria published by the National Cancer Institute (Table 4-2).[43]

Symptom Management

Patient education is an essential part of the nursing care plan. Patients must be prepared to recognize what is happening and have a plan to deal with the discomfort so their quality of life is minimally affected.

Symptom management and reassessment are the most productive ways of treating this condition. Inform patients about what to expect, what can be prevented, and when and to whom to report the side effects.[41] Nurses must educate patients regarding the potential for discomfort associated with arthralgias and myalgias. Patients may be reluctant to report adverse effects because of fear that their disease is progressing or that their treatment will be stopped. Reassurance can alleviate this concern. It is important to make patients understand that they may experience this side effect but that it is manageable and sometimes preventable with intervention. Providing concrete information about the finite period of time patients can expect to deal with this side effect can be reassuring.

A thorough nursing history and assessment must be done before the initiation of treatment as well as before each subsequent treatment because a patients' history can have a great impact on the adverse effects experienced. For example, patients with a history of arthritis or rheumatoid arthritis will be more complicated to assess. As patients start therapy, provide them with a verbal

TABLE 4-2 Toxicity Criteria for Arthralgias and Myalgias

Arthralgias (joint pain) Grade	0	1	2	3	4
	None	Mild pain, not interfering with function	Moderate pain; pain or analgesics interfering with function but not interfering with activities of daily living	Severe pain; pain or analgesics severely interfering with activities of daily living	Disabling
Myalgias (muscle pain) Grade	0	1	2	3	4
	None	Mild pain, not interfering with function	Moderate pain; pain or analgesics interfering with function but not interfering with activities of daily living	Severe pain; pain or analgesics severely interfering with activities of daily living	Disabling

Common Toxicity Criteria Version 2.0. Bethesda, MD: National Institutes of Health, National Cancer Institute, March 1998.[43]

and written explanation of this potential side effect, the delayed onset after the administration of the drug, the variation of discomfort (ranging from a mild ache to severe pain), and the duration of this side effect (i.e., that it ends in 4–7 days), and inform them that the problem does not continue after therapy has been completed or discontinued. For most patients, it is not necessary to discontinue or modify the dose of drugs because of this side effect.

Therapeutic Approaches

Antihistamines, corticosteroids, nonsteroidal antiinflammatory drugs, and opiates have been helpful in managing arthralgias and myalgias. After 24% of patients experienced grade 3 arthralgias and myalgias, Schiller et al.[16] started prednisone empirically in ten patients at 40 mg/day for 2 to 5 days. Patients reported a decrease in discomfort starting 2 to 4 hours after the first dose of the prednisone. Natale,[44] in a phase I/II study to determine the maximum tolerated dose of paclitaxel, treated grade 1 and grade 2 arthralgias and myalgias with nonsteroidal analgesics; grade 3 patients were given a 4-day course of dexamethasone at 4 to 8 mg bid.

Nonsteroidal analgesics are used because of their analgesics and antiinflammatory effects; they work peripherally to decrease prostaglandin synthesis. Corticosteroids are effective because of their ability to reduce the symptoms of inflammation reliably and rapidly. Corticosteroids inhibit a variety of proinflammatory genes and modify the leukocyte number at the inflammation site. Although arthralgias and myalgias are not associated with muscle inflammation, corticosteroids are effective in relieving the aches and pains associated with this symptom. With chronic high-dose use of corticosteroids, muscle weakness or steroid myopathy may occur.

Many institutions have found benefit in prophylactic use of some of these medications, with varying doses and schedules. Practitioners sometimes take a wait-and-see attitude, explaining to patients the possibility of the problem and providing instructions to call if this problem occurs. If the patient experiences arthralgias or myalgias, the practitioner will likely initiate a prophylactic regimen at the next cycle of treatment or provide the patient with instruction and prescriptions for intermittent use. Some examples of medications prescribed are listed in Table 4-3.

There have also been unsuccessful attempts to decrease or prevent neurotoxicity associated with vincristine by using various types of agents such as thiamine, vitamins (most frequently B6 or pyridoxine), and folic acid.[42] Neuropathy associated with the antitumor agent hexamethylmelamine has been ameliorated by the use of pyridoxine.[45] Despite the lack of documentation of success, when nurses were informally surveyed at a semi-annual meeting of the Gynecologic Oncology Group, some reported anecdotal use of either vitamins B6 or C for ar-

TABLE 4-3 Medications Used to Ameliorate Arthralgias and Myalgias

Extra strength Tylenol 1 to 2 tablets q4–6h
Naproxen 750–1500 mg/day, or given prophylactically the first 5 days after treatment
Tramadol 50–100 mg q4h prn
Prednisone 40 mg daily × 6 days (used days 2–7 following therapy)
Dexamethasone 4 mg bid × 3 days, decreasing to 4 mg daily × 3 days (start 2 days after treatment)
Methylprednisolone DOSE PAK (as per package instruction, start 24 hours after treatment)
Hydrocodone 1 tablet q3–4h prn
Oxycodone 5 mg q6h prn
Vicodin 1–2 tablets q4–6h prn

TABLE 4-4 Nursing Diagnosis in Arthralgias and Myalgias

Nursing Diagnosis	Expected Outcome	Intervention
Potential for pain or discomfort	Patient will verbalize relief or discomfort	Provide education on arthralgias and myalgias
		Assess discomfort
		Aid patient in identifying areas of discomfort
		Provide medication as ordered
		Instruct patient in nonpharmacologic intervention for comfort
		Provide written information and instructions about how to manage arthralgias and myalgias and when to notify healthcare professional

thralgias and myalgias associated with taxane therapy. The results were mixed—in some a decrease, some no effect, and a decreased incidence of arthralgias and myalgias was noted in a few patients. The antihistamine terfenadine was used to help ameliorate the side effects of paclitaxel, but the U.S. Food and Drug Administration (FDA) removed terfenadine drug from the market this year.

Exercise, warmth, and massage are part of the non-pharmacologic interventions recommended for these symptoms. Similar to supportive treatment for arthritis, all of these methods help to relieve the discomfort of joint and muscle aches. Warm baths and application of heating pads to affected areas for brief intervals provide relief to patients. Patients also report that remaining active and regular moderate walking are helpful to maintain normal activity function.

Educational Tools

The nursing diagnosis associated with arthralgia or myalgia is discomfort or pain. The expected outcome is that the patient will be free from discomfort or have the pain controlled (Table 4-4). The nursing intervention is to teach the patient about the potential for discomfort related to arthralgias or myalgias and to monitor the level of symptoms and the effectiveness of treatment for the problem.

Information must be provided to patients receiving therapy that may cause arthralgias and myalgias. Appendix 4A is a self-care guide that can be given to patients at risk for arthralgias and myalgias.

Conclusion

The oncology nurse providing education to patients undergoing chemotherapy regimens with drugs that cause arthralgias and myalgias is in a position to provide vital information regarding this potentially troublesome side effect. Nurses can educate patients to help them understand what is happening to them and can provide vital information for intervention and relief of this most distressing symptom. With adequate preparation and knowledge regarding their management, the arthralgias and myalgias associated with cancer treatment can be minimized and controlled.

References

1. Holism F, Walters R, Therauilt R, et al: Phase II trial of taxol—an active agent in the treatment of metastatic breast cancer. *J Natl Cancer Inst* 83:1797–1805, 1991
2. McGuire WP, Rowinsky EK, Rosenshein NB, et al: Taxol a unique antineoplastic agent with significant activity in advanced ovarian epithelial neoplasms. *Ann Intern Med* 111:273–279, 1989
3. Einhorn LH, Williams SD, Troner M, et al: The role of maintenance therapy in disseminated testicular cancer. *N Engl J Med* 305:727–731, 1981
4. D'Hondt V, Guillaume T, Humblit Y, et al: Tolerance of sequential or simultaneous administration of IL-3 and G-CSF in improving peripheral blood stem cell harvesting following multiple agent chemotherapy: A pilot study. *Bone Marrow Transplant* 13:261–264, 1994
5. Bishop MR, Tarantolo SR, Jackson JD: Allogenic-blood stem-cell collection following mobilization with low-dose granulocyte colony stimulating factor. *J Clin Oncol* 15:1601–1607, 1997
6. Rowinsky EK, Cazenave LA, Donehower RC: Taxol: A novel investigational agent. *J Natl Cancer Inst* 82:1247–1259, 1990
7. Rowinsky EK, Donohower RC: Paclitaxel (Taxol). *N Engl J Med* 332:1004–1014, 1995
8. Nakashima L: A review of taxol. Highlight on Antineoplastic Drugs 10:52–57, 1994
9. Einhorn LH, Donohue JP: Improved chemotherapy in disseminated testicular cancer. *J Urol* 117:65–69, 1977
10. Vogelzeng NJ, Fraley EE, Large PH, et al: State II nonseminatous testicular cancer: A 10 year experience. *J Clin Oncol* 1:171, 1983
11. Pizzocaro G, Zanni F, Milani A, et al: Retroperitoneal lymphadenectomy and aggressive chemotherapy in non-bulky clinic state II nonseminomatous germinal testis tumors. *Cancer* 53:1363, 1984
12. Weissbach L, Hartlapp JH: Adjuvant chemotherapy of metastatic state II nonseminomatous testes tumor. *J Urol* 146:1295, 1991
13. Williams SD, Birch R, Einhorn LH, et al: Treatment of

disseminated germ-cell tumors with cisplatin, bleomycin and either vinblastine or etoposide. *N Engl J Med* 316: 1435, 1987

14. Martoni A, Zamagni C, Gheka A, et al: Antihistamines in the treatment of taxol-induced paroxystic pain syndrome. *J Natl Cancer Inst* 85:676–677, 1993

15. Brown T, Havlin K, Weiss G, et al: A phase I trial of taxol given by 6-hour intravenous infusion. *J Clin Oncol* 9:1261–1267, 1991

16. Schiller JH, Storer B, Tutsch K: A phase I trial of 3-hour infusions of paclitaxel (Taxol) with or without granulocyte colony stimulating factor. *Semin Oncol* 21(suppl 8):9–14, 1994

17. Rowinsky EK, Eisenhauer EA, Chaudhry V, et al: Clinical toxicities encountered with paclitaxel (taxol). *Semin Oncol* 20(suppl 3):1–15, 1993

18. Donehower RC, Rowinsky EK, Grochow LB, et al: Phase I trial of taxol in patients with advanced malignancies. *Cancer Treat Rep* 71:1171–1177, 1987

19. Wiernik PH, Schwartz EL, Shauman JJ, et al: Phase I clinical and pharmacokinetic study of taxol. *Cancer Res* 47:2486–2493, 1987

20. Wiernik PH, Schwartz EL, Einzig A, et al: Phase I trial of taxol given as a 24 hour infusion every 21 days: Responses observed in malignant melanoma. *J Clin Oncol* 5:1232–1239, 1987

21. Langer CJ, Leighton JC, Comis RL, et al: Paclitaxel by 24 or 1 hour infusion in combination with carboplatin in advanced non-small cell lung cancer: The Fox Chase Cancer Center Experience. *Semin Oncol* 22(suppl 9):18–29, 1995

22. Evans EK, Earle CC, Stewart DJ: Phase II study of a one hour paclitaxel infusion in combination with carboplatin for advanced non-small cell lung cancer. *Lung Cancer* 18: 83–94, 1997

23. Donehower RC, Rowinsky EK: An overview of experience with Taxol (paclitaxel) in the USA. *Cancer Treat Rev* 19 (suppl C):63–78, 1993

24. Forastiere A, Rowinsky EK, Chaudhry V, et al: Phase I pharmacologic study of taxol and cisplatin and G-CSF. *Proc Am Soc Clin Oncol* 11A:117, 1992

25. Lipton RB, Apfel SC, Dutcher JP, et al: Taxol produces a predominantly sensory neuropathy. *Neurology* 39:368–373, 1989

26. Hitt R, Hornedo J, Colomer R, et al: Study of escalating doses of paclitaxel plus cisplatin in patients with inoperable head and neck cancer. *Semin Oncol* 24(suppl 2):S2-58–S2-64, 1997

27. Rowinsky EK, Gilbert M, McGuire WP, et al: Sequences of taxol and cisplatin: A phase I pharmacologic study. *J Clin Oncol* 9:1692–1703, 1991

28. Chaudhry V, Rowinsky EK, Sarzorious SE, et al: Peripheral neuropathy from taxol and cisplatin combination chemotherapy: Chemical and Electrophysiological studies. *Ann Neurol* 35:304–311, 1994

29. Rowinsky EK, Chaudhry V, Cornblath DR, et al: The neurotoxicity of taxol. *J Natl Cancer Inst Monogr* 15:107–115, 1993

30. Von Hoff, DD: The toxins: Same roots, different drugs. *Semin Oncol* 24(suppl 13):3–10, 1997

31. Einzig AI, Schuchter LM, Recio A: Phase II trial of docetaxel (Taxotere) in patients with metastatic melanoma previously untreated with cytotoxic chemotherapy. *Med Oncol* 13:111–117, 1996

32. Frances P, Schneider J, Hann L, et al: Phase II trial of docetaxel in patients with platinum-refractory advanced ovarian cancer. *J Clin Oncol* 12:2301–2308, 1994

33. Piccart MJ, Klijn J, Paridaens R, et al: Steroids do reduce the severity and delay the onset of docetaxel (DXT) induced fluid retention. Final results of a randomized trial of the EORTC Investigational Branch for Breast Cancer (IDBBC). *Eur J Cancer* 31A(suppl 5):575, 1995

34. D'Andrea GM, Seidman AD: Docetaxel and paclitaxel in breast cancer therapy: Present status and future prospectus. *Semin Oncol* 24(suppl 13):S13-27–S13-44, 1997

35. Quesada JR, Talpaz M, Rois M: Clinical toxicity of interferons in cancer patients: A review. *J Clin Oncol* 4:234–243, 1986

36. Loprinzi CL, Duffy J, Ingle JN: Postchemotherapy rheumatism. *J Clin Oncol* 11:768–770, 1993

37. Rowinsky EK, Onetto N, Canetta RM, et al: Taxol: The first of the taxanes, an important new class of antitumor agents. *Semin Oncol* 19:646–662, 1992

38. Rowinsky EK, Donehower RC: Antimicrotubule agents, in Chabner BA, Long DL (eds): *Cancer Chemotherapy and Biotherapy: Principles and Practice.* Philadelphia: Lippincott-Raven, 1996, pp. 263–296

39. American College of Rheumatology Ad Hoc Committee on Clinical Guidelines: Guidelines for the initial evaluation of the adult patient with acute musculoskeletal symptoms, in Kelley WN, Harris Jr ED, Ruddy S, Sledge CB (eds): *Textbook of Rheumatology.* (ed 5) Philadelphia: Saunders, 1997, pp. 1880–1887

40. Bennett RM: The fibromyalgia syndrome, in Kelley WN, Harris Jr ED, Ruddy S, Sledge CB (eds): *Textbook of Rheumatology* (ed 5). Philadelphia: Saunders, 1997, pp. 511–518

41. Walker F: Paclitaxel (Taxol): Side effects and patient education issues. *Semin Oncol Nurs* 9(suppl 2):6–10, 1993

42. Jackson DV, Pope EK, McMahan RA, et al: Clinical trial of pyridoxine to reduce vincristine neurotoxicity. *J Neurooncol* 4:37–41, 1986

43. Common Toxicity Criteria version 2.0. Bethesda, MD: National Institutes of Health, National Cancer Institute, March 1998

44. Natale RB: Preliminary results of phase I/II clinical trial of paclitaxel and carboplatin in non-small cell lung cancer. *Semin Oncol* 23(suppl 16):51–54, 1996

45. Smith JP, Rutledge FN: Random study of hexamethylmelamine, 5-fluorouracil and melphalan in treatment of advanced carcinoma of the ovary. *Natl Cancer Inst Monogr* 42:169–172, 1975

Arthralgias and Myalgias

Patient Name _____

It is very important that you read and understand the following information. If you have any questions or want more information, please contact the nurse or the physician.

Symptom and Description   Pain in the large joints of the arms and legs can occur any time from 48–72 hours after you receive chemotherapy. When in your joints, this pain is called *arthralgia,* when in your muscles, *myalgia.* It is a side effect of your chemotherapy. This discomfort occurs in the large joints such as the hips, the knees, or the shoulders and can range from a mild ache to severe pain. This muscle and joint pain can be more noticeable if colony stimulating factors or growth factors (G-CSF or GM-CSF) are a part of your treatment. You also may have trouble getting out of bed or a chair. This side effect may not occur with every treatment; you may experience pain during one treatment and not feel any aches after the next treatment.

You are at risk of having arthralgias and myalgias because of your cancer therapy, specifically the drug _____.

You are at risk for this side effect if you had treatment with a drug that caused numbness or tingling in your hands or feet such as the drugs:

- cisplatin
- vincristine
- vindesine
- etoposide

or

- if you have diabetes
- if you have a history of alcohol use
- if you have a history of arthritis

Learning Needs   You need to learn how to manage this side effect at home and understand when to notify the doctor or nurse. Your physician can prescribe medicines that will relieve this side effect.

Prevention   It is difficult to prevent this symptom. Remember the symptoms don't appear until 48–72 hours after treatment and can last from 4–7 days.

Some helpful hints to reduce the symptoms include:

- Medication can be taken if you experience this side effect. Your doctor has ordered the following to be taken after treatment:

_____

_____

- The following medication may also be taken if you experience additional pain:

  _____

  _____

Management   These are some ideas on how to manage these side effects at home.

- Take the medication prescribed by your doctor.
- Get plenty of rest, and plan your activities to include rest periods.
- A heating pad or hot water bottle may help give comfort to the achey area. Keep the pad or bottle covered with a towel when putting it next to your skin. Use for short periods, 5–10 minutes several times per day.
- Keep your nutrition up by eating healthy, regular meals.
- Relaxation techniques, such as guided imagery and biofeedback may be helpful.
- Taking a warm bath or whirlpool bath is comforting.
- Massage therapy to the affected areas may help.

Be sure to ask your doctor or nurse for more information if you are interested in trying any of these measures and you need additional information.

Follow-up   It may be helpful to keep a record of the muscle or joint pain, recording when it starts, what makes it better, and when it goes away. Bring this information with you when you visit the doctor or nurse.

If at any time you are uncomfortable and the discomfort does not go away, please call the doctor or nurse.

Comments:

Patient's Signature: _____ Date: _____
Nurses's Signature: _____ Date: _____

Source: Martin VR: Arthralgias and myalgias, in Yarbro CH, Frogge MH, Goodman M (eds): *Cancer Symptom Management* (ed 2). Sudbury: Jones & Bartlett, 1999.

CHAPTER 5

Dyspnea

Kerry V. Harwood, RN, MSN

The Problem of Dyspnea in Cancer

Dyspnea is defined as difficult or labored breathing. Dyspnea should be distinguished from *tachypnea* (increased respiratory rate) and *hyperpnea* (increased depth of ventilation). Objective signs may or may not indicate degree of dyspnea. As with pain, it is the person's perception of the sensation that is the most relevant indicator. No physiologic parameter is known to consistently predict the degree of dyspnea being experienced.

Dyspnea is a common problem in oncology. It has been estimated that 70% of patients with cancer experience dyspnea during the last six weeks of life.[1] Only pain and difficulty eating are reported more frequently for this population.[2] However, dyspnea is not limited to those with terminal disease. It may present as an acute symptom or persist as a chronic problem. Dyspnea may relate not only to cancer involving the lung but also to underlying medical conditions, an acute problem, or a side effect of cancer treatment. Considered through the spectrum of the cancer experience, dyspnea is undoubtedly one of the most common problems. Dyspnea is a distressing symptom that may evoke fear, anxiety, even panic.[3,4] It often limits the person's ability to engage in desired activities, social interaction, and even self-care activities.

For a variety of reasons, dyspnea may be less frequently recognized by healthcare providers than are other common symptoms. Roberts et al.[2] looked at the incidence of dyspnea in patients with cancer participating in a home-care hospice program. Significant discrepancies were found between the number of patients who identified dyspnea as a problem during the interview versus those for whom dyspnea had been identified as an issue in the medical record. Dyspnea was least frequently recognized by healthcare providers when the patient did not have lung involvement with cancer (78% dyspnea per interview vs. 26% dyspnea per chart review). Unlike pain, where dramatic advances in treatment have occurred, management of dyspnea frequently remains inadequate. This may result from inadequate identification of the problem or lack of familiarity with strategies to manage dyspnea.

Etiology

Dyspnea is commonly expected in the person with primary or metastatic cancer involving the lungs. However, the incidence of dyspnea extends far beyond this group, as numerous factors may contribute to dyspnea. In considering the causes of dyspnea, the warning of Campbell and Howell[5] is relevant: "a respiratory physiologist offering a unitary explanation for breathlessness should arouse the same suspicion as a tattooed archbishop offering a free ticket to heaven" (p. 868). Causes of dyspnea in persons with cancer may be attributable to the cancer itself, general debility, cancer treatments, and other concomitant medical conditions as listed in Table 5-1.

TABLE 5-1 Contributing Factors to Dyspnea in the Cancer Patient

Cancer effects
Large airway obstruction by tumor masses
Diffuse tumor infiltrating small airways or lymphatics
Pleural effusion
Postobstructive pneumonia
Pericardial effusion
Hepatomegaly
Ascites
Anorexia-cachexia syndrome

Cancer treatment effects
Surgery
   Decreased lung capacity
   Pneumothorax
Radiation therapy
   Radiation pneumonitis
Chemotherapy
   Drug-induced pneumonitis
   Cardiomyopathy
   Infection
   Anemia

Other medical, psychological, and situational effects
Chronic obstructive airway disease
Congestive heart failure
Asthma
Obesity
Anxiety, depression
Hot weather

Data from references 6–10.

Dyspnea Caused by the Cancer

Lung involvement

Tumor in the lung, either primary lung cancer or metastatic disease, is often the cause of dyspnea. Centrally located tumors may obstruct the bronchus or upper airways and inhibit air passage and may result in postobstructive pneumonia. Peripheral lesions frequently do not cause dyspnea. Diffuse tumor infiltration of small airways or pulmonary lymphatics can occur in carcinoma of the breast, leukemia, and lymphomas, and is more likely to result in dyspnea. Pleural involvement is most common with tumors of lung and breast origin, and resultant effusions may cause dyspnea.

Other organ involvement

Tumors involving organs other than the lungs may result in dyspnea. Pericardial involvement is not uncommon in patients with advanced cancer. Lung and breast cancers predominate as those most likely to cause myopericardial metastases, with incidence in autopsy studies of 35% and 25%, respectively.[11] Symptoms of pericardial effusion are usually nonspecific, and dyspnea is one of the most frequent symptoms.[11] Dyspnea may also result from diaphragmatic pressure, experienced with severe malignant ascites or gross hepatomegaly.

Anorexia-Cachexia Syndrome

Anorexia-cachexia syndrome, the combination of loss of appetite and physical wasting, results in muscle wasting and weakness, easy fatigability, and impairment of immune function. Respiratory muscle weakness appears to be an important contributing factor in dyspnea in patients with advanced cancer. In advanced cancer patients with no cardiothoracic disease, the National Hospice Study reported a prevalence of dyspnea of 24%, suggesting a more systemic correlate.[12] In cancer patients with cachexia, the maximal inspiratory pressure—used to test the strength of the diaphragm and other respiratory muscles—is severely impaired.[13] The reader may want to refer to Chapter 12 for additional information on this syndrome.

Dyspnea Caused by Cancer Treatment

Surgery

Dyspnea may occur due to decreased lung capacity after pneumonectomy for resection of primary lung cancer or isolated metastatic lesions. In most people, reduction in lung capacity is well compensated. However, in individuals with underlying respiratory impairment, which is typical of the primary lung cancer patient with significant smoking history, dyspnea may occur after lung resection. Dyspnea may also appear as an acute symptom of a surgical complication, such as pneumothorax following central-line insertion or liver biopsy.

Radiation therapy

The lung is radiosensitive, and most radiation doses and schedules will cause some reaction in the irradiated lung field. Irradiation of at least 10% of the lung is required to produce significant toxicity.[14] The clinical picture of radiation pneumonitis is noted in 5% to 15% of irradiated patients. Dyspnea, the classic sign of radiation pneumonitis, typically appears two to three months after completion of radiation treatment. Complete resolution of acute radiation pneumonitis is possible, but most individuals will develop some degree of permanent lung fibrosis. The incidence and severity of pneumonitis and fibrosis relate to the volume of lung irradiated, total dose and fractionation, and concomitant chemotherapy.[8] Persistent fibrosis of a large volume of lung may result in respiratory failure.

Chemotherapy

Many chemotherapeutic agents have the potential to cause pulmonary toxicity (Table 5-2). Of the agents listed, bleomycin most commonly causes pulmonary toxicity, with the incidence of clinical toxicity reported to be as high as 40% of recipients.[8] While a variety of mechanisms have been hypothesized for different drugs, the clinical

TABLE 5-2 Chemotherapy Agents Associated
with Dyspnea

Drugs causing pulmonary toxicity
Azathioprine
Bleomycin[a,b]
Busulfan
Carmustine[a]
Chlorambucil
Chlorozotocin
Cyclophosphamide
Cytosine arabinoside[b]
Etoposide
Lomustine
Melphalan
Mercaptopurine
Methotrexate[a]
Mitomycin[a,b]
Neocarzinostatin
Procarbazine[b]
Retinoic acid
Semustine
Vinblastine[b]
Vindesine[b]
VM-26
Drugs causing congestive heart failure
Amsacrine
Androgens
Daunorubicin
Doxorubicin
Estrogens
Mitoxantrone
Progestins

[a]Incidence >5%.

[b]Acute reactions observed.

Data from references 8,10.

picture of drug-induced pulmonary toxicity has several common features. Chemotherapy-induced pulmonary toxicity may become clinically evident weeks to years after treatment. Cardinal signs are dyspnea and dry cough. The symptoms tend to become progressively worse and prognosis for recovery is typically poor. Factors that increase risk and severity of chemotherapy-associated pulmonary toxicity include oxygen therapy (simultaneous or subsequent), radiation therapy (prior or simultaneous), and administration of multiple chemotherapy agents associated with pulmonary toxicity or high doses of these agents.

In addition to pulmonary toxicity, chemotherapy treatments may also result in dyspnea indirectly through other agent-related side effects such as anemia, infection, or cardiomyopathy. Symptomatic anemia, typically short-lived, is best relieved by transfusion. Infection and fever may increase oxygen demands, with an associated sense of dyspnea. Cardiotoxic drugs, such as doxorubicin, may cause a cardiomyopathy and subsequent respiratory symptoms. Hypersensitivity reactions to chemotherapy can result in acute dyspnea.

Other Conditions

Dyspnea is frequently associated with a variety of common medical conditions. Characteristics common to the oncology population, such as older age or history of smoking, also correlate with conditions typically associated with dyspnea such as chronic obstructive airway disease or congestive heart failure. Concurrent conditions that may affect respiratory reserve requirements, such as asthma or obesity, are important to consider in treatment planning.

The patient's emotions may contribute to the overall experience of dyspnea. The dyspnea-anxiety-dyspnea cycle is an often-observed phenomenon in which a panic reaction follows a dyspneic episode, worsening the severity. Environmental conditions such as temperature, humidity, and pollutants may also worsen sensations of dyspnea.

Pathophysiology

Dyspnea is a highly subjective sensation. The intensity of the experience cannot be adequately predicted by respiratory rate or the degree of lung dysfunction. The sensation of dyspnea encompasses both the sensation and the individual's response to the sensation. Gift[15] has developed a model of dyspnea that describes the multifactorial components of the dyspnea experience (Figure 5-1).

Sensation

Given the multitude of etiologic factors for dyspnea in the oncology population, it is not surprising that the sensation of dyspnea may arise from several different

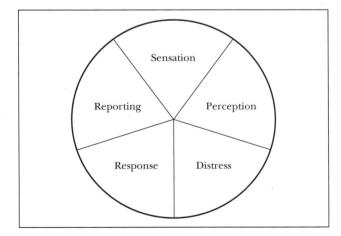

FIGURE 5-1 Components of dyspnea. (Source: Gift AG: Dyspnea. *Nurs Clin North Am* 25:956, 1990.[15]) Used with permission.

pathophysiologic conditions. Basic understanding of normal breathing control is necessary to understand the pathophysiologic basis of dyspnea. The balance of arterial oxygen and carbon dioxide is dependent on integration of respiratory control centers, sensors, and effectors (Figure 5-2). The brain-stem centers are responsible for automatic control of breathing but can be overridden by the cerebral cortex when voluntary control of breathing is needed. Sensors include chemoreceptors and sensory receptors. The effectors are the respiratory muscles that directly effect gas exchange.

Respiratory control centers

The role of voluntary and involuntary respiratory control centers in the sensation of dyspnea is unclear. Studies indicate that the degree of dyspnea can be very different in situations for which the information arising from the peripheral receptors should be the same, thereby suggesting an affective component.[16] The sensation of dyspnea can be decreased by voluntarily increasing venti-

lation, presumably bypassing or overriding the brain-stem respiratory center.[16]

Chemoreceptors

Central chemoreceptors respond primarily to changes in PCO_2. Peripheral chemoreceptors respond primarily to changes in PO_2. While hypoxia clearly can cause dyspnea, researchers report conflicting data regarding how well subjects can directly detect blood gas changes, as opposed to perceiving the distress caused by an increase in respiratory effort. Most investigators do not believe stimulation of chemoreceptors is the primary mechanism for the sensation of dyspnea.[16]

Sensory receptors

Sensory receptors in the airways, the lung parenchyma, and the chest wall respond to mechanical stimuli, such as stretch, pressure, or air flow.[16,17] The sensation of dyspnea has been shown to be affected by changes in air flow in the nose and mouth, stimulation of the trigeminal nerve, and changes in airway pressure gradients. These observations are the foundation for dyspnea management strategies described later in this chapter.

Respiratory muscle receptors

Studies of respiratory neurophysiology suggest that input from the respiratory muscles can be transmitted directly to the cerebral cortex and contribute to the sensation of dyspnea.[18] Findings conflict as to whether it is the diaphragm or the intercostal muscles that are primarily involved in the sensation of dyspnea related to respiratory effort.[16]

Perception, Distress, and Response

The perception of dyspnea is related to the base level of dysfunction and the degree of adaptation. Acute changes in PCO_2 produce immediate breathing changes, whereas chronically elevated levels of PCO_2 do not evoke a specific respiratory response.[15] The distress associated with dyspnea relates to both the symptom itself and the individual's interpretation. Exercise-induced dyspnea in the healthy individual, while evoking uncomfortable sensations of air hunger, does not elicit the panic, frustration, worry, anxiety, and anger described by those with illness-associated dyspnea.[4]

Psychological factors associated with dyspnea include anxiety and depression. Depression may be associated with chronic dyspnea and the resultant lifestyle limitations imposed by dyspnea.[19,20] A dyspnea-anxiety-dyspnea cycle has been suggested, wherein the response to the symptom exacerbates the symptom. The individual's response, i.e., the inability to use problem-focused or emotion-focused strategies to decrease dyspnea, clearly can become part of the dyspnea problem.[21–24]

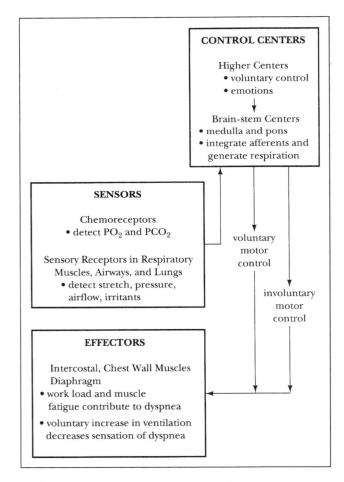

FIGURE 5-2 The integration of respiratory control centers, sensors, and effectors. (Source: Adapted from Cowcher K, Hanks GW: Long-term management of respiratory symptoms in advanced cancer. *J Pain Symptom Manage* 5:322, 1990.[6])

Reporting

The reporting of dyspnea is influenced by both the patient and the healthcare provider. Sociocultural norms influence what sensations are reported and to whom. If dyspnea is anticipated or believed to be untreatable, it may not be reported. Healthcare providers' expectations of the disease process may influence their level of inquiry. Dyspnea in individuals without cancer in the lungs is usually not anticipated and could subsequently go unrecognized by nurses and physicians.[2] If providers believe they cannot provide relief of dyspnea, they may not assess well for this symptom.

Assessment

Assessment of dyspnea is necessary to determine the cause(s) of the problem and to assess response to interventions. Thorough description of the dyspnea sensation, medical history, and physical assessment are all pertinent to assessing cause(s) and planning interventions. Ongoing use of dyspnea measurement tools is most appropriate for assessing dyspnea response to interventions or disease progression.

History and Physical Examination

Assessment of dyspnea begins with questions focusing on the characteristics of the symptom: onset, frequency, intensity, and nature of the respiratory changes. Stimuli that provoke dyspnea, both physical and emotional, are important, as well as strategies the individual uses to decrease the severity of the symptom. The meaning of the symptom to the individual is also relevant.

A medical history is an important part of the assessment, including other medical conditions or symptoms, previous and current cancer treatment, tobacco and alcohol use, allergies, medications, previous and current occupation, and family/living situation. Physical exam includes assessment of the heart, lungs, abdomen, and extremities, as well as assessment for fever, infection, or obesity. Diagnostic evaluation may include arterial blood gases, chest radiograph or computed tomography, pulmonary function tests, and ventricular function tests. While causes of dyspnea are frequently multifactorial, a thorough assessment can provide clues about primary etiology as well as direction for intervention.

Measurement Tools

A variety of instruments have been developed to measure various dimensions of dyspnea. A thorough review of the instruments has been completed by McCord and Cronin-Stubbs.[25] Some instruments are appropriate to guide initial assessment, whereas others are useful in measuring changes over time. Following are highlighted instruments.

Baseline assessment

The *American Thoracic Society Standardized Questionnaire (ATS-DLD-78)* was developed for an epidemiologic study.[26] It collects extensive data regarding respiratory symptoms, family history, occupational history, and medical history. "The Pulmonary Functional Status and Dyspnea Questionnaire (PFSDQ) was developed primarily for patients with chronic obstrive pulmonary disease and measures both the intensity of dyspnea with activity and changes in functional ability due to dyspnea."[27] The *Modified Baseline Dyspnea Index* scores functional impairment, with subscales for work and home.[28] The *Shortness of Breath Assessment Tool* also scores functional impairment, with subscales for body care, movement, eating, home management, and recreational and social activities.[29]

Ongoing assessment

The most commonly used method of measuring changes in dyspnea over time is the *visual analogue scale (VAS)*. This is done with a 100-mm horizontal or vertical line with markers representing "no dyspnea" and "dyspnea as bad as it can be."[3,30,31] This can be used to assess an individual's current dyspnea, worst dyspnea within a time frame, or dyspnea associated with a specific activity. An alternative is the *Transition Dyspnea Index,* an interview guide that assesses for deterioration versus improvement in dyspnea, using three subscales: functional impairment, intensity of activity, and magnitude of effort.[32]

The ability of healthcare providers to accurately assess changes in dyspnea is limited by the multitude of factors that may influence the perception of dyspnea. In a healthy population, anxiety, depression, anger, and cognitive disturbance were all associated with increased reporting of dyspnea and other respiratory symptoms.[19]

In patients with cancer, dyspnea may be only one of several troubling symptoms the patient is experiencing, and there may be significant overlap in symptom experience, particularly with fatigue. Assessment techniques must take into consideration the potential for multiple and overlapping symptoms, as well as the measurement burden imposed on patients.[33]

Symptom Management

Initial medical management is directed toward relieving the problem that resulted in dyspnea. If cancer is the underlying cause of dyspnea, treatment may include chemotherapy, radiotherapy, surgical resection, thoracentesis, paracentesis, or pleural sclerosing. Steroids may ameliorate lung toxicity of radiation therapy or chemotherapy. Other medical interventions directed toward primary treatment of dyspnea are red-cell transfusion for anemia, antibiotics for pneumonia, a chest tube for pneumothorax, and bronchodilators for asthma. The symptomatic management of dyspnea is needed concurrently with these therapies or when they fail to resolve the underlying cause.

Studies of individuals with chronic dyspnea indicate that they develop both problem-focused and emotion-focused coping strategies.[3,9] These strategies are often self-taught and include decreasing activity, positioning and breathing techniques, relaxation techniques, self-isolation, and distraction or diversion.[27] Some techniques are appropriate regardless of underlying cause, whereas other strategies are specific to certain etiologies of dyspnea. Patient education as follows can guide the individual to effective strategies for relieving or decreasing chronic dyspnea. (See also Appendix 5A.)

Breathing, Exercise, and Positioning Techniques

Pursed-lip breathing (PLB)

This technique has been used primarily with chronic obstructive pulmonary disease. During pursed-lip breathing training, participants are instructed to purse their lips during exhalation to apply a back pressure.[34] Researchers believe this technique may delay or prevent small airway collapse, thereby allowing better gas exchange.[35] Studies in this group of patients indicate that PLB can relieve the perception of dyspnea, increase tidal volume, decrease respiratory rate, and improve blood gas parameters.[34,36,37] To facilitate training, ear oximetry can be used to provide the participant with rapid feedback regarding arterial oxygen saturation.[34] The symptomatic relief of dyspnea, however, appears to be independent of improvement in arterial blood gases.[36]

Exercise training

Depending on the etiology, dyspnea may be improved by either specific breathing exercises to strengthen muscles associated with inspiration or general physical training. The ventilatory muscles include the diaphragm, the intercostal and accessory muscles, and the abdominal muscles. Breathing training to optimize the position of the diaphragm for maximal efficacy is particularly relevant with chronic obstructive pulmonary disease (COPD), because the diaphragm is typically shortened or flattened. Ventilatory muscle training can increase strength and endurance of ventilatory muscles in situations of chronic respiratory failure.[35] This type of training may be provided by a physical therapist, respiratory therapist, or nurse.

General physical training may reduce activity-associated dyspnea in the context of congestive heart failure.[38]

Exercise training in individuals with chronic heart failure should be individualized and used with caution. However, Coats et al.[39] conclude that simple, home-based training is a feasible and effective way to improve activity tolerance and symptoms in the face of moderate to severe heart failure. A pulmonary/cardiac rehabilitation program may be an appropriate referral for the individual with symptomatic, treatment-related heart failure.

Positioning

Positioning is the most common strategy individuals use to relieve dyspnea, regardless of its cause.[27] The typical position involves leaning forward with arms braced on a chair or knees and upper body supported. Banzett et al.[40] demonstrated that this position increases ventilatory capacity and attributed the capacity change to improved function of the accessory muscles that expand the rib cage. Long-term strategies used by individuals with dyspnea include sleeping in a chair or with the head elevated in bed and taking measures to avoid bending and stooping, such as wearing slip-on shoes. (Appendix 5A includes several illustrations for patient education.)

Oxygen and Air Therapy

Although oxygen therapy is an important component of treatment of hypoxemia, its role in symptomatic relief of dyspnea is not clearly established. Using a visual analogue scale as a measure, evaluation of oxygen therapy in patients with COPD did not demonstrate decreased dyspnea with oxygen therapy.[41] However, correction of hypoxia in a group of cancer patients having dyspnea at rest resulted in decreased dyspnea.[42,43] In a group of dyspneic cancer patients who were not necessarily hypoxic, oxygen therapy was found to significantly reduce the symptom of dyspnea.[44] There was no evidence that response was predicted by either history of lung disease or presence of hypoxia. In this same study, room air was administered by nasal cannula.[44] Similar improvement over baseline measurements was noted.

Other studies have also shown that alteration of air flow to the nares, mouth, or face may change the perception of dyspnea.[45,46] While having no effect on PO_2, air flow through a mask or nasal cannula accounted for 70% and 52% of oxygen therapy–associated improvement in dyspnea due to cancer and COPD, respectively.[41,47] While some consider this a placebo effect, others hypothesize that stimulation of the trigeminal nerve can alter the perception of breathlessness.[17] Bruera et al.[42] describe an effective method for assessing additive benefit of oxygen therapy over air flow in individual patients. By alternating O_2 and air at 5-minute intervals while assessing dyspnea and hypoxia using a VAS and PO_2 measurement, clinical decisions can be based on individual benefit. Other methods to stimulate this effect include a flow of cold air directed against the cheek[17] or cold compresses applied to the cheek.[48]

Coping Techniques

Individuals with dyspnea struggle to cope not only with the physical limitations induced by dyspnea but also with the accompanying anxiety, worry, and even panic. Activities are reduced to maintain a tolerable level of dyspnea. A variety of techniques have been identified to cope with the emotions associated with dyspnea. Progressive muscle relaxation (PMR) involves the sequential tightening and releasing of sixteen muscle groups, combining mental focus with physical relaxation. This can reduce dyspnea and the associated anxiety.[21] PMR instruction can be given through either recorded or live training.[49] PMR can be learned in a few sessions and performed at home with no expensive equipment. Desensitization and guided mastery techniques have also been reported to decrease fear and anxiety associated with dyspnea.[50] Desensitization involves exposing the person to greater than usual levels of dyspnea in a safe, monitored environment. The exposure to dyspnea with no adverse events may decrease the panic associated with the symptom. The addition of guided mastery may further increase tolerance of dyspnea and activity level. Guided mastery helps individuals identify and use coping strategies that are effective for them. Other coping strategies found to be effective include visual imagery, concentration, distraction, and breathing strategies. The nurse can provide coaching, including assistance in goal setting, feedback on physiologic parameters as appropriate, and encouragement and praise for improvement in performance and use of coping strategies.

Corner et al.[24] demonstrated the effectiveness of a combined approach. Twenty patients with advanced lung cancer and dyspnea were treated weekly in a nurse-led clinic with counseling, breathing retraining, relaxation, and education on coping and adaptation strategies. Distress from breathlessness was improved by a median of 53%, in comparison to the control group, in which breathlessness distress worsened by 10%.

Severe Dyspnea

The management of severe dyspnea in the terminal cancer patient follows standard symptom management principles. The treatment should be the most effective, simplest available that is appropriate for that patient at that time.[6] Several of the treatments previously described, such as positioning, oxygen or air therapy, and relaxation techniques, are very appropriate for severe dyspnea in the terminal phases. Others, such as exercise training and desensitization, are too time and energy consumptive. The use of narcotics, while limited by side effects

for long-term use, is very appropriate in the terminal phase.

Morphine

Narcotics are an important component of the management of severe dyspnea in the terminally ill. Narcotics may affect dyspnea through several actions: altered perception of breathlessness, reduced respiratory drive, and reduced oxygen consumption.[51] Researchers evaluating the efficacy of narcotics in dyspnea management have studied and used morphine in a variety of routes, including intravenous infusion,[51] subcutaneous injection,[52] and inhalation.[53,54] Morphine is highly effective in relieving dyspnea. Studies have demonstrated that 80% to 95% of terminal cancer patients receive significant relief with morphine treatment. The therapeutic challenge lies in balancing the relief of dyspnea with the side effects of morphine.

Somnolence is the primary side effect of morphine. Cohen et al.[55] caution, however, against making dose-modification decisions based on somnolence in the first few hours following initiation of morphine therapy, as deep sleep may occur in individuals who have been sleep-deprived due to dyspnea. Somnolence is best managed by dose reduction. Reversal agents, such as naloxone, are likely to precipitate severe dyspnea, anxiety, and agitation. Studies indicate that morphine can improve dyspnea at doses that do not significantly compromise respiratory function. Changes in arterial blood gas values may occur (PCO_2 increasing and pH decreasing); however, respiratory rate rarely drops below 10 breaths per minute and PO_2 changes are variable.[55]

Patients in the terminal stages of cancer are frequently receiving morphine or other narcotics for pain control. Increased morphine doses are required for management of dyspnea. Infusional doses of morphine are established by bolusing 1 to 2 mg of morphine every 5 to 10 minutes, until relief is noted.[55] Doses for injection can be estimated by increasing the established pain management dose by 50%.[56] Morphine may be combined with other drugs to improve response or alter the side effects. The addition of chlorpromazine may control psychomotor agitation as well as nausea and vomiting due to morphine.[57] In patients with tumor invasion of lung lymphatics, the addition of dexamethasone may improve symptoms.[6] Antianxiety drugs, such as diazepam or alprazolam, have been evaluated for dyspnea relief with little benefit noted.[55]

The application of nebulized morphine directly to the lung is a novel approach to minimizing toxicity. Small doses of morphine have been shown to significantly increase exercise endurance in a population with chronic pulmonary disease.[58] Participants in this study noted no side effects from the morphine. The authors describe anecdotal success in ameliorating dyspnea at rest through longer administration of nebulized morphine, also with no side effects, and hypothesize a direct effect on lung afferent nerves. This technique is being evaluated for efficacy in cancer patients.

Studies of cancer patients have shown mixed results. In a chart review study, Farncombe et al.[53] found nebulized morphine to be effective in relieving dyspnea in 34 of 54 (63%) patients referred to a palliative care service for dyspnea management.[53] These patients represented a mix of cancer and noncancer patients. Others described anecdotal benefits to nebulized morphine.[59,60] In contrast, Noseda et al.[54] reported that nebulized morphine was not more effective than placebo administration of nebulized normal saline. However, this study is limited in two ways. The sample consisted of 17 patients, 3 with cancer and the remainder with severe COPD. Fourteen of the patients completed the study, with 2 of 3 (67%) cancer patients dying before completion. Within this small sample, there were four arms: saline plus oxygen, 10 mg morphine plus oxygen, 20 mg morphine plus oxygen, and 10 mg morphine alone. Consequently, there was no comparison possible between morphine alone and saline alone.

Evaluation of Therapeutic Approaches

For several reasons, evaluating the effectiveness of dyspnea management strategies is challenging. First, dyspnea is often multifactorial in etiology; consequently, a combined therapeutic approach is more likely to be of benefit than a single-modality intervention. Evaluation of the combined therapeutic approach will provide much more helpful information than evaluation of each modality. Secondly, dyspnea is most prevalent in patients with advanced disease. The burden on the patient that is associated with diagnostics and evaluation must be considered when deciding on evaluation strategies. In addition, dyspnea is inherently a subjective symptom that does not correlate well with physiologic measures. It is the perspective of the patient that carries the most weight in dyspnea evaluation. Finally, investigators and clinicians must remember the potential effect of trigeminal nerve stimulation when evaluating the benefit of oxygen therapy.

For most patients, the use of either VAS or numerical rating of dyspnea will be the most reasonable method to evaluate therapeutic approaches. The various approaches described earlier in this chapter may be concurrently or sequentially implemented by a variety of healthcare providers, including nurses, respiratory therapists, physical therapists, social workers, psychologists, and physicians. The consistent use of a simple evaluation scale can facilitate communication between multiple healthcare providers involved in the patient's care.

Educational Tools and Resources

Research has shown that the breathing and positioning techniques used by patients with dyspnea are primarily self-taught.[27] The self-care guide for shortness of breath (Appendix 5A) is provided to facilitate early patient education in positioning, breathing, and coping techniques to reduce dyspnea. Patients in whom dyspnea is expected to be a chronic condition may certainly benefit through education and training provided within local and regional heart and lung rehabilitation programs. If these are not available, video exercise programs designed specifically for people with health problems, such as Gentle Fitness (1-800-566-7780) can be used. Organizations such as the American Lung Association (1-800-LUNGUSA) offer helpful pamphlets on managing shortness of breath.

Patients with advanced cancer and their families need education and support in order to maximize their ability to participate in activities they enjoy, given the constraints of dyspnea and, often, of other concomitant symptoms. They may also need educational resources regarding morphine or oxygen therapy used in dyspnea management. Resources on these topics may be available through local hospice organizations, as well as through the National Cancer Institute's Cancer Information Service (1-800-4CANCER).

Conclusion

Dyspnea is clearly one of the most prevalent and distressing symptoms individuals with cancer experience. An aggressive approach to managing dyspnea at all stages of illness can improve the quality of life of individuals with cancer.

References

1. Heyse-Moore LH, Ross V, Mulee M: How much of a problem is dyspnoea in advanced cancer? *Palliat Med* 5:27–33, 1991
2. Roberts DK, Thorne SE, Pearson C: The experience of dyspnea in late-stage cancer: Patients' and nurses' perspectives. *Cancer Nurs* 16:310–320, 1993
3. Brown ML, Carrieri V, Janson-Bjerklie S, et al: Lung cancer and dyspnea: The patient's perception. *Oncol Nurs Forum* 13:19–24, 1986
4. Janson-Bjerklie S, Carrieri VK, Hudes M: The sensation of pulmonary dyspnea. *Nurs Res* 35:154–159, 1986
5. Campbell EJM, Howell JBL: The sensation of dyspnea. *BMJ* 2:868, 1963
6. Cowcher K, Hanks GW: Long-term management of respiratory symptoms in advanced cancer. *J Pain Symptom Manage* 5:320–330, 1990
7. Farncombe M: Dyspnea: Assessment and treatment. *Support Care Cancer* 5:94–99, 1997
8. Stover DE, Kaner RJ: Pulmonary toxicity, in DeVita VT, Hellman SH, Rosenberg SA: *Cancer: Principles and Practice*

of Oncology (ed 5). Philadelphia: Lippincott, 1997, pp. 2729–2739

9. Gift AG, Pugh LC: Dyspnea and fatigue. Nurs Clin North Am 28:373–384, 1993

10. Dudgeon DJ: Management of dyspnea and cough in patients with cancer. Hematol Oncol Clin North Am 10:157–171, 1996

11. Pass HA: Malignant pleural and pericardial effusions, in DeVita VT, Hellman SH, Rosenberg SA: Cancer: Principles and Practice of Oncology (ed 5). Philadelphia: Lippincott, 1997, pp. 2586–2598

12. Reuben DB, Mor V: Dyspnea in terminally ill cancer patients. Chest 89:234–236, 1986

13. Ripamonti C, Bruera E: Dyspnea: Pathophysiology and assessment. J Pain Symptom Manage 13:220–232, 1997

14. Kimsey FC, Mendenhall NP, Edwald LM, Coons TS, Layon AJ: Is radiation treatment volume a predictor for acute or late effect on pulmonary function? Cancer 73:2549–2555, 1994

15. Gift AG: Dyspnea. Nurs Clin North Am 25:955–965, 1990

16. Tobin MJ: Dyspnea: Pathophysiologic basis, clinical presentation, and management. Arch Intern Med 150:1604–1613, 1990

17. Schwartzstein RM, Lahive K, Pope A, et al: Cold facial stimulation reduces breathlessness induced in normal subjects. Am Rev Respir Dis 136:58–61, 1987

18. Cherniak NS, Altose MD: Mechanisms of dyspnea. Clin Chest Med 8:207–214, 1987

19. Dales RE, Spitzer WO, Schechter MT, et al: The influence of psychological status on respiratory symptom reporting. Am Rev Respir Dis 139:1459–1463, 1989

20. Gift AG, Plant SM, Jacox A, et al: Pulmonary disease in critical care: Psychologic and physiologic factors related to dyspnea in subjects with chronic obstructive pulmonary disease. Heart Lung 15:595–601, 1986

21. Renfroe KL: Effect of progressive relaxation on dyspnea and state anxiety in patients with chronic obstructive pulmonary disease. Heart Lung 17:408–413, 1988

22. Gift AB, Moore T, Soeken K: Relaxation to reduce dyspnea and anxiety in COPD patients. Nurs Res 41:241–246, 1992

23. Bailey C: Nursing as therapy in the management of breathlessness in lung cancer. Eur J Cancer Care 4:184–190, 1995

24. Corner J, Plant H, A'Hern R, Bailey C: Non-pharmacological intervention for breathlessness in lung cancer. Palliat Med 10:299–305, 1996

25. McCord M, Cronin-Stubbs D: Operationalizing dyspnea: Focus on measurement. Heart Lung 21:167–179, 1992

26. American Thoracic Society: Recommended respiratory disease questionnaires for use with adults and children in epidemiological research. Am Rev Respir Dis 14:7–53, 1978

27. Lareau SC, Carrieri-Kohlman V, Janson-Bjerklie S, Roos PJ: Development and testing of the Pulmonary Functional Status and Dyspnea Questionnaire (PFSDQ). Heart and Lung 23:242–50, 1994

28. Stoller J, Ferranti R, Feinstein A: Further specification and evaluation of a new index for dyspnea. Am Rev Respir Dis 134:129–134, 1986

29. Lareau S, Kohlman-Carrieri V, Janson-Bjerklie S, et al: Functional levels and dyspnea in patients with COPD. Am Rev Respir Dis 133:163A, 1986

30. Wilson RC, Jones PW: A comparison of the visual analogue scale and modified Borg scale for the measurement of dyspnoea during exercise. Clin Sci 76:277–282, 1989

31. Gift AG: Validation of a vertical visual analogue scale as a measure of clinical dyspnea. Rehab Nurs 14:323–325, 1989

32. Mahler D, Weinberg D, Wells C, et al: The measurement of dyspnea: Contents, interobserver agreement, and physiologic correlates of two new clinical indexes. Chest 85:751–758, 1984

33. van der Molen B: Dyspnoea: A study of measurement instruments for the assessment of dyspnoea and their application for patients with advanced cancer. J Adv Nurs 22:948–956, 1995

34. Tiep BL, Burns M, Kao D, Madison R, Herrera, et al: Pursed lips breathing training using ear oximetry. Chest 90:218–221, 1986

35. Kigin ML: Breathing exercises for the medical patient: The art and the science. Phys Ther 70:700–706, 1990

36. Mueller RE, Petty TL, Filley GF: Ventilation and arterial blood gas changes induced by pursed-lips breathing. J Appl Physiol 28:784–789, 1970

37. Leith DE, Bradley M: Ventilatory muscle strength and endurance training. J Appl Physiol 41:508–516, 1976

38. Rossi P: Physical training in patients with congestive heart failure. Chest 101(suppl):350–353, 1992

39. Coats AJS, Adamopoulos S, Meyer TE, et al: Effects of physical training in chronic heart failure. Lancet 335:63–65, 1990

40. Banzett RB, Topulos GP, Leith DE, Nations CS: Bracing arms increases the capacity for sustained hyperpnea. Am Rev Respir Dis 138:106–109, 1988

41. Liss HP, Grant BJB: The effect of nasal flow on breathlessness in patients with chronic obstructive pulmonary disease. Am Rev Respir Dis 137:1285–1288, 1988

42. Bruera E, Schoeller T, MacEachern T: Symptomatic benefit of supplemental oxygen in hypoxemic patients with terminal cancer: The use of the N of 1 randomized controlled trial. J Pain Symptom Manage 7:365–368, 1992

43. Bruera E, de Stoutz N, Velasco-Leiva A, Schoeller T, Hanson J: Effects of oxygen on dyspnea in hypoxaemic terminal-cancer patients. Lancet 342:13–14, 1993

44. Booth S, Kely MJ, Cox NP, Adams L, Guz A: Does oxygen therapy help dyspnea in patients with cancer? Am J Respir Crit Care Med 153:1515–1518, 1996

45. Twycross RF, Lack SA: Therapeutics in Terminal Cancer (ed 2). Edinburgh: Churchill Livingstone, 1990

46. Heyes Moore L: Respiratory symptoms, in Saunders C (ed): The Management of Terminal Malignant Disease (ed 2). London: Edward Arnold, 1984, pp. 113–118

47. Waterhouse JC, Howard P: Breathlessness and portable oxygen in chronic obstructive airways disease. Thorax 38:302–306, 1983

48. Folgering H, Olivier O: The diving response depresses ventilation in man. Bull Eur Physiopathol Respir 21:143–147, 1985

49. Hiebert B, Cardinal J, Dumka L, et al: Self-instructed relaxation: A therapeutic alternative. Biofeedback Self Regul 8:601–617, 1983

50. Carrieri-Kohlman V, Douglas MK, Gormley JM, et al: Desensitization and guided mastery: Treatment approaches for the management of dyspnea. Heart Lung 22:226–234, 1993

51. Cohen MH, Anderson AJ, Krashow SH, et al: Continuous intravenous infusion of morphine for severe dyspnea. South Med J 84:229–234, 1991

52. Bruera E, Macmillan K, Pether J, et al: Effects of morphine on the dyspnea of terminal cancer patients. J Pain Symptom Manage 5:341–344, 1990

53. Farncombe M, Chater S, Gillin A: The use of nebulized morphine for breathlessness: A chart review. Palliat Med 9:306–312, 1994

54. Noseda A, Carpiauz JP, Markstein C, Meyvaert A, de Maertel-
aer V: Disabling dyspnoea in patients with advanced disease:
Lack of effect of nebulized morphine. *Eur Respir J* 10:
1079–1083, 1997
55. Cohen MH, Johnston-Anderson A, Krasnow SH, et al: Treatment of intractable dyspnea: Clinical and ethical issues.
Cancer Invest 10:317–321, 1992
56. Bruera E, MacEachern T, Ripamonti C, et al: Subcutaneous
morphine for dyspnea in cancer patients. *Ann Intern Med*
119:906–907, 1993
57. Ventafridda V, Spoldi E, De Conno F: Control of dyspnea
in advanced cancer patients. *Chest* 98:1544–1545, 1990 (letter to the editor)
58. Young IH, Daviskas E, Keena VA: Effect of low dose nebu-
lised morphine on exercise endurance in patients with
chronic lung disease. *Thorax* 44:387–390, 1989
59. MacLeod RD, King BJ: Relieving breathlessness with nebulized morphine. *Palliat Med* 9:169, 1995
60. Davis CL: The use of nebulized opioids for breathlessness.
Palliat Med 9:169–170, 1995

Shortness of Breath (Dyspnea)

Patient Name _____

Symptom and Description   Dyspnea, or shortness of breath, is the feeling of having trouble breathing. Most often, people have this feeling because their bodies are working hard to move air in and out of their lungs. Less often, dyspnea occurs because the body is not getting enough oxygen. Many things can contribute to dyspnea. Shortness of breath can be caused or worsened by:

- partial or complete removal of a lung
- some chemotherapy drugs
- radiation therapy to the lungs
- tumor blocking the airways or pushing on the lungs from the outside
- lung damage from smoking
- anemia (low blood count)
- infection
- obesity
- seasonal allergies

Feeling short of breath can cause anxiety, and anxiety can worsen the feeling, creating a vicious cycle that is hard to break. However, there are things you can do to make you feel less short of breath.

Learning Needs   You may be able to decrease your shortness of breath, which will help you do more and enjoy life. You will learn positioning, breathing, air flow, and relaxation techniques. Other things to try include:

- Plan your day to lessen those activities that increase your dyspnea, such as stair-climbing and bending over.
- Wear slip-on shoes. Pull sock and shoes on while sitting. Use special devices to pick up items on the floor or ground.
- Ask family and friends for help.
- Avoid things that make your breathing worse, such as cold air, humidity, pollen, or tobacco smoke.

Management

Positioning: These positions will help your lungs expand:

- Sitting upright in a chair, lean forward slightly, and rest your forearms on the arms of the chair, on another piece of furniture, or on your knees.

- Sleep with your head on several pillows or sitting up in a recliner.

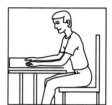 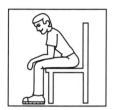 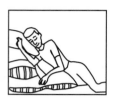 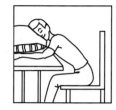 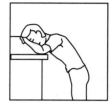

Breathing Techniques: *Pursed-lip breathing* slows the flow of air as you breathe out. This helps the smallest areas of your lungs open up. It is most helpful if you have chronic obstructive pulmonary disease (COPD).

- Breathe in through your nose, as you normally would.

- Breathe out for twice as long as you breathe in. Keep your lips tightly together, except for the very center. Blow out through this small opening.

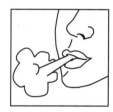

Abdominal breathing, also called diaphragmatic breathing, may lessen dyspnea by making the muscles that help you breathe more effective and stronger. If you have not been taught abdominal breathing, a variety of healthcare providers can help you learn this technique. To try it on your own:

- Find your diaphragm by placing your fingers just below your breastbone and sniffing. The muscle you feel moving is your diaphragm.

- Lie on your back as flat as is comfortable. Bend your knees and put a book on your abdomen. Breathe in deeply. As your diaphragm contracts, the book will rise. Continue to practice, with your goal being to move the book with each breath.

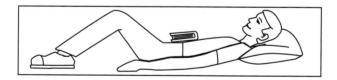

Air flow: Some people with shortness of breath feel better with oxygen treatments. Many people, however, will get the same results from cool air blowing on their cheek. Another way to reduce shortness of breath is to apply a cold cloth to your cheek.

Relaxation Techniques: Dyspnea can cause anxiety. Anxiety can worsen dyspnea. It is important to learn ways to break the cycle of dyspnea and anxiety.

- Concentration: Progressive muscle relaxation is a technique you can use at home to help you relax and reduce dyspnea. While live training may help you learn more quickly, audio and video taped training in progressive muscle relaxation is also helpful and can be found at many bookstores.

- Diversion: You may find activities that distract you from thinking about your breathing to be helpful.

Follow-up   There are other treatments for shortness of breath that can be tried, if your efforts aren't working well enough. Your healthcare provider may prescribe oxygen therapy or medications. In some cases, a lung or heart rehabilitation program may be suggested.

- Tell your healthcare team about the methods you are using at home and how well they are working.

- If you are unsure of any instructions you are given, tell your doctor or nurse.

- Be sure you understand when to call your doctor or nurse, and have both regular and emergency phone numbers handy.

Phone Numbers

Nurse: _____ Phone: _____

Physician: _____ Phone: _____

Respiratory Therapist: _____ Phone: _____

Physical Therapist: _____ Phone: _____

Pulmonary/Cardiac Rehab Program: _____ Phone: _____

Comments

Patient's Signature: _____ Date: _____

Nurse's Signature: _____ Date: _____

Source: Harwood KV: Dyspnea, in Yarbro CH, Frogge MH, Goodman M (eds): *Cancer Symptom Management* (ed 2). Sudbury: Jones & Bartlett, 1999. © Jones and Bartlett Publishers.

CHAPTER 6

Fatigue

Maryl L. Winningham, MSN, APRN, PhD, FACSM

The Problem of Fatigue in Cancer

Incidence in Cancer

People with cancer often say, "I don't have any energy," "Just thinking about work makes me tired," or "I just can't do many things I used to do." For many years, their comments were brushed off by healthcare professionals who said, "What do you expect . . . you've got cancer!" or "Get more rest." More recently, fatigue, the most common and distressing symptom associated with cancer and cancer therapies,[1-3] has been identified as significantly interfering with quality of life (QOL) in people of all ages who have cancer, regardless of diagnosis, treatment, or prognosis. Although there exist established medical interventions for most cancer-related symptoms, there are no standardized medical treatments for fatigue. For example, rest commonly is recommended by healthcare professionals. It is a common intervention used by many people with cancer. However, inappropriate or prolonged use of rest may predispose an individual to increased fatigue and decreased functioning! Clearly, understanding and managing the experience of fatigue in cancer presents one of the greatest challenges to oncology nursing today.

Recent studies have shown dramatic discrepancies between the seriousness with which patients, caregivers, and oncologists view fatigue. In a recent report by Vogelzang et al.,[4] patients reported that fatigue affected their daily lives more than pain, twice as often as their

physicians. On the other hand, oncologists were three times more likely than their patients to report pain as being a daily problem. Moreover, oncologists were far more likely to attribute fatigue to the illness, while patients and caregivers were more likely to attribute it to the treatment. Oncologists were also far more committed to treating pain (94%) than to treating fatigue (5%). It is clear that more needs to be done to improve communication between healthcare providers, caregivers, and patients.

In the past, few data were collected on the incidence or presentation of fatigue in people with cancer. Symptom surveys often ignored it, and it was not listed as a disease- or treatment-related side-effect in cancer educational material. Fatigue did not appear to be linked with morbidity, except when it was associated with anemia. Even now, most medical textbooks ignore the phenomenon of fatigue and its associated issues.

Early cancer researchers focused on objective functional performance rather than on symptom reports, and they were puzzled that decreases in functioning remained, despite improvements in disease state.[5] What they identified as decrements in functioning more likely reflected the long-term sequelae of profoundly decreased activity and bed rest. Unfortunately, they failed to identify and address the issue of deconditioning as a comorbid factor with disease and treatment. *Deconditioning* is the whole-body process, whereby the body adapts or deteriorates to a lower level of functioning.

National Aeronautics and Space Administration (NASA) researchers warned that morbidity resulting from disease and treatment should be distinguished from adaptive hypokinesia and bed rest–related problems. However, most symptoms experienced by people with cancer still are assumed to be disease- and treatment-related.[6] The perception of increased fatigue is an obvious and natural by-product of decreased activity, even in healthy individuals. A clear understanding of fatigue and the degree to which it may be prevented in patients with cancer is yet to be determined.

Like other symptoms, fatigue is subjective. Because of the multicausal and multidimensional nature of fatigue, it should be considered a syndrome or phenomenon rather than just a symptom. Reported descriptions of fatigue-related feelings are diverse and lend themselves to metaphors and combinations of words that may include "trouble breathing," "no energy," "weak and tired," or "can't get motivated." Hence, cancer survivors rarely choose the word "fatigue" to describe these feelings, unless health professionals suggest it (personal communication, Betty R. Ferrell, November 1994). To make things more difficult, there are no biophysical markers or laboratory tests commonly used that highly and exclusively correlate with perception of fatigue. Because there are no definite diagnostic indicators for detecting or monitoring fatigue, the clinician must accept the individual's report. Hence, feelings of fatigue are what the person says they are, and we are dependent on subjective reports for assessment and measurement.[3]

Background

Fatigue has been attributed to a host of biophysical/somatic and psychological manifestations and mechanisms.[3,7–9] For years, researchers have distinguished between *subjective* (perceived), *objective* (external and observable), and *biophysical* (cellular and mechanistic) fatigue. Bartley and Chute[10] assigned the effects of fatigue as a phenomenon to three categories. These categories are important because they provide a structural framework for clinicians in assessing fatigue in people with cancer, as will be discussed under the section on physical assessment. The categories are as follows:

Work output

Work output is performance data on overt activity, including occupational, recreational, and activities of everyday living. This category can be defined objectively in laboratories as well as in field studies with respect to the energetic value of physical work performed. Nurse researchers have obtained objective measures of work output in terms of energy in studies of women receiving chemotherapy for breast cancer.[11–13] More commonly, estimates of task-oriented work output in people with cancer are obtained through standard clinical functional status scales.

Impairment

This category includes biophysical changes at the tissue level, including changes in neural and motor functions. An example commonly cited in the literature is lactate accumulation. The terminal point of impairment with respect to work output is metabolic fatigue or exhaustion. Objective measures of fatigue-associated biophysical impairment are frequently obtained in conjunction with work-output studies. A few studies have validated measurement of both work output and impairment in cancer patients,[11,13] although this is not common practice. Pathologic processes contributing to fatigue-related impairment, such as dehydration and anemia, are evaluated through standardized laboratory tests and are amenable to routine treatment. Definitive biochemical indicators specific to fatigue remain largely unknown; for this reason, they are not part of the standard medical workup. Currently, the search is under way for specific biochemical markers of fatigue that may be used in research and clinical practice.

Fatigue proper

This category includes subjective sensations and feelings of bodily discomfort and aversion to effort. Note that this includes both sensory perception and motivation. Listening to patient descriptors of fatigue-related sensations and relating them to patient distress as well as to alterations in mobility and all-around functioning are critical assessment skills for clinicians to develop. Our understanding of perceived fatigue as a symptom complex is profoundly underdeveloped. Only recently have psychometric instruments been developed to investigate perception of fatigue specific to people with cancer.

The preceding three-part classification was rigid and ignored the probable interrelatedness of the three categories; however, the classifications clearly demonstrated the contrasting approaches to studying fatigue. Definition and descriptions of fatigue have advanced slowly since Bartley and Chute's early work.[14] The complexity of studying fatigue discouraged early researchers, leading one of them, in 1921, to argue for the abandonment of fatigue-related research altogether![15] Despite difficulties inherent in studying fatigue, the incidence, severity, and degree to which it so obviously affects the lives of people with cancer has stimulated renewed interest in this topic. Smets in the Netherlands and Piper in the United States have underlined the need for a continued multidimensional approach to fatigue in cancer.[2,8]

Impact of Fatigue on Quality of Life

It seems logical that having sufficient energetic resources to carry out the many activities and demands of everyday living would contribute to enhanced QOL in cancer patients. In fact, "energy level" has been identified as central to conceptualization of health in healthy women.[16] According to Orem,[17] the physical ability to engage in activity is a universal self-care requisite that depends entirely on the body's ability to produce energy. Although fatigue and "decreased energy" generally are reported to be associated with decreased activity and QOL, there is little research addressing intervention strategies that could maintain or increase feelings of "energy."

Looking at biological energy, a study of male Hodgkin's disease survivors indicated long-term decreases in energy expenditure related to leisure activities, which in turn negatively affected mood.[18] An unpublished study by the author noted that women with breast cancer receiving chemotherapy spent from 100 to 150 calories less in energy per day on activity than comparatively healthy women. There also appeared to be a trend toward increased psychological distress related to decreased energy expenditure in daily activity. Each QOL domain requires a certain amount of energetic effort or stamina. Unfortunately, the cancer experience often is characterized by progressive loss of actual as well as perceived energetic functioning, which often is limited by increased feelings of fatigue. The resulting psychological debilitation can limit functioning in any or all domains of QOL, with widespread interaction in all of life's activities.[19] Indeed, psychological well-being has been identified as critical to other QOL dimensions.[20]

Defining Fatigue

Fatigue is poorly understood. There is no definition for fatigue that satisfies all the clinical observations and subjective experiences associated with it. It is known to be multidimensional and multisensory. It is known to have both long-term and short-term characteristics. It clearly has biophysical and psychological components; indeed, attempts to establish a purely biophysical basis for fatigue were abandoned long ago as hopeless.

People with cancer usually define fatigue by describing their experiences. They often talk about how they feel, what they can't do that they used to do or want to do, and what that loss means to them. Descriptions identify fatigue as affecting all of life's aspects. The subjective reports of fatigue, then, are as multilayered and complex as the associated, objective biophysical phenomena.

Why it is so important to define fatigue? A definition can be used as a clinical guide in assessment of status and outcomes of people with cancer. It helps the clinician to distinguish between alternative phenomena and to determine appropriate interventions. It provides a theoretic framework from which research can be developed.

It is common to differentiate short-term (acute) from long-term (chronic) fatigue, which is *not* the same as "chronic fatigue syndrome." Although some authors have attempted to attach a temporal component (i.e., hours, weeks, months) to these terms,[8] time limits on experiences may be misleading. Recovery seems to be a

defining characteristic, with acute fatigue being akin to tiredness that can be relieved by rest. Chronic fatigue is not relieved by rest and is characterized by an unrelenting feeling of exhaustion.[3,7,8] This perceived chronic fatigue often is associated with other symptoms, including weakness, shortness of breath ("heaviness in my chest," "trouble breathing"), dizziness, trouble concentrating, and "no energy." It is important to note that "tiredness" may not be on a continuum with fatigue,[8] as some have suggested. Certainly the physiological mechanisms are not related, either by symptom induction or by how the state is resolved. Indeed, people with cancer often comment, "I used to think I was tired, but it was nothing like this . . . this is worse than anything I could imagine."

In defining as well as assessing fatigue, the following issues and phenomena must be addressed:

1. Short-term (acute) versus long-term (chronic) fatigue
2. Biophysical conditions versus psychosocial contributors in "normal" circumstances, particularly with respect to exertion or performance
3. Fatigue versus similar symptoms such as weakness, dizziness, or shortness of breath
4. Relative contribution of pathologic conditions to fatigue
5. Pharmacologic influences on fatigue
6. The relative influences of rest and recovery processes on fatigue
7. Nutritional influences on fatigue
8. Environmental influences on fatigue
9. Maturational processes in fatigue
10. Cultural differences in perception of fatigue and affecting fatigue
11. Individual differences in perception of fatigue
12. Interaction of fatigue with other symptoms such as pain
13. The influence of such states as excitement and anxiety on perception of fatigue
14. Spiritual values or meaning of fatigue to the individual

Obviously, it is an ambitious person who will attempt to define this most puzzling symptom complex! Currently, no one has included all of these characteristics in any one definition of fatigue. However, Piper,[8] Smets,[2] and others have provided excellent reviews on delimiting and defining fatigue.

Etiology

More than any other symptom, fatigue is characterized by multiple and interacting causes. These include biophysical-, functional-, psychological-, social-, occupational-

(including economic), disease-, treatment-, and symptom- (regardless of the source) related causes interacting over time. The pattern of fatigue in relation to disease and treatment events may help us identify causative or aggravating situations. Generally, fatigue becomes progressively worse as treatment continues and as the malignancy progresses. Periodic exacerbations can be treatment related, worsening with each course of treatment but rarely returning to normal between cycles. In many cases, the fatigue does not end with the conclusion of treatment and improvement in health. The term "post-cancer fatigue" (PCF) has been suggested for that fatigue that remains after all treatable causes of fatigue have been ruled out.[21] (These issues will be developed further in the section on pathophysiologic and pathopsychological mechanisms.)

Although fatigue may be addressed in terms of specific cause or contributions, there is a compelling "big-picture" approach that is helpful in understanding how fatigue affects the cancer experience. Aistars[9] pointed to exertion or stress, as defined by Selye, to be the common categorical cause of fatigue. This theory is useful to oncology nurses because of the clear presentation of multitudes of stressors in the lives of those with whom we work every day.

Fatigue and Energetics

Understanding fatigue requires an understanding of the relationship between fatigue and energetics. Biophysical energy, food combining with oxygen to produce energy, is the basis for functioning in every aspect of life. As limitations in body energetic resources are reached, fatigue-related metabolic and perceptual changes become overwhelming. These are measurable under laboratory conditions. While subjective measures of fatigue are underdeveloped, objective measures of "energy" are well defined in the research literature. Because physiologic fatigue is the metabolic experience corresponding to terminal energy expenditure, perceived as well as actual energetic output may constitute an objective measurement that can be used to define fatigue. One nursing study measured metabolic changes in response to a series of progressive workloads as a means of evaluating the outcome of an experimental exercise program for women receiving chemotherapy for breast cancer. Findings indicated that women in the exercise group could produce more energy while experiencing less metabolic stress.[13]

Adaptation Energy and Stress

In his general adaptation syndrome (GAS) or "stress" theory, Selye[22] proposed fatigue to be the process of exhausting energetic resources. He differentiated between energy as a physical/metabolic/caloric phenomenon (preceding) and *adaptation energy*, the energy an individual needs for dealing with stressors. As localized energetic resources are depleted, he said, the organism is forced to either slow down or stop to recover or draw on energetic resources found elsewhere. Selye stated, "It may be said without hesitation that for man the most important stressors are emotional, especially those causing distress."[22] Selye then added, "We still have no precise concept of what this [adaptation] energy might be"; he went on to suggest that "it touches on the fundamentals of fatigue."[22]

Selye was not the first to speak of a nonphysiologic "energy." Reflecting a common belief in her day called "vitalism," Nightingale referred to it as "vital force."[23] Many of her interventions focused on preserving and promoting this vital force in those suffering from illness. Although we have yet to define and measure Selye's adaptation energy, the GAS strongly contributed to Lazarus's development of coping theory with respect to emotions. Coping theory introduced the concept of meaning with respect to perceived stressors. In exertional/physiologic stress, protective techniques like rest and pacing are adaptations to minimize exhaustion. Coping influences psychological/emotional stress through a process called *appraisal*.[24] Coping includes a variety of mechanisms by which we make things less stressful to us. Lazarus suggested the immune system to be the means by which we may someday elucidate the difference between biological/metabolic energy and emotionally related energy.[24] Currently, researchers in psychoneuroimmunology are attempting to identify key variables that explain the link between stress, fatigue/exhaustion, and health.[25]

The Fatigue-Inertia Spiral

Healthy individuals maintain their energetic basis for their functional status by activities of living: occupational, social, recreational, and leisure activities. During periods of disease- and treatment-imposed hypodynamia, these normal activities are decreased. Contrary to popular belief, the individual on bed rest is not in a state of homeostasis. The resting individual is subject to the adaptive physiologic effects of entropy. Hence, the inactive individual tends to gravitate toward a state of less available energy. This is the previously mentioned deconditioning. Because the body works on a "use it or lose it" basis, the energetic basis for functional status decreases. Feelings of fatigue often are interpreted by patients as a signal to rest, resulting in accelerating fatigue and decreased functioning. The fatigue-inertia spiral (Figure 6-1), also known in rehabilitation medicine as the disability spiral, illustrates the relationship of fatigue and other symptoms to diminished activity and physiologic changes.

The Psychobiological-Entropy Model of Fatigue

The Winningham Psychobiological-Entropy Model of fatigue demonstrates the relationships among loss of en-

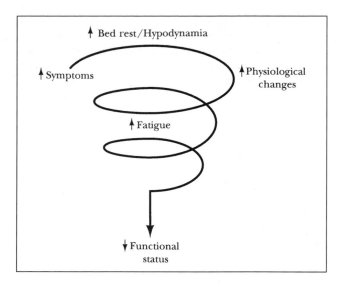

FIGURE 6-1 The fatigue-inertia spiral. Copyright 1991, 1994 by Maryl L. Winningham. Used with written consent of the author.

ergy, fatigue, other symptoms, and decreased functioning. Not only can fatigue be a *primary* symptom (i.e., a direct consequence of preexisting conditions, disease, or treatment), but it can be a *secondary* symptom (i.e., a result of the individual's pathophysiologic and pathopsychological response to other symptoms). This concept is illustrated in Figure 6-2. Failure to understand this

relationship may account for the dearth of effective nursing interventions to mitigate fatigue.

The biological sources of energy are summarized as follows. There are four sources of biological energy for living. These are related to the Winningham Psychobiological Entropy Model and are shown in the upper left hand corner of Figure 6-2. Anything that affects one of those sources affects the body's ability to function. They can be explained as follows:

1. Oxygen is required to "burn the fuel." Individuals who are anemic must, of necessity, make adjustments in their lifestyle to accommodate the decreased energetic resources. The problem of oxygen delivery and anemia is discussed below.

2. Adequate nutrition and hydration provide the fuel for living cells; the hydration also assists keeping muscles at the optimal "stretch" for effective and strong contractions.

3. Energy expenditure in kilocalories per day is the greatest predictor of energy for functioning. In other words, "Use it or lose it." Even small increments or decrements in activity each day can have a profound effect over a longer period of time, such as someone would experience with surgery, a bone marrow transplant, immunotherapy, chemotherapy, or radiation therapy. Unfortunately, individuals who feel profoundly fatigued may find it difficult or impossible to maintain their precancer activity levels. This explains the success of the strategic "activity-rest" intervention. When ex-

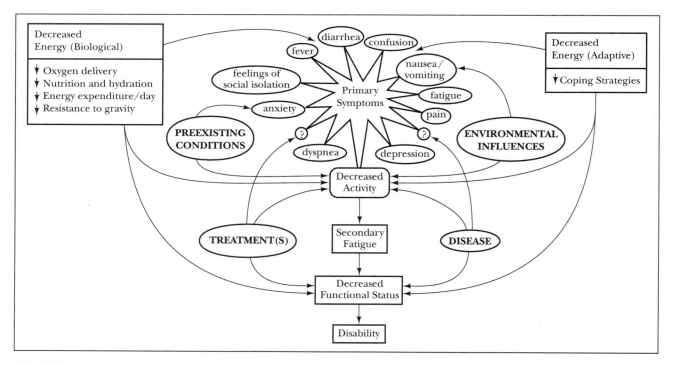

FIGURE 6-2 The Winningham Psychobiological-Entropy Model of functioning. Copyright 1995, 1998 by Maryl L. Winningham. All rights reserved. Used with written consent of the author.

tremely deconditioned individuals do a little, then rest awhile, then do some more, they are able to actually "burn" more energy than those who push themselves to exhaustion.

4. Resistance to gravity is a critical component of maintaining energetic capacity. NASA researchers referred to this as the "horizontal-vertical equation. That is, when you start to spend more time in the horizontal (or resting) position than previously, however subtle, your body starts to deteriorate. Research has demonstrated that inappropriate bed rest can be hazardous to your health!

In conjunction with the Winningham Psychobiological-Entropy Model, Ten Propositions ("Ten Commandments") of Cancer Fatigue have been developed (Table 6-1). These propositions clarify the intimate relationships among activity, energy, fatigue, symptom management, and functional status.

Testing these propositions in research and clinical practice can provide a rich source of intervention ideas. Unfortunately, many standard medical interventions for disease- and treatment-related symptoms have a sedating effect and serve to decrease spontaneous (everyday) activ-

TABLE 6-1 Ten Propositions Explaining Fatigue in Cancer

The relationships among activity, energy, fatigue, symptom management, and functional status in people with cancer can be summarized in the following propositions:

1. Too much rest as well as too little rest contributes to increased feelings of fatigue.
2. Too little activity as well as too much activity contributes to increased feelings of fatigue.
3. A relative balance between activity and rest promotes restoration; an imbalance promotes fatigue and deconditioning.
4. Deconditioning is the adaptive energetic response, whereby an organism's biological work potential is decreased over time.
5. Everyday energy expenditure in activity is the most potent known regulator of the body's energy systems. ("Use it or lose it.")
6. Any symptom/condition that contributes to decreased activity will lead to deconditioning—increased fatigue and decreased functional status.
7. Any intervention that provides relief of a symptom/condition that contributes to decreased activity may simultaneously serve to mitigate fatigue and promote functioning, provided that intervention does not have a sedating or catabolic effect.
8. The experience of fatigue potentiates distress associated with other symptoms/conditions.
9. The experience of other symptoms/conditions potentiates feelings of fatigue.
10. Deconditioning and perceived fatigue interact to make every aspect of life more stressful and negatively impact quality of life, thus contributing to increased suffering.

ity, promote feelings of fatigue, and contribute to a long-term decrease in functional status. Of these, the most common is the advice to "get more rest."

Normally, functional *status* is defined according to task-oriented questionnaires. It also can be defined in terms of energy required (i.e., calories burned) to perform everyday activities. Functional *capacity* can be defined as the highest energy expenditure an individual can accomplish, one's maximal physical exertion level (Figure 6-3).[26,27] Functional *reserve* is the buffer between the energy required for everyday activity and the energy required for life's extra demands. The less the functional reserve, the more easily a person tires. As we age, functional capacity and functional status decrease and the functional reserve narrows, manifesting in a lack of energy to do the extraordinary things in life. When cancer (or any chronic pathologic process) is diagnosed, surgery and other treatments usually follow (precipitating event). There is a tendency for both functional status and functional capacity to decrease overall during this period. If the decreases are subtle and people have altered their lifestyle to be less vigorous, they may suffer a considerable loss before they become aware of it. Sometimes people with cancer will say, "The other day I tried to do [X], but try as I might, I couldn't do it. I don't understand, I used to do that all the time!" This is called the *functional capacity crisis* and is often accompanied by emotional distress. It means that people no longer can function at their accustomed energetic level. If they continue to decline, they eventually come to a point at which they no longer can care for themselves and require assistance. This functional status crisis in which people lose their independence is not only a crisis for the individual, but it usually constitutes a crisis for the family and society. Resources must be sought to help in the care and to redistribute the family tasks. Two other phenomena can be observed in fatigued individuals. Compromised people will sometimes experience a sudden, overwhelming

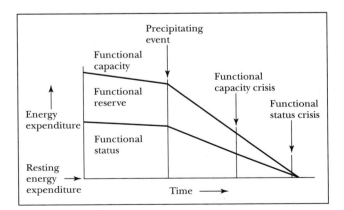

FIGURE 6-3 The energetics of functioning. Copyright 1992, 1994 by Maryl L. Winningham. Used with written consent of the author.

exhaustion. This is a transient fatigue attack (TFA), a very frightening experience. At other times, compromised individuals will feel surges of what has been described as "nervous energy." This transient energy attack (TEA) is short lived and usually is followed by 24 hours or more of extreme exhaustion. The reasons for these phenomena are unknown.

Pathophysiologic and Pathopsychological Mechanisms

No single cause or mechanism is responsible for the sensation of fatigue identified by most people with cancer. It is important to understand that "normal" fatigue, both physical and psychological, exerts a protective effect to prevent injury. It is safe to assume that people with cancer still experience normal fatigue mechanisms like those of any human being. Unfortunately, in cancer there are pathologic processes that are superimposed on normal mechanisms and that limit both activity and recovery.

Physiologic Basis

There are several general physiologic mechanisms related to fatigue in healthy individuals. Extensive research has examined the influence of peripheral (peripheral nerve or contracting muscle) fatigue as a limiting factor to exertion. Peripheral mechanisms are powerfully influenced by the central nervous system, particularly with respect to motivation and metabolic disturbances.[28] These disturbances usually are described by various *accumulation/depletion* hypotheses that relate to the buildup or accumulation of waste products or to the depletion of energetic substrates.[29] In reality, both are involved and interrelated in high levels of exertion. In exercise-fatigue research, however, it must be remembered that the exertional intensity is very high and of long duration and does not represent activity characteristic of most people with cancer. Several specific chemical substances that have been linked to fatigue in healthy subjects include lactate, glycogen, and neurotoxins. It is likely that lactate plays only a small role in clinical fatigue. On the other hand, glycogen depletion in the liver and muscles as a result of exhaustive activity, extended lack of nutritional intake, and stressful experiences may play important roles in acute fatigue exacerbations lasting no more than 48 hours. Neurotoxins such as ammonia inhibit central nervous system functioning in healthy individuals[28] and probably play a more significant role in cancer-related fatigue than has heretofore been suggested.

Pathophysiologic Basis

Although knowledge about the specific mechanisms linking physiologic variables to perceptions of fatigue is vague at best, researchers are examining the impact of biochemical factors on the etiology of fatigue. Cytokines such as tumor necrosis factor (TNF) and interleukin-1 (IL-1) have been associated with muscle loss and muscle contractility.[3,30] Tumor necrosis factor appears to be involved in numerous chronic disease processes, in addition to cancer, in which fatigue is a major complaint.

As a rule, any process, treatment, or pathology that interferes with oxygen uptake and delivery, nutritional and hydration status, or carbon dioxide elimination will contribute to increased fatigability and decreased energy production. Anemia, for example, is a pathologic impairment of oxygen delivery that is a predictable and common sequela to many treatment protocols. The problem of anemia in cancer, whether as a primary or secondary condition, is legendary. The contribution of treatment for cancer, especially chemotherapy, to cyclic states of relative anemia is often predictable. In the past, when hemoglobin levels dropped to dangerously low levels (often as low as 7 or 8 g/dL), it was treated by blood transfusions.

From a physiologic perspective, any deviation of an individual's hemoglobin (often estimated as 14 g/dL in women and 16 g/dL in men) from that which was necessary for normal, everyday functioning prior to the onset of their cancer jeopardizes functioning. Because people compensate for decreased hemoglobin by slowing down or altering their lifestyle, there is a humane, QOL biological imperative to keep hemoglobin levels as near normal as possible. Clinical studies on anemia, QOL, and clinical conditions have virtually ignored issues such as the immunological threat of blood transfusions, impaired lifestyle, and physiologic alterations such as decreased myoglobin and related recovery time. Given the predictability of decreased hemoglobin levels in select treatment protocols, there is no excuse for not treating anemia prophylactically and aggressively.

Cancer patients at risk for or experiencing anemia should be assessed for nutritional status (particularly iron status) and whether they are appropriate candidates for treatment with erythropoietin. Loss of functioning from progressive and untreated anemia can be devastating, especially in the elderly.

Disease factors

In addition to disease-related cytokines and anemia, metabolic and electrolyte imbalances as a result of tumor products induce disorders such as hypercalcemia, tumor lysis syndrome, syndrome of inappropriate antidiuretic hormone secretion, and hemostatic alterations.[31] Although individual experiences vary, reports of weakness often accompany many of these disorders; sudden-onset weakness and fatigue may indicate an impending crisis and should be evaluated.

Surgery

In one study, fatigue was described as the "most surprising and troublesome symptom" following surgery. The author went on to state that reports of fatigue were often related to sleep disruption.[32] This is not surprising considering the cumulative effect of such variables as metabolic responses to stress, anesthetics, pain and pain medications, missed meals,[33] forced convalescence, and bed rest–related dehydration.

Chemotherapy

The fatigue-promoting characteristics of chemotherapy are legendary. The general cytotoxic characteristics of chemotherapy contribute to fatigue through cellular mechanisms (such as pancytopenia and immune suppression), through pathophysiologic side effects (fluid volume deficits, electrolyte imbalance, nutritional deficits), and through psychological factors such as generalized stress.[3,8] Although it is generally thought that the fatigue pattern is related to chemotherapy administration,[3,8,34] this is not always the case.[35] With mixed protocols, nadirs may overlap with effects of radiation treatment, creating a confounding effect and a puzzling pattern.

Radiation therapy

Fatigue is also a significant clinical problem for those undergoing radiation therapy[36] and may be a significant predictor of functional changes.[37] There are contradictory reports as to whether there is improvement in perceived fatigue over the weekend in the absence of treatment.[3,38,39] Faithful[40] reported on a "somnolence syndrome" in adults going through cranial radiation therapy as separate from radiation-related fatigue. She noted two distinct posttreatment stages, the first occurring between days 13 and 26, the second between days 32 and 36.

Biotherapy

Fatigue patterns are reported as varying widely with various biotherapeutic agents.[41] Sensations of profound fatigue are confounded by the "flulike syndrome," which usually includes fever, chills, myalgias, headache, malaise, and cognitive impairment.[3,41]

Deconditioning

As mentioned previously, one of the most remarkable and most demonstrated pathophysiologic mechanisms of fatigue in human beings involves deconditioning, a catabolic process resulting from decreased daily energy expenditure and bed rest. The relationship between purposeful activity and fatigue frequently is misunderstood:

Individuals with cancer and other chronic illnesses frequently imagine that rest will help them feel better and activity or exercise will make them feel more fatigued. Indeed, the desire for rest or decreased activity is an automatic response to fatigue.

Pathologic states arising from even a few days of bed rest or hypokinesia included relative dehydration, sensory deficits, hyperglycemia, loss of energetic capacity, negative mood states, weakness and fatigue, fluid and electrolyte shifts, balance impairments, and immunologic impairment.[6]

Pathopsychological Basis

Cognitive dysfunction

Early researchers recognized cognitive and motivational issues in fatigue that included variables such as anxiety, fatigue, and sleep disturbances. Cimprich studied development of attentional fatigue, which involves loss or decline in the capacity to direct attention. This type of mental fatigue may have an effect on such activities as learning, planning, problem solving, and performing tasks of everyday living.[42,43]

Emotional pathopsychology

In a recent study of women's responses to environmental demands in their lives, it was found that internal states such as depression or anxiety were more significantly related to fatigue and vitality than external stressors such as negative life events or situations.[44] However, the experience of cancer involves many issues that immeasurably complicate an already complex everyday life. The turmoil of dealing with a potentially fatal disease and toxic treatments, complex economic and legal issues, grieving, and loss, all while carrying on everyday family responsibilities and roles, is potentially overwhelming. It is now recognized that depression and fatigue share many similar characteristics.[3,29] Although it was once assumed that many people with cancer were depressed, an unpublished study of women receiving chemotherapy for breast cancer noted that anxiety, fatigue, and confusion better described their emotional state and that depression did not seem to play a role.

Individuals with preexisting illnesses, whether physical or mental, are at extremely high risk for morbidity. They must cope with symptoms from their preexisting illness in addition to the stress of dealing with cancer and treatment regimens, all the while trying to carry on everyday life. It is critical to be aware of the existence of major depression and to monitor for suicide risk. As one exhausted individual receiving biotherapy for metastatic disease whispered, "If this is what life is like, it's not worth living." It is essential to differentiate fatigue from depression or other conditions so the appropriate treatment may be initiated.

Recently, attention has been called to the PCF phenomenon. As previously stated, this is characterized by lingering fatigue after cancer diagnosis and treatment are completed, and after all treatable causes have been resolved.[21] For most individuals, there is delayed (up to 3 years) partial to complete recovery. Some, however, never recover the functional ability they once had. It is important to reassure people that this usually is *not* evidence that they still have cancer but may be evidence of posttreatment residual impairment.

Assessment

Measurement Tools

Although fatigue is a multidimensional concept, it often has been assessed by a single item on a general symptom checklist.[5] According to Varricchio, "The assessment and/or measurement of the presence and level of fatigue require that a definition of fatigue be agreed upon."[45] The ideal fatigue measurement tool is reliable, valid, and short enough that it isn't a burden to subjects. The time of day when it is administered is important because fatigued people generally feel better in the morning (an exception is people with lung cancer who often feel terrible in the morning). Smets[46] presents a concise presentation of the issues related to fatigue in cancer with her 20-item Multidimensional Fatigue Inventory (MFI) that identifies at least five dimensions to fatigue: general fatigue, physical fatigue, mental fatigue, reduced motivation, and reduced activity. The Piper Fatigue Scale (PFS) has 41 items with four dimensions of subjective fatigue: temporal, affective, sensory, and severity.

Recently the Revised Piper Fatigue Scale, a multidimensional scale that includes scoring instructions, was published.[47] Piper's work in evaluating and measuring fatigue has a history in excess of 10 years and has benefited from a variety of advisers and clinical insights. Another new scale, the Multidimensional Fatigue Symptom Inventory (MFSI), may be useful for assessing fatigue on a weekly basis in individuals as well as in evaluating treatment modalities.[48] Other fatigue scales are also in development. It is important to remember that however elegant the psychometrics, any fatigue scale that is not sensitive to individual differences in patients is clinically worthless. Critical questions for clinicians to ask when selecting a scale are, "Does this scale appear to reflect the complaints I hear from the patients? Does it capture the phenomenon?"

Other instruments that have been widely used include the Profile of Mood States, the Rhoton Fatigue Scale, the Symptom Distress Scale, and the Fatigue Symptom Checklist. For a quick clinical (not research) assessment of fatigue that is easy to monitor, the unidimensional item on the Rhoton Fatigue Scale is pragmatic and permits comparisons over time. It is also similar to pain evaluation tools that use a 0 to 10 scale. Ask the person with cancer to use words to describe how their fatigue feels.

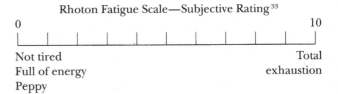

Rhoton Fatigue Scale—Subjective Rating[33]

Physical Assessment

In her book *Notes on Nursing*, Florence Nightingale gave several admonitions about assessing patients. She said, "It is the highest folly to judge of the sick . . . during a period of excitement."[23] To summarize her recommendations:

1. *Do not jump to conclusions about people's status when you see them in the clinical setting.* Most people become excited when they see their physicians, whether in the clinic or in the hospital. In this excitement, they may appear more energetic than they are. People should be observed when they are unaware that they are being observed, such as in the waiting room or waiting for the car. Observe the difference in their behavior when they're alone versus when they're with others. Many individuals rise to the occasion when stimulated by the presence of others. Assume that most people will look much better in the clinic than they will look the next day. If a person is judged based on appearances, the person's functional status and perceived well-being will nearly always be overestimated.

2. *To see how they really are, come back afterward and see how they did.* People suffering extreme fatigue often "crash" after appointments and threatening, exhaustive, or painful procedures. This has both psychological and physical components. Psychologically, there is the let-down after the excitement has passed. Some individuals describe feeling depressed afterward. Physically, exhaustion can relate to muscle glycogen depletion, dehydration, and electrolyte imbalance. Individuals usually tighten muscles during painful procedures, resulting in metabolic exhaustion and glycogen usage. It is not uncommon for them to suffer from concomitant muscle soreness 1 to 2 days afterward. There are many contributing factors to this postevent fatigue.

There is an old physiologic maxim, "Shivering costs the same as jogging." While we would never think of asking an individual undergoing treatment to jog, we often see them dressed in thin examination gowns, shivering as a result of treatments and widespread cold exposure during diagnostic and surgical procedures and radiation treatments. Metabolically, this is very expensive as well as stressful. There is a second physiologic maxim, "Micturition precedes shivering." Human beings vasoconstrict in a cold environment. To aggravate their condition, we often give them intravenous fluids that are at room temperature. When vasoconstriction occurs, there is an increase in urine production. In addition, they often are positioned supine on tables, beds, or gurneys, which further contributes to urine production through atrial natriuretic factor activity. All this contributes to dehydration, a critical contributor to physical fatigability as well as weakness. It also can contribute to subclinical hypothermia, a condition especially threatening to the elderly. One of the cardinal signs associated with this condition is mental confusion.

3. *Carefully and exactly ask how they spent the night.* People who are extremely stressed and fatigued often report that their sleep is unrestful, unrestorative, and disrupted. During nocturnal wake periods, other symptoms appear to be magnified and the loneliness, anxiety, and confusion can be overwhelming. Furthermore, people may feel exhausted and vulnerable up to several days after the prior period of excitement. Clinical observation seems to show that the individuals who suffer most from profound periods of stress and excitement are those who are the most fatigued and weakened. Using Nightingale's admonitions will help the nurse identify the more vulnerable individuals and gain a more accurate assessment of their status.[23]

Older functional assessment techniques such as the Karnofsky scale (zero equals dead, 100% means fully active) and objective portions of the Rhoton Fatigue Scale depended on observations made by health professionals. While professional observations are important, they must be balanced with self-reports from the person experiencing fatigue. The Clinical Assessment Guide for Fatigue and Functioning (Table 6-2) can help the nurse obtain effective and systematic information on an individual's fatigue, as well as on how it relates to their clinical status and how it affects their life. It uses the three categories of fatigue identified by Bartley and Chute as an organizational framework. Prompting for specific information may also help the person communicate more effectively about their fatigue. Further material may be found in

TABLE 6-2 Clinical Assessment Guide for Fatigue and Functioning

Background

Brief history of individual

1. Age
2. Gender
3. Cultural/lifestyle orientation
4. Role expectations
   - Occupation
   - Home
   - Social
   - Economic (insurance coverage)
   - Breadwinner?
   - Living with? Responsible for?
5. Normal activity patterns
6. Normal sleep patterns
7. Preexisting conditions
8. Diagnosis
9. Treatment regimen

Functional Work Output

Focus on changes

1. Are routine tasks getting harder?
2. Have you slowed down?
3. Have you stopped doing some things because of fatigue or any other symptom?

Changes in everyday activities

1. Are you capable of complete self-care?
2. Have you changed your bedtime? How much time do you spend in bed, resting, napping?
3. Are your activity-rest patterns changing?
4. Are you able to participate in family activities?
5. Are you making occupation-related changes?
6. Have you changed your social activities?
7. Have you changed your eating habits? Drinking habits?
8. Do you have any other health problems? Anything that affects your activity? (Consider need for referrals.)

Impairment/Pathophysiology

Diagnostic and laboratory tests

1. Decreased hemoglobin?
2. Hydration status?
3. Electrolyte imbalance? (potassium and magnesium!)

Preexisting conditions or disabilities?

Physical assessment—look for changes in:

1. Alertness and focus? Confusion, irritability, or short attention span?
2. Posture (slumped or erect)?
3. Gait, coordination, and balance (shuffle? steady pace? moving slowly and deliberately?)
4. Ability to arise from seated position?
   - Needs to use hands?
   - Able to rise rapidly from seated to standing position and keep balance?

Feelings Related to Fatigue

Describe sensation of fatigue

1. Ask specifically about no energy, tiredness, or exhaustion.
2. Ask about other symptoms (weakness, depression, dyspnea, pain, etc.).

Establish symptom burden

1. Check intensity of fatigue and related symptoms. (Get rating on fatigue and other prominent symptoms such as dyspnea, depression, weakness, pain.)

0 |__|__|__|__|__|__|__|__|__|__| 10

Patterns of fatigue (ask to see patient diary or chart).

Evaluate meaning of perceived symptom burden.

How do any of the above affect your quality of life?

the Self-Care Guide: Talking about Fatigue (Appendix 6A).

In questioning people about their fatigue, remember that answering questions is fatiguing for most people. If necessary, ask a few questions while performing other tasks (vital signs, starting IV, etc.), and elicit information from a spouse or significant other if possible. This will also help them understand how fatigue is affecting their loved one. After a while, you will learn to select the questions from the list that are pertinent to understanding that individual's status. This also will help you learn to identify patterns and problems associated with fatigue and will help you sharpen your assessment skills.

Symptom journals, graphs, and even art or poetry can help people communicate their feelings of fatigue and fatigue-related symptoms (FRS) to you and others. For those with high fatigability and symptom burden, a family member may be able to keep some record. Subjective reports of fatigue are as complex to assess as the objective biophysical phenomena; but by using a systematic approach, you will be able to become proficient at evaluating fatigue.

Diagnostic Evaluation

A basic physical assessment will include watching for posture, gait, coordination, ability to focus, and level of consciousness. Likewise, elicit the individual's thoughts about satisfaction in life: Consider grief, hopelessness, spiritual distress, depression, or suicidal ideation. Depression in cancer often goes untreated because it mimics other conditions. People with cancer have a right to appropriate mental healthcare, and appropriate treatment may contribute to improved overall functioning. Make sure individuals with a history of mental illness continue receiving their appropriate medications in the inpatient setting and when other oral intake is restricted. Abrupt withdrawal of such medications may result in hallucinations, confusion, and agitation.

Evaluate symptom burden. What can be relieved? Often, if people can get help with one or two symptoms, the others become less distressing. Watch for sudden changes in dyspnea, weakness, dizziness, or other symptoms often associated with fatigue, and look for physiologic reasons. Do they seem to be spending a lot of time in bed, on a recliner, or on the sofa? How many batteries have they replaced in TV remote-control devices in the past month? What is their attitude toward bed rest? Refer to the Dangers of Bed Rest Self-Care Guide, Appendix 6B.

Symptom Management

Prevention begins at home in the bedroom: Going to bed at a regular time is critical to maintaining circadian rhythms. Short naps during the day with ambulation in between help prevent many of the negative consequences of bed rest or decreased activity. Work the energy cycle: Low-intensity exercise such as walking can boost energy and should be attempted during "good times" of the day. Rest during the energy lows. Power walks and power naps are an excellent combination. Good overall symptom management will encourage the person to maintain regular activities and role commitments.

Nutrition and adequate hydration are important, but fatigued individuals tend to overestimate how much they are eating and drinking. Encourage them to get help in meal preparation if necessary. Help people with special nutritional needs obtain the consulting services of a registered dietitian. Monitor hydration status and electrolytes (particularly potassium and magnesium). One of the symptoms associated with bed rest is anorexia. Ambulation may help maintain appetite and nutritional intake. Understanding the many causes of fatigue can help identify appropriate interventions.

Therapeutic Approaches

Because research on fatigue in cancer is still in its infancy, it is difficult to say with certainty which interventions will have therapeutic benefits for which persons. In controlling fatigue and functional ability, it is important to focus on two things: (1) *Maintain what you can,* and if you can't, (2) *minimize loss.*

It is critical to identify interventions that appropriately respect the individual's abilities and interests. Individuals with preexisting pathologies may need a referral to a physical therapist or occupational therapist to help them with specific activities or in energy conservation. In addition to nutrition, hydration, and appropriate rest, the following interventions may be beneficial.

1. Attentional deficit fatigue is identified as a source of major distress for people with cancer. It rarely appears alone but is associated with other general characteristics of the fatigue symptom complex. Research is demonstrating that distraction may be a helpful source of relief.[45,46] Gardening, quietly listening to soft music, watching beautiful scenery, and taking quiet walks all may help attentional deficit fatigue. It is important to note that such interventions are effective only if the individual enjoys them. Often people with cancer can identify those things that are beneficial to them and take charge of managing their own symptoms.

2. Fatigue from uncertainty and anxiety is related to coping. Education may also be of some benefit.[49] It stands to reason that understanding what is happening or is going to happen may help an individual adjust and minimize losses in "adaptation energy." People with cancer are highly variable and set their own cues. Some want to know all the details. Others don't want to know

anything. Let them be the teachers and let them set the pace.

3. Exercise may be one of the most potent interventions, but it also carries risks. Several clinical trials have investigated the benefits of individualized exercise programs on functioning, energy, symptom management (including fatigue), and mood.[50] One author showed how to develop a walking program for people with cancer.[51]

Not all exercise is created equal. We would never tell a person with diabetes to "take some insulin," but we often tell people with cancer to "get some rest" or "get some exercise." To be effective and safe, exercise should be prescribed. Exercise prescriptions include five basic criteria:

1. Status of the individual: the exercise should be adapted to the age, gender, condition, risk factors, disease, and treatment of the individual.

2. Type of exercise: rhythmic, repetitive movement of large muscle groups, as in walking, swimming, or cycling.

3. Intensity of exercise: exercise should never be so hard that the person is out of breath.

4. Frequency of exercise: for a walking program or some other moderate activity such as gardening, several days a week (up to six) is sufficient.

5. Duration of exercise: start with what the person can do comfortably and work up *very* gradually from there. If a 10-minute walk is exhausting, the person should walk 7 minutes and slow down. And last, if the exercise is appropriate, the person should never be stiff, sore, or fatigued as a result.

Contraindications to low-intensity exercise include cardiac irregularities, recurring and unexplained pain in any part of the body, onset of nausea with exercise, confusion, cyanosis, febrile illness, and sudden onset of muscular weakness or unusual fatigability. Specific guidelines and precautions regarding exercise have been published elsewhere.[51,52]

Recently, a number of nursing studies have focused on "self-paced" exercise programs. Although such programs may have recreational value, it is difficult to predict any kind of outcome when the process is nonspecific. Enough work relating to cancer and exercise has been done to demonstrate that some cancer populations can benefit from appropriate exercise in terms of physiologic status as well as in broad dimensions of quality of well-being, QOL, and general psychosocial status. Exercise has been demonstrated to be a powerful intervention; hence, it may be harmful if not done correctly. Too little may not benefit; too much may exhaust. Exercise protocols that are not quantified are of limited value in developing repeatable and reimbursable rehabilitation and intervention programs.

Nurses who are interested in learning more about exercise for cancer patients can contact the American College of Sports Medicine (ACSM) in Indianapolis, Indiana. The ACSM is the international organization that is most influential in developing interdisciplinary guidelines for exercise programs and practice. This organization sponsors excellent workshops and certification programs for both healthy and chronic-illness populations.

Although there are few studies evaluating additional symptom-management techniques for fatigue in cancer, individuals often report other things that help them. Common interventions include guided imagery; laughter; work redistribution; environmental changes; limiting social obligations; establishing priorities; keeping a journal; working on art, poetry, and music; scheduling of activity and rest; getting help for housework; or using prescribed medication (such as for depression).[3,53] A small notebook with the following information can help individuals record their fatigue on a periodic basis and evaluate their own progress (use a different set of descriptors for each symptom):

Date: _____ Time: _____

Symptom: _____

Scale (0–10): _____

Feels like: _____

It affected me: _____

What I did: _____

Result (0–10): _____

Helping people with cancer understand their symptoms, particularly one as mysterious and paradoxical as fatigue, can help them develop ways to live according to their choices rather than as victims.

Resources

Because the study of fatigue is still relatively basic, nurses can supplement their cancer-specific knowledge by applying information from other disciplines. The following are excellent references representing both nursing and interdisciplinary works of importance to fatigue-related clinical issues.

Review References on Fatigue

- Irvine DM, Vincent L, Bubela N, et al: A critical appraisal of the research literature investigating fatigue in the individual with cancer. *Cancer Nurs* 14:188–199, 1991

- Piper BF: Fatigue, in Carrieri-Kohlman V, Lindsey AM, West CM (eds): *Pathophysiological Phenomena in Nursing: Human Responses to Illness* (ed 2). Philadelphia: Saunders, 1993, pp. 279–302

- Smets EMA, Garssen B, Schuster-Uitterhoeve ALJ, de Haes JCJM: Fatigue in cancer patients. *Br J Cancer* 68:220–224, 1993

- Winningham ML, Nail LM, Barton Burke M, et al: Fatigue and the cancer experience: The state of the knowledge. *Oncol Nurs Forum* 21:23–36, 1994

Review References on Bed Rest

- Corcoran PJ: Disability consequences of bed rest, in Stolov WC, Clowers MR (eds): *Handbook of Severe Disability*. Washington, DC: US Department of Education Rehabilitation Services Administration, 1981, pp. 55–63

Review References on Exercise in Cancer

- Winningham ML: A walking program for people with cancer: Getting started. *Cancer Nurs* 14:270–276, 1991

- Winningham ML: Exercise and cancer, in Goldberg L, Elliot DL (eds): *Exercise for Prevention and Treatment of Illness*. Philadelphia: FA Davis, 1994, pp. 301–315

Review Reference on Fatigue Relief in Cancer

- Piper BF: Alteration in comfort: Fatigue, in McNally JC, Somerville ET, Miaskowski C, Rostad M (eds): *Guidelines for Oncology Nursing Practice* (ed 2). Philadelphia: Saunders, 1991, pp. 155–162

Conclusion

Florence Nightingale emphasized the need to create an environment in which self-healing could occur. An important challenge to researchers as well as clinicians in oncology nursing is to create a "therapeutic milieu" in the clinical setting in which individuals can focus their energies on effective coping and healing. The current milieu in cancer treatment is loaded with threats, stressors, and risks. Economic changes in the healthcare environment are making this worse, not better. Because there are so few medical and "high-tech" solutions, fatigue presents a special challenge to nurse clinicians. The effective management of fatigue can help individuals focus their energies on physiologic and psychological healing. By providing respite for the mind, information to lessen the threat of the unknown, and effective symptom management, by minimizing fatigue, and by promoting functional status, we too can help people to heal themselves.

References

1. Meyerowitz BE, Watkins IK, Sparks FC: Quality of life for breast cancer patients receiving adjuvant chemotherapy. *Am J Nurs* 83:232–235, 1983
2. Smets EMA, Garssen B, Schuster-Uitterhoeve ALJ, deHaes JCJM: Fatigue in cancer patients. *Br J Cancer* 68:220–224, 1993
3. Winningham ML, Nail LM, Barton Burke M, et al: Fatigue and the cancer experience: The state of the knowledge. *Oncol Nurs Forum* 21:23–36, 1994
4. Vogelzang NJ, Breitbart W, Cella D, et al: Patient, caregiver, and oncologist perceptions of cancer-related fatigue: Results of a tripart assessment survey. *Semin Hematol* 34(suppl 2): 4–12, 1997
5. Karnofsky DA, Burchenal JH. The clinical evaluation of chemotherapeutic agents in cancer, in McCleod CM (ed): *The Clinical Evaluation of Chemotherapeutic Agents*. New York: Columbia University Press, 1949, pp. 191–205
6. Greenleaf JE, Kozlowski S: Physiological consequences of reduced physical activity during bed rest, in Terjung R (ed): *Exercise and Sports Science Review*. Philadelphia: Franklin Institute Press, 1982, pp. 84–119
7. Taber's *Cyclopedic Medical Dictionary* (ed 17). Philadelphia: FA Davis, 1993, pp. 713–714
8. Piper BF: Fatigue, in Carrieri-Kohlman V, Lindsey AM, West CM (eds): *Pathophysiological Phenomena in Nursing: Human Responses to Illness* (ed 2). Philadelphia: Saunders, 1993, pp. 279–302
9. Aistars J. Fatigue in the cancer patient: A conceptual approach to a clinical problem. *Oncol Nurs Forum* 14:25–30, 1987
10. Bartley SH, Chute E: *Fatigue and Impairment in Man*. New York: McGraw-Hill, 1947
11. Winningham ML: Effects of a bicycle ergometry program on functional capacity and feelings of control in women with breast cancer. Unpublished doctoral dissertation, The Ohio State University, 1983
12. MacVicar MG, Winningham ML, Nickel JL: Effects of aerobic interval training on cancer patients' functional capacity. *Nurs Res* 38:348–351, 1989
13. Winningham ML: Defining functional capacity through three-dimensional triangulation: A cancer model. Unpublished master's thesis, The Ohio State University, 1991
14. Holding DH: Fatigue, in Hockey GRJ (ed): *Stress and Fatigue in Human Performance*. New York: Wiley, 1983, pp. 145–167
15. Moscio B: Is a fatigue test possible? *Br J Physiol* 12:31–46, 1921
16. Dixon JK, Dixon JP, Hickey M: Energy as a central factor in the self-assessment of health. *Adv Nurs Sci* 15:1–12, 1993
17. Orem DE: *Concepts of Practice* (ed 2). New York: McGraw-Hill, 1980
18. Bloom JR, Hoppe RT, Fobair P, et al: Effect of treatment on the work experiences of long-term survivors of Hodgkin's disease. *J Psychosoc Oncol* 6:65–80, 1988

19. Winningham ML: Fatigue: The missing link to quality of life. *Quality of Life: A Nursing Challenge* 4:2–7, 1995

20. Ferrell BR: Overview of psychological well-being and quality of life. *Quality of Life: A Nursing Challenge—Psychological Well-Being* 1(2):1–3, 1991

21. Harpham WS: *After Cancer: A Guide to Your New Life.* New York: Norton, 1994

22. Selye H: *The Stress of Life* (ed 2). New York: McGraw-Hill, 1978, p. 370

23. Nightingale F: *Notes on Nursing.* London: Harrison and Sons, 1859. Reprinted in 1946 by Edward Stern & Co., Inc., Philadelphia PA

24. Lazarus RS: From psychological stress to the emotions: A history of changing outlooks. *Annu Rev Psychol* 44:1–21, 1993

25. Chrousos GP, Gold PW: The concept of stress and stress-system disorders. *JAMA* 267:1224–1252, 1992

26. Valbonna C: Bodily responses to immobilization, in Kottke FJ, Stillwell GK, Lahman JF (eds): *Krusen's Handbook of Physical Medicine and Rehabilitation* (ed 3). Philadelphia: Saunders, 1982, pp. 963–976

27. MacVicar MG, Winningham ML, Nickel JL: Effects of aerobic interval training on cancer patients' functional capacity. *Nurs Res* 38:348–351, 1989

28. Sahlin K: Metabolic factors in fatigue. *Sports Med* 13:99–107, 1992

29. Nail LM, Winningham ML: Fatigue, in Groenwald SL, Frogge MH, Goodman M, Yarbro CH (eds): *Cancer Nursing: Principles and Practice* (ed 4). Sudbury: Jones and Bartlett, 1997, pp. 640–654

30. St Pierre B, Kasper C, Lindsey A: Fatigue mechanisms in patients with cancer: Effects of tumor necrosis factor and exercise on skeletal muscle. *Oncol Nurs Forum* 19:421–425, 1992

31. Dietz KA, Flaherty AM: Oncologic emergencies, in Groenwald SL, Frogge MH, Goodman M, Yarbro CH (eds): *Cancer Nursing: Principles and Practice* (ed 3). Sudbury: Jones and Bartlett, 1993, pp. 801–839

32. Oberle K, Allen M, Lynkowski P: Follow-up of same day surgery patients. *AORN J* 59:1016–1025, 1994

33. Rhoton D: Fatigue and the postsurgical patient, in Norris CM (ed): *Concept Clarification in Nursing.* Rockville, MD: Aspen Publications, 1982, pp. 277–300

34. Richardson A, Ream EK: The experience of fatigue and other symptoms in patients receiving chemotherapy. *Eur J Cancer Care* 5(suppl 2):24–30, 1996

35. Green D, Nail LM, Fieler VK, et al: A comparison of patient-reported side-effects among three chemotherapy regimens for breast cancer. *Cancer Pract* 2:57–62, 1994

36. Irvine DM, Vincent L, Bubela N, et al: A critical appraisal of the research literature investigating fatigue in the individual with cancer. *Cancer Nurs* 14:188–199, 1991

37. Irvine D, Vincent L, Graydon JE, et al: The prevalence and correlates of fatigue in patients receiving treatment with chemotherapy and radiotherapy. *Cancer Nurs* 17:367–378, 1994

38. Haylock P, Hart L: Fatigue in patients receiving localized radiation. *Cancer Nurs* 2:461–467, 1979

39. Nail LM: Coping with intracavitary radiation treatment for gynecologic cancer. *Cancer Pract* 1:218–224, 1993

40. Faithful S: Patients' experiences following cranial radiotherapy: A study of the somnolence syndrome. *J Adv Nursing* 16:939–946, 1991

41. Skalla KA, Rieger PT: Fatigue, in Rieger PT (ed): *Biotherapy: A Comprehensive Review.* Sudbury: Jones and Bartlett, 1995, pp. 221–242

42. Cimprich B: Attentional fatigue following breast cancer surgery. *Res Nurs Health* 15:199–207, 1992

43. Cimprich B: Developing an intervention to restore attention in cancer patients. *Cancer Nurs* 16:83–92, 1993

44. Lee KA, Lentz MJ, Taylor DL, et al: Fatigue as a response to environmental demands in women's lives. *Image* 26:149–154, 1994

45. Varricchio CG: Selecting a tool for measuring fatigue. *Oncol Nurs Forum* 12:122–127, 1985

46. Smets EM, Garssen B, Bonke B, deHaes JC: The Multidimensional Fatigue Inventory (MFI): Psychometric qualities of an instrument to assess fatigue. *J Psychosom Res* 39:315–325, 1995

47. Piper BF, Dibble SL, Dodd MJ, et al: The Revised Piper Fatigue Scale: Psychometric evaluation in women with breast cancer. *Oncol Nurs Forum* 25:677–684, 1998

48. Stein PM, Martin SC, Hann DM, et al: A multidimensional measure of fatigue for use with cancer patients. *Cancer Pract* 6:143–152, 1998

49. Johnson JE, Nail LM, Lauver D, et al: Reducing the negative impact of radiation therapy on functional status. *Cancer* 61:46–51, 1988

50. Mock V, Barton Burke M, Sheehan P, et al: A nursing rehabilitation program for women with breast cancer receiving adjuvant chemotherapy. *Oncol Nurs Forum* 21:899–907, 1994

51. Winningham ML: Walking program for people with cancer: Getting started. *Cancer Nurs* 14:270–276, 1991

52. Winningham ML: Exercise and cancer, in Goldberg L, Elliot DL (eds): *Exercise for Prevention and Treatment of Illness.* Philadelphia: FA Davis, 1994, pp. 301–315

53. Nail LM, Jones LS, Greene D, et al: Use and perceived efficacy of self-care activities in patients receiving chemotherapy. *Oncol Nurs Forum* 18:883–887, 1991

Talking about Fatigue

Patient Name: _____

Symptom and Description   Fatigue is a difficult side effect of cancer and cancer treatment. Fatigue may be difficult to talk about. Weakness, dizziness, difficulty thinking, and tiredness may be part of the feeling. People sometimes think they are just being lazy or depressed. They may tell themselves, "I can snap out of this if I really try." There are no medical tests to measure fatigue. Sudden changes in feelings of fatigue may mean there is a serious problem. Slow development of fatigue may not allow you to do everyday activities. You need to report your feelings to the nurse or physician. Here are some suggestions to help you talk about your feelings of fatigue:

1. How do you *feel*? Describe the *kind* of fatigue feelings. *When* do you feel better or worse? *What* makes you feel better or worse? People often use words such as no energy, weak, confused, trouble thinking, shaky, always tired, dragged out, and no motivation.

2. How does fatigue *affect your life*? Compare what you can do now with what you did before your cancer. What activities in your life have changed? For example, can you still work like you used to? Are you able to spend time with people as before? Do you have trouble thinking clearly? Does your fatigue make you anxious with people around you?

3. What does fatigue mean to you? If there have been changes in your lifestyle, how important are those changes to you? How satisfied are you with what you are able to do? Are there things you want to do but can't? Do you feel guilty that you should be doing more?

Talk with your nurse or physician about your fatigue. Ask whether there are things you can do to help you feel better. Your fatigue is often related to your treatment. Understanding more about your fatigue can help your better plan your activity and rest periods. This can help you feel more in control of your life.

Learning Needs   You and your family need to understand that fatigue is a real problem. It is *not* the same as being lazy or depressed. Keep a record or diary of your fatigue patterns. Day of the week, treatment cycles, activities, and time of day all may be important. Draw a straight line in your diary. On the left end, write "No fatigue at all (0)." On the right, write "Worst fatigue I can imagine (10)." This is your fatigue scale. Place an X on that line to describe how bad your fatigue is now. If you want to, use a number between 0 and 10 to tell how bad your fatigue is. If you rate your fatigue on a line like this, it will help you learn how to plan your activity and rest.

```
        0 ———————X——————— 10
     No fatigue        Worst fatigue
       at all          I can imagine
```

Try to rest when you feel the worst. Use better times to stay as active as possible. Try writing down what kinds of things make you feel more or less fatigued, how often you feel fatigue, how bad your fatigue is, and how long the fatigue feelings last. What helps you feel better or worse? If you have difficulties managing your fatigue, ask your nurse to explain to your family members how they can help.

Prevention and Management   Keep a diary of your fatigue. Know when your fatigue probably will be better or worse. Write down words that describe what kind of fatigue you are feeling (such as fatigue—tired, fatigue—dragged out, etc.). Talk with others about your fatigue. It helps to know you are not alone.

Follow-up   Bring your fatigue record to the clinic to show your nurse or physician. Tell your nurse or physician how fatigue is affecting your life. Ask them to help you develop a special care plan if your fatigue becomes overwhelming.

Phone Numbers

Nurse: _____ Phone: _____

Doctor: _____ Phone: _____

Other: _____ Phone: _____

Comments

Patient's Signature: _____ Date: _____

Nurse's Signature: _____ Date: _____

Source: Winningham ML: Fatigue, in Yarbro CH, Frogge MH, Goodman M (eds): *Cancer Symptom Management* (ed 2). Sudbury: Jones and Bartlett, 1999. © Jones and Bartlett Publishers.

The Dangers of Bed Rest

Patient Name: _____

Symptom and Description   Cancer often forces you to get more rest. Many people think resting in bed or lying on the sofa will help them feel better. This leads to a problem: The more bed rest they get, the worse they feel. Too much bed rest can be dangerous. To feel and do your best, your body needs to be in the upright position and moving around at least several hours each day. Some of the problems that can result from bed rest include the following:

- Too little fluid or water in your body
- Changes in hearing and eyesight (eyeglass prescription may change)
- Muscle weakness
- Blood clots
- Dizziness, especially with movement
- Poor balance
- Blood sugar changes
- Feelings of nausea
- Depression
- Feelings of helplessness and hopelessness
- Irritability

Rest is important. But too much rest, as well as too little rest, can make you feel more tired. Activity also is important. But too much activity, for too long, may lead to exhaustion. A balance between activity and rest can keep you from feeling worse. Another benefit of trying to balance rest with activity during the day is that you may sleep better at night. When people with cancer are in a hospital, they usually spend more time in bed. Every day you are in bed, more of your strength and energy are being lost. And every day in bed will make it harder for you to get up and move the next day. Your nurse will encourage you to do as much as possible for yourself. There is no medicine that can help you regain what you lose through inactivity. Your family and friends may help you get up and walk around. This is an important way they can show their concern for you.

Learning Needs   You and those close to you should know that bed rest can be harmful as well as helpful. Lack of activity and bed rest can make your recovery longer. Medical tests and treatments can be very tiring. Fatigue often is made worse by too much bed rest. When you sleep more during the day, you will have a difficult time sleeping at night. Even walking around your room is better than lying in bed or sitting in a chair. Activity or exercise that leads to exhaustion is also bad for you. Family and friends should know that you may not be able to do your usual activities and need more rest. They should help protect your rest and recovery periods or "power naps" from interruption. A balance between rest and activity is necessary to keep you feeling as well as possible.

Prevention and Management

- Don't lie in bed or sit in a chair more than you must. Try to increase your activity by little amounts every day. If you can walk for 5 minutes today, try walking for 6 minutes tomorrow.
- Balance activity with rest. Alternate activities (including diagnostic tests, eating, and going to the clinic) with rest periods.
- Keep a regular sleep schedule. Go to bed the same time each night even if you don't feel sleepy. If you never watched late-night TV before, don't start now. Don't sleep or nap after supper. Don't "sleep in" more or longer than you used to.
- Keep a regular schedule. If you are easily fatigued, try to rest for 10 to 15 minutes before and after meals.
- "Power naps" can be good if they are brief (not longer than 30 to 40 minutes at a time) and if you get up and move around between them.
- If you are so ill that you can't get out of bed for very long, a family member can help you with bed exercises. This can help you keep some of your muscle strength. Ask your doctor whether a physical therapist can work with you. This requires a special order but is an important part of your treatment plan.
- Drink plenty of fluids. This will help your balance when you get up. It also will help your muscles feel stronger.

Follow-up

- Keep a regular schedule.
- Tell your nurse or physician if you need more rest than usual during the daytime.
- Ask your nurse or physician to explain to your family if they do not seem to understand your need for both rest and activity.

Phone Numbers

Nurse: _____ Phone: _____

Doctor: _____ Phone: _____

Other: _____ Phone: _____

Comments

Patient's Signature: _____ Date: _____

Nurse's Signature: _____ Date: _____

Source: Winningham ML: Fatigue, in Yarbro CH, Frogge MH, Goodman M (eds): *Cancer Symptom Management* (ed 2). Sudbury: Jones and Bartlett, 1999. © Jones and Bartlett Publishers.

CHAPTER 7

Flulike Syndrome

Brenda K. Shelton, RN, MS, CCRN, AOCN
Lisa Turnbough, RN, AA

The Problem of Flulike Syndrome (FLS) in Cancer

In cancer care, there are many disease states and therapies that produce a group of symptoms described as "constitutional" symptoms. *Constitutional symptoms* are those comprising "the physical make-up of the body, including the mode of performance of its functions, the activity of its metabolic processes, the manner and degree of its reactions to stimuli, and its power of resistance to the attack of pathogenic organisms."[1p.462] Constitutional symptoms are related to the physiologic effects resulting from a nonspecific immunologic response and tend to involve lymph nodes, the skin, and the musculoskeletal system. The literature reports interchangeable definitions for constitutional symptoms and flulike syndrome (FLS),[2,3] but no specific definition of FLS. These definitions probably evolved from the descriptions of influenza epidemics in the early 1900s.[4] Descriptions of FLS have also been associated with chronic postviral fatigue syndrome[5] and acute HIV infection (asymptomatic AIDS),[6] and are cited as a consequence of cancer therapies such as radiation therapy, antineoplastic chemotherapy, and biotherapy.[7,8] There is wide disparity of opinion regarding the components of this syndrome, with the broadest definitions including fever, chills/rigors, headache, myalgias, arthralgias, fatigue, malaise, anorexia, nausea, vomiting, diarrhea, nasal stuffiness, cough, and bone pain. See Table 7-1 for more details regarding different authors' interpretations of the inclusive symptoms of FLS.[1–3,9–19]

The lack of agreement regarding a definition of the symptom grouping stems in part from the lack of research on this clinical topic. For the purposes of this chapter, we have defined the constellation of symptoms in FLS as fever, chills/rigors, headache, myalgias, arthralgias, malaise, and nasal stuffiness. Although the symptoms are often found in tandem with one another, there are some circumstances in which some symptoms may be absent. Because fatigue is a common symptom independent of other associated findings, it is discussed separately (see Chap. 6). Gastrointestinal symptoms such as anorexia, nausea, vomiting, and diarrhea are also common symptoms that occur in isolation and are addressed separately in other chapters (see Chaps. 12, 14, and 28, respectively).

Incidence in Cancer

FLS occurs with varying frequency, severity, and duration depending on dosage, route of administration, and treatment schedule. FLS associated with biological therapy and fluorouracil is dose dependent and reversible with discontinuation of the agent. It has also been shown that tachyphylaxis occurs with the prolonged use of interferon alfa.[7,20,21] Different methods of delivery (subcutaneous versus intramuscular) and timing of administration (morning versus evening) have been investigated in an effort to demonstrate strategies to reduce the adverse effects of FLS[22] but have been inconclusive thus far.

TABLE 7-1 Components of FLS

Author	Chills	Fever	Arthralgia	Myalgia	Headache	Bone Pain	Nasal Stuffiness	Fatigue	Malaise	Cough	Anorexia	Nausea	Vomiting	Diarrhea
Brophy L, Reiger PT[9]	X	X	X	X	X									
Haeuber D[2]	X	X	X	X	X		X		X	X	X	X	X	
Shelton BK[10]	X	X	X	X	X		X		X	X	X		X	X
Hood LE, Abernathy E[11]	X	X		X					X					
Berkow R[4]	X	X			X		X			X				
Reiger PT[12]	X	X	X	X	X			X						
Rumsey K, Reiger PT[13]	X	X	X	X	X	X		X						
Roche Laboratories[14]		X	X	X	X			X						
Schering Corporation[15]	X	X		X	X									
Sergi JS[16]	X	X	X	X	X		X		X	X	X	X	X	
Shelton BK, Belcher AE[17]	X	X	X	X	X			X			X	X	X	X
Hensyl WR[1]	X	X		X	X					X				
Strauman JJ[18]	X	X		X		X		X						
White CL[19]	X	X							X					

78

Although the physical manifestations of FLS stem from a central organic etiology, each of the constellation symptoms is often assessed and managed separately. An overview of the identifying characteristics of each of these symptoms is included in Table 7-2. It is acceptable to report the presence of FLS even if only some symptoms are noted. When reporting FLS as a toxicity, it may be more accurate to describe each symptom individually.

Impact on Quality of Life

By definition, FLS implies that the symptoms are subtle and not life-threatening. Symptom distress is defined as the physiologic symptom patterns that "hamper self-care and threaten independence."[23 p.242] There are many subjective variables that influence perception of symptom distress, and the degree to which FLS is the cause or exacerbates perceptions of distress is unclear. Patients have reported that FLS is distressing because symptoms interfere with activities of daily living.[19,24] FLS has also has been

identified as one of the most common dose-limiting toxicities of biological therapy.[18,25–27] Clinical research studies are needed to address the impact of FLS on quality of life.[28]

Etiology

FLS in the cancer patient may occur as the result of localized or metastatic disease, cancer chemotherapy, biotherapy, other medications, or concomitant problems such as sepsis.[10,27–31] Many physical disorders have accompanying symptoms that resemble FLS. For this reason, only FLS that is cancer treatment–induced is addressed in this text. Even among pharmacologic references, there is considerable variability in whether FLS or its component symptoms are identified as adverse effects. Compiled with Micromedex, a pharmacologic search system,[32] Table 7-3 lists the biotherapeutic agents, chemotherapeutic agents, and other medications that are associated with FLS or at least three of its component symptoms.[2,3,7,8,10,12–16,29–46] The severity of FLS with each agent is ill-defined, but some newer agents have FLS listed in the manufacturer's package insert as a potential toxicity.[14,15,46] It is also clear that certain agents are more frequently linked with this side effect than others. Studies report more than 90% occurrence of FLS with some biotherapy regimens,[20] particularly in combination therapies (e.g., interferon and interleukin-2).[25] It also seems that biotherapy combined with chemotherapy agents known to produce FLS (e.g., 5-fluorouracil) may enhance this adverse effect.[8]

Pathophysiology

The precise physiologic mechanism of FLS is unknown, but due to its immunostimulant features, it is postulated that the release of immune mediator substances (or exogenous administration of immune mediators, as in biotherapy) triggers normal inflammatory mechanisms.[2,45,46] The variations in FLS associated with the use of different agents are a reflection of the different mechanisms triggering the symptoms or of the levels and locations of mediator substances.[2,16] Cytokine biotherapy agents (e.g., interferons, interleukins) and multilineage growth factors are most likely to trigger the inflammatory mediators that cause FLS.[10]

The pathophysiologic mechanism of FLS is closely associated with fever pathology, a model that will be used to describe FLS. A configuration of this process is summarized in Figure 7-1.[2,10,16,49–51] Pyrogens are fever-producing substances that have the capacity to affect the temperature regulation center in the preoptic anterior hypothalamus. Pyrogens may be *exogenous*—produced outside the body—and include bacterial endotoxins, other microbes,

TABLE 7-2 Identifying Characteristics of FLS

Symptom	Identifying Characteristics
Headache	Usually upper frontal or retrobulbar Often accompanied by photosensitivity May include visual disturbances
Fever	May be greater than 39°C, but subsides with continued exposure to some biologic response modifiers (BRMs) Sudden onset, often temporally related to therapy-causing syndrome Accompanied by chills
Chills/rigors	Often precede fever and coincide with headache Have a crescendo pattern until fever occurs Involves upper body first
Arthralgias	Pervasive, aching pain poorly localized in a joint area May have throbbing quality May be accompanied by joint swelling Discomfort may be exacerbated by weight bearing
Myalgias	Large muscle groups involved (e.g., thighs, pectorals) Nonlocalized discomfort May or may not be relieved by rest Accompanied by sensation of weakness
Malaise	Fatigue, weariness Accompanied by sense of apathy Lack of energy or motivation
Cough	Dry, hacking, and persistent Rarely productive
Nasal congestion	Stuffiness of the nose Rhinitis—usually clear, watery, persistent Difficulty breathing

TABLE 7-3 Etiologies of FLS (medications commonly used in cancer patients and included in Micromedex system[32])

Medication*	Dose Related: Y/N	Headache	Fever	Chills	Arthralgias	Myalgias	Malaise	Nasal Stuffiness
Biotherapy								
Antithymocyte globulin (ATG)	N	+	+	+	+	+	+	+
Cytomegalovirus (CMV)–IgG	N	+	+ Rate-related	+ Rate-related	+	+ Rate-related	+	+
Erythropoeitin	N	+	+	NR	+	UK	NR	NR
Granulocyte colony-stimulating factor (G-CSF)	N	+	+ Mild	+	+	+	+	NR
Granulocyte-macrophage colony-stimulating factor (GM-CSF)	N	++ Mild	++ Mod-Sev	++	++	++ Mod-Sev	++	+
Immune globulin (IgG)	N	+	+	+	+	+	+	NR
Interferon	Y	+++ Vary	+++ Severe	+++	++	+++ Severe	+++ Severe	+
Interleukin-2	Y	++	+++	+++	++	++	+++	+
Interleukin-3 (IL-3)	UK	+++ Mild	+++ Mild	+++	UK	+	UK	UK
Levamisole	N	+	++	+	+	+	++	NR
All-trans-retinoic acid (tRA)	Y	+++	+	+	+++	+	NR	UK
Monoclonal antibodies (in general)	N	+	++	+	++	+	NR	NR
Plasma proteins: plasma protein fraction, albumin, plasmanate	N	+	+	+	+	+	+	+
Rituximab	N	++	+++	+++	NR	+	NR	+
Tumor necrosis factor (TNF)	Y	+++	+++	+++	+	+++	+++	UK
Vaccines: influenza, pneumococcal, measles	N	+	+	+	+	+	+	UK
Chemotherapy								
Bleomycin	N	NR	+++	+++	NR	NR	+	NR
Cladribine	UK	UK	+	+	UK	UK	+	NR
Cytarabine/cytosine arabinoside	N	NR	++	NR	+	+	+	NR
Dacarbazine (may occur up to 7 days after first dose, last 7–21 days, and recur with subsequent doses)	N	++	++	++	NR	++	++	NR
5-Fluorouracil	Y	NR	+	+	++	++	++	NR
L-asparaginase (less often with IM route)	N	NR	++	++	NR	NR	+	NR
Procarbazine	N	NR	+	+	NR	++	++	NR
Trimetrexate	UK	NR	+	+	NR	NR	+	NR
Others								
Amphotericin B	N	+++	+++	+++	++	++	++	UK
Azathioprine	N	+	++	+	+	++	UK	UK
Aztreonam	N	+	+	+	NR	+	+	+ (with sneezes)
Cyclosporine	N	+	+	+	+	NR	+	NR
Foscarnet	N	++	+++	+	NR	+	+	NR
Ganciclovir	N	+	+	+	NR	+	+	NR
Paclitaxel	N	NR	+	+	+	+	+	NR
Pentoxifylline	UK	NR	+	+	NR	+	UK	NR
Procainamide hydrochloride	UK	NR	+	+	+	+	+	NR
Fluoxetine	NR	UK	+	+	NR	NR	+	NR
Rifampicin	NR	+	+	+	UK	UK	+	NR

+++ = Frequent; ++ = Occasional; + = Rare; UK = Unknown; NR = Not reported as an adverse effect in product information; Mild = Mild; Mod = Moderate; Sev = Severe; Vary = Variable severity.
*Criteria for inclusion were medications that listed FLS or ≥ 3 symptoms.

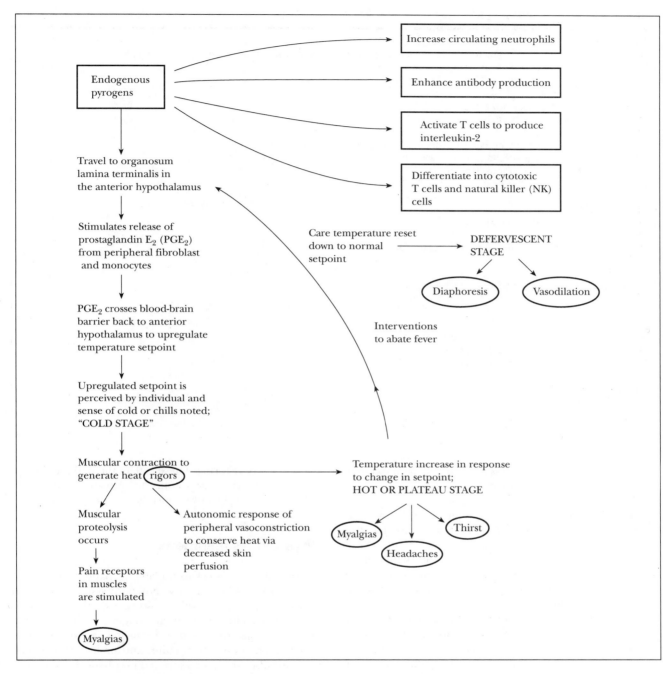

FIGURE 7-1   The pathophysiologic mechanism of FLS.

and certain drugs. Endogenous pyrogens are substances produced by the body and are also known as cytokines. Cytokines may be triggered by natural immunologic responses or administered as an antitumor agent. Well-known cytokines that act as endogenous pyrogens include interferon-alfa, interferon-beta, interleukin-1 (IL-1), interleukin-2 (IL-2), interleukin-6 (IL-6), and tumor necrosis factor-alfa (TNF-α).[2,10] In addition to their effects on the temperature regulation center, they have significant vascular effects, causing profound vasodilation such as

that seen with sepsis and as manifested in headaches, hypotension, and rhinitis.[2,10,18] Pyrogens act further to increase the circulating pool of neutrophils, enhance antibody production, and activate T cells to produce IL-2 and to differentiate into cytotoxic T cells and natural killer (NK) cells.[10] Neutrophil activation may contribute to bone pain in individuals undergoing therapy. Introduction of the pyrogen and its subsequent triggering of white blood cell responses causes the release, from fibroblasts and monocytes, of prostaglandin E (PGE), which crosses

TABLE 7-4 Assessment of FLS

Neurosensory

Headache pain—intensity or character (throbbing or dull ache), timing (continual or exacerbated with exertion), location (usually frontal)
Visual disturbances—blurred vision, diplopia, photophobia
Dizziness/vertigo—position when it occurs, other associated symptoms
Mental status changes
Emotional lability—dysphoria, euphoria

Musculoskeletal

Joint discomfort—at rest or with weight bearing, accompanying swelling, crepitus
Muscle aches—cramping, spasmotic or dull, location, exacerbating factors, alleviating factors
Inability to stand without lower back or leg pain
Degree of shivering

Dermatologic

Increased skin temperature, erythema
Skin dry or moist
Rash characteristics—color, raised or flat, pruritus, distribution

General

Body temperature—fever or subnormal temperature
Sensation of cold—chills, rigors

Laboratory Findings

Increased lactate dehydrogenase (LDH) with rigors
Increased creatine kinase (CPK) with rigors
Elevated erythrocyte sedimentation rate (ESR)
Hyperglycemia
Increased blood urea nitrogen (BUN)
Increased creatinine
Leukocytosis

the blood-brain barrier to the thermoregulatory center and "resets" the base temperature.

The body responds to the reset base temperature by trying to generate heat. When the thermoregulatory center demands heat production, the body generates it in the most rapid way possible—muscular contraction. These contractions are seen as the chills and rigors that often precede the rise in temperature.[10,47–51] This is accompanied by vasoconstriction to prevent heat loss; however, predominant features of warmth and vasodilation may be present due to circulating mediator substances. Runaway mediator substances in this syndrome also produce generalized symptoms of fatigue and malaise. Muscular contraction and PGE released into the muscles stimulate pain receptors, producing myalgias.[47] It is probable that arthralgias have a similar pathophysiologic etiology in this syndrome.

Assessment

Measurement Tools

There are no standardized tools to measure FLS. Most clinicians recommend general physical exam criteria or symptom report forms. These reflect the patient perception of the severity of symptoms, an appropriate approach to reporting a subjective constellation of symptoms.

Physical Assessment

Performing a physical exam on the patient at risk for FLS involves assessment of several body systems with both subjective and objective measures. Certain symptoms, such as headache, myalgias, arthralgias, and malaise, are primarily subjective in nature, requiring patient participation in evaluation. Fever, chills, and nasal stuffiness can be more objectively measured. The physical assessment for FLS includes evaluation of vital signs and laboratory findings, assessment of neurologic/cognitive/emotional parameters and the respiratory system, and a thorough skin/musculoskeletal exam. Parameters to be assessed are included in Table 7-4.

Diagnostic Evaluation

Confirmation of FLS is made by clinical suspicion in the face of known risk factors. There are no diagnostic studies specifically directed at detection of FLS. It is presumed that there should be elevated levels of inflammatory mediators, although the value in monitoring them has not been described. Other diagnostic tests, such as creatine phosphokinase (CPK) or lactate dehydrogenase (LDH) enzymes and potassium levels, reflect the severity of tissue or muscle damage.

Degrees of Toxicity

There is no consistent language describing FLS and levels of toxicity; however, the National Cancer Institute's (NCI) toxicity-grading criteria encompass most symptoms grouped in this constellation and have the advantage of rating severity. The NCI toxicity grading for fever, chills, headache, and myalgias/arthralgias are included in Table 7-5.[52]

Holtzclaw[53] has also developed a scale for chills/rigors that has been used for clinical research in this area; it also proves useful for determining a threshold for pharmacologic treatment of rigors.

Symptom Management

Prevention

It may be impossible to prevent FLS for individuals with cancer, as it is a side effect of many treatment modalities. However, there are management strategies that can decrease the severity of the symptoms, including prophylactic measures (see under Therapeutic Approaches).

With regimens that are highly associated with FLS, a cocktail of prophylactic medications before and several hours after therapy may prevent or lessen the incidence and severity of FLS. Common prophylactic medications include (1) acetaminophen, (2) nonsteroidal antiinflammatory drugs (NSAIDs), (3) diphenhydramine, and (4) diazepam, morphine, or meperidine.[3,11,12,17,18,36] The selection preventive medications depends on individual variables and the anticipated severity of FLS.

Education of the patient and significant others regarding the underlying causes of FLS helps to reduce fear and anxiety and allows the individual to plan daily activities so that there is minimal interference by symptoms experienced. Some patients alleviate FLS symptoms with pharmacologic preventive measures combined with activity restrictions.

Therapeutic Approaches

Management of FLS centers on comfort measures.[12] Understanding that FLS is an adverse effect of treatment with predictable patterns, rather than a sign of disease progression, is important information to impart because some individuals may have experienced similar symptoms with disease onset or recurrence. Their concerns may influence attitudes or compliance with therapy.[27,54] Those who are knowledgeable about their therapy feel more comfortable and confident of their ability to manage this syndrome.

Differences in definitions of quality of life and values need to be discussed before initiation of therapy to ensure maximal patient cooperation and satisfaction with symp-

---

TABLE 7-5 National Cancer Institute Common Toxicity-Grading Criteria for FLS

Toxicity	Grade				
	1	2	3	4	5
Headache	None	Mild	Moderate or severe but transient	Unrelenting and severe	—
Aching pain (muscle or bone)	None	Mild, transient; does not interfere with casual daily activity	Moderate; interferes with usual daily activity	Severe; interrupts usual daily activity	Intractable
Fever	None	>38.5°C	>39°C	>40°C	—
Chills	None	Mild, transient	Moderate	Severe	Intractable
Malaise	None	25% of time	50% of time	75% of time	100% of time
Fatigue/asthenia	None	25% of time	50% of time	75% of time	100% of time
Anorexia	None	Able to eat normal meals, loss of hunger	Able to eat 2 meals/day with loss of hunger	Able to eat 1 meal/day with loss of hunger	Unable to eat a meal, some nutritional fluids tolerated

Source: NCI Common Toxicity Criteria, in *Investigators Handbook*. National Institutes of Health—National Cancer Institute, October 1993, Appendix 12.[52]

tom control. An outcome acceptable to the nurse may not be tolerable to the person experiencing the adverse effect. For example, when narcotics are used to control chills/rigors, the fear and discomfort experienced with the rigor and subsequent fever must be weighed against the sedation and possible nausea caused by the narcotic. In addition, individuals and their care settings (e.g., inpatient vs. ambulatory care) are considered when choosing strategies for symptom control. With planning, education, and a mutual willingness to try and to modify various options, the negative effect of FLS on lifestyle can be minimized.

There is no perfect formula for management of FLS. Because FLS is an adverse effect of most biological response modifiers (BRMs) and specific chemotherapeutic agents, there are three general approaches to take: (1) Manipulate the treatment; (2) administer medications to prevent or treat the individual symptoms; and (3) provide education on expected side effects, causes, and self-care.[2,10]

A treatment protocol may dictate the dosages, timing, and route of administration of the therapy, limiting its manipulation. It is possible in some circumstances to reduce the symptoms of FLS by changing administration times or methods. For example, IL-2 administered in a 2-hour IV infusion produces less severe FLS than when given as a 24-hour infusion.[2] Likewise, subcutaneous injection sites of BRMs may absorb at different rates, and site rotation could alter symptoms experienced.[16] Chills, fever, headache, and myalgias are predictable in the first 2 to 4 hours after a BRM is given, lasting up to 24 hours.[2,10] If the dose is given in the evening, the patient may be able to sleep through some of the most uncomfortable symptoms.[15,18]

For ease of clinical application, it is important to realize that some interventions are designed to manage the entire syndrome, whereas others focus on relieving the discomfort of one or a few symptoms. There are a number of pharmacologic and nonpharmacologic interventions to consider, and these interventions tend to have overlapping therapeutic effects. For example, acetaminophen may control fever and relieve the discomfort of headaches and myalgias; heat packs help relieve muscle discomfort as well as warm the chilling patient. The following text discusses the management of each symptom individually.

Fever

The fevers associated with FLS usually peak at 39.0°C to 40.0°C and often spike after a rigor. This can mimic the clinical picture of sepsis, which necessitates evaluation for infection with each fever. Cultures of blood, urine, and any possible source of infection are obtained when new fevers are experienced. Chest x-ray films or CT scans are followed to rule out pulmonary infections. Individuals with neutropenia are at particular risk for infection; therefore, broad-spectrum antibiotics may be started before culture results are obtained.[11] Establishing an individualized fever curve after the administration of a BRM provides a comparison against a new fever spike or a fever unresponsive to antipyretics. Fever and chills may also be

symptoms of blood product reactions or administration of amphotericin B.

Antipyretics are the primary therapy for fevers, although some advocate not treating mild to moderate fevers because they may enhance immune responses.[10,50,51] Antipyretics act by lowering the hypothalamic setpoint, which then allows for heat loss. Acetaminophen is most commonly used and may need to be given around the clock to prevent an uncomfortable cycle of fever spikes with chills, followed by defervescence and sweating.[3,10] Aspirin and NSAIDs interfere with platelet aggregation and hence may be contraindicated for some patients. Corticosteroids are usually avoided with biotherapy, because they may block the effects of these drugs on the immune system.[3,11,18,32]

Severe or dangerous fevers exceeding 40°C that are unresponsive to antipyretics may be relieved with cooling measures such as tepid sponging, ice packs, or hypothermia (cooling) blankets.[3,12,51,55] Hypothermia blankets, however, may worsen the chills and rigors because shivering is the body's mechanism to generate warmth when the central thermoregulatory setpoint has been changed.[10,50,51,56] Thus, this treatment is reserved as a last resort to treat life-threatening fever. There is controversy regarding the effectiveness of these measures in fever, as they do not alter the hypothalamic setpoint.[56] Moreover, they may cool the patient rapidly, causing chills that result in an even higher temperature or tissue injury.[56] However, in the heat-dissipating stage of fever, these cooling measures do offer some comfort.

Attention needs to be given to the fluid and electrolyte status of a febrile patient. Significant losses of potassium, sodium, chloride, and magnesium can occur with perspiration, and fluid intake should be encouraged unless otherwise contraindicated. Water or other nonalcoholic beverages may be taken in liberal amounts (e.g., 3–4 liters/day).[18,36] Patients are cautioned against alcohol intake, as this increases dehydration. Serum electrolytes should be monitored and replenished as needed. In the hospital setting, intravenous fluids are provided, but outpatients can be encouraged to drink high-electrolyte solutions such as Pedialyte and Gatorade.

Chills

The body generates heat through the muscle activity of shivering, usually resulting in a temperature elevation. Chills associated with FLS are usually self-limiting but may range from feeling cold to teeth-chattering rigors. Pallor and difficult-to-palpate pulses often accompany rigors due to peripheral vasoconstriction. Rigors are frightening and uncomfortable and often leave a person feeling "washed out."[11] The muscle activity of rigors can exacerbate myalgias; increase creatine, creatinine kinase (CPK), phosphorus, and potassium liberation; and enhance red blood cell or platelet lysis.

Adequate clothing and a warm environment free of drafts are provided to prevent chills. As soon as the patient begins to feel cold, warm blankets should be added. Increased body temperature will occur from shivering, if not supported by nursing interventions to warm the patient. The initial provision of warmth does not decrease temperature elevation; it merely stops the shivering method of obtaining increased body temperature. An electric heating pad, hot water bottle, or chemical heat packs may be used. Caution should be used to avoid burns by never applying these sources directly to the skin, by checking to be sure that they are not too hot and that heat packs are free of leaks. Extremity wraps (three layers of terry cloth fashioned into mittens or boots) have been used with some success in decreasing rigors experienced with amphotericin B.[53] There may be some justification for their use in those experiencing chills with FLS.

Persistent rigors may require the use of narcotics or benzodiazepines to alleviate this symptom. The literature recommends meperidine most consistently, but the dosage ranges from 10–25 mg every 1 to 5 minutes up to 75–100 mg total dose.[2,3,7,9,11,16–18] The authors' experience has supported the use of meperidine 10 mg intravenously every 5 minutes up to 100 mg. It is unclear how meperidine relieves rigors, but it is usually quite effective. However, nausea and vomiting may occur with rapid intravenous push of meperidine, and sedation and hypotension are side-effects requiring frequent monitoring of vital signs and oxygen saturation. Premedicating with diazepam 10 mg orally has been reported to be effective in minimizing chills associated with interferon therapy, possibly through its muscle-relaxant properties.[2,18] There are also reports of using morphine[11] and hydromorphone[57] to treat chills. Oral meperidine may also be given to patients receiving BRMs to offset chills.[19]

Myalgias and arthralgias

Little has been written about the muscle and joint pain associated with FLS. It may be related to mediator release, and chills and rigors worsen this problem. Benzodiazepines or other muscle relaxants can be given to relax muscles[18] and analgesics may be necessary for pain relief. NSAIDs are effective for managing bone and joint pain but may not be allowed by certain protocols. The application of heat or cold may be soothing, and based on literature addressing arthritic discomfort, warmth would be recommended.[58,59] Rest, relaxation techniques, and diversional activities should also be explored.

Headaches

There is little research regarding headaches associated with FLS. Experience with headaches in general indicates that fever and muscle tension may cause or at least potentiate them. Onset of headaches is often noted within a few hours of initiating BRM therapy. The headaches associated with influenza are retrobulbar and associated with photosensitivity,[4] but it is unknown whether the same symptomatology occurs with therapies causing FLS. Because headaches are also a cardinal symptom of more serious complications such as intracranial bleeding or meningitis, other disorders may need to be ruled out when the etiology is unclear.

Analgesics are appropriate for relief of headache pain, which may be severe. The use of a pain rating scale of 0 to 10 (0 being pain-free and 10 being the worst pain imaginable) gives clearer feedback regarding the effectiveness of analgesics or other pain-relieving measures. A dark and quiet environment and cool cloths on the forehead are usually soothing to the headache sufferer. Frontal headaches may also be secondary to sinus congestion, for which warmth and steam are the best interventions to relieve discomfort.[58,59] Headaches originating at the back of the head or neck may be related to muscle tension, and heat application and massage may help.[60] Massage, acupressure, and reflexology (massage limited to the feet or hands only) have also shown benefit.[61,62] Referrals to those trained in such therapies can be made.

Malaise and fatigue

The overwhelming sense of weariness and lethargy associated with the flu are referred to as *malaise* or fatigue.[19] Fatigue is one of the most common universal symptoms reported by cancer patients undergoing antineoplastic therapy[63] and is one of the most profound and persistent symptoms in patients receiving biotherapy.[64] These symptoms are often linked to the schedule (more common with continuous infusions) and duration of therapy.[3,12,13,16,65] Patients are not always able to articulate the symptoms by name but describe a lack of motivation, inability to waken, and feelings of apathy or depression. Some report worsening of these symptoms throughout the day. Rest periods and limitation of activities are frequent self-interventions for these symptoms. Dose reduction rarely eliminates the symptom, and in many instances the only management may be a break in therapy. (These symptoms and their management are described in greater detail in Chapter 6, Fatigue.)

Cough and congestion

Any respiratory symptoms experienced by the individual with cancer require serious evaluation. Some patients experiencing FLS will have a stuffy nose and cough; however, adventitious breath sounds, a productive cough, and sore throat all indicate need for further diagnostic tests. Throat, sputum, and blood cultures may be indicated. Chest x-ray films and CT scans are often used to elucidate early pulmonary abnormalities. Antihistamines and cough suppressants may provide relief of simple upper respiratory complaints; however, cough suppressants should be used cautiously in immunocompromised patients with a productive cough. Suppressing the cough may enhance the risk of serious infection. Steroid nasal sprays should be avoided as they may block the therapeutic effects of biotherapeutic agents.[3,32]

TABLE 7-6   Nursing Diagnoses in FLS

Nursing Diagnosis	Expected Outcomes	Nursing Interventions
Knowledge deficit related to FLS: adverse effect of medication	1. Patient will be able to discuss expected side-effects and reportable symptoms. 2. Patient will be able to state at least one self-care measure for each symptom.	1. Instruct patient on expected side-effects of therapy and on measures to control such side-effects. 2. Instruct patient on potential complications if symptoms are not controlled—dehydration, dysrhythmias, angina, low urine output. 3. Assess patient's understanding of when and whom to call for reportable symptoms as well as rationale for self-care measures. 4. Use written, audiovisual, and oral methods of instruction at the appropriate level of understanding for patients. 5. Make necessary referrals for the use of massage, relaxation techniques, etc. 6. Encourage rest periods to coincide with peak of symptoms. 7. Encourage use of social support systems to cope with FLS.
Hyperthermia related to therapy	1. Patient will be able to identify at least one measure to manage body temperature. 2. Patient will gain acceptable control of temperature.	1. Measure and document temperature at least two times per shift; check every hour when febrile. Have outpatients take temperature at least twice daily, timed 2–6 hours after SQ injections. 2. Monitor and document hydration status daily: • Assess intake and output (I&O) • Assess skin and mucous membranes • Monitor for tachycardia, tachypnea, orthostasis, hypotension • Check urine specific gravity against I&O if dehydration is suspected 3. Initiate patient education for managing body temperature: • Document teaching and patient's understanding of at least one management strategy 4. Administer antipyretics as ordered. 5. Tepid sponge baths or other cooling measures if severely febrile and unresponsive to antipyretic medications. 6. Ensure cool comfortable environment. When patient feels hot: • Remove heat sources such as blankets, unnecessary electrical equipment, etc. • Use indirect fans • Encourage increased fluid intake during fever 7. Control chills/rigors as needed: • Keep chilling patient warm • May need to medicate with meperidine or benzodiazepine 8. Monitor for CNS changes with prolonged or very high temperature.

TABLE 7-6 Nursing Diagnoses in FLS (continued)

Nursing Diagnosis	Expected Outcomes	Nursing Interventions
Alteration in comfort related to headache, muscle, or joint pain	Patient will report relief of pain to acceptable level; patient will be able to describe/demonstrate pain-control measures.	1. Administer analgesics as ordered. 2. Offer heat application to areas of muscle tension or joint pain. 3. Offer cool compresses for headache. 4. Document patient responses to pain relief measures. 5. Discuss with patient what measures work, and begin education for self-management at discharge.

In summary, FLS is an adverse effect of many anticancer and supportive therapies. Tachyphylaxis is a common occurrence, with symptoms usually occurring during the first few days of therapy, but decreasing in severity over time.[9,11,16] Symptoms may reappear or worsen if treatment is interrupted and then resumed or if the dose is increased.[15] ln most cases, the symptoms and their severity are largely dependent on dose and route of administration of the FLS-causing drug. Severe FLS may include malignant hyperthermia, rigors sufficient to cause metabolic abnormalities, aches or pain that incapacitate the patient, and prostration. Severe symptoms usually warrant a break in therapy, with consideration of resuming treatment at a lower dose or different therapy schema. Dose reduction is not a recommended strategy, possibly because it often requires a total absence of drug for a period of time in order to resolve FLS.

Evaluation of Therapeutic Approaches

An assessment plan, to detect symptoms early and provide a system of follow-up for interventions employed to alleviate symptoms, is essential for quality care. The mechanisms used will depend on the anticipated incidence and severity of FLS and the practice setting. Therapies provided in the inpatient setting often require daily or every-shift physical assessments and interviews. In the ambulatory care setting, maintenance of symptom logs or diaries by the patient is an ideal method of tracking symptoms and effective preventive or management strategies. The frequency of evaluation may be individualized according to the specific therapy regimen and expected outpatient visits. For example, patient visits may be scheduled to capture the peak of symptoms, so that physical assessment data may be used along with subjective complaints to develop a comprehensive symptom management plan.

Documentation tools

Nursing flow sheets and plans of care are the best tools to document the patients' responses to interventions used to alleviate the symptoms of FLS. Individualized plans of care communicate to staff the problems and the interventions that have been used to provide patient care. The record also indicates when diagnostic tests have been completed, such as x-ray films and laboratory tests. The onset of symptoms should be documented on the flow sheet so that any patterns can be followed and the effectiveness of prophylaxis or treatment strategies for FLS can be evaluated. Evaluation of responses to interventions is ongoing, so that the plan of nursing care can be adapted as necessary. Anticipated nursing diagnoses and expected outcomes of FLS are outlined in Table 7-6.[13,17] This information can also be used as a nursing-care guide to provide a quick reference for management strategies and to educate nurses in care of these patients.

Evaluation tools

Symptoms are subjective and are difficult if not impossible for the nurse to measure accurately. There is also the risk of altered interpretation by caregivers, as evidenced in a study by Robinson and Posner[64] comparing patient and health care provider perceptions of fatigue from biotherapy. It is therefore useful for patients to record objective data, such as temperature, along with subjective perceptions, such as the severity of FLS symptoms, timing of onset, duration, interventions attempted, and response to interventions.[19,23] This information provides a better picture of the efficacy of management strategies. A symptom documentation log may be given to patients to report these symptoms and interventions (Appendix 7A).

Educational Tools and Resources

The interventions identified in Table 7-6 may be a useful guide for nurses caring for individuals with FLS. This nursing-care guide can be used for planning care and providing the patient with innovative suggestions to manage FLS.

Information about medications, expected side-effects, and management strategies must be provided to patients receiving therapy that may cause FLS. Education of the patient and significant others can reduce anxiety and fear and help them gain confidence in their ability to safely manage some of their symptoms. Prescriptions for appropriate prophylactic medications and those used to mitigate adverse effects are provided, and on occasion first doses are given while the patient is in the health care setting. Patients are provided information on how to get in touch with a doctor or nurse during the day, night, and weekends or holidays.

There are a variety of methods for educating the patient. Information can be provided in oral, written, or audiovisual form. (See Appendix 7B for a sample patient self-care guide that can be given to those likely to experience FLS.) Evidence of learning may be manifested by appropriate behaviors or the ability to discuss concepts. Several manufacturers have patient videos and information booklets describing FLS and management strategies that can be reviewed for their appropriateness for specific patient populations.[14,15,32]

Nonpharmacologic measures, such as relaxation techniques, imaging, biofeedback, and self-hypnosis, may be explored with the patient and family. A trial-and-error period may be necessary to see what works best for the individual. Patients should not feel pressured into using these activities and must be reminded that these measures may not alleviate the need for more traditional methods of symptom relief.

Conclusion

Nursing care of patients likely to experience FLS involves a comprehensive assessment plan and general interventions as well as those specific to particular symptoms. The literature includes a variety of definitions for this constellation of symptoms and is often contradictory in its recommendations for management. FLS in patients with cancer is common and influences their health and well-being, but it has not been well researched. This text offers a definition based on the available minimal research data, anecdotal reports, and scientific principles. Our suggested management strategies are built on consistent recommendations, and those are based on pathophysiologic principles. Until more research is available, it is essential for nurses to explore the effects of nature, severity, and perception of FLS on patients' quality of life.

References

1. Hensyl WR (ed): *Stedman's Medical Dictionary* (ed 26). Baltimore: Williams & Wilkins, 1995
2. Haeuber D: Recent advances in the management of biotherapy-related side-effects: Flu-like syndrome. *Oncol Nurs Forum* 16(suppl):35–41, 1989
3. Oncology Nursing Society: *Recommendations for Nursing Course Content and Clinical Practicum Related to Biotherapy,* Pittsburgh, PA: Oncology Nursing Society, 1995
4. Berkow R (ed): *The Merck Manual* (ed 16). Rahway, NJ: Merck Sharp and Dohme, 1992
5. Komaroff AL: Chronic fatigue syndromes: Relationship to chronic viral infections. *J Viral Methods* 2:3–10, 1988
6. Fan H, Connor RF, Villareal LP (eds): *The Biology of AIDS* (ed 3). Sudbury: Jones & Bartlett, 1994
7. Sandstrom SK: Nursing management of patients receiving biological therapy. *Semin Oncol Nurs* 12:152–162, 1996
8. Pazdur R, Jackson D, Shepard B, et al: 5-Fluorouracil and recombinant interferon alfa-2a: Review of activity and toxicity in advanced colorectal carcinomas. *Oncol Nurs Forum* 18(suppl):11–17, 1991
9. Brophy L, Reiger PT: Implications of biological response modifier therapy for nursing, in Clark JC, McGee RF (eds): *Core Curriculum for Oncology Nursing* (ed 2). Philadelphia: Saunders, 1992, pp. 346–358
10. Shelton BK: Flu-like syndrome, in Rieger PT (ed): *Biotherapy: A Comprehensive Overview.* Sudbury: Jones & Bartlett Publishers (in press)
11. Hood LE, Abernathy E: Biologic response modifiers, in McCorkle R, Grant M, Frank-Stromborg M, Baird SB (eds): *Cancer Nursing: A Comprehensive Textbook* (ed 2). Philadelphia: Saunders, 1996, pp. 434–457
12. Reiger PT: Biotherapy, in Otto SE (ed): *Oncology Nursing* (ed 2). St. Louis: Mosby, 1997
13. Rumsey KA, Reiger PT: *Biologic Response Modifiers: A Self-Instruction Manual for Health Professionals.* Chicago: Precept Press, 1992
14. Roche Laboratories: *Step-by-Step Injection with Roferon-A Interferon Alfa-2a Recombinant.* Nutley, NJ: Roche, 1993
15. Schering Corporation: *Intron A Interferon Alfa-2b Patient Guide.* Kenilworth, NJ: Schering, 1992
16. Sergi JS: Issue 1. The physiology of the flu-like syndrome and the cardiopulmonary and renal symptoms associated with BRM therapy, in *Biologic Response Modifiers: Perspectives for Oncology Nurses.* San Francisco: Professional Healthcare, 1991, pp. 4–10
17. Shelton BK, Belcher AE: Biologic therapy: Therapies which hold great promise for patients with cancer, in Ashwanden P, Belcher AE, Mattson EAH, et al (eds): *Advances, Treatments and Trends in Oncology Nursing into the 21st Century.* Rockville, MD: Aspen Publications, 1990, pp. 78–96
18. Strauman JJ: Issue 3. Strategies for managing symptoms, in *Biologic Response Modifiers: Perspectives for Oncology Nurses.* San Francisco: Professional Healthcare, 1992, pp. 4–10
19. White CL: Symptom assessment and management of outpatients receiving biotherapy: The application of a symptom report form. *Semin Oncol Nurs* 8(suppl 1):23–28, 1992
20. Quesada JR, Talpaz M, Rios A, et al: Clinical toxicity of interferons in cancer patients: A review. *J Clin Oncol* 4: 234–239, 1986
21. Skalla K: The interferons. *Semin Oncol Nurs* 12:97–105, 1996
22. Abrams PG, McClamrock E, Foon KA: Evening administration of alpha interferon, *N Engl J Med* 312:443–444, 1985
23. Rhodes VA, Watson PM: Symptom distress—the concept: Past and present. *Semin Oncol Nurs* 3:242–247, 1987
24. Jackson BS, Strauman J, Frederickson K, et al: Long-term biopsychosocial effects of interleukin-2 therapy. *Oncol Nurs Forum* 18:683–690, 1991
25. Brophy L, Sharp EJ: Physical symptoms of combination bio-

therapy: A quality of life issue. *Oncol Nurs Forum* 8(suppl): 25–30, 1992

26. Jassak PF: Nursing considerations for patients receiving biologic response modifiers. *Semin Oncol Nurs* 9(suppl 1):32–35, 1993

27. Craig TJ, Moecki JK, Donnelly A: Noncompliance with immunotherapy secondary to adverse effects (letter, comments). *Ann Allergy, Asthma Immunol* 75:290, 1995

28. Farrell M: Nursing opportunities in biotherapy. *Semin Oncol Nurs* 12:82–87, 1996

29. American Hospital Formulary Service: *AHFS 96 Drug Information.* Bethesda, MD: American Society of Hospital Pharmacists, 1996

30. Murren JR, Ganpule S, Sarris A, et al: A phase II trial of cyclosporin A in the treatment of refractory metastatic colorectal cancer. *Am J Clin Oncol* 14:208–210, 1991

31. Rosenthal E: Azathioprine shock. *Postgrad Med J* 62:677–678 1986

32. Micromedex, Inc.: Vol 84:1975–1998. Denver CO, Micromedex, Inc. Clinical Information System.

33. Chiron Corporation: *Proleukin™ Aldesleukin for Injection.* Emeryville, CA: Chiron Therapeutics, 1992

34. Dukes MNG: *Meyler's Side Effects of Drugs* (ed 11). Amsterdam, The Netherlands: Elsevier, 1988

35. Dorr RT: *Cancer Chemotherapy Handbook.* East Norwalk, CT: Appleton-Lange, 1994

36. Podrasky DL: Amphotericin B: The nurse's role in controlling adverse reactions. *Focus Crit Care* 16:194–198, 1989

37. Anderson M, Faulkner N: Amphotericin B: Effective management of adverse reactions. *Cancer Nurs* 5:461–464, 1982

38. Rutledge DN, Holtzclaw BJ: Use of amphotericin B in immunosuppressed patients with cancer. I. Pharmacology and toxicities. *Oncol Nurs Forum* 17:731–736, 1990

39. Holtzclaw BJ, Rutledge DN: Use of amphotericin B in immunosuppressed patients with cancer. II. Pharmacodynamics and nursing implications. *Oncol Nurs Forum* 17:737–740, 1990

40. Gallis HA, Drew RH, Pickard WW: Amphotericin B: 30 years of clinical experience. *Rev Infect Dis* 12:308–328, 1990

41. Burke MB, Wilkes GM, Ingerson K, (eds): *Cancer Chemotherapy: A Nursing Process Approach* (ed 2). Sudbury: Jones & Bartlett, 1996

42. Gahart BL: *Intravenous Medications* (ed 9). St. Louis: Mosby, 1992

43. Sutton JD, Thalken DW, Powell MC: *Nurses' IV Drug Manual.* Norwalk, CT: Appleton-Lange, 1993

44. Shelton BK. Medications used in organ transplantation, in Kuhn MM (ed): *Pharmacotherapeutics: A Nursing Process Approach* (ed 4). Philadelphia: FA Davis, 1998, pp. 922–935

45. Pillon LR: Cyclosporine: A nursing focus on immunosuppressive therapy. *Dimen Crit Care Nurs* 10:68–73, 1987

46. IDEC Pharmaceuticals Corporation and Genetech Inc. Rituxan Rituximab (G48097-RO [544]). San Diego: IDEC Pharmaceuticals Corporation; and South San Francisco: Genetech, Inc. 1997

47. Baracos V, Rodemann HP, Dinarello CA, et al: Stimulation of muscle protein degradation and prostaglandin E_2 release by leukocytic pyrogen (interleukin-1). *N Engl J Med* 308: 553–558, 1983

48. Dinarello CA, Cannon JG, Wolff SM: New concepts on the pathogenesis of fever. *Rev Infect Dis* 10:128–189, 1988

49. Carpenter R: Fever, in Chernecky CC, Berger BJ (eds): *Advanced and Critical Care Oncology Nursing: Managing Primary Complications.* Philadelphia: Saunders, 1998, pp. 156–171

50. Henker R, Kramer D, Rogers S: Fever. *AACN Clin Iss Crit Care* 8:351–367, 1997

51. Shaffer C: The chilling truth about fever. 1997 AACN National Teaching Institute Proceedings (audiotape). Aliso Viejo, CA: AACN Corporation

52. NCI Common Toxicity Criteria, in *Investigators Handbook.* National Institutes of Health—National Cancer Institute, October 1993, Appendix 12

53. Holtzclaw BJ: Effects of extremity wraps to control drug-induced shivering: A pilot study. *Nurs Res* 39:280–283, 1990

54. Germino BB: Symptom distress and quality of life. *Semin Oncol Nurs* 3:299–302, 1987

55. Rosenthal TC, Silverstein DA: Fever: What to do and what not to do. *Postgrad Med J* 83:75–84, 1988

56. Bruce JL, Grove SK: Fever: Pathology and treatment. *Crit Care Nurs* 12:40–49, 1992

57. Herzog PJ, Lorenzi VG, Sandstrom KS, Sergi JS: Biotherapy, in Gross J, Johnson BL (eds): *Handbook of Oncology Nursing* (ed 2). Sudbury: Jones & Bartlett, 1994, pp. 94–122

58. Suddarth LS, Brunner DS (eds): *Textbook of Medical-Surgical Nursing* (ed 13). New York: Lippincott, 1992

59. Larson DE (ed): *Mayo Clinic Family Health Book.* New York: William Morrow, 1990

60. Turin A: *No More Headaches.* Boston: Houghton Mifflin, 1981

61. Ashley M: *Massage: A Career at Your Fingertips.* Barrytown, NY: Station Hill Press, 1992

62. Ehrmantraut HC: *Headaches.* Brookline, MA: Autumn Press, 1980

63. Winningham ML, Nail LM, Burke MB, et al: Fatigue and the cancer experience: The state of the knowledge. *Oncol Nurs Forum* 21:23–33, 1994

64. Robinson KD, Posner JD: Patterns of self-care needs and interventions related to biologic response modifier therapy: Fatigue as a model. *Semin Oncol Nurs* 8(suppl 1):17–22, 1992

65. Viele CS, Moran TA: Nursing management of the nonhospitalized patient receiving recombinant IL-2. *Semin Oncol Nurs* 9:20–24, 1993

Symptom Documentation Log

Patient Name: _____

Instructions   Use this chart daily to record the symptoms that you are experiencing. Rate the symptoms according to severity using a scale of 1 to 4 (see below). Under "Interventions," record what you did for relief, and under "Comments," whether or not it helped. Share this log with your nurse or physician each week.

Date	Symptoms	Rating	Interventions	Comments

Codes for symptoms present

F = Fever
C = Chills
HA = Headache
M = Muscle aches
J = Joint pain
NC = Nasal congestion/cough

Severity rating for symptoms

1 = Able to carry on daily activities normally
2 = Symptoms mildly affect my day
3 = Severe symptoms, but gained relief after intervention
4 = Severe symptoms; no relief gained

Phone Numbers

Nurse: _____   Phone: _____

Physician: _____   Phone: _____

Home-Care Nurse: _____   Phone: _____

Other: _____   Phone: _____

Comments

Patient's Signature: _____   Date: _____

Nurse's Signature: _____   Date: _____

Source: Shelton BK, Turnbough L: Flu-like syndrome, in Yarbro CH, Frogge MH, Goodman M (eds): *Cancer Symptom Management* (ed 2). Sudbury: Jones and Bartlett, 1999. © Jones and Bartlett Publishers.

Flulike Syndrome

Patient Name: _____

Symptom and Description   Except for the cause, flulike syndrome (FLS) is much like the flu. Your symptoms of fever, chills, headaches, body aches, and nasal stuffiness are expected side-effects of your treatment. Any or all bones, joints, and muscles may hurt. Fever may be mild or severe. Chills may occur—especially when the fever begins—that may range from feeling cold to your teeth chattering or body shaking. These shakes usually don't last more than a few minutes, but your temperature will almost always increase afterward. You may feel washed out or sweaty afterward. Muscle soreness is also a problem after severe shaking. Usually, the worst symptoms happen in the first few days after treatment has been started. As your body adjusts, your symptoms will probably be less severe. You are at risk of having FLS because of your cancer therapy, specifically the drug _____ .

Learning Needs   You need to learn how to manage these side-effects at home. You also need to know when to call your doctor or nurse.

Prevention   It is difficult to prevent this syndrome. The symptoms are usually at their worst 4 to 8 hours after you receive _____ . Some helpful hints to reduce the symptoms include:

- Getting your drug in the evening, which allows you to be active before treatment.
- Getting your drug late, which can help you sleep through some symptoms.
- Taking medications before or after treatment to help prevent these side-effects. Your doctor has ordered the following to be taken before your therapy:

  _____

  _____

  _____

- Your doctor has ordered the following to be taken after your therapy:

  _____

  _____

  _____

- Making sure that you wear comfortable clothing to bed.
- Wearing layers of clothing, so that if you feel warm you can remove some.
- Having plenty of blankets and a heating pad nearby, in case you feel cold at night.

Management   For side-effects that cannot be prevented, here are some ideas on how to manage them at home.

General guidelines:

- Some people find that relaxation techniques, mental imaging, biofeedback, or massage help them to relax and better tolerate the symptoms of FLS.
- Plan your activities before you receive your medicine, so there is less to do when you have side-effects.
- Keep your nutrition up by eating regular, healthy meals.
- Get plenty of rest.
- Ask your doctor or nurse for more information if you are interested in trying relaxation exercises.

Fever:

- Have an easy-to-read thermometer.
- Take and record your temperature in the morning, at bedtime, after a chill, and any time you feel warm.
- Acetaminophen, 650 mg, can be taken every 4 hours until your temperature returns to below 38.3°C (101°F).
- Notify your doctor or nurse if your temperature stays at 40.0°C (104°F) or greater and does not come down with acetaminophen.
- Avoid chilling yourself.
- You may apply cool compresses or ice packs or take tepid baths to feel refreshed and lower your temperature.

Chills:

- Keep yourself as warm as possible during these episodes.
- A heating pad or hot water bottle may help.
- Notify your doctor or nurse if these episodes last longer than usual, or if you feel any shortness of breath during a shaking period or afterward.

Aches (headaches, joint aches, muscle aches):

- Taking medication for pain as prescribed by your doctor *or* acetaminophen— 650 mg every 4 to 6 hours—should give some relief.
- A dark and quiet environment is often helpful.
- Applying cool compresses to your forehead or warm compresses to the back of your neck may also help, depending on where the pain is located.
- Notify your doctor or nurse if you notice any visual changes or dizziness with your headaches.
- Also call the doctor if the pain is in the neck and you can't touch your chin to your chest.
- Get plenty of rest—don't overdo when you are having these aches.
- Sometimes fun activities will help get your mind off the pain. Reading, sewing, listening to music, and watching TV are a few ideas you may try.
- Notify your doctor or nurse if you notice increased stiffness or difficulty in walking or in getting up or sitting or lying down.

Cough/nasal congestion:

- Antihistamines and cough preparations are usually helpful. Ask your doctor to suggest medicines you can take if needed.
- Drink plenty of fluids—try to drink at least eight glasses of fluid per day.

- Avoid excess dryness in the home, but be certain that humidifiers are cleaned every few days.
- If you are coughing up yellow or green phlegm, notify doctor or nurse.

Follow-up   Be sure you understand what to expect, what to do about it, and when to call your doctor or nurse. Have emergency phone numbers available. Be able to discuss these plans with your nurse before you go home. If you are unsure of any of the instructions, be sure to clarify them with your doctor and nurse.

Keep a log or diary of your symptoms, how long they last, what you did about them, and how well the methods worked to get rid of the symptoms. Bring this log with you to the doctor or the clinic visits.

Nurse: _____ Phone: _____

Physician: _____ Phone: _____

Home-Care Nurse: _____ Phone: _____

Other: _____ Phone: _____

Comments

Patient's Signature: _____ Date: _____

Nurse's Signature: _____ Date: _____

Source: Shelton BK, Turnbough L: Flu-like syndrome, in Yarbro CH, Frogge MH, Goodman M (eds): *Cancer Symptom Management* (ed 2). Sudbury: Jones and Bartlett, 1999. © Jones and Bartlett Publishers.

CHAPTER 8

Menopausal Symptoms

Michelle Goodman, RN, MS

The Problem of Menopausal Symptoms in Cancer

The prevention and management of menopausal symptoms can have a significant impact on a woman's current quality of life as well as provide protection from serious threats to her long-term health. With an understanding of the physiologic consequences of estrogen deprivation and with knowledge of the current research concerning the management of the symptoms of menopause and related health issues, the nurse may more appropriately interpret the estrogen replacement therapy and cancer-risk controversy to clients and colleagues, particularly as it concerns the potential role and safety of hormone replacement therapy in the woman with a history of cancer.

Incidence in Cancer

The U.S. Census Bureau[1] estimates that by the year 2010, more than 20 million women in the United States will be at least 50 years old and menopausal. As such, 33% of the female population will then be menopausal or postmenopausal, compared with about 10% of the current female population. With life expectancy approaching 80 years, these women can expect to spend more than one-third of their lives without the benefits of ovarian hormones.

For some women the symptoms of menopause may be mild, but for others they are disabling. In general, estrogen deficiency causes two types of symptoms: (1) effects attributed to vasomotor instability, specifically hot flashes, insomnia, and increased irritability, and (2) effects attributed to urogenital atrophy. The latter include thinning of the vaginal wall and glandular atrophy, leading to persistent vaginal dryness, itching, irritation, dyspareunia (pain during intercourse), and postcoital bleeding. Vaginal atrophy precipitates vaginitis and problems related to sexual function. Urinary symptoms include urgency, stress incontinence, and frequent urinary tract infections. Specific behavioral changes at the time of menopause include changes in mood, memory, decision making, and the ability to concentrate. Quality of life has been shown to diminish as a result of menopausal symptoms.[2]

The current interest and concern regarding estrogen deprivation derives from the impact this syndrome has, whether natural or medically induced, on the incidence and severity of such disabling and life-threatening conditions as osteoporosis and heart disease. Current research indicates that estrogen deprivation contributes to heart disease and to bone loss resulting in osteoporosis. Epidemiologic evidence indicates that estrogen therapy is associated with a 40% to 50% reduction in the risk of cardiovascular disease, which is known to cause the greatest number of deaths in women over 55 years of age.[3,4]

Table 8-1 depicts a woman's lifetime risk of developing certain serious illnesses, her risk of death, and deaths per year attributed to each.[5-7]

Hormone replacement therapy (HRT) is associated

TABLE 8-1 Lifetime Risk, Risk of Death and Deaths per Year for Women According to Selected Medical Conditions[5-7]

Medical Condition	Lifetime Risk (%)	Risk of Death (%)	Deaths per Year (approx.)
Cardiovascular disease	46.1	31.0	376,000
Hip fracture	15.3	1.5	40,000
Breast cancer	10.2	3.0	44,000
Endometrial cancer	2.6	0.3	6,000
Alzheimer's disease	28.0	N/A	65,000

with certain risks and benefits. It is important for the nurse to have an understanding of what these risks and benefits are in order to counsel the woman who is approaching menopause or is postmenopausal.

Some women turn to their family physician or gynecologist for management of their menopausal symptoms, but many women do not seek medical counsel for what is perceived as a natural and unavoidable consequence of aging. Only about 15% of women who are eligible for HRT receive it; in lower socioeconomic groups, it is only 5% to 6%. There may be many reasons for this, but most relate to physician and patient attitudes, a lack of access to information and health care, particularly of a preventive nature, or concern about the risk of cancer (breast and endometrial) and the fact that cyclic regimens cause monthly menstrual bleeding.[8-10] While postmenopausal HRT is becoming more widely accepted, due to increased public and professional awareness of benefits to the overall health of the aging female, issues of compliance with therapy and cancer risk with prolonged therapy remain important areas for research.

Etiology

The Climacteric and the Phases of Menopause

Natural menopause (as opposed to surgical menopause resulting from removal of the ovaries) is due to the exhaustion of the remaining ovarian follicles that contain the germ cells that produce the steroid hormones estrogen and progesterone. Follicular depletion, then, is the actual cause of menopause.

Menopause is defined as the absence of menses for 12 months. While it can occur anywhere from 40 to 60 years of age, the average age of menopause is 52. The premenopausal state is usually characterized by a shortened cycle and skipped menses. During this time, the woman may also experience sleeplessness, irritability, loss of concen-

tration, vaginal dryness, mild depression, and increased avoidance of social contact. Onset of the premenopausal era occurs on the average at 47.5 years, and this era usually lasts for 4 years.

"Climacteric" is not synonymous with menopause. *Climacteric* means a period of major change and implies passage of time, which includes the premenopausal state, the period of acute menopausal symptoms, and a period of years following the menopause. *Perimenopause* is used to describe the last few years of the climacteric and the first year after menopause.[11]

Premature ovarian failure is defined as the cessation of ovarian function prior to the age of 40, which occurs naturally in only about 1% of women.[12] Premature ovarian failure can also occur following abdominal hysterectomy, possibly due to compromise in the blood supply to the ovary.

Ovarian failure may also be induced by exposure to external radiation, cytotoxic chemotherapy, viral infection, or surgery. Chemotherapy, especially with the alkylating agents cyclophosphamide and busulfan, has been reported to cause irreversible gonadal damage in the majority of patients. More than two-thirds of women over age 30 who receive chemotherapy develop complete ovarian failure. Horning et al.[13] report a high incidence of menopausal symptoms (68%) and menstrual irregularity (79%) in women over age 30 treated with irradiation and chemotherapy. Total body irradiation usually leads to irreversible ovarian failure. Fifty percent of women who receive radiation to the abdomen as treatment for Hodgkin's lymphoma will receive a dose to the ovaries sufficient to produce permanent hypergonadotropic amenorrhea. For any given dose of radiation, the older the woman, the greater her risk of developing amenorrhea. It is now common practice to transpose the ovaries surgically outside the field of irradiation as an attempt to preserve ovarian function.

Menstrual cycle changes

In terms of menstrual function, 10% of women experience sudden amenorrhea, 70% experience oligomenorrhea (abnormally sparse menstrual periods with intervals of 36 to 90 days between periods) or hypomenorrhea (regular menses but a decrease in the amount of bleeding). Eighteen percent of women will experience menorrhagia (bleeding of excess duration), metrorrhagia (bleeding irregularly between cycles), or hypermenorrhea (excessive bleeding). These menstrual symptoms decline in severity as time passes.[14]

Hormonal changes

The primary biological marker for the onset of menopause is an elevated level of follicle-stimulating hormone (FSH). As ovarian failure progresses, the decreased level of hormone is detected by the hypothalamus, which signals the pituitary gland to secrete FSH and luteinizing hormone (LH). As levels of estradiol, the predominant estrogen, fluctuate, cycle length may vary, ovulation may or may not occur, and menstrual bleeding becomes irregular. As the ovaries fail to respond to the effects of the gonadotropins (FSH and LH), estrogen deficiency results in anovulation and amenorrhea.

Postmenopausal women have serum estradiol levels of about 15 pg/mL and mean estrone (the weaker estrogen) levels of about 30 pg/mL.[15] Estrone is derived from peripheral aromatization of androstenedione, 95% of which comes from the adrenal gland and 5% from the ovaries. With increasing weight, there is increased conversion of androstenedione to estrogen, resulting in elevated estrogen levels in obese women compared with slender women. The major source of circulating estradiol in postmenopausal women comes from the peripheral aromatization of androgens. The ovarian secretion of androgens decreases during menopause, as does the secretion of androstenedione.

Pathophysiology

Hormonal changes during menopause result in physiologic changes that are manifested in various acute symptoms such as vasomotor instability and genitourinary changes, as well as in more long-term problems such as bone loss and changes in lipid profiles. The more predominant menopausal symptoms and long-term complications of ovarian failure are discussed individually.

Vasomotor Instability

Estrogen plays a role in the stability of a woman's thermoregulatory system and in the functioning of the vascular system. The firing rate of the thermosensitive neurons in the preoptic area of the hypothalamus are influenced by serum estrogen levels. Likewise, estrogen affects the responsiveness of the vascular smooth muscle to vasoactive substances such as epinephrine and norepinephrine.[16]

Endocrine instability occurs when estrogen is depleted and is manifested in numerous clinical sequelae. The predominant clinical sequela is vasomotor instability, also referred to as "hot flashes" (or "hot flushes"). Vasomotor instability is thought to be caused by a disruption of the function of the thermoregulatory center in the hypothalamus, as a consequence of enhanced hypothalamic activity secondary to the loss of critical triggers in the ovarian hormonal feedback mechanisms. This disruption in the function of the thermoregulatory center is associated with a sharp rise in blood levels of epinephrine, a potent stimulator of heart function.[17] Kronenberg et al.[16] measured serum catecholamines in women during hot flashes and found an increase in epinephrine, accompanied by a sharp decrease in norepinephrine. These authors conclude that the hot flash occurs most likely from an alteration in peripheral vascular control and that the classic vascular response of vasodilation, intense heat, and profuse perspiration is caused by adrenergic factors. This explains why drugs that decrease central adrenergic activity (e.g., clonidine) may be useful in lessening hot flashes.[18] Women commonly report that their heart "pounds," and in fact clinical measures show that the heart rate increases. In addition, the increase in cardiac output and rise in systolic blood pressure result in headache and dizziness. While a woman's core temperature does not increase, the woman will report feeling intense warmth throughout the upper body, with flushing of the neck, face, and chest—which may or may not be accompanied by profuse perspiration, followed by chills.

Between 65% and 76% of women suffer from hot flashes. Fifteen to 25% of women will experience severe or frequent hot flashes (more than 10 per day). The duration of a hot flash varies anywhere from a few seconds to minutes. Frequency will vary from person to person and even in the same individual. Hot flashes can be rare or occur every few minutes. The average frequency is 10 or more occurrences per day, with the greatest number of hot flashes occurring during the night. Night sweats are generally described by many as being more intense than hot flashes that occur during the day. Nocturnal sweats interfere with efficient sleep patterns. REM sleep is longer in women with hot flashes compared to those with no hot flashes. This disturbed sleep leads to fatigue, irritability, memory loss, nervousness, and anxiety during the day. The majority of women (80%) will experience symptoms for longer than 1 year, and 25% to 85% of these women complain of episodes for longer than 5 years.[19] For women who experience surgical removal of the ovaries, symptoms may be more severe and longer lasting.

In summary, the physiologic events in a hot flash are thought to be manifestations of the effects of the body's thermoregulatory center, as it activates mechanisms for heat loss (vasodilation, heat dissipation) at the onset of the hot flash and then for body heat conservation (vasoconstriction and shivering) at the completion of the hot flash.

Genitourinary Symptoms

Within 5 years of estrogen deprivation, women will begin to experience clinical symptoms due to atrophic changes in the vagina, urethra, and bladder. The cells of the vagina and urethra contain among them the highest concentration of estrogen receptors anywhere in the body. During the climacteric, atrophic changes of the vagina occur and are accompanied by vaginal dryness, infections, burning, itching, dyspareunia, discharge, and occasionally bleeding. Urinary symptoms include dysuria, urinary frequency, urgency, nocturia, urinary stress incontinence, and frequent urinary tract infections. Estrogen receptors in the urethra, bladder, and pelvic floor are sensitive to fluctuations in estrogen levels. When circulating estrogen levels fall, there is urogenital atrophy and a gradual increase in the incidence of the aforementioned urinary symptoms. The genitourinary symptoms worsen with time, unlike the symptoms of vasomotor instability, which tend to improve over time.[20]

Estrogen increases arterial blood flow. Thus, in the estrogen-deprived state, there is a decrease in blood flow to the vagina and vulva, resulting in atrophy of Bartholin's glands, cellular atrophy and thinning of the vaginal wall, flattening of the epithelial glands, and loss of water-retaining ability. These atrophic changes result in a lack of lubrication as well as a shortening and narrowing of the vaginal vault and dyspareunia. The protective covering of the clitoris usually atrophies such that the clitoral glans becomes more irritated with any type of contact.[21]

With estrogen deficiency, the vaginal secretions are altered, both in quantity and composition.[22] The pH and sodium content of the vagina changes, and normal microflora (lactobacilli) diminish, permitting overgrowth of contaminating organisms from the vagina and perineum, which increases the incidence of infection (e.g., candidal, trichomonal). Burning and irritation are generally caused by a chronic discharge because of the elevation in pH and changes in bacterial flora. The itching commonly interferes with sleep and occurs because of thinning and inflammation of the vulvovaginal epithelial layer.

Urinary tract infections are also more common, because as the vagina shortens, the urethral meatus is closer to the introitus, causing increased urinary discomfort, frequency, and infection. As mentioned above, urinary stress incontinence worsens with time; and it is more common in women who have had a vaginal hysterectomy. The actual prevalence of postmenopausal urinary incontinence is not known but has been estimated to be about 30% in women over 60 years of age.[23]

About 30% to 50% of menopausal women complain of a problem in one or more aspects of sexual functioning.[24,25] As would be anticipated, a decrease in vaginal lubrication, atrophic vaginitis, and frequent infections can result in dyspareunia. In a study by Bachmann et al.[26] of 887 gynecologic outpatients, dyspareunia was found to be the most common sexual problem (identified by 100%), followed by decreased sexual desire, partner problems or dysfunctions, vaginismus, and anorgasmia. There is a direct correlation between increased dyspareunia and decreasing levels of estradiol. The lower the estradiol levels, the worse the dyspareunia.[25]

Dyspareunia occurs for many reasons. Bartholin's glands and endocervical glands atrophy over time, resulting in a lack of lubrication that does not improve as sexual activity continues. Because of loss of epithelial cells in the vagina, tissues become friable and pale. The vagina becomes more narrow and shortens as it loses its rugation, and the muscular layer is replaced by fibrous tissue, resulting in a loss of elasticity. This condition accelerates if the woman is sexually abstinent.

Low estradiol levels correlated with decreased blood flow to the vagina, such that vaginal engorgement, which is necessary for comfortable coitus, is not physiologically possible. Coital pain, sensations of burning and pressure, and postcoital bleeding lead to apprehension, loss of sexual desire, and decreased coital frequency due to the fear of pain. Women who stop having sexual relations, regardless of the cause (loss of libido, dyspareunia), appear to develop more atrophic vaginal changes than women who continue to be coitally active.[26]

Libido, or sexual motivation, is influenced by many factors, but the general consensus is that it is primarily due to the synergistic effect of both estrogen and androgen. Loss of ovarian function eliminates approximately 34% of circulating serum androgens.[27]

Mood Changes

Psychic changes occurring at menopause may be due at least in part to the alteration in hormonal milieu.[28] Symptoms commonly reported include mood swings, nervousness, depression, and anxiety, as well as memory loss.[28–30] The results of research concerning the occurrence of depression as a consequence of menopause are conflicting. Of interest is the fact that estrogen increases the rate of degradation of monoamine oxidase, the enzyme that catabolizes the neurotransmitter serotonin. Serotonin deficiency is thought to be a causal factor in depression. However, some studies,[31,32] particularly one by McKinlay et al.,[33] fail to document an increase in depressive symptoms around the time of menopause compared with other times during a woman's lifetime. Depression appears to correlate more directly with the problems associated with aging (stress in interpersonal relationships and decline in physical health) rather than with menopause. In a rather large study, Hunter et al.[34] found an increased incidence of depressive symptoms in menopausal and postmenopausal women. Of further significance are the findings of a longitudinal survey of 2500 middle-aged women: Those who had undergone a surgical menopause had high and clinically significant depression scores compared with women experiencing a natural menopause.[35]

Women who are menopausal commonly complain of memory loss. While the exact mechanism responsible for this is not known, it appears that estrogen enhances adrenergic function, which has been linked to cognitive abilities, particularly short-term memory.[36] Estrogen may stimulate the growth of nerve cells; inhibit levels of the fatty acid apolipoprotein E, which is closely linked to heart disease and Alzheimer's disease (AD); act as an antioxidant; and increase the levels of acetylcholine, an important transmitter of nerve messages in the brain.

Estrogen is a critical inducer of choline acetyltransferase, the enzyme needed to synthesize acetylcholine. A deficiency of brain acetylcholine concentrations may be directly associated with AD. Further, estrogen receptors are in abundance throughout the central nervous system, especially the hypothalamus. Research conducted by Kawas et al.[37] indicates that estrogen replacement therapy (ERT) may yield as much as a 54% reduction in risk of AD. ERT has also been found to protect against AD; specifically, the age at onset has been found to be significantly later in women who have taken estrogen.[38,39] Sherwin and Phillips[40] demonstrated in a prospective study of surgically menopausal women that those who were given estrogen postoperatively maintained their scores on several tests of memory and abstract reasoning, whereas the performance scores of those who were given placebos decreased.

Bone Loss

The skeleton consists of two types of bone: cortical bone, which forms the shafts of the long bones, and trabecular bone, which resists compressive stress. Bone remodeling is like a restorative maintenance process in which old bone is continually replaced by new bone. Until about age 40, bone resorption roughly equals formation. Beyond age 40, resorption begins to exceed formation, with a net loss of bone (osteopenia). This imbalance accelerates after menopause, and about 3% to 5% of total bone loss will occur per year for the 5 to 10 years that follow menopause.[41] This loss of bone in the aging female can lead to osteoporosis, which is characterized by low bone mass with micro-architectural deterioration of bone tissue, leading to enhanced bone fragility and an increased risk of fracture.

The amount of bone in the skeleton is a function of one's genetic inheritance, dietary calcium, vitamin D consumption, the peak amount of bone mass, and the rate of loss of bone mass thereafter. However, the principal determinant of skeletal status in the aging woman is ovarian function. Estrogen deprivation results in critical alterations in skeletal homeostasis that cause net loss of bone tissue. The precise mechanism by which estrogen influences bone remodeling is not known; however, specific receptors for estrogens have been identified in cells of osteoblast lineage.

Bone mass and osteoporosis are related more to the loss of estrogen than to chronologic age. Women 50 years of age who have had their ovaries removed 20 years earlier have levels of bone density comparable to 70-year-old women who experienced a natural menopause at age 50. Women who have had a hysterectomy are also more likely to develop osteoporosis, compared with women who experience a natural menopause.[42] For women entering menopause, the lifetime risk of suffering a hip fracture is approximately 15%.[42] Hip fractures alone occur in about 240,000 women per year, with a mortality of 40,000 annually. Approximately 25% of caucasian women over the age of 70 and 50% over the age of 80 will have vertebral fractures. African-American women have hip fracture rates one-third that of Caucasian women in the U.S., presumably due to the difference in skeletal density.[42]

Estrogen deprivation also appears to have a negative influence on calcium homeostasis, in that calcium depletion increases after menopause.[43] Calcium absorption through the intestine decreases and calcium loss from the kidney increases, resulting in an increased utilization of skeletal calcium to maintain serum calcium levels within physiologic parameters. Other factors that increase risk for osteoporosis include:

- therapeutic use of glucocorticoids, which decrease osteoblast activity and increase osteoclast activity; chronic heparinization
- high consumption of caffeine and some animal proteins, which accelerate urinary calcium excretion
- alcohol consumption
- cigarette smoking, which interferes with estrogen metabolism
- prolonged bed rest
- the use of thyroid hormone replacement
- positive family history

It is thought that parathyroid hormone is responsible for recruitment of new remodeling sites, which can accelerate bone loss in the otherwise estrogen-deprived state. Table 8-2 summarizes the risk factors for osteoporosis and bone fractures.

Cardiovascular Disease

Coronary artery disease accounts for 23% of all deaths and is the leading cause of death among women in the United States.[3,44] The risk of cardiovascular disease in women is less than that in men until the woman reaches menopause, after which a woman's risk doubles.[45] The problem of cardiovascular disease in women has only been addressed to any significant degree in the last 16 years. While considerable effort and resources have been devoted to the study of risk factors and to the development of programs to prevent cardiovascular disease in men, until recently, few studies have included women. In a series of research reports,[46–48] findings indicate that when women present with symptoms of cardiovascular disease, their symptoms are managed differently compared to men. Women were found to undergo less aggressive diagnostic and curative procedures than men, and the overall mortality and morbidity following a cardiac event were worse in women than in men. Thirty-nine percent of women who have an acute myocardial infarction die within a year, compared with 31% of men.[49]

In women, the risk of cardiovascular disease correlates with estrogen deficiency. The protective effect of estrogen

TABLE 8-2 Risk Factors for Osteoporosis and Bone Fracture

Predictive Factors for Loss of Peak Bone Mass

Age: peak bone mass occurs by age 40
Genetic factors:
   Prevalence in family
   White
   Asian
   Small frame
   Low weight
Nulliparity
Dietary factors:
   Low calcium intake
   Low vitamin D consumption
   High caffeine consumption
   Red meat consumption
   Eating disorders
Lifestyle:
   Alcohol use
   Cigarette smoking
   Bed rest, lack of exercise
   Low exposure to sunlight
   Amenorrhea/athletic women
   Glucocorticoid therapy
   Thyroid hormone therapy

→

Factors That Accelerate Bone Loss

Estrogen deprivation:
   Surgical ovariectomy
   Radiation
   Chemotherapy
   Physiologic stress
   Immobilization
Aging: Bone loss occurs at an
   average rate of 1–2% per year

→

Osteoporosis

Low bone density:
   Increasing bone fragility
   Impaired protective mechanisms

→

Fracture

Trauma and bone fracture:
   Vertebral fractures
   Hip fractures
   Colles' fractures

lies in its impact on the plasma total cholesterol and lipid profile. Plasma total cholesterol is an important risk factor for coronary artery heart disease.[50] A favorable plasma lipid profile includes an increased high-density lipoprotein (HDL) cholesterol and a decreased low-density lipoprotein (LDL) cholesterol. Estrogens lower the levels of LDL cholesterol and raise the concentration of HDL cholesterol.

LDLs are produced in the liver and carried to the peripheral tissues, where they provide a major source of energy for cardiac muscle cells. The uptake of LDLs by macrophages is inhibited locally by HDLs. Lower levels of HDL (the "good" cholesterol) result in a net increase in LDL (the "bad" cholesterol). Estrogen lowers LDL by increasing LDL catabolism and clearance. It decreases hepatic HDL receptors and therefore decreases HDL catabolism. The overall effect is reduced accumulation of cholesterol in peripheral tissues and an increased concentration in the biliary fluid with subsequent elimination. In addition to its effect on plasma lipid proteins, estrogens inhibit lipid accumulation in the coronary arteries and improve arterial blood flow.[51]

In the United States, 27% of all women aged 20 to 74 have plasma total cholesterol levels higher than 240 mg/dL.[52] As women age they have a reduced capacity to remove LDL cholesterol due to a reduction in hepatic LDL receptors. Within 6 months after menopause, total cholesterol levels increase by about 6%. LDL cholesterol levels increase by 10%, whereas HDL cholesterol levels decrease by about 6% over a period of 2 years following menopause.[53] A 1% increase in plasma total cholesterol or LDL increases the risk of coronary artery disease by 2%. Likewise, a 1% decrease in HDL increases the risk of coronary disease by 2 to 4%. Postmenopausal women have greater increases in LDL cholesterol levels and greater decreases in HDL cholesterol levels than age-adjusted premenopausal women.[50]

Obesity and a sedentary lifestyle are significant risk factors for coronary artery disease. Seventy percent of heart disease in obese women and 40% of heart disease in all women is attributed to being overweight, and it is therefore potentially preventable.[54] Obesity also contributes to hypertension, which is a significant and independent risk factor for heart disease. Diabetes mellitus accelerates atherosclerosis and increases the risk of acute coronary ischemia, particularly in women.[55] Hypertension, obesity, and diabetes mellitus often occur concomitantly in the aging female, contributing to an overall high-risk profile in the estrogen-deprived female.

Lastly, cigarette smoking will contribute to a woman's risk for heart disease. Cigarette smoking is the single most important preventable risk factor for cardiovascular disease in women. Cigarette smoking is directly responsible for 21% of all mortality from cardiovascular disease and for 50% of all acute coronary events before the age of 55.[56] The mechanism of the relationship between heart disease and cigarette smoking is known to involve nicotinic release of catecholamines, which stimulate the sympathetic nervous system, thereby increasing plasma levels of LDL cholesterol. Smokers are known to have an unfavorable plasma lipid profile, specifically increased levels of total cholesterol and triglycerides and decreased levels of HDL cholesterol. Cigarette smoking may eliminate the protective effect of estrogens on the cardiovascular system and is associated with a risk of early natural menopause.

Symptom Management

Prevention

As the majority of women born during the postwar era enter the menopausal years and thereby become more at risk for health problems, there will be a rise in cancer incidence, heart disease, and osteoporosis. The number of women with breast cancer has increased at a rate of 3% per year since 1980. The disease effected more than 183,000 new women in 1998.[57] Fortunately, as a result of early detection, most women have breast cancer that is amenable to treatment, and for the first time the mortality rates for breast cancer have begun to decline.[58,59]

Adjuvant chemotherapy is increasingly being incorporated into the treatment plan of women with localized breast cancer. Therefore, more women who have an excellent survival prognosis and whose disease has been detected at an earlier age will develop early menopause after treatment. For these women, the decision regarding HRT is likely to affect the quality and quantity of their lives for several decades.[60]

The controversy surrounding the issue of HRT for menopausal women in general and for women with a history of breast and other hormone-related cancers in particular centers around the question of whether such therapy provides more good than harm. Definitive information on the effect of HRT on breast cancer risk will likely be obtained from the Women's Health Initiative Clinical Trial, which is now in its early stages. Definitive information will be available in 2005.

Historically, the concerns regarding the risks of HRT were based on (1) epidemiologic and biological evidence that suggested a potential association of estrogens with increased breast cancer risk, (2) studies that reported complications with high-dose oral contraceptive use, and (3) an observed increase in the incidence of endometrial cancers in women treated with unopposed estrogens to relieve menopausal symptoms. As more is learned about each of these areas of concern, and as the incidence of heart disease and osteoporosis rises and they become recognized as even greater risks to a woman's health, physicians are likely to view the prospects of HRT as therapeutically more valuable than just a treatment for hot flashes.

The problem of increased incidence of endometrial cancer has been attributed to the effect of estrogen on the endometrium, which causes stimulation and hyperplasia of the endometrial cells. The risk of endometrial cancer with estrogen therapy has been mitigated by the use of supplemental progestational agents, which cause shedding of the endometrium (in women who have not had a hysterectomy). However, the belief that HRT causes endometrial cancer remains a concern for physicians and is a primary factor in why many physicians do not readily prescribe HRT.

Scientific scrutiny and review of the impact of exogenous estrogens on the risk of breast cancer is currently under way. While much will be learned from the Women's Health Initiative, a number of studies concerning this issue have already shed valuable light on this important and controversial subject. One study reported that women with a history of HRT had significantly better survival rates overall and less relative risk of dying between the ages of 50 and 60 years compared with women with no history of HRT.[61] A lower mortality rate from breast cancer in women who were taking HRT at the time they were diagnosed has been previously reported.[62]

In the Nurses's Health Study, the largest longitudinal study of estrogen and breast cancer, it was reported that the risk of breast cancer was moderately elevated among current users of HRT who drink alcohol. The Harvard researchers also found that current hormone users had a lower risk of death due to breast cancer than subjects who had never taken hormones. The benefit decreased with long-term use, that is after 10 or more years.[10] In a study by the Centers for Disease Control, the risk of breast cancer did not appear to increase until at least 5 years of estrogen use. A 30% increase in the risk of breast cancer was reported in women who had 15 years or more of estrogen replacement. In this study, women with a family history of breast cancer and a positive history of estrogen use had a significantly higher risk of breast cancer.[63]

While the results of individual studies are inconsistent, especially in regard to certain subgroups, the results of a metaanalysis of the literature concerning breast cancer and estrogen replacement therapy suggest that low-dose estrogen (0.3–0.625 mg/day of conjugated estrogen) does not increase the risk of breast cancer.[64,65] Cobleigh[66] further concludes, following an extensive review of the literature, that collectively the studies concerning HRT and risk for breast cancer among women who have used HRT do not show an increased risk. Evidence demonstrates that short-term (<10 years) HRT does not appear to cause breast cancer in healthy women. However, it is possible that women with a personal history of breast cancer may be more susceptible to the tumor-promoting effects of estrogen. Long-term use (10–15 years) may increase risk of breast cancer. Tamoxifen reduces the risk of contralateral breast cancer. Therefore, taking tamoxifen with HRT may eliminate any possible cancer-promoting effect of estrogen on breast cells.

Therapeutic Approaches

Cardiovascular disease (CVD)

The lifetime risk that a 50-year-old woman will die of coronary artery disease is 31%. This is much greater than her risk of dying from either osteoporotic fractures or breast cancer.[67] A recent review of 20 studies spanning a period of approximately 15 years indicates that HRT reduces the risk of cardiovascular disease by 40%–60% in HRT users compared to nonusers.[45] The Nurses' Health Study, which included 48,470 postmenopausal women, reported that the overall relative risk of major coronary disease in women currently taking estrogen was significantly reduced among those women with either natural or surgical menopause. In this prospective study, it was found that when current postmenopausal estrogen users were compared with women who had never used estrogen, the estrogen users had about half the risk of major coronary disease or a fatal CVD event.

The beneficial effects of estrogen replacement therapy include its ability to reduce LDL cholesterol levels, increase HDL cholesterol levels, and slightly decrease serum total cholesterol levels.[4,68] Estrogens may also exert a protective effect on vascular function by directly enhancing the activity of the endothelium and stimulating blood flow, thereby lessening the potential for coronary vasoconstriction and thrombosis. There is no evidence that estrogen therapy increases risk of venous thrombosis in postmenopausal women. In women who are at risk for vascular thrombosis or embolism, transdermal estrogen administration is associated with less hepatic production of clotting factors, thus theoretically posing less risk of thromboembolic disease. Angiographic studies have consistently found less coronary artery disease in women who receive estrogen replacement.[69,70]

Smoking is a known risk factor for cardiac disease in women. Postmenopausal women who smoke more than one pack of cigarettes per day may need estrogen replacement even more than their nonsmoking age-matched cohorts. Postmenopausal smokers may need a higher dose of estrogen to overcome the antiestrogen metabolic effects of nicotine. Counseling on the effects of smoking and education regarding smoking cessation strategies are appropriate.

Women who have preexisting hypertension may still receive estrogen therapy. There is no evidence that estrogen either exacerbates or induces hypertension in the postmenopausal woman. For those women who experience a rise in blood pressure during HRT, the use of appropriate antihypertensives and the transdermal hormone replacement patch may be prescribed. There is overwhelming evidence that estrogen induces a fall in blood pressure when administered to postmenopausal women. Any rise in blood pressure is thought to be more related to the effects of progestin therapy. In women who experience an increase in blood pressure, the dose of progestin is titrated down to the lowest acceptable level to avoid any potential progestin-induced change in vessel wall response.[71]

Elevated levels of both systolic and diastolic blood pressure are independent risk factors that directly correlate with acute coronary events as well as increased mortality from CVD. Elevated blood pressure commonly occurs in women in conjunction with other risk factors for CVD, such as obesity, unfavorable lipid profiles, and diabetes. Roughly one-third of postmenopausal women are at moderate risk and one-fourth are at high risk of coronary artery disease as indicated by a high total cholesterol level (>200 mg/dL), but particularly HDL cholesterol levels below 45 mg/dL. A high intake of dietary fat and the presence of abdominal fat, together with a sedentary lifestyle, place a woman at higher cardiac risk as she approaches menopause. These women can benefit not only from hormone replacement therapy but from dietary counseling to reduce their intake of fat, and more importantly an exercise program that reduces weight, particularly abdominal fat. Dieting alone has not been shown to be effective over time without exercise, which increases energy expenditure and metabolic rate and effectively alters body composition.

As each year of estrogen deprivation passes and as the woman ages, her risk for CVD increases. The research concerning the beneficial effects of HRT in the postmenopausal woman seems compelling, if not convincing; yet, each woman must be evaluated and advised by her physician based on her medical history. Decisions made for or against HRT are then based on the woman's understanding of the risk/benefit ratio. The American Heart Association currently recommends consideration of HRT for postmenopausal women, particularly those at increased risk for coronary heart disease and osteoporosis.[72] Table 8-3 summarizes risk factors for coronary artery disease.

Osteoporosis

Osteoporosis is more easily prevented than treated. Among the causes of postmenopausal bone loss, estrogen deficiency is clearly the most important, but it is also perhaps the easiest risk factor to alter, potentially reversing bone loss and subsequent risk for fracture. Inadequate exercise also contributes to bone loss. The same exercises that enhance muscle strength are beneficial for enhancing bone density, in particular weight-bearing exercises (stair climbing, jogging, tennis, dancing, baseball) for 30 minutes three times per week. Swimming, cycling, and walking are beneficial from a cardiovascular perspective but have no effect on slowing bone loss. More intense skeletal loading is needed to slow bone loss. A combination of aerobic exercise and weight training is more beneficial than either one of these activities alone. However, exercise alone independent of HRT will not suffice to prevent bone loss.

Nutritional factors, specifically calcium intake, can have an impact on the incidence and severity of osteoporosis. While it is impossible to identify the precise level of calcium intake below which osteoporosis is increased, some general guidelines are available. Total calcium intake should be 1000 mg/day for premenopausal women and 1500 mg/day for postmenopausal women. Calcium is a nutrient and can be obtained from nutritional sources; however, such sources are generally high in calories and fat and are avoided by health-conscious individuals. The average intake of calcium in most adults is 400–500 mg/day. Therefore, 500–1000 mg/day of calcium supplements should be adequate. Calcium supplements should be taken with food to enhance absorption. Calcium carbonate has the highest percentage of elemental calcium (40%), whereas calcium gluconate has 9% elemental calcium and is therefore less likely to be absorbed. Calcium carbonate chewable tablets supply 500 mg of elemental calcium. Most generic oyster-shell calcium preparations are adequate, although a few have been shown to be poorly absorbed because of an insoluble coating. A tablet should dissolve in household vinegar after 30 minutes; otherwise, it probably is not being absorbed when consumed.

The true benefit of calcium in the retardation of bone loss in menopausal women is unclear. Some studies have suggested that calcium supplementation might be useful,[73] while others have shown no real benefit except in women who are at least 6 years postmenopausal.[74] Of particular interest is the finding that calcium supplementation exerted no appreciable effect on spinal bone loss, suggesting no benefit of calcium augmentation in the prevention of vertebral crush fractures. However, a beneficial effect of calcium supplementation on the neck of the femur was shown.

To appropriately counsel a woman regarding HRT and prevention of osteoporosis, it is important to be able to determine her risk for fracture in later years. Estimates of bone density are reflective of the strength of the bone and can predict the future risk of fracture. The most accurate single technique for measurement of bone mineral density is quantitative digital radiography. Women with a bone mineral density less than .85 g/cm² are considered at high risk for bone fracture. Women with a bone mineral density of greater than 1.0 g/cm² are at low risk of fracture. Quantitative digital radiography is a painless, risk-free test that in some cases may be performed initially to establish a baseline and repeated 1 or 2 years later to determine the pace of bone loss. Bone density at a given age is predictive of bone density in that individual in later years.[75] Bone loss occurs on the average at a rate of 1% to 2% per year following cessation of ovarian function. Thus in a very short time a woman may be at risk for fracture, especially if she is receiving glucocorticoids, which further accelerate bone loss. For any woman this can be devastating, but particularly for women who experience estrogen deprivation due to premature menopause (as early as their 30s or early 40s) as a result of cancer treatment. Prevention of bone loss in these women is particularly challenging, as current medical practice

TABLE 8-3 Risk Assessment and Prevention of Cardiovascular Disease in Women

Risk Factor	Goal	Strategy	Estimated Risk
Estrogen deficiency	Equivalent of plasma E_2 50–200 pg/mL	Estrogen replacement unless contraindicated	50% lower risk in users compared to nonusers
Diet: high fat, high cholesterol	Balanced diet Moderate alcohol consumption	Lifestyle modifications Low-fat diet	24%–45% higher risk for those who consume alcohol daily
Cigarette smoking	Cessation of smoking	Prevention Education	50%–70% reduced risk in nonsmokers compared with current smokers
Obesity, especially abdominal fat	Achieve and maintain ideal body weight	Balanced diet Exercise	35%–55% lower risk compared to obese ($\geq 30\%$ above desirable weight) women
Lipids: unfavorable lipid profile	Total cholesterol ≤ 200 mg/dL HDL-C ≥ 55 mg/dL LDL-C ≤ 130 mg/dL	Low-fat diet Lipid- and cholesterol-lowering medications Weight reduction Modifications in lifestyle	2%–4.7% reduction per 1% decrease in total cholesterol or 1% increase in HDL-cholesterol
Sedentary lifestyle	Active lifestyle	Aerobic exercise 3–5 times per week at 60%–90% of the maximum heart rate for 20–30 minutes (running, walking, stair climbing, swimming)	45% lower risk
Acute thrombosis	Reduce the risk	Prophylactic low-dose aspirin	33% lower risk of heart disease

Data from Gorodeski GI, Utian WH. Epidemiology and risk factors of cardiovascular disease in post-menopausal women, in Lobos RA (ed): *Treatment of the Post-Menopausal Woman: Basic and Clinical Aspects.* New York: Raven Press, 1994, p. 215.[50]

recommends the use of alternatives to HRT for the treatment of menopausal sequelae. Bisphosphonates are being evaluated for their efficacy and safety as a nonhormonal option for the prevention of bone loss in women with breast cancer and premature menopause.[76,77] Findings suggest that bisphosphonates may prevent both trabecular and cortical bone loss in women whose menopause was induced by chemotherapy for breast cancer.[78]

Selective estrogen receptor modulator agents represent a new therapeutic avenue to treat the postmenopausal syndrome, potentially without the same cancer risks associated with HRT. One such medication, raloxifene, has been approved for the prevention of postmenopausal osteoporosis.[79] The drug also decreases total and LDL cholesterol levels. Because of raloxifene's estrogen antagonistic properties in uterine and breast tissues, preliminary data suggest that this potentially may be a safe HRT alternative for breast cancer survivors.[80] As with tamoxifen, there is a substantial reduction in the development of breast cancers in patients treated with raloxifene when compared to placebo.[81] Tamoxifen and raloxifene share estrogen antagonistic properties in the breast, vaginal tissues, and central nervous system. They also share estrogen agonistic properties in bone and liver. They differ in their estrogenicity in the uterus. Tamoxifen stimulates the endometrium, while raloxifen has no effect.[80]

Estrogen replacement therapy, usually with the addition of progestogen in women who still have their uterus, is the only established means of preventing bone loss in menopausal women. The nonsynthetic form of estrogen (conjugated estrogen) taken as an oral, percutaneous, subcutaneous, or transdermal preparation is beneficial in preventing bone loss. Estrogen's effect is most beneficial if started early in menopause. When continued for a period of up to at least 6 years, estrogen has demonstrated a 50%–70% reduction in osteoporosis-related fractures.[82] The benefit to the spine is less certain; however, long-term use (>10 years) reduces the incidence of vertebral deformity in postmenopausal women by about 90%.[83] If estrogen treatment is discontinued, bone loss begins again at an accelerated rate compared with average postmenopausal bone loss.

While estrogen therapy has been shown to be effective in preserving bone mass in elderly women, data from the Framingham study showed that estrogen therapy had little protective effect on bone density in women over 75 years of age, unless it was taken for 10 years or more.[84] In a prospective study of 9704 women aged 65 and older, Cauley et al.[85] determined that current use of estrogens reduces the risk for hip, wrist, and all nonspinal fractures, but estrogen is more effective if begun within 5 years of menopause and if used for longer than 10 years. HRT has also been noted to be associated with less radiologic evidence of osteoarthritis in the hips of users compared to nonusers.[86,87] (See Self-Care Guide, Osteoporosis: Maximizing the Health of Your Bones, Appendix 8A.)

Vasomotor instability

Hot flashes commonly occur in menopausal women and are the most common side effect of the antiestrogen tamoxifen. Women may experience headache or head pressure, sleep disturbances, and physical symptoms such as a flushed appearance with or without profuse perspiration on the forehead and chest. Initially, many women do not understand what is causing their symptoms. Some think they are having a heart attack if they wake up drenched with perspiration and with their heart pounding. This can be a frightening experience and is one that for many can be repeated ten or more times in a night. Given the option of HRT, relieving these symptoms has been found to be a stronger motivation for use than the long-term health advantages of reducing the risks of heart disease and osteoporosis.[88] HRT effectively eliminates the symptoms of vasomotor instability and bothersome hot flashes within the first cycle of treatment. For some, symptoms abate within days of beginning therapy. Valuing one's quality of life over quantity of life has implications for the approach to teaching and for probable compliance with therapy. Once the symptoms abate, motivation to be compliant with therapy diminishes. Emphasizing the long-term benefits of HRT is critically important to minimize the risk of noncompliance.

The combination of estrogen and progestin is the preferred approach to management of symptoms in the women with an intact uterus. The addition of progestin virtually eliminates the risk for endometrial cancer. In women who have undergone hysterectomy, the progestin is not needed.

Withdrawal bleeding may be a significant factor in a woman's decision to begin, continue, or discontinue HRT. Women on cyclic combination estrogen-progestin therapy commonly experience withdrawal bleeding on days 21 to 30 of the treatment cycle. In addition, the progestin is associated with increased complaints of depression and mood changes. In women who object to these symptoms, estrogen alone is safe, provided they are adequately monitored with yearly endometrial biopsies to assess for early endometrial hyperplasia. With continuous combination regimens, the incidence of breakthrough bleeding decreases with increased duration of treatment. Table 8-4 includes examples of estrogen and progestin replacement therapies.

HRT is generally contraindicated in a number of medical conditions, including recent stroke, recent myocardial infarction, breast cancer, acute liver disease, pancreatic disease, gallbladder disease, recent thromboembolic event, and undiagnosed vaginal bleeding. Relative contraindications include hypertension, endometrial hyperplasia, endometriosis, and pancreatitis. Table 8-5

includes alternative therapies for management of menopausal symptoms. These alternative measures, particularly those related to vasomotor instability such as hot flashes, sleeplessness, and mood swings are gaining in popularity.[89,90] A pilot study recently conducted by Loprinzi[91] demonstrated that the antidepressant venlafaxine (12.5 mg PO bid) reduced the incidence of hot flashes by 55% compared to placebo. The use of natural therapies such as diet, herbs, and homeopathy often appeals to women. The concern, of course, is that none of these alternative therapies has been studied scientifically, nor are the herbal remedies regulated in any way by the U.S. Food and Drug Administration. Herbs and other "natural" remedies falsely reassure some women, as they assume something natural cannot be harmful. What they do not realize is that most drugs and controlled substances come from natural sources, predominantly plants. Additionally, there is always concern regarding drug interactions and the bioavailability of phytoestrogens and their potential effect on quiescent estrogen receptor–positive breast cancer cells.

While management of vasomotor instability is the most common reason a woman may choose HRT, other benefits include reversal of genitourinary atrophy and dyspareunia. Vaginal dryness and dyspareunia affect nearly 40% of women in the decade following the menopause. Postmenopausal women have reduced levels of vaginal and vulva blood flow, and estrogen replacement therapy increases blood flow, which correlates with increased lubrication and decreased frequency and severity of dyspareunia. (See the Self-Care Guide, Managing the Symptoms of Menopause, Appendix 8B.)

HRT in the woman with a history of cancer

Women with cancer may develop estrogen deficiency as a result of natural menopause or prematurely as a consequence of surgery and cancer therapy. Although menopause in these women carries health risks similar to those in the general population, women who experience premature menopause will suffer longer with more risk for osteoporosis and heart disease, because risk is reactive to the age at which estrogen loss occurs. For women with a primary cancer that is not associated with hormonal dependence (e.g., lung cancer, colon cancer, leukemia, lymphoma), the use of HRT is not contraindicated. However, because they may fear cancer, they may be reluctant to inquire regarding the benefits of HRT or may stop taking their estrogens altogether. If the woman is currently taking HRT, she should continue unless there is a contraindication, such as obvious liver dysfunction, which warrants medical review in terms of her overall health risk.

Breast cancer Women with breast cancer are generally advised against receiving HRT because of concerns that estrogen may activate dormant cancer cells or micrometastases in hormone-sensitive breast tissue, or increase

TABLE 8-4   Hormone Replacement Therapy

Preparation	Dosage/Schedule	Side Effects	Comments
Oral Estrogens (natural)			
• Conjugated equine estrogen	0.625–2.5 mg/day: 3 weeks on, 1 week off	Breakthrough menstrual bleeding	• Estrogen may be poorly metabolized in impaired liver function.
• Piperazine estrone sulfate	0.625–2.5 mg/day	Premenstrual-like syndrome	• There is a 2-fold to 3-fold increase in gallbladder disease in women receiving oral estrogens.
• Micronized estradiol	1.2 mg/day 0.5 mg/day 1 mg/day 2 mg/day 3 weeks on, 1 week off	Vaginal candidiasis Nausea, vomiting, Bloating Cholestatic jaundice Intolerance to contact lenses Headache Dizziness Increase or decrease in weight Change in libido Unopposed estrogens can cause endometrial hyperplasia	• Photosensitivity may occur; encourage use of sunscreen and protective clothing. • Drug interactions may occur with anticoagulants, tricyclic antidepressants, barbiturates, and corticosteroids. • Endometrial surveillance is indicated in women with an intact uterus (every 2 years indefinitely). • Combining estrogen and progesterone in women with intact uteri prevents endometrial hyperplasia.
Vaginal Estrogens			
• Conjugated equine estrogen	0.625 mg/g 0.1 mg/g	Breast tenderness Bloating PMS-type symptoms Depression Weight gain Uterine bleeding	• Vaginal cream results in serum levels 25%–50% of those obtained with comparable oral doses. • Vaginal conjugated estrogens have diminished hepatic effects compared with oral preparations. • Vaginal preparations are most useful in the treatment of atrophic vaginitis.
• Premarin with methyltestosterone			
• Micronized estradiol			
Transdermal Estrogens			
• Transdermal estradiol	0.05 mg–0.1 mg applied to the skin twice weekly. Place adhesive side on a clean, dry area, preferably the abdomen. Rotate sites. Avoid the waistline and breasts.	Redness and irritation may occur at site of application	• Transdermal estrogens have minimal effect on clotting factors and are the preferable route of estrogen administration when procoagulant activity is increased. • Therapy may be continuous in women who do not have an intact uterus. In patients with an intact uterus therapy is given on a cyclic schedule (3 weeks on, 1 week off). • Estradiol levels drop after 2 days and may cause increased vasomotor instability. • Skin sensitivity may occur due to an allergic response to the adhesive or due to occlusion. • Compliance may be enhanced with transdermal application. • Decreases urinary excretion of calcium. • Estradiol transdermal patch affects serum LDL, HDL, and cholesterol very little.

the risk for a new primary breast cancer. This concern has yet to be clearly demonstrated by existing clinical evidence.[66]

At issue is whether there are subgroups of breast can-cer survivors for whom HRT is irrelevant to the course of their disease, yet who are denied the benefit of HRT because of historic and unproven hypotheses. The possibility that HRT may be safe in breast cancer survivors

TABLE 8-5 Alternative Methods for Management of Menopausal Symptoms

Agent or Application	Dosage/Schedule	Side Effects	Comments
Clonidine			
Alpha-2 adrenergic agonist • Reduces peripheral vasodilation • Marketed as an antihypertensive	0.05–0.15 mg/day at time of sleep or 1 mg tid	Dizziness Dry mouth Headache Nausea Fatigue Insomnia Potassium loss Irritability	• Avoid alcohol. • Associated with a 46% reduction in hot flashes. • Avoid excessive exercise in hot weather. • Take potassium supplement or drink orange juice.
Catapres transdermal patch	Catapres TTS 1, 2, or 3: 0.1, 0.2, or 0.3 mg/day; every 7 days apply to hairless area (back or arm)		
Venlafaxine	12.5 mg bid		• Has antidepressant properties.
Megestrol Acetate			
Progestational agent	20–40 mg/day PO	Bloating Irregular vaginal bleeding Breast tenderness Mood changes	• Significantly reduces incidence and frequency of hot flashes, lowers serum gonadotropins; does not improve vaginal atrophy.
Bellergal and Bellergal-S (long-acting)			
Combination of bella-donna alkaloids, ergotamine tartrate, phenobarbital	1 tablet in morning, 1 tablet in evening	Sedative effects Mouth dryness Blurred vision Potentially addictive	• Associated with a 60% reduction in hot flashes. • Because it decreases circulation to skin, fingers, and toes, women should dress warmly and avoid cigarette smoking. • Do not exercise excessively in hot weather; may cause overheating and dizziness. • If a dose is missed, do not take double dose.
Propranolol			
Beta-receptor blocking agent	60–80 mg/day PO	Light-headedness Fatigue Nausea occurs in 24% of patients	• Only slightly reduces hot flashes.
Lofexidine			
Alpha agonist and alpha methyldopa	1.6 mg bid	Dry mouth Fatigue Headache	• Can significantly reduce hot flashes. • Side effects limit usefulness.
Vitamin E	400 IU bid	Fatigue Weakness Nausea Headache Blurred vision Flatulence Diarrhea	• Avoid overdosing. • May relieve vaginal dryness. • Other vitamins (B and C) may also help relieve symptoms.
Ginseng			
A root; a source of plant estrogen	Capsule Tea Powder Syrup Root		• No clinical studies are available to evaluate effectiveness. Reports on efficacy are anecdotal. • Vitamin C may inactivate ginseng.

(continued)

TABLE 8-5 (continued)

Agent or Application	Dosage/Schedule	Side Effects	Comments
Black cohash, wild yams, dong quai, licorice root, evening primrose oil	variable		• contain plant estrogens • balancing hromones
Isoflavones	Variable	None	• Plant estrogens, soybeans
Biofeedback and Exercise Hypnotherapy/acupuncture			• Effect may be in stress reduction, lowering blood pressure, and reduction of headache.
Diet: avoid caffeine, alcohol, spicy foods			• Exercise is also beneficial to prevent bone loss.

is particularly important in the current management of the woman with a history of breast cancer. Adjuvant chemotherapy is prescribed more often now, based on favorable outcomes for women with small invasive but node-negative disease, even though it causes premature ovarian failure.[92] There is an increased incidence of breast cancer related to better screening techniques. The incidence of noninvasive and small, invasive axillary node–negative breast cancers has increased as well. With the known benefits of HRT and the lack of evidence suggesting a harmful effect of HRT on previously treated breast cancer, it is imperative that prospective trials be conducted to resolve the issue of the use of HRT in women with a history of breast cancer.[93,94]

Endometrial cancer Although endometrial cancer is commonly listed as a contraindication to estrogen replacement therapy, there is no evidence to substantiate this admonition. Many women who are cured of adenocarcinoma of the endometrium have frequent vasomotor symptoms secondary to bilateral oophorectomy. In addition, in postmenopausal women, vasomotor symptoms can develop following bilateral oophorectomy due to the removal of the androgens produced by the ovarian stroma. Estrogen therapy, either oral or as a transdermal patch, effectively relieves symptoms of menopause and can safely be given to most women with a history of endometrial cancer.[95,96]

Conclusion

Women's health issues are rapidly gaining attention in the professional as well as lay literature. Many women are also recognizing that, as they age, they are at risk for serious health problems such as osteoporosis and heart disease and that these diseases can threaten their long-term survival. Only recently have these issues begun to

receive the appropriate attention of health-care providers. Many menopausal women are turning to lay publications for information and advice for management of their menopausal symptoms, because their health-care providers have not inquired regarding their symptoms or have not recognized them as important problems that have a significant impact on quality of life. For others, the abundance of unproven methods are more attractive than the medicinal approach, which may be perceived as potentially harmful and less natural. Nurses must try to provide appropriate educational information that permits women to make informed decisions regarding their health.

The need for more women's health centers and menopause clinics is obvious. Women may feel embarrassed to speak about their menopausal symptoms with their physicians, especially male physicians, and prefer the comfort and perhaps the reassurance of women-only clinics.

A multidisciplinary approach to the problems of the aging woman includes:

- wellness through health promotion and early detection of disease

- prevention of heart disease and stroke through cardiovascular fitness and weight reduction

- education regarding lifestyle changes, such as smoking reduction and moderate alcohol consumption

- counseling regarding mental well-being, stress reduction, and sexual health

Oncology nurses are in a unique position to identify women at risk for the symptoms of menopause and for the serious health problems that may occur as a consequence of cancer treatment and the aging process. Recognizing the problems of menopausal women and the need to institute a multidisciplinary approach is the first step in the prevention and management of women's health issues.

References

1. U.S. Bureau of the Census: *Statistical Abstract of the United States: 1993* (ed 113). Washington, DC: Government Printing Office, 1993
2. Daly E, Gray A, Barlow D, et al: Measuring the impact of menopausal symptoms in quality of life. *BMJ* 307:836–840, 1993
3. Barrett-Connor E, Bush TL: Estrogen and coronary heart disease in women. *JAMA* 265:1861–1867, 1991
4. Belchetz PE: Hormonal treatment of post-menopausal women. *N Engl J Med* 300:1062–1071, 1994
5. Advance report of final mortality statistics 1989. *Monthly Vital Stat Rep* 40(suppl):1–47, 1992
6. DeSaia PJ: Hormone replacement therapy in patients with breast cancer. *Cancer* 71(suppl 4):1490–1500, 1993
7. Seshadri S, Wolf PA, Beiser A, et al: Life time risk of dementia and Alzheimer's disease. *Neurology* 49:1498–1504, 1997
8. Gambrell R: Endometrial cancer from ERT: An unfounded fear. *Menop Management* 11:13–15, 1989
9. DeSaia PJ, Grosen EA, Kurosaki T, et al: Hormone replacement therapy in breast cancer survivors: A cohort study. *Am J Obstet Gynecol* 174:1494–1498, 1996
10. Grodstein F, Stampfer MJ, Golditz GA, et al: Postmenopausal hormone therapy and mortality *N Engl J Med* 336:1769–1775, 1997
11. Barber HRK: Gynecologic problems, in Eskin BA (ed): *The Menopause: Comprehensive Management* (ed 3). New York: McGraw-Hill, 1994, pp. 183–210
12. Coulam CB, Adamson SC, Anneagers JF: Incidence of premature ovarian failure. *Obstet Gynecol* 67:604, 1986
13. Horning SJ, Negrin RS, Chao JC, et al: Fractionated total body irradiation, etoposide, and cyclophosphamide plus autografting in Hodgkin's disease and non-Hodgkin's lymphoma. *J Clin Oncol* 12:2552–2558, 1994
14. Seltzer VL, Benjamin F, Deutsch S: Perimenopausal bleeding patterns and pathologic findings. *J Am Med Wom Assoc* 45:132–134, 1990
15. Levrant SG, Barnes RB: Pharmacology of estrogens, in Lobos RA (ed): *Treatment of the Post-Menopausal Woman: Basic and Clinical Aspects.* New York: Raven Press, 1994, pp. 57–68
16. Kronenberg F, Cote LT, Linkie DM, et al: Menopausal hot flushes: Thermoregulatory, cardiovascular and circulating catecholamine and LH changes. *Maturitas* 6:31–43, 1984
17. Ravnikar V: Physiology and treatment of hot flushes. *Obstet Gynecol* 75(4 suppl):3S–8S, 1990
18. Ginsburg J, O'Reilly B, Swinhoe J: Effect of oral clonidine on human vascular responsiveness: A possible explanation of the therapeutic action of the drug in menopausal flushing and migraine. *Br J Obstet Gynaecol* 92:1169–1175, 1985
19. U.S. Congress Office of Technology Assessment: Menopause, Hormone Therapy, and Women's Health (OTA-BP-BA-88). Washington, DC: US Government Printing Office, May 1992
20. Formosa M, Brincat MP, Cardozo LD, et al: Collagen—The significance in skin, bones, and bladder, in Lobos RA (ed): *Treatment of the Post-Menopausal Woman: Basic and Clinical Aspects.* New York: Raven Press, 1994, pp. 143–149
21. Bachmann GA: Vulvovaginal complaints, in Lobos RA (ed): *Treatment of the Post-Menopausal Woman: Basic and Clinical Aspects.* New York: Raven Press, 1994, pp. 137–141
22. Leiblum SR, Bachmann GA: The sexuality of the climacteric woman, in Eskin BA (ed): *The Menopause: Comprehensive Management* (ed 3). New York: McGraw-Hill, 1994, pp. 137–154
23. Iosif CS, Beckassy Z: Prevalence of genito-urinary symptoms in the later menopause. *Acta Obstet Gynecol Scand* 63:257–260, 1984
24. Hallstrom T, Samuelsson S: Changes in women's sexual desire in middle life: The longitudinal study of women in Gothenberg. *Arch Sex Behav* 19:259–268, 1990
25. Nachtigall LE: Sexual function in the menopause and postmenopause, in Lobos RA (ed): *Treatment of the Post-Menopausal Woman: Basic and Clinical Aspects.* New York: Raven Press, 1994, pp. 301–306
26. Bachmann G, Leiblum S, Grill J: Brief sexual inquiry in gynecologic practice. *Obstet Gynecol* 73:425–427, 1989
27. Burger HG, Hailes J, Nelson J, et al: Effect of combined implants of estradiol and testosterone on libido in postmenopausal women. *Lancet* 294:936–937, 1987
28. Schmidt PJ, Rubinow DR: Menopause-related affective disorders: A justification for further study. *Am J Psychol* 148:844–852, 1991
29. Sherwin BB: Impact of the changing hormonal milieu on psychological functioning, in Lobos RA (ed): *Treatment of the Post-Menopausal Woman: Basic and Clinical Aspects.* New York: Raven Press, 1994, pp. 119–124
30. Teran AZ, Gambrell RD: Menopause, comprehensive management, in Eskin BA (ed): *The Menopause: Comprehensive Management* (ed 3). New York: McGraw-Hill, 1994, pp. 307–327
31. Goldman L, Tosteson ANA: Uncertainty about postmenopausal estrogen: Time for action not debate. *N Engl J Med* 325:800–802, 1991
32. Hunter MS: Emotional well-being, sexual behavior and hormone replacement therapy. *Maturitas* 12:299–314, 1990
33. McKinlay SM, Brambilla DJ, Pasher JG: The normal menopausal transition. *Maturitas* 14:103–115, 1992
34. Hunter M, Battersby R, Whitehead M: Relationships between psychological symptoms, somatic complaints and menopausal status. *Maturitas* 8:217–228, 1986
35. McKinlay JB, McKinlay SM, Brambilla D: The relative contribution of endocrine changes and social circumstances to depression in mid-aged women. *J Health Soc Behav* 28:345–363, 1987
36. Phillips S, Serwin BB: Effects of estrogen on memory function in surgically menopausal women. *Psychoneuroendocrinology* 17:485–495, 1992
37. Kawas C, Resnick S, Morrison A, et al: A prospective study of estrogen replacement therapy and risk of developing Alzheimer's disease: The Baltimore Longitudinal Study of Aging. *Neurology* 48:1517–1521, 1997
38. Tang MX, Jacobs D, Stern Y, et al: Effect of estrogen during menopause on risk and age at onset of Alzheimer's disease. *Lancet* 348:429–432, 1996
39. Baldereschi M, DiCarlo A, Lepore V, et al: Estrogen replacement therapy and Alzheimer's disease in the Italian Longitudinal Study on Aging. *Neurology* 50:996–1002, 1998
40. Sherwin BB, Phillips S: Estrogen and cognitive functioning in surgically menopausal women. *Ann NY Acad Sci* 592:474–475, 1990
41. Peck WA: Estrogen therapy after menopause. *J Am Med Wom Assoc* 45:87–90, 1990

42. Lindsay R, Cosman F: Osteoporosis: The estrogen relationship, in Swartz DP (ed): *Hormone Replacement Therapy*. Baltimore: Williams & Wilkins, 1992, pp. 17–28

43. Lindsay R: Pathophysiology of bone loss, in Lobos RA (ed): *Treatment of the Post-Menopausal Woman: Basic and Clinical Aspects*. New York: Raven Press, 1994, pp. 175–182

44. Grady D, Rubin SM, Petitti DB, et al: Hormone therapy to prevent disease and prolong life in postmenopausal women. *Ann Intern Med* 117:1016–1037, 1992

45. Smith HO, Kammerer-Doak DN, Barbo DM: Hormone replacement therapy in menopause: A pro opinion. *CA Cancer J Clin* 46:343–363, 1996

46. Ayanian JZ, Epstein AM: Differences in the use of procedures between women and men hospitalized for coronary heart disease. *N Engl J Med* 325:222–225, 1991

47. Steingart RM, Packer M, Hamm P, et al: Sex differences in the management of coronary artery disease. *N Engl J Med* 325:226–230, 1991

48. Maynard C, Litwin PE, Martin JS, et al: Gender differences in the treatment and outcome of acute myocardial infarction. *Arch Intern Med* 152:972–976, 1992

49. American Heart Association: *1993 Heart and Stroke Facts*. Dallas: American Heart Association National Center, 1993

50. Gorodeski GI, Utian WH: Epidemiology and risk factors of cardiovascular disease in post-menopausal women, in Lobos RA (ed): *Treatment of the Post-Menopausal Woman: Basic and Clinical Aspects*. New York: Raven Press, 1994, pp. 199–221

51. Gilligan DM, Badar DM, Panza JA, et al: Acute vascular effects of estrogen in postmenopausal women. *Circulation* 90:786–791, 1994

52. Isles CG, Hole DJ, Hawthorne VM, et al: Relation between coronary risk and coronary mortality in women of the Renfrew and Paisley Survey: Comparison with men. *Lancet* 339:702–706, 1992

53. Jensen J, Nilas L, Christiansen C: Influence of menopause on serum lipids and lipoproteins. *Maturitas* 12:321–331, 1990

54. Manson JE, Tosteson H, Ridker PM, et al: The primary prevention of myocardial infarction. *N Engl J Med* 326:1406–1416, 1992

55. Kannel WB, Wilson PWF, Zhang TJ: The epidemiology of impaired glucose tolerance and hypertension. *Am Heart J* 121:1268–1273, 1991

56. LaCroix AZ, Lang J, Scherr P, et al: Smoking and mortality among older men and women in three communities. *N Engl J Med* 324:1619–1625, 1991

57. Landis S, Murray J, Bolden S, et al: Cancer Statistics 1998. *CA Cancer J Clin* 48:6–29, 1998

58. Newcomb PA, Lantz PM: Recent trends in breast cancer incidence, mortality and mammography. *Breast Cancer Research and Treatment* 28:97–106, 1993

59. Bonadonna G, Valagussa P, Moliterni A, et al: Adjuvant cyclophosphamide, methotrexate and fluorouracil in node-positive breast cancer. *N Engl J Med* 332:901–906, 1995

60. Vassilopoulou-Sellin R: Estrogen replacement therapy in women at increased risk for breast cancer. *Breast Cancer Research and Treatment* 28:167–177, 1993

61. Bergkvist L, Hoover R, Persson I, et al: Risk of cancer in women receiving hormone replacement therapy. *Int J Cancer* 44:833–839, 1989

62. Gambrell RD: Use of progesterone therapy. *Am J Obstet Gynecol* 156:1304–1313, 1987

63. Steinberg KK, Thacker SB, Smith SJ, et al: A meta-analysis of the effect of estrogen replacement therapy on the risk of breast cancer. *JAMA* 265:1985–1990, 1991

64. Dupont WD, Page DL: Menopausal estrogen replacement therapy and breast cancer. *Arch Intern Med* 151:67–72, 1991

65. Zumoff B: Biological and endocrinological insights into the possible cancer risk from menopausal estrogen replacement therapy. *Steroids* 58:196–204, 1993

66. Cobleigh A: Hormone replacement therapy in breast cancer survivors. *Dis Breast* 1:1–10, 1997

67. Cummings SR, Black DM, Rubin SM: Lifetime risks of hip, Colles' or vertebral fracture and coronary heart disease among white post-menopausal women. *Arch Intern Med* 149:2445–2448, 1989

68. Walsh BW, Schiff I, Rosner B, et al: Effects of postmenopausal estrogen replacement on the concentration and metabolism of plasma lipoproteins. *N Engl J Med* 325:1196–1204, 1991

69. Hong MK, Romm PA, Reagan K, et al: Effects of estrogen replacement therapy on serum lipid values and angiographically defined coronary artery disease in post-menopausal women. *Am J Cardiol* 69:176–178, 1992

70. Lieberman EH, Gerhard MD, Uehata A, et al: Estrogen improves endothelium-dependent flow-mediated vasodilation in post-menopausal women. *Ann Intern Med* 121:936–941, 1994

71. Wren BG: Effects of estrogen and management of hypertension in women, in Lobos RA (ed): *Treatment of the Post-Menopausal Woman: Basic and Clinical Aspects*. New York: Raven Press, 1994, pp. 283–285

72. Eaker ED, Chesebro JH, Sacks FM, et al: Cardiovascular disease in women. *Circulation* 88:1999–2009, 1993

73. Aloia JF, Vaswani A, Yeh JK, et al: Calcium supplementation with and without hormone replacement therapy to prevent postmenopausal bone loss. *Ann Intern Med* 120:97–103, 1994

74. Dawson-Hughs B, Dallal GE, Krall EA, et al: A controlled trial of the effect of calcium supplementation on bone density in postmenopausal women. *N Engl J Med* 323:878–883, 1990

75. Lindsay R, Cosman F: Osteoporosis: The estrogen relationship, in Swartz DP (ed): *Hormone Replacement Therapy*. Baltimore: Williams & Wilkins, 1992, p. 17

76. Bachmann GA: Non-hormonal alternatives for the management of early menopause in younger women with breast cancer. *Monogr Natl Cancer Inst* 16:161–171, 1994

77. Singer FR, Minoofar PN: Bisphosphonates in the treatment of disorders of mineral metabolism. *Adv Endocrinol Metab* 6:259–288, 1995

78. Delmas PD, Balena R, Confravreux E, et al: Bisphosphonate Risedronate prevents bone loss in women with artificial menopause due to chemotherapy of breast cancer: A double blind placebo controlled study. *J Clin Oncol* 15:955–962, 1997

79. Bryant HU, Dere WH: Selective estrogen receptor modulators: An alternative to hormone replacement therapy. *Proc Soc Exper Biol Med* 217:45–52, 1998

80. Delmas PD, Bjarnason BH, Mitlak AC, et al: Effects of raloxifene on bone mineral density, serum cholesterol concentrations, and uterine endometrium in postmenopausal women. *N Engl J Med* 337:1641–1647, 1997

81. Cummings SR, Norton L, Eckert S, et al: Raloxifene reduces the risk of breast cancer and may decrease the risk of endometrial cancer in post-menopausal women. Two year findings from raloxifene evaluation (MORE) trial. *Proc Am Soc Clin Oncol* (abstract 3):2, 1998

82. Roy JA, Sawka CA, Pritchard DE: Hormone replacement therapy in women with breast cancer: Do the risks outweigh the benefits? *J Clin Oncol* 14:997–1006, 1996

83. Consensus Development Conference: Prophylaxis and treatment of osteoporosis. *Am J Med* 90:107–110, 1991

84. Felson DT, Zhang Y, Hannon MT, et al: The effect of postmenopausal estrogen therapy on bone density in elderly women. *N Engl J Med* 329:1141–1146, 1993

85. Cauley JA, Seeley DG, Ensrud K, et al: Estrogen replacement therapy and fractures in older women. *Ann Intern Med* 122:9–16, 1995

86. Mayeaux E, Johnson C: Current concepts in postmenopausal hormone replacement therapy. *J Fam Pract* 43:69–75, 1996

87. Nevitt MC, Cummings SR, Lane NE, et al: Association of estrogen replacement therapy with the risk of osteoarthritis of the hip in elderly white women. *Arch Intern Med* 156:2073–2080, 1996

88. Rothert M, Rovner D, Holmes M, et al: Women's use of information regarding hormone replacement therapy. *Res Nurs Health* 13:355–366, 1990

89. Soffa VM: Alternatives to hormone replacement for menopause. *Altern Ther Health Med* 2:34–39, 1996

90. Soltes BA: Therapeutic options for menopause in cancer survivors. *Cancer Nursing Updates.* 4:1–12, 1997

91. Loprinzi CL, Pisansky TM, Fonseca R, et al: A pilot evaluation of venlafaxine HCL for the therapy of hot flashes in cancer survivors. *J Clin Oncol* 16:2377–2381, 1998

92. Early Breast Cancer Trialists' Collaborative Group: Systemic treatment of early breast cancer by hormonal, cytotoxic or immune therapy: 133 randomized trials involving 31,000 recurrences and 24,000 deaths among 75,000 women. *Lancet* 399:1–15, 71–85, 1992

93. Wile AG, Opfell RW, Margileth DA: Hormone replacement therapy in previously treated breast cancer patients. *Am J Surg* 165:372–375, 1993

94. Cobleigh MA, Berris RF, Bush T, et al: Estrogen replacement therapy in breast cancer survivors: A time for change. *JAMA* 272:540–545, 1994

95. Baker DP: Estrogen replacement therapy in patients with previous endometrial carcinoma. *Compr Ther* 16:28–35, 1990

96. *Committee Opinion, Number 80.* Washington, DC: American College of Obstetricians and Gynecologists, Feb 1990

Osteoporosis—Maximizing the Health of Your Bones

Patient Name: _____

Symptom and Description   Before menopause, the body naturally replaces old bone with new bone. With the change of life the body begins to lose estrogen, and there is a rapid loss of bone mass. The bone becomes more thin and frail. A woman's risk for bone fracture in the hips, spine, and wrist increases each year after the change.

As a woman ages, the body is also less able to absorb calcium. At the same time there is a loss of calcium from the bones. This further weakens the bones. Low calcium can cause osteoporosis. Steroid therapy can also cause osteoporosis because steroids increase bone loss, reduce calcium absorption, and make bones more frail and likely to break. Thyroid hormone therapy is also associated with increased risk.

All causes of estrogen loss—change of life, removal of the ovaries, chemotherapy, or radiation therapy—result in loss of bone, usually in the first 2 years after loss of estrogen. Even though hormone replacement is the only way to restore bone strength, there are some things you can do to help maintain or even partially restore healthy bone.

Learning Needs   To maintain or restore bone strength, you need to know whether you are at significant risk for bone loss and fracture.

1. White and Asian women with small frames who are at or below their ideal weight are at risk for bone loss. Black women have less risk because their bones are more dense.
2. Bone mineral density studies are painless and can predict risk for fracture and may be advised if you are approaching the change or having symptoms. Your doctor may recommend a baseline bone test with a repeat of the test in 2 years to determine your rate of bone loss.
3. Women who have eating disorders or who eat foods low in calcium, drink high-caffeine beverages, drink alcohol, or smoke cigarettes are at high risk for bone loss and bone fracture with aging.
4. Lack of physical exercise can lead to bone loss and calcium loss.
5. Women who for personal or health reasons are unable to take hormone replacement therapy are at high risk, depending on their other risk factors.

Management

1. If hormone therapy is prescribed, it must be continued as ordered by your doctor. When hormone therapy is stopped, bone loss resumes. Do not stop your hormone therapy before consulting with your doctor.
2. Tamoxifen, because of its estrogen-like action helps to prevent the bone loss that occurs with menopause. It also helps prevent breast cancer.
3. Raloxifene is proven to prevent osteoporosis in postmenopausal women. It may also prevent breast cancer.

(continued) 113

4. Aredia is given to prevent bone loss, promote bone healing, and perhaps prevent bone metastases.

5. Most women take in only 400–500 mg of calcium daily. Premenopausal women should supplement their diet with 500-1000 mg of calcium a day. Postmenopausal women should add 1500 mg of calcium a day because of reduced calcium absorption. Two Tums 500 supplies 2500 mg calcium carbonate, which provides 1000 mg of calcium. Three tablets provide 3750 mg calcium carbonate, which provides 1500 mg of calcium.

6. Alendronate sodium (Fosamax) may be taken in combination with calcium citrate (Citracal) if osteoporosis is present. Calcium supplements should be taken with food. Orange juice or other acidic foods are especially helpful in aiding absorption.

7. For most people, the average diet and some sunlight exposure provide adequate vitamin D, which is necessary to absorb calcium. Multivitamins with vitamin D, 400 IU daily, may be taken if necessary.

8. Most generic oyster-shell calcium is absorbed. If your calcium tablet does not dissolve in household vinegar after 30 minutes with gentle stirring, select one that does.

9. If you have a history of renal stones, consult your doctor before taking added calcium.

10. Try to eat calcium-rich, low-fat foods, yogurt, cottage cheese, skim milk (with vitamin D), and juices and cereals with added calcium. Minimize caffeine intake. Avoid cola drinks and chocolate as well as red meats, which contain high levels of phosphorus, which affects calcium absorption.

11. Exercise may help to increase bone strength. Stair climbing, racket sports, impact aerobics, jogging, weight training, and dancing are advised. Swimming, walking, and cycling help your heart but do not increase bone strength.

12. If you have weak bones or have had a bone fracture consult your doctor regarding an exercise program.

13. Thirty to 60 minutes of exercise 3 to 4 times a week helps to strengthen bone.

14. Exercise may also help to improve coordination, balance, and muscular strength, which help to decrease the likelihood of falls.

15. If you smoke cigarettes or drink alcohol daily, ask your nurse or doctor about ways you can learn to stop smoking or to drink alcohol in moderation.

Follow-up   Consult your doctor if you experience any unpleasant side effects from your medications such as stomach upset or diarrhea.

Phone Numbers

Nurse: _____ Phone: _____

Physician: _____ Phone: _____

Other: _____ Phone: _____

Comments

Patient's Signature: _____ Date: _____

Nurse's Signature: _____ Date: _____

Source: Goodman M: Menopausal symptoms, in Yarbro CH, Frogge MH, Goodman M, (eds): *Cancer Symptom Management.* (ed 2) Sudbury: Jones and Bartlett, 1999 © Jones and Bartlett Publishers.

Managing the Symptoms of Menopause

Patient Name: _____

Symptom and Description   As menopause approaches, whether it is a natural process of aging, the result of surgical removal of the ovaries, or the effects of radiation or chemotherapy, many women will have symptoms of estrogen loss.

While every woman will experience menopause in her own way, most will have hot flashes—ranging from rarely to more than ten times a day. Hot flashes are often worse at night and can disrupt sleep, causing mood changes and difficulty making decisions. Some women will complain of anxiety and even periods of depression. These symptoms will improve over time.

Other problems can occur because of estrogen loss. The vagina becomes shortened and more dry. These changes can cause itching and burning and can interfere with comfortable sexual intercourse. A woman may also experience more vaginal and bladder infections.

Other symptoms include headache, dizziness, skin changes, and thinning of the scalp and pubic hair.

Management   The best way to manage the symptoms of menopause is to restore the body's level of estrogen. This can be done by taking a pill (e.g., Premarin), by applying an estrogen patch to the skin twice a week, or by using a vaginal cream. However, estrogen therapy is not for every woman. Some women prefer to try other means of learning to live with the change of life. Your doctor will help you make the choice that is best for you. The following suggestions may help you with your symptoms of menopause.

1. *Hormone replacement:* Estrogen therapy is given for menopause symptoms but also to prevent heart disease, stroke, and frail bones. If estrogen therapy has been prescribed for you, it is important that you continue therapy as prescribed. If you have not had a hysterectomy, you may also need to take progesterone. The purpose of this drug is to shed the lining of the uterus once a month, which means you will once again start to menstruate. This is normal and helps to prevent uterine cancer. If you choose not to take progesterone (as some women do because it can cause mood changes and depression), you will need to be examined regularly to ensure a healthy uterus. If you have had your uterus removed you do not need to take progesterone.

2. *Vitamin E:* Vitamin E, 400 IU twice a day, has been found by some women to increase energy and help minimize hot flashes and vaginal dryness.

3. *Venlafaxine:* 12.5 mg twice a day may help to minimize hot flashes and is an antidepressant.

4. *Clonidine:* Clonidine is a drug taken to manage high blood pressure. It can also help to relieve hot flashes in some women. It should be taken at nighttime,

(continued)

because it can cause light-headedness. This drug is also available as a patch. It requires a prescription from your doctor (0.1 mg patch once a week).

5. *Bellergal:* Bellergal is sometimes used to minimize hot flashes but can cause mouth dryness, blurred vision, and sedation. Do not use with alcohol. It requires a prescription from your doctor.

6. *Diet, vitamins, and herbs:* A multivitamin may be added each day to your diet, but large doses can be harmful. Ask your doctor before starting higher doses of vitamins. Try to limit caffeine from all sources (colas, coffee, and chocolate) and avoid hot, spicy foods and alcohol. All can trigger hot flashes.

   Ginseng root is a natural plant estrogen and is available as a tea, capsule, powder, or syrup. Some women feel it helps to control their hot flashes. Other possibly helpful but unproven methods to minimize hot flashes include garlic, hops, catnip, chamomile, passion flower, black cohash, wild yams, dong quai, licorice root, and evening primrose oil.

7. *Biofeedback and relaxation:* Stress has been known to increase the frequency and intensity of hot flashes and tension headaches. Learning biofeedback techniques can help to reduce stress. Relaxation tapes have helped some women to ease the severity of their hot flashes and to cope with the normal tensions of life.

8. *Exercise:* Many women are sedentary and do not exercise regularly. No matter what a woman's age, there is an exercise to enhance well-being and general health. Consult your doctor before engaging in strenuous sports, but begin a program that fits your lifestyle and abilities.

9. *Vaginal lubricants:* It is not uncommon for women to notice a lack of sexual desire and passion during the menopausal years. Some women have pain during sex and may even notice bleeding afterward. Orgasm may occur less often, especially in women who also are diabetic. The male partner may also abstain from sexual intercourse for fear of hurting the woman. While other factors such as stress, fatigue, and each other's general health will play a role in sexual relationships, most women prefer to maintain a healthy sexual relationship with their partner. Women who continue to have sexual intercourse throughout menopause experience fewer vaginal changes than women who abstain or have sex only infrequently.

   - Vaginal estrogen creams are useful to reverse vaginal changes. A start-up dose of estrogen cream, 2–4 grams nightly for 1 to 2 weeks, followed by 2 grams once or twice a week will help to restore vaginal health.

   - Personal lubricant, Lubrin, K-Y Jelly, or Astroglide will temporarily relieve vaginal dryness during sexual intercourse. Apply liberally and as often as necessary to prevent discomfort and irritation during sexual intercourse.

   - Replens is applied 2 to 3 times per week and restores vaginal moisture and comfort but should not be used as a lubricant during sexual intercourse.

   - Sitz baths followed by Burrow's solution applications help to relieve itching and irritation.

   - Cotton undergarments should be worn and tight garments made of synthetic materials (girdles) and pantyhose should be worn only if necessary.

   - Kegel exercises may help to strengthen the muscles that control bladder relaxation and can help reduce urinary accidents when you laugh, cough, or strain. Ask your nurse or doctor for information.

Many women will benefit from counseling with a trained professional. Women's health centers are available throughout the country and help women to both understand and cope with menopause. Occasionally, women will find that antidepressants and antianxiety drugs help to improve their mood and level of anxiety. A woman should speak openly about her concerns regarding her health during menopause and in general. Seeking help and guidance from your physician and members of your health team will help you make informed decisions regarding your health.

Follow-up   Report the following symptoms to your doctor or nurse:

Chronic vaginal discharge

Vaginal itching, burning, and irritation

Urinary frequency and burning

Depression

Anxiety

Insomnia

Light-headedness

Headaches

Symptoms of gallbladder disease:

Right upper quadrant pain

Indigestion

Burping

Nausea

Phone Numbers

Nurse: _____ Phone: _____

Physician: _____ Phone: _____

Psychologist/Social Worker: _____ Phone: _____

Women's Health Center/Menopause Clinic: _____ Phone: _____

Comments

Patient's Signature: _____ Date: _____

Nurse's Signature: _____ Date: _____

Source: Goodman M: Menopausal symptoms, in Yarbro CH, Frogge MH, Goodman M (eds): *Cancer Symptom Management.* Sudbury: Jones and Bartlett, 1999. © Jones and Bartlett Publishers.

CHAPTER 9

Pain

Judith A. Paice, RN, PhD, FAAN

The Problem of Pain in Cancer

Of the many symptoms associated with cancer, pain is the most feared. Although it is relatively common, the majority of those persons experiencing cancer-related pain can and do obtain relief. Healthcare professionals caring for these individuals must be cognizant of the incidence of cancer pain, barriers to its relief, and assessment and management techniques, as well as resources for providing optimal care.

Incidence of Pain in Cancer

Pain is experienced by approximately one-third of persons receiving treatment for cancer and two-thirds of those with advanced disease.[1-7] More recent studies have evaluated the characteristics of those individuals at risk for poor pain control. Cleeland et al.[8] interviewed 1308 outpatients with metastatic cancer treated at 54 oncology centers affiliated with the Eastern Cooperative Oncology Group (ECOG). Physicians were also interviewed regarding their assessment of their patient's pain intensity, the treatment used to relieve pain, and the impact of pain on the patient's ability to function. Of those persons studied, 67% had experienced pain during the week preceding the interview and 36% had pain significant enough to decrease functioning. Using the World Health Organization guidelines for cancer pain management to determine whether analgesic regimens were appropriate,

42% of these outpatients studied received inadequate analgesic therapy.

Several factors in this study were predictive of poor pain control, including discrepancies between the physician's and patient's assessment of pain intensity, and the presence of pain that was perceived by the physician to be unrelated to the cancer. Furthermore, minorities, the elderly, females, and those with better performance levels were individuals at risk for poor pain relief.

The benefits of such studies include heightened awareness of those individuals at risk for unrelieved cancer pain. However, the reasons for these inadequacies also demand further investigation so that this problem may be corrected. Many studies have identified barriers to adequate pain relief, including those related to the healthcare professional, the patient, and the healthcare system.

Barriers to Adequate Analgesia

The reasons for unrelieved pain are many, including lack of knowledge by healthcare professionals regarding pain and its management and misguided fears and attitudes about the use of opioids. Compounding these professional-related barriers are obstacles related to the individual and to the healthcare system (Table 9-1).

Barriers related to healthcare professionals

Numerous studies have documented the lack of basic pain education received by nurses and physicians, as well

TABLE 9-1 Barriers to Cancer Pain Management

Problems Related to Healthcare Professionals

Inadequate knowledge of pain management
Poor assessment of pain
Concern about regulation of controlled substances
Fear of patient addiction
Concern about side effects of analgesics
Concern about patients becoming tolerant to analgesics

Problems Related to Patients

Reluctance to report pain
    Concern about distracting physicians from treatment of underlying disease
    Fear that pain means the disease is worse
    Concern about not being a "good" patient
Reluctance to take pain medications
    Fear of addiction or of being thought of as an addict
    Worries about unmanageable side effects
    Concern about becoming tolerant to pain medications

Problems Related to the Healthcare System

Low priority given to cancer pain treatment
Inadequate reimbursement
The most appropriate treatment may not be reimbursed or may be too costly for patients and families
Restrictive regulation of controlled substances
Problems of availability of treatment or access to it

Reprinted from Jacox A, Carr DB, Payne R, et al: *Management of Cancer Pain. Clinical Practice Guideline No. 9.* AHCPR Publication No. 94-0592. Rockville, MD: Agency for Health Care Policy and Research, Public Health Service, U.S. Department of Health and Human Services, March 1994.[9]

as the resultant lack of knowledge regarding pain and its management expressed by these professionals.[10–20] Misconceptions regarding side effects of opioids, particularly respiratory depression, and overestimating the incidence of addiction are particularly troublesome, as these fears lead to reduced delivery of medication to individuals with cancer.[21]

Another barrier related to healthcare professionals is the lack of systematic assessment of pain, leading to discrepancies between patient reports and professional observations.[2,22–24] For example, professionals may expect the person in pain to exhibit physical findings—such as altered vital signs, grimacing, or guarding behaviors—that are unusual in chronic pain. The professional's own past pain experiences may also affect their assessment of another's pain. Nurses who had experienced intense pain were more likely to report higher pain scores for their patients.[25]

Barriers related to the individual

The public perceives cancer as a very painful disease, yet believes that taking opioids to relieve pain will lead to addiction.[26] Therefore, it is not surprising that when these individuals become patients, they are reluctant to admit to having pain and may take less medication than ordered. A recent study of patient-related barriers to adequate analgesia found that older, less educated, lower-income individuals were more likely to have concerns regarding pain and using pain medication.[27] In a study

of oncologists, 62% cited patient reluctance to report pain as an obstacle to adequate relief.[28]

Barriers related to the healthcare system

Access to necessary medications may be limited in some regions. Regulatory barriers to obtaining essential medications, specifically the need for special, multiple-copy prescriptions, lead to the prescribing of fewer opioids. Prescribers fear that regulatory agencies will judge prescribing large doses of opioids to be inappropriate and that the prescriber will be punished for such behavior.[29] Ambiguity in the laws regarding opioid prescription further compound the problem.

Impact of Pain on Quality of Life

Unrelieved pain resulting from the numerous barriers to treatment affects all aspects of an individual's life. Several studies indicate that cancer pain is significantly correlated with fatigue, anxiety, emotional distress, mood disorders, depression, fewer social interactions, and altered family activities.[3,30–32] As a result, people experiencing cancer-related pain report reduced quality of life when compared with those individuals free of pain.[33]

In an examination of suffering in the advanced cancer patient, a phenomenon that occurs when quality of life is diminished, Cherny et al.[34] describe the interrelation-

TABLE 9-2 Etiology of Chronic Cancer Pain

Pain Association with Tumor

Bone pain due to primary or metastatic lesions
Headache and facial pain related to primary or metastatic lesions of the brain, skull, or cranial nerves
Plexopathies and neuropathies due to tumor involvement of the peripheral nervous system
Visceral pain due to invasion of tumor within abdominal organs or to obstruction
Paraneoplastic syndromes such as tumor-related gynecomastia

Pain Associated with Cancer Therapy

Postchemotherapy pain syndromes
   Chronic painful peripheral neuropathy
   Avascular necrosis of femoral or humeral head
   Plexopathy associated with intraarterial infusion
   Peripheral neuropathy after vinca alkaloids or taxol therapy
Hormonal therapy–associated pain
   Gynecomastia with hormonal therapy for prostate cancer
Postsurgical pain syndromes
   Postmastectomy pain syndrome
   Postradical neck dissection pain
   Postthoracotomy pain
   Postoperative frozen shoulder
   Phantom pain syndromes
   Stump pain
   Postsurgical pelvic floor myalgia
Postradiation pain syndromes
   Plexopathies
   Chronic radiation myelopathy
   Chronic radiation enteritis and proctitis
   Burning perineum syndrome
   Osteoradionecrosis

Pain Unrelated to Cancer or Its Treatment (selected examples)

Musculoskeletal disorders, such as arthritis, activity-induced strains
Chronic headaches

Reprinted from Cherny NI, Portenoy RK: Principles of assessment and syndromes, in Wall PD, Melzack R (eds): *Textbook of Pain* (ed 3). Pp. 798–799, 1994, by permission of the publisher Churchill Livingstone.[36]

ship of the distress experienced by patient, family, and healthcare provider. When multiple factors, predominantly pain, contribute to the patient's distress, the distress of family members and healthcare providers also increases as a result of witnessing this discomfort. Over time, this may lead to caregiver fatigue in family members and burnout in healthcare professionals. Thus, the devastating effects of suffering and unrelieved pain extend beyond the patient, affecting family and professionals involved in their care. A qualitative study of cancer pain management in the home revealed that family members report intense physical and psychological burdens when caring for loved ones in pain, and home-care nurses describe emotional and spiritual pain while managing patients' pain in this setting.[35]

Etiology

Cancer pain can result from three primary etiologies. The majority of pain experienced by individuals with cancer originates directly from the tumor[36] (Table 9-2). Pain can also occur as a result of therapy aimed at reducing the tumor, including surgery, chemotherapy, radiation therapy, immunotherapy, and biological therapy. For example, anthracycline chemotherapeutics can produce a painful flare reaction,[37] and hormonal therapy often leads to an acute onset of generalized bone pain in those being treated for prostate cancer.[38] Finally, people with cancer can develop pain totally unrelated to the cancer or its treatment. Examples include the development of appendicitis or strained muscles from lifting a heavy object.

Pain can further be categorized as acute or chronic in duration. *Acute pain,* generally defined as occurring less than 1 to 3 months, is typically associated with some type of warning sign and is more closely associated with anxiety.[39] *Chronic pain* persists long past its potential usefulness and is more commonly correlated with depression.[40]

Finally, pain can be classified as nociceptive or neuropathic, according to the terms people use to describe the sensation, often suggesting an etiology. *Nociceptive pain* can be somatic or visceral in nature.[36] For example, localized somatic pain described as aching or throbbing may be due to musculoskeletal changes. Squeezing, gnawing, or cramping pain in the abdomen may be due to pressure on organ capsules or stretching of the mesentery or other visceral structures. *Neuropathic pain,* referred to as tingling, burning, electrical, or shooting, suggests nerve damage.[41]

Pathophysiology

Much remains unknown regarding the pathophysiology of cancer pain, and research continues to explore changes that occur within the nervous system as well as therapies that might reduce pain. The pathophysiology of pain associated with acute trauma is better understood; however, chronic pain elicits long-term changes within the nervous system that perpetuate the sensation long after the stimuli are removed.

Acute Pain

During an acute episode of mechanical trauma, such as the scalpel blade cutting through skin during surgery, substances that excite or sensitize sensory nerve endings are released in the periphery. These include prostaglandins, serotonin, histamine, bradykinin, substance P, and others.[42] The rationale for using corticosteroids and nonsteroidal antiinflammatory drugs (NSAIDs) is based on the release of prostaglandins: these agents work by different mechanisms to block the formation of prostaglandins, thereby blocking pain[43] (Figure 9-1).

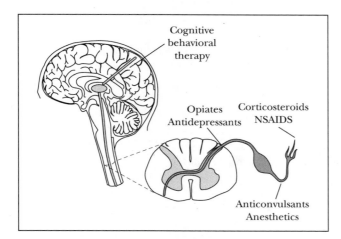

FIGURE 9-1 Pain pathophysiology and primary location of action of analgesic therapies. Pain is transmitted by sensory neurons through the periphery to the dorsal horn of the spinal cord, where they synapse with ascending nerve tracts. These tracts continue transmission to the thalamus and various areas of the cortex. Analgesics act at various points in this pathway to reduce pain.

With intense stimulation of the sensory nerve endings, the neurons involved are excited; they depolarize and transmit the painful message through the peripheral nervous system to the spinal cord. Anticonvulsants and local anesthetics act to block the transfer of ions across the neuronal membrane, preventing depolarization, or firing, of these sensory nerves.[44]

Transmission along the nerve fiber continues to, and terminates within, the dorsal horn of the spinal cord. In the spinal cord, neurotransmitters, excitatory amino acids, and other substances are released.[45] This causes excitation within other nerve tracts that ascend to the brain stem and thalamus, continuing transmission of the message to higher centers. Administering opioids blocks the release of neurotransmitters, preventing continuation of pain transmission.[46] The message is then blocked at the level of the spinal cord and does not reach the brain, where it is believed perception of painful events occurs.

The body can diminish pain perception through modulatory systems, often called descending systems, that project downward from various areas within the brain. For example, neurons within the pons and medulla project axons caudally to the dorsal horn of the spinal cord, where they release substances such as serotonin and norepinephrine.[47] The rationale for giving epidural or intrathecal clonidine, an α_2-noradrenergic agonist, is based on the analgesic action of norepinephrine within the spinal cord. Unfortunately, the systemic effects of such a drug can lead to vascular dilatation and orthostatic hypotension.[48] Another method for relieving pain based on the modulatory system increases the availability of endogenous norepinephrine and serotonin. Tricyclic antidepressants block the reuptake of these substances, making more available within the synapse in the dorsal horn.[49]

Chronic Pain

Occasionally, pain persists long after the initial stimulus has diminished. For example, in postmastectomy pain syndrome an individual continues to experience pain months, and possibly years, after the incision has healed. Research is beginning to reveal several mechanisms that may explain the persistence of pain after the organic cause is removed. Direct damage along the neuron may lead to sites that generate ectopic impulses.[50] Prolonged activation of sensory neurons, with continued release of excitatory amino acids, leads to increased intracellular calcium.[51] This can also lead to irreversible neuronal damage and may be a mechanism for neuropathic pain. Many other mechanisms are currently under study for their possible role in chronic pain; once the underlying pathophysiology is understood, treatment can more effectively be designed.

Assessment

The first essential step in providing relief is to assess the individual's pain. The Agency for Health Care Policy and Research (AHCPR) *Management of Cancer Pain Clinical Practice Guideline*[9] reflects the importance of pain assessment in the following "ABCDE" mnemonic:

A   Ask about pain regularly.
     Assess pain systematically.
B   Believe the patient and family in their reports of pain and what relieves it.
C   Choose pain-control options appropriate for the patient, family, and setting.
D   Deliver interventions in a timely, logical, and coordinated fashion.
E   Empower patients and their families.
     Enable them to control their course to the greatest extent possible.

Components of the pain assessment include the use of unidimensional tools that measure intensity along with multidimensional instruments that determine various aspects of the pain, such as the quality of the sensation, duration, and the effect pain has had on other aspects of the person's life. These tools are used to obtain a complete pain history. Other essential components of assessment include a comprehensive physical examination and diagnostic evaluation (Table 9-3).

Measurement Tools

Unidimensional measures

Several simple tools are available to quantify the intensity of pain, including a numeric rating scale (NRS), a visual analog scale (VAS), and a verbal descriptor scale (VDS) (Figure 9-2).[52] Although the VAS is frequently used in research studies of pain and its treatment, it may be difficult for some patients to complete due to motor

TABLE 9-3 Initial Pain Assessment

Assessment of Pain Intensity and Character

1. **Onset and temporal pattern**—When did your pain start? How often does it occur? Has its intensity changed?
2. **Location**—Where is your pain? Is there more than one site?
3. **Description**—What does your pain feel like? What words would you use to describe your pain?
4. **Intensity**—On a scale of 0 to 10, with 0 being no pain and 10 being the worst pain you can imagine, how much does it hurt right now? How much does it hurt at its worst? How much does it hurt at its best?
5. **Aggravating and relieving factors**—What makes your pain worse? What makes your pain better?
6. **Previous treatment**—What types of treatments have you tried to relieve your pain? Were they and are they effective?
7. **Effect**—How does the pain affect physical and social functions?

Psychosocial Assessment Should Include the Following:

1. Effect and understanding of the cancer diagnosis and cancer treatment on the patient and the caregiver.
2. The meaning of the pain to the patient and the family.
3. Significant past instances of pain and their effect on the patient.
4. The patient's typical coping responses to stress or pain.
5. The patient's knowledge of, curiosity about, preferences for, and expectations about pain management methods.
6. The patient's concerns about using controlled substances such as opioids, anxiolytics, or stimulants.
7. The economic effect of the pain and its treatment.
8. Changes in mood that have occurred as a result of the pain (e.g., depression, anxiety).

Physical and Neurologic Examination

1. Examine site of pain and evaluate common referral patterns.
2. Perform pertinent neurologic evaluation.
   - Head and neck pain—cranial nerve and funduscopic evaluation.
   - Back and neck pain—motor and sensory function in limbs; rectal and urinary sphincter function.

Diagnostic Evaluation

1. Evaluate recurrence or progression of disease or tissue injury related to cancer treatment.
   - Tumor markers and other blood tests.
   - Radiologic studies.
   - Neurophysiologic (e.g., electromyography) testing.
2. Perform appropriate radiologic studies and correlate normal and abnormal findings with physical and neurologic examination.
3. Recognize limitations of diagnostic studies.
   - Bone scan—false negatives in myeloma, lymphoma, previous radiation therapy sites.
   - CT scan—good definition of bone and soft tissue but difficult to image entire spine.
   - MRI scan—bone definition not as good as CT; better images of spine and brain.

Reprinted from Jacox A, Carr DB, Payne R, et al: *Management of Cancer Pain. Clinical Practice Guideline No. 9.* AHCPR Publication No. 94-0592. Rockville, MD: Agency for Health Care Policy and Research, Public Health Service, U.S. Department of Health and Human Services, March 1994.[9]

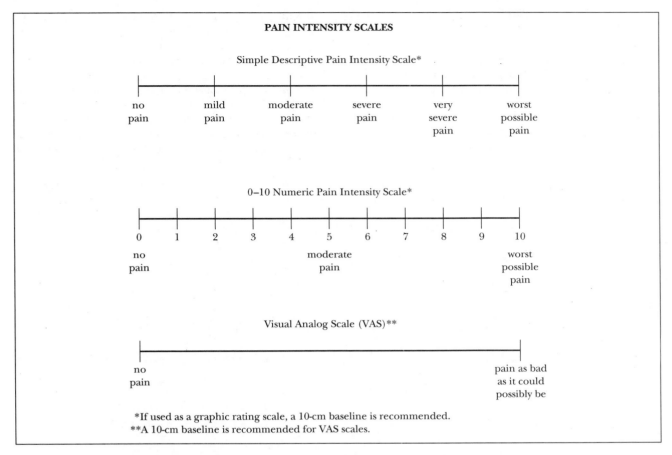

PAIN INTENSITY SCALES

Simple Descriptive Pain Intensity Scale*

no	mild	moderate	severe	very	worst
pain	pain	pain	pain	severe	possible
				pain	pain

0–10 Numeric Pain Intensity Scale*

0 1 2 3 4 5 6 7 8 9 10

no   moderate   worst
pain   pain   possible
                                             pain

Visual Analog Scale (VAS)**

no   pain as bad
pain   as it could
                                            possibly be

*If used as a graphic rating scale, a 10-cm baseline is recommended.
**A 10-cm baseline is recommended for VAS scales.

FIGURE 9-2 Measures of pain intensity. Three simple tools are used to measure pain intensity. Factors to consider when choosing the appropriate tools include the patient's age, developmental status, and physical, emotional, or cognitive condition. (Source: Acute Pain Management Guideline Panel: *Acute Pain Management: Operative or Medical Procedures and Trauma. Clinical Practice Guideline.* AHCPR Publication No. 92-0032. Rockville, MD: Agency for Health Care Policy and Research, Public Health Service, U.S. Department of Health and Human Services, 1992.[52])

handicaps, visual deficits, or inabilities to conceptualize their pain as a line.[53] The VDS is a reasonable alternative; however, the tool is not quite as sensitive and persons with poor command of the English language may experience difficulties in selecting an adjective that best describes their pain intensity.[54]

The simplest tool requires simply rating the pain from 0 to 10, with 0 indicating "no pain" and 10 indicating "the worst pain imaginable." One can use a line with numbers underneath or merely ask patients to verbally rate their pain without any visual cues. This is especially useful when managing pain problems over the telephone or when patients cannot speak or see well. Investigations of these tools indicate that the use of the NRS is highly correlated with the VAS and does not suffer the same obstacles as the 10-cm line drawing.[53,55,56] Researchers generally prefer to use the VAS, however, because it is believed to be more sensitive and because data generated from the use of this tool can be analyzed by parametric statis-

tics.[57] For a complete review of these self-report measures, see Jensen and Karoly.[58]

Pediatric tools include a faces scale,[59] with faces illustrating a range of emotions from happy to very distressed, and the Eland color scale,[60] which uses four colors on a gender-neutral figure drawing to indicate the intensity and location of pain. A comprehensive review of pediatric pain measures can be found in several texts.[61,62]

Multidimensional tools

A large number of tools have been developed to measure the various components of a complete pain assessment; however, many of these instruments are primarily intended to be used in research. One of the first tools developed to measure multiple dimensions was the McGill Pain Questionnaire (MPQ), which uses multiple descriptors to evaluate the sensory and affective component of pain.[63] This tool is frequently used in both pain research and clinical practice but may be cumbersome to complete for patients with limited vocabulary.[64] The long form is more comprehensive, yet the short form is valid and reliable and more palatable for patients due to the reduced time required to complete it.[65]

Another multidimensional pain instrument is the Brief Pain Inventory (BPI),[66] measuring location, quality, and the effect pain has had on various aspects of the patient's life (Figure 9-3). The tool also measures worst, least, average, and present pain, as well as relief obtained from the current regimen. Additionally, the tool has been translated into Spanish, French, Vietnamese, and Mandarin Chinese. This tool is particularly useful in the clinical setting, because most patients can complete the BPI without difficulty.

Other instruments include the Memorial Pain Assessment Card, an 8½-by-11-inch card folded into four sections, measuring intensity using a VAS, intensity using randomly placed descriptors, relief using a VAS, and mood measured by a VAS anchored by "worst mood" and "best

---

B1. Brief Pain Inventory (Short Form)

Date: _____ / _____ / _____

Time: _____

Name: _____ _____ _____
                    Last   First   Middle Initial

1) Throughout our lives, most of us have had pain from time to time (such as minor headaches, sprains, and toothaches). Have you had pain other than these everyday kinds of pain today?   1. Yes   2. No

2) On the diagram, shade in the areas where you feel pain. Put an X on the area that hurts the most.

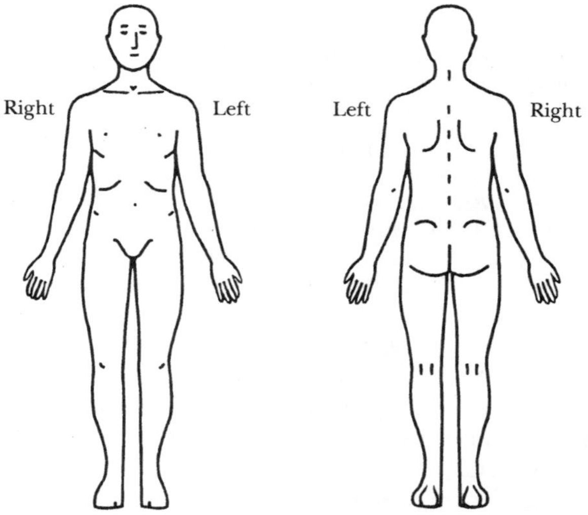

3) Please rate your pain by circling the one number that best describes your pain at its **worst** in the past 24 hours.
   0   1   2   3   4   5   6   7   8   9   10
   No   Pain as bad as
   pain   you can imagine

4) Please rate your pain by circling the one number that best describes your pain at its **least** in the past 24 hours.
   0   1   2   3   4   5   6   7   8   9   10
   No   Pain as bad as
   pain   you can imagine

(continued)

FIGURE 9-3 Brief Pain Inventory. (Source: Daut RL, Cleeland CS, Flanery RC: Development of the Wisconsin Brief Pain Questionnaire to assess pain in cancer and other diseases. *Pain* 17:197–210, 1983.[66] © CS Cleeland and the University of Wisconsin. Reprinted with permission)

mood."[67] Simple one-page instruments, most based on the tool developed by McCaffery and Beebe,[68] are useful in clinical practice, incorporating the essential components of a complete pain assessment (Figure 9-4). Clinicians are advised to examine these and other available instruments and to determine the unique needs of their patients and settings when selecting a tool.

Medication history

Although not included in many standardized pain assessment tools, a complete analgesic history is essential. This includes determining: (1) what has been ordered for pain, (2) what the patient is actually taking, and (3) why any disparity between the two exists. Patients may take less medication than ordered due to adverse effects, lack of efficacy, cost, fears of addiction or tolerance, or other concerns. Clarifying these barriers provides an excellent opportunity for patient teaching. In addition to the medications ordered by the physician, patients may be taking over-the-counter drugs. Many of these compounds are labeled "non-aspirin pain killers," and patients may be unaware that they contain acetaminophen. Evaluate the total acetaminophen content of both ordered and

FIGURE 9-3 (continued)

5) Please rate your pain by circling the one number that best describes your pain on the **average.**

| 0 | 1 | 2 | 3 | 4 | 5 | 6 | 7 | 8 | 9 | 10 |

No pain   Pain as bad as you can imagine

6) Please rate your pain by circling the one number that tells how much pain you have **right now.**

| 0 | 1 | 2 | 3 | 4 | 5 | 6 | 7 | 8 | 9 | 10 |

No pain   Pain as bad as you can imagine

7) What treatments or medications are you receiving for your pain?

_____

8) In the past 24 hours, how much **relief** have pain treatments or medications provided? Please circle the one percentage that most shows how much relief you have received.

| 0% | 10% | 20% | 30% | 40% | 50% | 60% | 70% | 80% | 90% | 100% |

No relief   Complete relief

9) Circle the one number that describes how, during the past 24 hours, **pain has interfered** with your:

A. General activity

| 0 | 1 | 2 | 3 | 4 | 5 | 6 | 7 | 8 | 9 | 10 |

Does not interfere   Completely interferes

B. Mood

| 0 | 1 | 2 | 3 | 4 | 5 | 6 | 7 | 8 | 9 | 10 |

Does not interfere   Completely interferes

C. Walking ability

| 0 | 1 | 2 | 3 | 4 | 5 | 6 | 7 | 8 | 9 | 10 |

Does not interfere   Completely interferes

D. Normal work (includes both work outside the home and housework)

| 0 | 1 | 2 | 3 | 4 | 5 | 6 | 7 | 8 | 9 | 10 |

Does not interfere   Completely interferes

E. Relations with other people

| 0 | 1 | 2 | 3 | 4 | 5 | 6 | 7 | 8 | 9 | 10 |

Does not interfere   Completely interferes

F. Sleep

| 0 | 1 | 2 | 3 | 4 | 5 | 6 | 7 | 8 | 9 | 10 |

Does not interfere   Completely interferes

G. Enjoyment of life

| 0 | 1 | 2 | 3 | 4 | 5 | 6 | 7 | 8 | 9 | 10 |

Does not interfere   Completely interferes

INITIAL PAIN ASSESSMENT TOOL   Date_____

Patient's Name_____ Age_____ Room_____

Diagnosis_____ Physician_____

                                        Nurse_____

I.   LOCATION: Patient or nurse mark drawing.

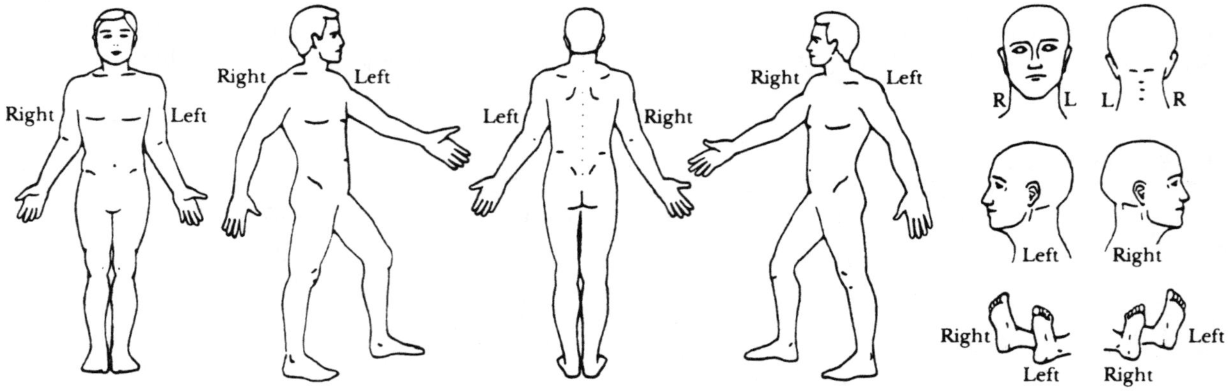

II. INTENSITY: Patient rates the pain. Scale used _____

     Present:_____

     Worst pain gets:_____

     Best pain gets:_____

     Acceptable level of pain_____

III. QUALITY: (Use patient's own words, e.g. prick, ache, burn, throb, pull, sharp)_____

IV. ONSET, DURATION VARIATIONS, RHYTHMS:_____

V.   MANNER OF EXPRESSING PAIN:_____

VI. WHAT RELIEVES THE PAIN:_____

VII. WHAT CAUSES OR INCREASES THE PAIN?_____

VIII. EFFECTS OF PAIN: (Note decreased function, decreased quality of life.)

     Accompanying symptoms (e.g. nausea)_____

     Sleep_____

     Appetite_____

     Physical activity_____

     Relationship with others (e.g. irritability)_____

     Emotions (e.g. anger, suicidal, crying)_____

     Concentration_____

     Other_____

IX. OTHER COMMENTS:_____

X.   PLAN:_____

FIGURE 9-4   Pain assessment tool. (Source: McCaffery M, Beebe A: *Pain: A Clinical Manual for Nursing Practice.* St. Louis: Mosby, 1989.[68])

over-the-counter drugs; the recommended daily maximum dose is approximately 4000 mg in persons with a functioning liver.

Patients should also be questioned regarding their past and current use of recreational drugs and alcohol. Patients with a past history may be particularly reluctant to take opioids, believing that the drugs may cause them to lose control. Patients with a current history of abuse present more complex challenges. Psychologists, substance abuse experts, and others may be consulted when developing a plan of care.

Physical Assessment

A complete physical assessment follows the pain history. Inspection, palpation, and manipulation of the affected area are essential, with particular attention to the neurologic examination. Assess the area of the pain, considering dermatomal distribution and evaluating sensory and motor changes occurring in this region.[9] Reflexes may also be obtained.

Although vital signs, including heart rate, blood pressure, respirations, and temperature, are components of a complete physical assessment and should be obtained, these findings are not valid measures of pain.[69] Also invalid as measures of pain in alert, verbal individuals are behavioral changes, such as guarding or facial grimacing.

Diagnostic Evaluation

Radiographic studies and laboratory analyses can contribute essential information to the pain assessment.[36] For example, bone scans can identify the presence of metastases causing rib pain. In this circumstance, radiation therapy may be warranted. Tumor markers may provide evidence for the existence or spread of a malignancy, suggesting the origin of the pain. Moreover, laboratory data may reveal other conditions that can complicate pain therapy, including calcium levels to rule out hypercalcemia as a cause of confusion in patients receiving opioids.

This complete pain assessment should be conducted with each new complaint of pain, and regularly after initiating a new treatment plan.[9] Intensity and relief scores should be obtained after administering a pharmacologic intervention, with the timing of the assessment based on the estimated onset of action of the drug. After assessment, documentation is essential to ensure continuity of care (see Evaluation of Management Interventions).

Degrees of Toxicity (Staging Systems)

Clinical staging systems have provided major advancements to the science of oncology by systematically categorizing the stages of various malignancies. In doing so,

clinical trials can be more accurately interpreted, and individual patients can be treated with greater specificity. These same benefits would apply to cancer pain management, should such a classification system exist. The only cancer pain staging system developed to date, the Edmonton staging system for cancer pain,[70,71] is extremely comprehensive and is reliable but unfortunately is not widely used. In part, this may be due to the complexity of the system, incorporating five features of pain (i.e., mechanisms of pain, pain characteristics, psychological distress, tolerance, history) into a two-stage clinical staging system (i.e., good or poor prognosis). Future studies of this and other systems are needed.

Symptom Management

The goals of pain management include relief of pain, prevention and alleviation of side effects of pain treatment, and enhanced quality of life. Reducing tumor bulk through the use of cancer therapies, including chemotherapy, radiation therapy, and in some cases surgery, will be effective in many situations. Other pain management techniques entail two primary interventions: pharmacologic therapy and nonpharmacologic interventions. Pharmacologic therapy can be classified into three primary categories: (1) nonopioids, including NSAIDs and acetaminophen; (2) opioids; and (3) adjunct drugs, such as tricyclic antidepressants, anticonvulsants, corticosteroids, local anesthetics, and others. Nonpharmacologic approaches include cognitive-behavioral techniques and invasive procedures.

Prevention

Prevention of cancer pain may not be practical in all situations, particularly when it is the presenting symptom of the disease for many individuals; however, attempts can be made to block or reduce pain associated with invasive procedures or inhibit recurrence of pain once it is alleviated.[72] Although the efficacy of these techniques is controversial,[73] preemptive analgesia entails premedicating before and during invasive procedures to prevent the changes that occur within the nervous system during activation of pain pathways. Examples of this technique include the administration of analgesic agents (NSAIDs, opioids, tricyclic antidepressants) prior to surgery, the application of local anesthetic within the area to be incised, and the delivery of a nerve block before making the surgical incision.[74]

Less controversial is the recognition that once pain is under control, prevention of the recurrence of pain is an essential goal. This is achieved by using the agents and techniques described in the following section.

Interventions

Anticancer therapies

Treating the tumor with surgery, chemotherapy, or radiation therapy may produce a reduction in mass sufficient to alleviate pain, although the individual's risks for complications or adverse effects must be carefully weighed.

Surgery may be indicated to relieve pain in certain cases. For example, pain caused by complete intestinal obstruction secondary to colorectal cancer may be effectively relieved through formation of a colostomy.[9] Care must be taken to prevent complications when performing surgery within a previously irradiated area, and patient factors, such as diminished white blood cell and platelet counts, reduced plasma proteins, and generalized infection, may preclude use of this therapy.[9]

Antineoplastic therapies, including chemotherapy, hormonal therapy, and biological response modifiers, may provide palliation by decreasing tumor burden.[75] Unfortunately, little research has been directed at evaluating the analgesic effect of various chemotherapeutic regimens, focusing instead primarily on tumor regression. Hormonal therapy has been documented to produce analgesia, specifically in the relief of pain due to bone metastases.[76]

Radiation therapy is extremely effective in the management of several pain states, particularly pain associated with bone metastases.[77] Approximately 75% of patients treated for pain due to bone metastases obtain some level of relief, and almost half become pain free.[78]

Pharmacologic interventions

Although antitumor therapies can be useful in treating pain, the foundation of cancer pain management is based on pharmacologic treatment. The World Health Organization three-step analgesic ladder provides a guide to the use of pain-relieving drugs based on the patient's reported pain intensity (Figure 9-5).[79] This model employs nonopioids, opioids, and adjuvant drugs.

Nonopioids Nonopioids include NSAIDs and acetaminophen. NSAIDs interfere with the enzyme cyclooxygenase (prostaglandin synthetase), which blocks the conversion of arachidonic acid to prostaglandins (PGE_1, PGE_2, and PGF_2), prostacyclins (PGI_2), and thromboxane (TXA_2) (Figure 9-6). Prostaglandins are known to sensitize tissues to the effects of inflammatory mediators such as bradykinin. Thus, inhibition of prostaglandin synthesis leads to relief of inflammation and pain.[43] Additionally, these agents are antipyretic. Finally, although these agents have been believed to exert their analgesic effects primarily through peripheral mechanisms, newer research suggests that the NSAIDs may also have central pain-relieving effects.[80]

The toxicities associated with these agents are also

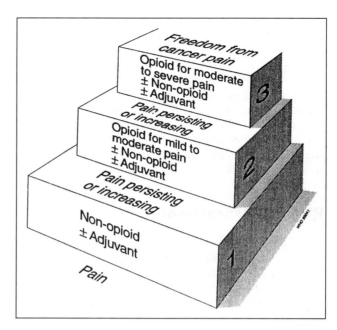

FIGURE 9-5 World Health Organization three-step analgesic ladder. The World Health Organization three-step analgesic ladder incorporates nonopioids, opioids, and adjuvant drugs in the treatment of mild, moderate, and severe pain. (Source: WHO Expert Committee: *Cancer Pain Relief and Palliative Care* (ed 2). Geneva: World Health Organization, 1996.[79] Reprinted with permission.)

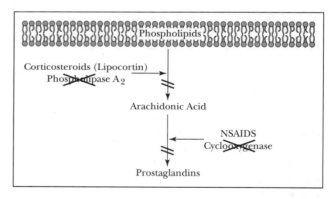

FIGURE 9-6 Mechanisms of action of NSAIDs.

related to prostaglandin inhibition. Gastrointestinal effects, ranging from upset to hemorrhage, result from increased gastric acid secretion, inhibition of gastric mucin production, and reduced sphincter tone, leading to reflux.[81,82] Prevention of gastrointestinal toxicity includes the administration of prostaglandin analogs, such as misoprostol, to replace the action of prostaglandin in the stomach.[83]

Prolonged bleeding, due to the decrease in thromboxane, is another adverse effect associated with the NSAIDs.[43] Platelet numbers are not affected; rather, aggregation is inhibited and bleeding time is increased, as evidenced by an elevated prothrombin time (PT) and activated partial thromboplastin time (APTT). NSAIDs may be discontinued approximately 1 week before planned invasive procedures to limit the potential complications associated with prolonged bleeding.

Renal prostaglandin inhibition leads to vasoconstriction in kidney blood vessels and, potentially, renal failure.[84] This effect occurs more often during the first month of therapy, in the elderly, with higher doses, or when used concomitantly with other nephrotoxic drugs.[85] This effect is generally reversible after discontinuing the NSAID. Hydration may prevent this effect.

Central nervous system toxicities with NSAIDs are generally mild, including headache and minor cognitive impairment, particularly in the elderly.[43] Alternative NSAIDs should be tried before abandoning therapy.

A large number of NSAIDs are available for use, with varying side effect profiles and alternative delivery forms. The nonacetylated salicylates (such as choline magnesium trisalicylate or sodium salicylate) produce less effect on platelet aggregation and may cause fewer episodes of gastrointestinal bleeding.[86] Previously, the majority of NSAIDs were available only in oral formulations. Currently, one parenterally administered NSAID, ketorolac tromethamine, is available for short-term (5 days or less) intramuscular or intravenous administration at maximum daily doses of 120 mg.[87] Only indomethacin is commercially available in suppository form; however, pharmacists can often compound other NSAIDs for rectal administration.

Drug interactions can occur when administering NSAIDs, particularly in individuals diagnosed with cancer. Because NSAIDs are metabolized in the liver, conditions or therapies that alter hepatic function may modify NSAID bioavailability.[43] For example, reduced hepatic function as a result of disease, chemotherapy, or radiotherapy will result in impaired NSAID metabolism, necessitating a reduction in dose. NSAIDs are excreted by the kidneys and may inhibit the renal tubular secretion of other compounds. This is of critical importance when methotrexate is given in conjunction with fenoprofen, naproxen, or tolmetin, which have been shown to increase the toxicity of this chemotherapeutic agent.[88] These and other drug interactions are listed in Table 9-4.

Acetaminophen is another nonopioid, with much less effect on prostaglandin inhibition compared with the NSAIDs. Having both analgesic and antipyretic properties, acetaminophen has little antiinflammatory activity. Because acetaminophen concentrates in the liver, and in large doses (10 g) can lead to hepatic necrosis, maximum daily doses should not exceed 4 g or 4000 mg.[43] This becomes a concern when administering admixtures of opioids and acetaminophen (Table 9-5), particularly if patients are taking additional over-the-counter preparations containing acetaminophen.

Nonopioids used alone or in conjunction with adjuvant agents provide significant relief of mild pain; how-

TABLE 9-4   Drug Interactions and NSAIDs

Effects of Other Drugs on NSAIDS

Decreases NSAID metabolism (causing decreased clearance and increased duration of effect—generally requires lengthening frequency of administration):

- Anabolic steroids
- Dipyridamole
- Salicylates
- Sulfinpyrazone

Increases NSAID metabolism (leading to decreased effect—usually necessitating increased dose of NSAID):

- Phenobarbital
- Antihistamines

Effects of NSAIDs on Other Agents

NSAIDs increase activity of agents highly bound to plasma proteins by competitive displacement:

- Corticosteroids
- Coumadin
- Oral hypoglycemics
- Penicillin
- Sulfonamides

NSAIDs increase activity of these agents through competition at renal binding sites:

- Lithium
- Methotrexate (specifically fenoprofen, naproxen, or tolmetin)

TABLE 9-5 Selected Oral Opioid Admixtures and Acetaminophen Content

Preparation	Content		Maximum Daily Intake
Codeine and Acetaminophen[a]			
Tylenol #1	7.5 mg codeine	+ 300 mg acetaminophen	13 tablets
Tylenol #2	15 mg codeine	+ 300 mg acetaminophen	13 tablets
Tylenol #3	30 mg codeine	+ 300 mg acetaminophen	13 tablets
Tylenol #4	60 mg codeine	+ 300 mg acetaminophen	13 tablets
Hydrocodone and Acetaminophen			
Vicodin	5 mg hydrocodone	+ 500 mg acetaminophen	8 tablets
Vicodin ES	7.5 mg hydrocodone	+ 750 mg acetaminophen	5 tablets
Lortab	5 mg hydrocodone	+ 500 mg acetaminophen	8 tablets
Lortab ES	7.5 mg hydrocodone	+ 500 mg acetaminophen	8 tablets
Lorcet	10 mg hydrocodone	+ 650 mg acetaminophen	6 tablets
Oxycodone and Acetaminophen[b]			
Percocet	5 mg oxycodone	+ 325 mg acetaminophen	12 tablets
Roxicet	5 mg oxycodone	+ 500 mg acetaminophen	8 tablets
Tylox	5 mg oxycodone	+ 500 mg acetaminophen	8 tablets

[a] Codeine is available without acetaminophen in numerous preparations.
[b] Oxycodone without acetaminophen is sold as Roxicodone tablets, oral solution, or Intensol (Roxane Laboratories, Columbus, Ohio).

ever, as pain increases, opioids must be added to the treatment regimen.

Opioids The treatment of moderate to severe cancer pain requires the addition of opioids such as morphine. Three major categories of opioids are available for clinical use:

- agonists (codeine, morphine, hydromorphone, methadone, fentanyl, and others)
- partial agonists (buprenorphine)
- and mixed agonist-antagonists (butorphanol, dezocine, nalbuphine, and pentazocine)[86]

Because partial agonists have a ceiling effect, meaning that there is little additional analgesia after attaining a certain dose, they have little use in chronic cancer pain management.[9] The role of mixed agonist-antagonists is also minor, since the use of these agents in persons already on agonist opioids may precipitate withdrawal.[9] Furthermore, these drugs often cause significant psychomimetic effects and, therefore, are rarely used in cancer pain management.[86]

Opioids relieve pain primarily by binding to opioid receptors in the dorsal horn of the spinal cord to block neurotransmitter release, although newer research findings suggest that opioids may also have a peripheral mechanism of action.[46,89] Opioid use is associated with several phenomena, including tolerance, physiologic dependence, and psychological dependence, that lead to an enormous amount of misunderstanding regarding these drugs. *Tolerance* is the need for higher doses of opioid to maintain the original analgesic effect.[90] Often mistaken for addiction, this is a known pharmacologic effect of these drugs. Tolerance is easily overcome by increasing the dose of the opioid; because there is no maximum

dose or ceiling effect of agonist opioids, this can be safely accomplished by careful titration. In fact, the dose necessary to relieve pain is highly variable and should be based on the patient's self-report of pain severity.[91]

Physiologic dependence is also an effect of chronic opioid use. If the agent is abruptly withdrawn, or if an antagonist is given, the individual will experience agitation, abdominal cramping and diarrhea, rhinorrhea, piloerection, and return of pain.[90] Although these are symptoms commonly manifested by drug addicts in movies or TV, the onset of these symptoms does not imply the patient is addicted. In the majority of cases, physiologic dependence is not a clinical problem. If an opioid is to be withdrawn, for example after obtaining relief from radiation therapy or a neurolytic procedure, it should be done so gradually, reducing approximately 10% to 25% daily to prevent the abstinence syndrome.[9]

The use of opioid antagonists (such as naloxone) will also lead to an abrupt onset of the abstinence syndrome; therefore, these agents should be used cautiously in persons on chronic opioid therapy.[9] Furthermore, naloxone is not an innocuous drug, having been associated with hypertension, ventricular arrhythmias, pulmonary edema, and sudden death in healthy individuals.[92-95] In those rare circumstances for which naloxone is indicated, it can be mixed in 10 mL of saline and administered slowly in 1-mL increments to antagonize the respiratory depressant effects without precipitating an acute episode of the abstinence syndrome.

Psychological dependence, or addiction, is greatly feared by healthcare professionals and the public alike. An overwhelming obsession to obtain and use a drug for nonmedically approved purposes, *addiction* is extremely rare, occurring in less than 1% of those treated with opioids.[96] Thus, fear of this effect is unjustified and should not serve as a barrier to adequate cancer pain relief. Education of healthcare professionals and lay persons is essential.

Misunderstandings regarding side effects of opioids also serve as obstacles to adequate analgesia. The side effects associated with opioid use are related to binding of the drug to opioid receptors in various parts of the body. Constipation occurs as a result of binding to opioid receptors distributed throughout the gastrointestinal tract, leading to three disturbances in function: (1) peristalsis is slowed, (2) the release of enzymes and substances that digest food is inhibited, and (3) resorption of water from fecal contents into the colon is enhanced.[90] The result of these changes is constipation, which in most cases can be treated with stool softeners in combination with laxatives. Tolerance does not develop to these effects of opioids; therefore, a bowel program must be continued during opioid therapy and intensified when opioid doses are increased.[9] (See Chapter 27 for a complete discussion of the management of constipation.)

Respiratory depression is a feared consequence of opioid therapy; however, the incidence of this adverse effect is quite small and is exceptionally rare in persons tolerant to the opioid.[90] Nausea and vomiting are known effects of opioid administration, particularly during initial exposure to the drug; approximately 40% of postoperative patients given opioids will vomit. Antiemetic therapy administered continuously during the first 24 to 48 hours after introducing opioids will often relieve these effects. In those rare persons who continue to experience nausea and vomiting, changing to a different opioid may provide relief. Other causes of nausea and vomiting should also be considered (see Chapter 14).

Sedation can occur when opioids are initially introduced, but tolerance to this effect generally builds rapidly. If persistent, the dose of opioid may be reduced and the frequency of administration increased.[9] An alternative opioid may also be tried. Finally, psychostimulants, such as methylphenidate, 5 to 10 mg, or dextroamphetamine, 2.5 to 7.5 mg, upon arising and in the early afternoon, may provide relief.[97] Doses should not be repeated in the late afternoon or evening, to avoid sleep alterations.

Other adverse effects of opioid therapy include pruritus and urinary retention.[91] Mediated in part by histamine release, pruritus can be managed by the administration of antihistamines, such as diphenhydramine. Tolerance generally develops to this effect within several days after initial exposure to the opioid. Urinary retention usually occurs in elderly males with prostatic hyperplasia or in those individuals who have preexisting disturbances in urinary system function. Intermittent bladder catheterization may be warranted within the initial exposure period; however, tolerance also develops to this effect and the usual urinary flow returns 24 to 48 hours after beginning opioid therapy.

Myoclonic jerking is a known effect of high-dose opioids, although particularly sensitive individuals may experience this at lower doses.[91] Clonazepam, beginning at doses of 0.5 mg orally twice daily and titrated upward, can be given to reduce this effect.[9] Hallucinations can occur but are rare, and are more often due to other organic disorders.[98] Sexual dysfunction as a result of chronic opioid use, including amenorrhea, reduced libido, and difficulty obtaining and maintaining an erection, have all been reported.[99,100]

The treatment of some adverse effects involves changing to an alternative pure agonist opioid. This is done by converting the daily dose of one opioid, such as morphine, to the equivalent dine of an alternative opioid, such as hydromorphone, using equianalgesic tables as a guide (Table 9-6). The 24-hour equianalgesic dose is usually reduced by approximately 20% to 25% due to incomplete cross-tolerance and is titrated as needed.[9] Ongoing evaluation of the efficacy of any analgesic regimen is essential, and doses of drug must be titrated based on the patient's self-report of pain.

Of the many pure agonist opioids available for clinical use, one in particular should be avoided in chronic cancer pain management. Meperidine is metabolized in the liver to normeperidine, which is then excreted through the urinary system.[91] Excretion is altered in those individuals with renal disorders, leading to excess levels of circulating normeperidine, resulting in central nervous system toxicity such as seizures.[106,107] Its use is contraindicated in those persons also taking monoamine-oxidase (MAO) inhibitors.[91] Meperidine use in chronic cancer pain is also complicated by the poor oral bioavailability of the drug; 50 mg of oral meperidine is approximately equianalgesic to two aspirin tablets (650 mg). Finally, intramuscular injections of meperidine are quite painful and can lead to sterile abscess formation.

Various routes of administration are available to enhance opioid use in the person with chronic cancer pain (Table 9-7). Although the majority of persons with cancer can obtain adequate relief using oral analgesics,[9] occasionally alternative routes, including rectal, sublingual, buccal, transdermal, or parenteral administration, may be required. Although 66% of patients in one hospice were able to take oral medication during their last day of life,[123] many patients may require more than one route of administration. When these are not commercially available, pharmacists can often compound solutions, suppositories, and other formulations.[124]

In addition to alternative routes of administration, sustained-release oral morphine preparations have allowed greater convenience and improved quality of life.[125] When using these sustained-release formulations, as well as transdermal fentanyl, several principles should be considered: (1) titration should first occur with a short-acting product, such as immediate-release morphine, and the 24-hour dose effective in relieving pain can then be converted to the sustained-release product; (2) immediate-release opioids should be available for breakthrough pain; (3) if the patient consistently requires more than two doses of breakthrough medication in a 4-hour period or more than six rescue doses in a 24-hour period, that

TABLE 9-6 Equianalgesic Conversion Table

	Mild to moderate pain	Oral dose (mg)[a]
	Codeine	30
	Meperidine	50
	Propxyphene	65
	Acetaminophen	650
	Sodium salicylate	1000

Severe Pain	IM (mg)[b]	PO (mg)[b]	Plasma Half-life (hr)	Average Duration of Action (hr)
Codeine	130	200	2.5–3	3–5
Meperidine	75	300	3–5	2–4
Oxycodone	15	30	2–3	3–5[c]
Hydromorphone	1.5	7.5	2–3	3–6
Morphine	10	60[d]	2–3.5	4–5[c,e]
Fentanyl[f]	0.1	——	3–4	1–2
Levorphanol	2	4	11–16	4–5
Methadone	10	20	15–30	4–6
Oxymorphone	1	——	2–3	4–5

[a] Approximately equal to aspirin 650 mg.

[b] Approximately equivalent to morphine 10 mg IM. These values were determined from and based on clinical experience and single-dose studies of patients in acute pain.

[c] Refers to immediate-release short-acting preparations; also available in q12h preparations.

[d] For chronic dosing, some pain experts believe that the oral morphine dose is approximately 20–30 mg, but this has not been demonstrated in any controlled trial.

[e] Available in a q24h preparation.

[f] Available as a transdermal patch, with a 72-hour duration of action.

From McGuire DB, Sheidler VR: Pain, in Groenwald SL, Frogge MH, Goodman M, Yarbro CH (eds): *Cancer Nursing: Principles and Practice* (ed 4). Sudbury: Jones and Bartlett, 1997, p. 557.[101] Based on information from references [90] and [102–105]. Reprinted with permission.

amount should be added to the sustained-release dose; and (4) the immediate-release dose must be increased as the dose of the sustained-release product is also increased.[9,126]

The dose of opioid necessary to relieve pain is the correct dose for that individual. Unlike many other pharmacologic interventions, there are no maximum accepted doses for pure agonist opioids, and larger doses may be needed in some pain states, such as neuropathic pain.[127] Although opioids are the mainstay of cancer pain treatment, other agents, referred to as adjuvant drugs, provide additional relief, particularly for neuropathic pain.

Adjuvant drugs Adjuvant analgesics include several categories of drugs that are used to provide pain relief. These include antidepressants, anticonvulsants, local anesthetics and oral analogs, corticosteroids, and others (Table 9-8).

Antidepressants are known to provide relief, probably by blocking the reuptake of serotonin and norepinephrine, thereby enhancing activation of the monoamine pain modulatory systems described earlier. These agents provide analgesia independent of their mood-elevating effect. The majority of analgesic efficacy trials have been conducted using amitriptyline; therefore, many recommend using this agent first, unless contraindicated. Cardiac arrhythmias, conduction abnormalities, narrow-angle glaucoma, and clinically significant prostatic hyperplasia are relative contraindications to the use of these agents.[9,128]

Sedation is the most frequent side effect; therefore, tricyclic antidepressants are generally given at bedtime to enhance sleep. Doses can be increased every other day by approximately 25 mg, with an analgesic effect occurring within approximately 4 to 7 days. The dose-limiting side effects are anticholinergic, including dry mouth, constipation, urinary retention, and orthostatic hypotension.

Anticonvulsants act as membrane stabilizers and are effective in relieving episodic lancinating pains, such as trigeminal neuralgia and other neuropathies.[9] Carbamazepine may produce nausea, sedation, and confusion if the dose is increased too rapidly; therefore, lower doses are used initially and increased gradually to prevent these adverse effects. Bone marrow suppression may be an unacceptable side effect in the person receiving concomitant antitumor therapies. Clonazepam is a benzodiazepine that should be withdrawn slowly to prevent an abstinence syndrome. Although the mechanism of action of gabapentin, a newer anticonvulsant, is unclear, this compound has been found to be useful in relieving various types of neuropathic pain.[129] Because there are few data evaluating the efficacy of anticonvulsants in cancer pain, the choice should be based on patient factors as well as on clinician familiarity with a particular agent.

Corticosteroids can be useful in relief of pain associated with compression of nervous system structures and reduction of the edema associated with this mechanical trauma. These agents inhibit prostaglandin synthesis and may reduce ectopic impulses generated by damaged nerves.[130] Adverse effects include hypertension, hyperglycemia,

TABLE 9-7 Routes of Opioid Administration

Route	Benefits	Limitations
Enteral		
Oral[9]	• Convenient • Economical • Safe	• Subject to first-pass effect • Absorption may be affected by gastrointestinal disturbances and other factors
Transmucosal (buccal/sublingual)[108–110]	• Can be used when patient unable to swallow • Provides rapid onset	• Primary effect probably due to both oral uptake and absorption through mucous membranes • Prevent aspiration if patient has limited consciousness or difficulty swallowing
Rectal[111–113]	• Useful alternative to oral route • Can be placed in stoma if not actively functioning • Sustained-release tablets have been used rectally with delayed time to peak plasma level and approximately 90% of bioavailability of oral administration of the tablets	• Absorption dependent on placement within rectum; lower aspect of rectum avoids first-pass effect, yet difficult to control • Not indicated if patient has diarrhea, thrombocytopenia, or painful rectal lesions • Can be difficult to self-medicate
Vaginal[112,113]	• Alternative to rectal route if that route is contraindicated	• Lack of sphincter may lead to discharge of drug, especially if patient ambulatory; can be kept in place with a tampon covered with a condom • No dosing studies are available and no commercial preparations are available for this route
Parenteral		
Intravenous[114,115]	• Rapid effect • Permits rapid titration of doses • Can be given via bolus, continuous infusion, or patient-controlled analgesia (PCA)	• Requires vascular access • Potential for infection • Complex care • Increased cost
Intramuscular[9]		• Erratic absorption • Contraindicated in thrombocytopenia and during anticoagulant therapy • Limited volume • Requires syringes, needles, special knowledge to administer • Sterile abscess formation
Subcutaneous[116,117]	• Useful alternative when enteral routes not available • Can be given as continuous infusion • Slower absorption than IM • Hyaluronidase speeds absorption • May be preferred over IV route	• Volumes greater than 10 mL/hour often poorly tolerated • Not to be used with irritating substances • Continuous infusions require special equipment, infusion pumps, and expertise
Other Routes		
Epidural[118,119]	• Effective when patients unable to tolerate side effects associated with other routes of administration • Provides route of administration for local anesthetics for neuropathic pain • Allows greater volume than intrathecal routes delivered by implanted pumps.	• Requires expensive equipment and knowledgeable personnel • Risk of infection • Cost
Intrathecal[118,119]	• Usually delivered by implanted pump, also by reservoirs • Bypasses blood-brain barrier	• Requires expensive equipment and specialized, knowledgeable personnel • Potentially reduced risk of infection when compared with epidural; however, when infection occurs, may be more serious (meningitis) • Cost

(continued)

TABLE 9-7 Routes of Opioid Administration (continued)

Route	Benefits	Limitations
Transdermal[120]	• Useful if patient unable to swallow or cognitive impairment leads to noncompliance • Currently only transdermal opioid is fentanyl	• Expensive • Difficult to titrate • Onset delayed (often 17 hours to therapeutic plasma levels) • Prolonged effect after discontinuing due to subcutaneous reservoir (may take 17 hours for plasma levels to diminish) • Absorption may be affected by diaphoresis, elevated temperature, variation in fat stores, and other factors
Inhalation[121]	• Nebulized morphine used to treat severe air hunger associated with lung cancer and end-stage pulmonary or cardiac disease	• Absorption, mechanisms of action, and dosing unclear • Slight potential for uptake of drug by caregivers in the immediate area
Nasal[9,122]	• Useful route if patient unable to swallow • Rapid onset	• Only agent currently available is butorphanol, a mixed-agonist antagonist, that may precipitate withdrawal in persons currently taking agonist opioids • May cause irritation, bleeding of nasal mucosa • Cost

Based on information from the references cited.

immunosuppression, and psychiatric reactions. Although corticosteroids were previously believed to cause peptic ulcers, this effect probably occurs only with the concomitant use of NSAIDs.[130] Long-term use can lead to Cushing's syndrome and osteoporosis. As with all medications, the potential benefits of therapy must be weighed against the possible adverse effects.

Local anesthetics have been used as alternative therapy for neuropathic pain when opioids, antidepressants, and anticonvulsants have failed to provide relief.[131] Mexiletine is started at low doses of 150 mg/day and gradually titrated to levels as high as 900 mg/day in divided doses. Adverse effects include cardiac arrhythmias; therefore, electrocardiogram monitoring is essential before and during higher-dose administration. Other adverse effects include nausea and vomiting, constipation, and tremor. Tocainide is considered only after mexiletine has failed to provide analgesia, due to its more pronounced side effect profile.

Methotrimeprazine is the single phenothiazine demonstrated to be analgesic.[132] Available only in an intramuscular formulation, 15 mg of methotrimeprazine is approximately equivalent to 10 mg of parenterally administered morphine. Indications for the use of this agent include moderate to severe pain unrelieved by opioids or the presence of severe side effects to opioids. Sedation and orthostatic hypotension as well as the onset of extrapyramidal signs may limit its use.

Other agents provide analgesia in specific pain states. *Baclofen* is a γ-aminobutyric acid (GABA) agonist that has been used extensively in the treatment of spasticity and in the relief of pain associated with trigeminal neuralgia. Baclofen appears to be most effective in reducing episodic pain, and therefore may be indicated in lancinating-type pain states. Adverse effects include sedation and gastrointestinal upset. Gradually tapering the dose when discontinuing the drug is essential to prevent hallucinations and seizures.[133]

Capsaicin is a naturally occurring substance derived from chili peppers of the Solanaceae family and is available as a topical cream in two concentrations (0.025% and 0.075%).[134] The initial mechanism of action of capsaicin is believed to be due in part to opening of nonspecific ion channels in the skin, airways, oral mucosa, and visceral organs, leading to release of substance P.[135] Substance P, a peptide stored in the terminals of sensory neurons, is a neuromodulator known to sensitize nociceptive neurons involved in pain transmission. This initial release leads to an increased perception of pain. Repeated, regular topical application, however, leads to further release and eventual depletion of substance P from the terminals of primary afferent neurons, reducing transmission of pain.

Approved for the relief of pain due to rheumatoid arthritis or osteoarthritis and neuropathic pain related to herpes zoster or diabetic neuropathy, capsaicin's effect on other cancer pain syndromes has also been examined. A randomized, parallel trial of 0.075% capsaicin topically applied to the incision in women with postmastectomy pain syndrome demonstrated that capsaicin produced superior relief.[136] A more recent randomized controlled clinical trial in patients with neuropathic pain due to cancer surgery also revealed significant relief obtained by capsaicin.[137]

Agents used to treat bone pain include calcitonin, gallium nitrate, pamidronate disodium (a bisphosphonate),

TABLE 9-8 Adjuvant Analgesics

Agent	Usual Daily Starting Dose	Approximate Daily Dose Range
Antidepressants		
Tricyclic		
Amitriptyline	10–25 mg PO qhs	75–150 mg
Clomipramine	10–25 mg PO qhs	10–150 mg
Desipramine	10–25 mg PO qhs	75–200 mg
Doxepin	25–50 mg PO qhs	75–150 mg
Imipramine	10–25 mg PO qhs	50–200 mg
Nortriptyline	10–50 mg PO qhs	75–100 mg
Non-tricyclic antidepressants		
Maprotiline	25 mg PO qhs	75–100 mg
Paroxetine	20 mg PO qd	50 mg
Trazodone	50 mg PO tid	150–250 mg
Anticonvulsants		
Carbamazepine	100–200 mg bid	600–1600 mg
Clonazepam	0.5 to 1.5 mg/day	3–4 mg
Gabapentin	(usual) 100–300 mg/day	(approx) 900–2400 mg
Phenytoin	150–200 mg/bid	300–500 mg
Valproic acid	15 mg/kg	3000 mg
Corticosteroids		
Dexamethasone (PO, IV)	4–10 mg bid	16–96 mg
Local Anesthetics		
Lidocaine (IV, SQ)	1 mg/kg	5 mg/kg
Mexiletene	150 mg/day	900 mg
Phenothiazines		
Methotrimeprazine (IM)	10–20 mg IM qid	40–80 mg
Others		
Baclofen	5 mg bid	50–60 mg
Capsaicin cream	Apply 4 times/day	
(0.025% or 0.075%, topical)		

Data compiled from references[9,128–134].

and strontium-89 (a radionuclide).[9] Calcitonin, gallium nitrate, and pamidronate are used to treat hypercalcemia, by reducing osteoclast activity, believed to also be responsible for pain associated with bone metastases. Few studies have evaluated the analgesic efficacy of these agents, although some clinical trials suggest reduction in pain.[9] Strontium-89 is a radiopharmaceutical that has produced palliation of pain, with myelosuppression the major adverse effect.[138]

Other agents are being investigated for the treatment of refractory cancer pain, particularly pain that does not respond completely to opioids, and will undoubtedly enter clinical use within the coming years. Applying various principles of analgesic use will improve outcomes associated with existing pharmacologic therapies.

Principles of analgesic use To deliver effective relief, the individual's pain and response to therapy must be constantly assessed, and changes in the treatment plan should reflect these assessments.[9] The regimen should incorporate the simplest dosage schedule using the least invasive route, usually oral administration. Around-the-clock administration is essential—rather than an as-needed, or prn, approach—to maintain therapeutic plasma levels and reduce the potential for adverse effects. Keeping in mind these principles, the treatment plan should be individualized to meet the patient's needs. Side effects should be prevented whenever possible and treated promptly when they do occur.

Patients should be given a written copy of the pain management plan, including contingencies should side effects occur.[9] This written plan designates the responsible healthcare professional along with methods for contacting that individual when problems occur. Copies of this plan can be shared with all those involved in the patient's care to ensure continuity.

Placebos have no role in the management of cancer pain. Their use is unethical, impairing trust between patients and healthcare professionals. Furthermore, because a large number of individuals will report some analgesia when given placebo, their utility in diagnosing psychological components to pain is grossly limited.[9]

Nonpharmacologic interventions

Nondrug treatments such as cognitive-behavioral therapies may be effective adjuncts to pharmacologic interventions. Generally well-tolerated by patients, these therapies tend to be inexpensive and often incorporate family members and support systems. Invasive procedures such as nerve blocks and ablative neurosurgical techniques are indicated for those persons not obtaining pain relief with appropriate analgesic therapy, estimated to be 1% to 5% of those with cancer pain.

Cognitive-behavioral techniques Cognitive-behavioral techniques decrease pain-intensity scores and reduce distress associated with pain.[139,140] Part of the effect of these therapies is due to increased control; however, mental and physical relaxation also leads to reduced muscle tension, a contributing factor in pain.[141] Relaxation, guided imagery, distraction, and other interventions are useful when used in conjunction with, rather than as a replacement for, pharmacologic therapies.

People with cancer should be taught these techniques early in the course of their illness, as practice is necessary and may be impossible when fatigue is excessive.[9] Several audiotapes are available, or a tape can be made that is customized to the individual, and scripts provide structure for those wishing to use these interventions.[68]

Behavioral therapies include massage, heat, cold, and vibration. As with cognitive interventions, these techniques must be individualized to the needs of each patient. Both cognitive and behavioral exercises can be taught to individuals and their support persons, incorporating and empowering loved ones to participate in the person's care. Much remains unknown regarding the mechanism of action, specific indications, and additional effects of these therapies; this is an area in which nurses are uniquely prepared to conduct the research necessary to answer these questions.

Invasive neurolytic or neurosurgical procedures When standard analgesic therapy is unsuccessful, nerve blocks may be of benefit, particularly when pain is well localized. For example, a recent metaanalysis of celiac plexus block for abdominal pain due to pancreatic cancer or other malignancies indicated that this procedure is very effective and generally well tolerated.[142] Of particular concern, after any neurolytic procedure produces relief of pain, is the gradual reduction of opioid doses to prevent the onset of withdrawal.

Neurosurgical procedures are generally reserved for the small number of individuals who do not obtain relief with any of the previous therapies.[143] Life expectancy is another essential consideration, as regeneration may produce significantly elevated pain intensity with a change in quality that may exacerbate pain management difficulties. Ablative procedures include commissural myelotomy, dorsal rhizotomy, hypophysectomy, neurectomy, and percutaneous or open anterolateral cordotomy.

Evaluation of Management Interventions

Evaluation of the effectiveness of therapy is essential. Clinicians must know whether a chosen regimen is successful in alleviating the pain of an individual patient. Furthermore, clinicians and administrators concerned about the quality of care within their setting must also know whether pain management is effective in their population of patients.

Individual evaluation

When evaluating the efficacy of a treatment regimen, serial intensity measures can reflect the degree of change in pain scores. This information assists in titrating the dose of analgesics. When measured regularly after administering a treatment, intensity scores can also reveal how long the therapy relieves pain. This is vital information when determining the frequency of drug administration, particularly because wide variability exists in opioid dose and timing among individuals.[91] Pain relief scores, using a 0% to 100% relief scale, can also assist in the evaluation of a treatment regimen.

To visualize these changes and any resultant adverse effects, documentation is essential. The use of systematic pain documentation, incorporating standardized assessment forms and flow sheets, can reduce pain intensity, presumably through greater awareness on the part of healthcare professionals of the individual's pain. In fact, the American Pain Society and other organizations advocate making pain the "fifth vital sign."[144,145] An example of a flow sheet is included in Figure 9-7.

Institutional evaluation: Quality improvement

The American Pain Society has published quality assurance (QA) standards for acute and cancer pain relief to assist in the institutional evaluation of pain treatment.[146] The AHCPR *Management of Cancer Pain Clinical Practice Guideline* incorporates these standards when developing recommendations for all practice settings (Table 9-9). One of these recommendations includes surveying patient satisfaction with pain management.

Using a survey adapted from recommendations advanced by the American Pain Society Quality Assurance Committee, investigators have found that although patients may report significant pain and experience long delays in obtaining attention to the pain, most indicate satisfaction with pain management (Table 9-10).[47,148] Adaptation of the existing patient satisfaction surveys and interviewing techniques is essential, including using independent observers and asking patients about the discrepancies between pain reports and satisfaction (Table 9-11). Although measuring satisfaction has proved somewhat difficult, these obstacles can be overcome. Measuring the effectiveness of pain management along with patient satisfaction with the treatment is the first step in developing measures to improve the quality of care.

FLOW SHEET—PAIN

Patient _____ Date _____

Pain rating scale used [a] _____

Purpose: To evaluate the safety and effectiveness of the analgesic(s).

Analgesic(s) prescribed: _____

Time	Pain rating	Analgesic	R	P	BP	Level of arousal	Other[b]	Plan & comments

[a] Pain rating: A number of different scales may be used. Indicate which scale is used and use the same one each time. For example: 0–10 (0 = no pain, 10 = worst pain).
[b] Possibilities for other columns: bowel function, activities, nausea and vomiting, other pain relief measures. Identify the side effects of greatest concern to patient, family, physician, nurses.

FIGURE 9-7 Flow sheets for the documentation of pain and its treatment. (Source: McCaffery M, Beebe A: *Pain: A Clinical Manual for Nursing Practice.* St. Louis: Mosby, 1989.[68])

TABLE 9-9 AHCPR Recommendations for Monitoring the Quality of Pain Management

1. Promise patients attentive care.
2. Assign responsibility for pain management.
3. Document the assessment of pain and its relief.
4. Define pain and relief levels to trigger a review.
5. Survey patient satisfaction.
6. Analgesic drug treatment should comply with two basic principles:

   - Oral analgesics and other noninvasive routes are used whenever possible and administered in accordance with the principles expressed in the WHO analgesic ladder.

   - Analgesics are titrated to maximally effective doses or to the appearance of dose-limiting side effects before specialized invasive analgesic approaches are used.

7. Monitor use of specialized analgesic technologies.
8. Offer nonpharmacologic interventions.
9. Monitor the efficacy of pain treatment.

Jacox A, Carr DB, Payne R, et al: *Management of Cancer Pain. Clinical Practice Guideline No. 9.* AHCPR Publication No. 94-0592. Rockville, MD, Agency for Health Care Policy and Research, Public Health Service, U.S. Department of Health and Human Services, March 1994.[9]

TABLE 9-10 Patient Satisfaction Survey

1. At any time during this hospital stay have you needed treatment for pain?
2. How long have you been in pain?
3. Have you experienced pain in the last 24 hours?
4. Did you tell the doctors or nurses you were having pain?
5. On a scale of 0 to 10, with 0 representing "no pain" and 10 representing the "worst pain imaginable," what was the worst pain you had in the past 24 hours?
6. On a scale of 0 to 10, with 0 representing "no pain" and 10 representing the "worst pain imaginable," how much pain do you have right now?
7. On a scale of 0 to 10, with 0 representing "no pain" and 10 representing the "worst pain imaginable," where did the pain go after you got pain medication?
8. How satisfied are you with the amount of pain relief you received?
9. How satisfied are you with how the staff responded to your reports of pain?
10. Who do you believe is responsible for your pain relief while you are in the hospital?
11. Of the following health team members (i.e., doctor, nurse, social worker, physical therapist, pharmacist, other), who has been helpful to you when you were in pain?
12. When you asked for pain medication, what was the longest time you had to wait to get it?
13. Was there a time when the medication you were given for pain didn't help and you asked for something more or different to relieve the pain?
14. If your answer is yes, how long did it take before your doctor or nurse changed your treatment to a stronger or different medication and you got it?
15. If longer than one hour, why do you think it took so long?
16. Did your doctors or nurses ask you to be sure to tell them when you have pain?
17. Did your doctors or nurses tell you we consider treatment of pain very important?

Reprinted by permission of Elsevier Science from: Assessment of patient satisfaction utilizing the American Pain Society's quality assurance standards on acute and cancer-related pain, by Miaskowski C, Nichols R, Brody R, et al. *Journal of Pain and Symptom Management* 9:6. Copyright 1994 by the U.S. Cancer Pain Relief Committee.[147]

TABLE 9-11 Recommendations for Patient Satisfaction Surveys

1. Use a surveyor who is not directly involved in the patient's care, or conduct the survey after the patient has been discharged from the facility.
2. Evaluate analgesic prescriptive practices (i.e., number of analgesics ordered, types of analgesics ordered, frequency, route of administration, and dose).
3. Evaluate patient satisfaction with pain management practices and satisfaction with care providers using a descriptive, numeric rating scale.
4. Explore with the patient, in a nonthreatening manner, the incongruity between their pain intensity ratings and the level of satisfaction with pain relief or the staff's response to reports of pain.
5. Use additional survey responses (e.g., ratings of pain relief, waiting time for pain medications, and requests for changes in pain management plan) to determine patient satisfaction with pain management practices.
6. Ask patients to rate how much pain they expect to have following surgery or as a result of a procedure and how much pain relief they expect to be provided to them.
7. Ask patients direct questions about what they would change about pain management in the institution.

Reprinted by permission of Elsevier Science from: Assessment of patient satisfaction utilizing the American Pain Society's quality assurance standards on acute and cancer-related pain, by Miaskowski C, Nichols R, Brody R, et al. *Journal of Pain and Symptom Management* 9:11. Copyright 1994 by the U.S. Cancer Pain Relief Committee.[147]

Educational Tools and Resources

Self-care guide

Many tools are available to assist nurses and other healthcare professionals in educating patients and caregivers about cancer pain (Table 9-12). Teaching guides must be chosen based on the individual needs of each person and their family members.[149] The *Managing Cancer Pain* consumer guide that accompanies the AHCPR's *Management of Cancer Pain Clinical Practice Guideline* provides a general discussion of the causes of pain, methods for assessing and relieving pain, and tools to assist in documenting the daily pain scores and drug effects.[150] Appendix 9A contains a shorter self-care guide for use with persons experiencing cancer-related pain.

Resources

Numerous organizations are available to assist the individual with cancer-related pain, as well as the nurse caring for those persons. In addition to those resources listed for patients in Table 9-12, numerous pharmaceuti-

TABLE 9-12 Teaching Tools and Educational Resources for Individuals in Pain and Their Support Persons

Organizations:
American Cancer Society, Inc.
1599 Clifton Road, N.E.
Atlanta, GA 30329-4251
(800) ACS-2345
Check the phone book for the number of your local unit
 	
American Chronic Pain Association
P.O. Box 850
Rocklin, CA 95677
(916) 632-0922   FAX (916) 632-3208
Although not specifically directed to the needs of people with cancer, this organization has literature that assists the person in chronic pain.
 	
National Cancer Institute
Office of Cancer Communications
Building 31, Room 10A24
Bethesda, MD 20892
(800) 4-CANCER
Includes CancerFax: dial (301) 402-5874, using the telephone receiver on the FAX machine
 	
National Chronic Pain Outreach Association
7979 Old Georgetown Road, Suite 100
Bethesda, MD 20814-2429
(301) 652-4948
 	
Literature (Booklets):
Cancer Pain Can Be Relieved
Children's Cancer Pain Can Be Relieved
Jeff Asks About Cancer Pain
Wisconsin Cancer Pain Initiative
3675 Medical Sciences Center
University of Wisconsin Medical School
1300 University Avenue, Room 4720
Madison, WI 53706
(608) 262-0978
 	
Get Relief from Cancer Pain, NIH Publication No. 94-3735
Available from the National Cancer Institute and the American Cancer Society by calling (800) 4-CANCER
 	
Managing Cancer Pain/Patient Guide
   English: AHCPR Pub. No. 94-0595
   Spanish: AHCPR Pub. No. 94-0596
	Pain Control After Surgery: A Patient's Guide
	   AHCPR Pub. No. 92-0021
	AHCPR Publications Clearinghouse
	P.O. Box 8547
	Silver Spring, MD 20907
	(800) 4-CANCER (for individual copies of the cancer pain guide), (800) 358-9295
	
	Questions and Answers About Pain Control: A Guide for People with Cancer and Their Families
	Available from the American Cancer Society and the National Cancer Institute by calling (800) 4-CANCER or (800) ACS-2345
	
	Literature (Books):
	Cowles J: *Pain Relief: How to Say No to Acute, Chronic & Cancer Pain!*
	New York: Mastermedia Ltd., 1993
	Call (800) 334-8232 to order.
	
	Haylock PJ, Curtiss CP: *Cancer Doesn't Have to Hurt: How to Conquer the Pain Caused by Cancer and Cancer Treatment.*
	Alameda, CA: Hunter House Publishers, 1997
	(510) 865-5282
	
	Long SS, Patt RB: *You Don't Have to Suffer.*
	New York: Oxford Press, 1994
	Call (713) 792-6911 to order.
	
	Stacy CB, Kaplan AS, Williams G: *The Fight Against Pain*, 1993
	Consumer Reports Books
	101 Truman Avenue
	Yonkers, NY 10703
	(212) 741-6680
	
	Wall PD, Jones M: *Defeating Pain: The War Against a Silent Epidemic.*
	New York: Plenum Press, 1991
	
	Journals:
	Coping
	2019 N. Caruthers
	Franklin, TN 37064
	(615) 790-2400/FAX (615) 791-4719
	
	Audiocassettes:
	The Cancer Pain Education Program: A Comprehensive Approach to Pain Management in the Home.
	The Marketing Department
	City of Hope National Medical Center
	1500 East Duarte Road
	Duarte, CA 91010-0269
	(818) 301-8346

cal firms have specialized programs to assist the financially needy in obtaining medications at reduced cost or, in some cases, free of charge. Resources for nurses provide educational enrichment and materials useful for clinical practice, such as position statements and practice guidelines, as well as networking opportunities (Table 9-13).

Conclusion

Of the many symptoms affecting those with cancer, pain is widely believed to be inevitable and is greatly feared. Numerous barriers exist to the delivery of adequate relief;

TABLE 9-13 Resources for Professionals Interested in Cancer Pain

Organizations:
American Pain Society
4700 West Lake Avenue
Glenview, IL 60025
(847) 375-4715
Journal: *Pain Forum*

American Society of Pain Management Nurses
7794 Grow Drive
Pensacola, FL 32514
(888) 34-ASPMN

International Association for the Study of Pain
909 NE 43rd Street, Suite 306
Seattle, WA 98105
(206) 547-6409
Journal: *Pain*

National Cancer Institute
Office of Cancer Communication
Bethesda, MD 20892
(800) 4-CANCER

National Hospice Organization
1901 North Moore Street, Suite 901
Arlington, VA 22209
(703) 243-5900

Oncology Nursing Society
501 Holiday Drive
Pittsburgh, PA 15220-2749
(412) 921-7373
Journal: *Oncology Nursing Forum*
Members can join the pain special interest group (SIG) for a minor additional fee.

Resource Center for State Cancer Pain Initiatives
1300 University Avenue, #3671
Madison, WI 53706
(608) 265-4013

Journals (in addition to those available to members of organizations listed above):
Clinical Journal of Pain
Raven Press, Ltd.
1140 Avenue of the Americas
New York, NY 10036
(212) 930-9500

Journal of Pain and Symptom Management
Elsevier Science Inc.
P.O. Box 945
New York, NY 10010
(212) 633-3730

Pharmaceutical Care in Pain & Symptom Control
The Haworth Press, Inc.
10 Alice Street
Binghamton, NY 13904-1580
(607) 722-5857

Monographs:
American Pain Society: *Principles of Analgesic Use in the Treatment of Acute Pain and Cancer Pain* (ed 4), 1998
American Pain Society
4700 West Lake Avenue
Glenview, IL 60025
(847) 375-4715

World Health Organization: Cancer Pain Relief and Palliative Care: Report of a WHO Expert Committee, 1990
World Health Organization Publications Center USA
49 Sheridan Avenue
Albany, NY 12210
or: World Health Organization, Distribution and Sales
1211 Geneva 27
Switzerland

Position Papers and Clinical Practice Guidelines:
Jacox A, Carr DB, Payne R, et al: *Management of Cancer Pain, Clinical Practice Guideline* No. 9, AHCPR Publication No. 94-0592 Rockville, MD: Agency for Health Care Policy and Research, U.S. Department of Health and Human Services, Public Health Service, March 1994.
Also includes:
Management of Cancer Pain: Adults/Quick Reference Guide for Clinicians, AHCPR Publication No. 94-0593
Managing Cancer Pain/Patient Guide
   English: AHCPR Pub. No. 94-0595
   Spanish: AHCPR Pub. No. 94-0596
AHCPR Publications Clearinghouse
P.O. Box 8547
Silver Spring, MD 20907
(800) 4-CANCER (for individual copies)
(800) 358-9295

Spross JA, McGuire DB, Schmitt RM: Oncology Nursing Society position paper on cancer pain
   Part I. *Oncology Nursing Forum* 17:595–614, 1990
   Part II. *Oncology Nursing Forum* 17:751–760, 1990
   Part III. *Oncology Nursing Forum* 17:943–955, 1990

however, those with cancer and their support persons working in concert with educated healthcare professionals can, and do, obtain relief from pain in the majority of cases. Ongoing assessment, in combination with the appropriate use of pharmacologic and nonpharmacologic therapies, is essential. Greater professional and public awareness of the problem of cancer pain has led to the development of educational and supportive resources for those in pain and for those responsible for their care. Through these efforts, pain and unnecessary suffering will be diminished and the quality of life of those with cancer will be improved.

References

1. Daut RC, Cleeland CS: The prevalence and severity of pain in cancer. *Cancer* 50:1913–1918, 1982
2. Donovan MI, Dillon P: Incidence and characteristics of pain in a sample of hospitalized cancer patients. *Cancer Nurs* 10:85–92, 1987
3. Dorrepaal KL, Aaronson NK, van Dam FSAM: Pain experience and pain management among hospitalized cancer patients. A clinical study. *Cancer* 63:593–598, 1989
4. Coyle N, Adelhardt J, Foley KM, et al: Character of terminal illness in the advanced cancer patient: Pain and other symptoms during the last four weeks of life. *J Pain Symptom Manage* 5:83–93, 1990
5. Paice JA, Mahon SM, Faut-Callahan M: Factors associated with adequate pain control in hospitalized postsurgical patients diagnosed with cancer. *Cancer Nurs* 14:298–305, 1991
6. Portenoy RK: Cancer pain: Epidemiology and syndromes. *Cancer* 63:2298–2307, 1989
7. Twycross RG: Incidence of pain. *Clin Oncol* 3:5–15, 1984
8. Cleeland CS, Gonin R, Hatfield AK, et al: Pain and its treatment in outpatients with metastatic cancer. *N Engl J Med* 330:592–596, 1994
9. Jacox A, Carr DB, Payne R, et al: *Management of Cancer Pain. Clinical Practice Guideline No. 9.* AHCPR Publication No. 94-0592. Rockville, MD: Agency for Health Care Policy and Research, Public Health Service, U.S. Department of Health and Human Services, March 1994
10. Diekmann JM, Wassem RA: A survey of nursing students' knowledge of cancer pain control. *Cancer Nurs* 14:314–320, 1991
11. Ferrell BR, McCaffery M, Rhiner M: Pain and addiction: An urgent need for change in nursing education. *J Pain Symptom Manage* 7:117–124, 1992
12. Ferrell BR, McGuire DB, Donovan MI: Knowledge and beliefs regarding pain in a sample of nursing faculty. *J Prof Nurs* 9:79–88, 1993
13. Grossman SA, Sheidler VR: Skills of medical students and house officers in prescribing narcotic medications. *J Med Educ* 60:552–557, 1985
14. Hamilton J, Edgar L: A survey examining nurses' knowledge of pain control. *J Pain Symptom Manage* 7:18–26, 1992
15. Marks RM, Sachar EJ: Undertreatment of medical inpatients with narcotic analgesics. *Ann Intern Med* 78:173–181, 1973
16. McCaffery M, Ferrell B, O'Neil-Page E, et al: Nurses' knowledge of opioid analgesic drugs and psychological dependence. *Cancer Nurs* 13:21–27, 1990
17. Sheehan DK, Webb A, Bower D, et al: Level of cancer pain knowledge among baccalaureate student nurses. *J Pain Symptom Manage* 7:478–484, 1992
18. Sheidler VR, McGuire DB, Grossman SA, et al: Analgesic decision-making skills of nurses. *Oncol Nurs Forum* 19:1531–1534, 1992
19. Vortherms R, Ryan P, Ward S: Knowledge of attitudes toward, and barriers to pharmacologic management of cancer pain in a statewide random sample of nurses. *Res Nurs Health* 15:459–466, 1992
20. Weissman DE, Dahl JL: Attitudes about cancer pain: A survey of Wisconsin's first-year medical students. *J Pain Symptom Manage* 5:345–349, 1990
21. Cleeland CS, Cleeland LM, Dar R, et al: Factors influencing physician management of cancer pain. *Cancer* 58:796–800, 1986
22. Grossman SA, Sheidler VR, Sweden K, et al: Correlation of patient and caregiver ratings of cancer pain. *J Pain Symptom Manage* 6:53–57, 1991
23. Taylor AG, Skelton JA, Butcher J: Duration of pain condition and physical pathology as determinants of nurses' assessments of patients in pain. *Nurs Res* 33:4–8, 1984
24. Teske K, Daut RL, Cleeland CS: Relationships between nurses' observations and patients' self-reports of pain. *Pain* 16:289–296, 1983
25. Holm K, Cohen F, Dudas S, et al: Effect of personal pain experience on pain assessment. *Image J Nurs Schol* 21:72–75, 1989
26. Levin DN, Cleeland CS, Dar R: Public attitudes toward cancer pain. *Cancer* 56:2337–2339, 1985
27. Ward SE, Goldberg N, Miller-McCauley V, et al: Patient-related barriers to management of cancer pain. *Pain* 52:319–324, 1993
28. Von Roenn J, Cleeland CS, Gonin R, et al: Physician attitudes and practice in cancer pain management. A survey from the Eastern Cooperative Oncology Group. *Ann Intern Med* 119:121–126, 1993
29. Hill CS: Relationship among cultural, educational, and regulatory agency influences on optimum cancer pain treatment. *J Pain Symptom Manage* 5(suppl):37–45, 1990
30. Blesch KS, Paice JA, Wickham R, et al: Correlates of fatigue in people with breast or lung cancer. *Oncol Nurs Forum* 18:81–87, 1991
31. Spiegel D, Sands S, Koopman C: Pain and depression in patients with cancer. *Cancer* 74:2570–2578, 1994
32. Strang P: Emotional and social aspects of cancer pain. *Acta Oncol* 31:323–326, 1992
33. Ferrell BR, Rhiner M, Cohen MZ, et al: Pain as a metaphor for illness. Part I: Impact of cancer pain on family caregivers. *Oncol Nurs Forum* 18:1303–1309, 1991
34. Cherny NI, Coyle N, Foley KM: Suffering in the advanced cancer patient: A definition and taxonomy. *J Palliat Care* 10:57–70, 1994
35. Ferrell BR, Taylor EJ, Grant M, et al: Pain management at home: Struggle, comfort, and mission. *Cancer Nurs* 16:169–178, 1993
36. Cherny NI, Portenoy RK: Cancer pain: Principles of assessment and syndromes, in Wall PD, Melzack R (eds): *Textbook of Pain* (ed 3). Edinburgh: Churchill Livingstone, 1994, pp. 787–823

37. Curran CF, Luce JK, Page JA: Doxorubicin-associated flare reactions. *Oncol Nurs Forum* 17:387–389, 1990

38. Thompson IM, Zeidman EJ, Rodriguez FR: Sudden death due to disease flare with luteinizing hormone-releasing hormone agonist therapy for carcinoma of the prostate. *J Urol* 144:1479–1480, 1990

39. *Principles of Analgesic Use in the Treatment of Acute Pain and Cancer Pain* (ed 4). Skokie, IL: American Pain Society, 1998

40. Bonica JJ: Definitions and taxonomy of pain, in Bonica JJ (ed): *The Management of Pain* (ed 2). Philadelphia: Lea & Febiger, 1990, pp. 18–27

41. Bennett GJ: Neuropathic pain, in Wall PD, Melzack R (eds): *Textbook of Pain* (ed 3). Edinburgh: Churchill Livingstone, 1994, pp. 201–224

42. Rang HP, Bevan S, Dray A: Nociceptive peripheral neurons: Cellular properties, in Wall PD, Melzack R (eds): *Textbook of Pain* (ed 3). Edinburgh: Churchill Livingstone, 1994, pp. 57–78

43. Insel PA. Analgesic-antipyretics and antiinflammatory agents: Drugs employed in the treatment of rheumatoid arthritis and gout, in Gilman AG, Rall TW, Nies AS, et al (eds): *Goodman and Gilman's The Pharmacological Basis of Therapeutics* (ed 8). New York: Pergamon 1990, pp. 638–681

44. Tanelian DL, MacIver MB: Analgesic concentrations of lidocaine suppress tonic A-delta and C-fiber discharges produced by acute injury. *Anesthesia* 74:934–936, 1991

45. Dray A, Urban L, Dickenson A: Pharmacology of chronic pain. *Trends Pharmacol Sci* 15:190–197, 1994

46. Yaksh TL, Jessell TM, Gamse R, et al: Intrathecal morphine inhibits substance P release from mammalian spinal cord in vivo. *Nature* 286:155–156, 1980

47. Proudfit HK: Pharmacologic evidence for the modulation of nociception by noradrenergic neurons, in Fields HL, Besson JM (eds): *Progress in Brain Research*, vol 77. Amsterdam: Elsevier, 1988, pp. 357–370

48. Eisenach JC, Rauck RL, Buzzanell C, et al: Epidural clonidine analgesia for intractable cancer pain: Phase I. *Anesthesiology* 71:647–652, 1989

49. Monks R: Psychotropic drugs, in Bonica JJ (ed): *The Management of Pain* (ed 2). Philadelphia: Lea & Febiger, 1990, pp. 1676–1689

50. Wall PD, Gutnick M: Ongoing activity in peripheral nerves: The physiology and pharmacology of impulses originating from a neuroma. *Exp Neurol* 43:580–593, 1974

51. Coderre TJ, Katz J, Vaccarino AL, et al: Contribution of central neuroplasticity to pathological pain: Review of clinical and experimental evidence. *Pain* 52:259–285, 1993

52. Acute Pain Management Guideline Panel: *Acute Pain Management Operative or Medical Procedures and Trauma. Clinical Practice Guideline.* AHCPR Publication No. 92-0032. Rockville, MD: Agency for Health Care Policy and Research, Public Health Service, U.S. Department of Health and Human Services, 1992

53. Jensen MP, Karoly P, Braver S: The measurement of clinical pain intensity: A comparison of six methods. *Pain* 27:117–126, 1986

54. Ferraz MB, Quaresma MR, Aquino IRI, et al: Reliability of pain scales in the assessment of literate and illiterate patients with rheumatoid arthritis. *J Rheumatol* 17:1022–1024, 1990

55. Jensen MP, Karoly P, O'Riodan EF, et al: The subjective experience of acute pain: An assessment of the utility of 10 indices. *Clin J Pain* 5:153–159, 1989

56. Kremer E, Atkinson JH, Ignelzi RJ: Measurement of pain: Patient preference does not confound pain measurement. *Pain* 10:241–248, 1981

57. Scott J, Huskisson EC: Graphic representation of pain. *Pain* 2:175–184, 1976

58. Jensen MP, Karoly P: Measurement of cancer pain via patient self-report, in Chapman CR, Foley KM (eds): *Current and Emerging Issues in Cancer Pain: Research and Practice.* New York: Raven Press, 1993, pp. 193–218

59. McGrath PA: *Pain in Children: Nature, Assessment, and Treatment.* New York: Guilford, 1990

60. Eland J: Minimizing pain associated with prekindergarten intramuscular injections. *Issues Compr Pediatr Nurs* 5:361–372, 1981

61. McGrath PJ, Unruh AM: Measurement and assessment of paediatric pain, in Wall PD, Melzack R (eds): *Textbook of Pain* (ed 3). Edinburgh: Churchill Livingstone, 1994, pp. 303–313

62. Beyer JE, Wells N: Assessment of cancer pain in children, in Patt RB (ed): *Cancer Pain.* Philadelphia: Lippincott, 1993, pp. 57–84

63. Melzak R: The McGill Pain Questionnaire: Major properties and scoring methods. *Pain* 1:277–299, 1975

64. McGuire DB: Assessment of pain in cancer in patients using the McGill Pain Questionnaire. *Oncol Nurs Forum* 11:32–37, 1984

65. Melzak R: The short-form McGill Pain Questionnaire. *Pain* 30:191–197, 1987

66. Daut RL, Cleeland CS, Flanery RC: Development of the Wisconsin Brief Pain Questionnaire to assess pain in cancer and other diseases. *Pain* 17:197–210, 1983

67. Fishman B, Paternak S, Wallenstein SL, et al: The Memorial Pain Assessment Card: A valid instrument for the evaluation of cancer pain. *Cancer* 60:1151–1158, 1987

68. McCaffery M, Beebe A: *Pain: A Clinical Manual for Nursing Practice.* St. Louis: Mosby, 1989

69. Beyer JE, McGrath PJ, Berde CB: Discordance between self-report and behavioral pain measures in children aged 3–7 years after surgery. *J Pain Symptom Manage* 5:350–356, 1990

70. Bruera E, MacMillan K, Hanson J, et al: The Edmonton staging system for cancer pain: Preliminary report. *Pain* 37:203–209, 1989

71. Bruera E, Schoeller T, Wenk R, et al: A prospective multicenter assessment of the Edmonton Staging System for cancer pain. *J Pain Symptom Manage* 10:348–355, 1995

72. Katz J, Kavanagh BP, Sandler AA, et al: Preemptive analgesia: Clinical evidence of neuroplasticity contributing to postoperative pain. *Anesthesiology* 77:439–446, 1992

73. Yaksh TL, Abram SE: Preemptive analgesia: A popular misnomer, but a clinically relevant truth? *APS J* 2:116–121, 1993

74. Kehlet H, Dahl JB: Preemptive analgesia: A misnomer and a misinterpreted technique. *APS J* 2:122–124, 1993

75. Kurman MR: Systemic therapy (chemotherapy) in the palliative treatment of cancer pain, in Patt RB (ed): *Cancer Pain.* Philadelphia: Lippincott, 1993, pp. 251–274

76. Stoll BA: Hormonal therapy—Pain relief and recalcification, in Stoll BA, Parbhoo S (eds): *Bone Metastasis: Monitoring and Treatment.* New York: Raven Press, 1983, pp. 321–342

77. Ashby M: Radiotherapy in the palliation of cancer, in Patt RB (ed): *Cancer Pain.* Philadelphia: Lippincott 1993, pp. 235–249

78. Nielsen OS, Munro AJ, Tannock IF: Bone metastases: Pathophysiology and management policy. *J Clin Oncol* 9: 509–524, 1991

79. WHO Expert Committee: *Cancer Pain Relief and Palliative Care* (ed 2). Geneva: World Health Organization, 1996

80. Malmberg AB, Yaksh TL: Antinociceptive actions of spinal nonsteroidal antiinflammatory agents on the formalin test in the rat. *J Pharmacol Ther* 263:136–146, 1992

81. Allison MC, Howatson AG, Torrance CJ, et al: Gastrointestinal damage associated with the use of nonsteroidal antiinflammatory drugs. *N Engl J Med* 327:749–754, 1992

82. Kaufman DW, Kelly JP, Sheehan JE, et al: Nonsteroidal antiinflammatory drug use in relation to upper gastrointestinal bleeding. *Clin Pharmacol Ther* 53:485–494, 1994

83. Koch M, Dezi A, Ferrario F, Capurso I: Prevention of nonsteroidal anti-inflammatory drug-induced gastrointestinal mucosal injury. A meta-analysis of randomized controlled clinical trials. *Arch Intern Med* 156:2321–2332, 1996

84. Sandler DP, Smith JC, Weinberg CR, et al: Analgesic use and chronic renal disease. *N Engl J Med* 320:1238–1243, 1989

85. Perez Gutthann S, Garcia Rodriguez LA, Raiford DS, et al: Nonsteroidal anti-inflammatory drugs and the risk of hospitalization for acute renal failure. *Arch Intern Med* 156: 2433–2439, 1996

86. Levy MH: Pharmacologic treatment of cancer pain. *N Engl J Med* 335:1124–1132, 1996

87. *Physicians' Desk Reference*. Montvale, NJ: Medical Economics Data, 1997

88. Thyss A, Milano G, Kubar J, et al: Clinical and pharmacokinetic evidence of a life-threatening interaction between methotrexate and ketoprofen. *Lancet* 8475:256–258, 1986

89. Stein C: Peripheral mechanisms of opioid analgesia. *Anesth Analg* 76:182–191, 1992

90. Jaffe JH, Martin WR: Opioid analgesics and antagonists, in Gilman AG, Rall TW, Nies AL, et al (eds): *Goodman and Gilman's The Pharmacological Basis of Therapeutics* (ed 8). New York: Pergamon, 1990, pp. 485–521

91. Brescia FJ, Portenoy RK, Ryan M, et al: Pain, opioid use, and survival in hospitalized patients with advanced cancer. *J Clin Oncol* 10:149–155, 1992

92. Schwartz JA, Koenigsberg MD: Naloxone-induced pulmonary edema. *Ann Emerg Med* 16:1294–1296, 1987

93. Flacke JW, Flacke WE, Williams GD: Acute pulmonary edema following naloxone reversal of high-dose morphine anesthesia. *Anesthesiology* 47:376–378, 1977

94. Michaelis LL, Hickey PR, Clark TA, et al: Ventricular irritability associated with the use of naloxone hydrochloride. *Ann Thorac Surg* 18:608–614, 1974

95. Burke DF, Dunwoody CJ: Naloxone: A word of caution. *Orthop Nurs* 9:44–46, 1990

96. Porter J, Jick H: Addiction rare in patients treated with narcotics. *N Engl J Med* 302:123, 1980

97. Bruera E, Watanabe S: Psychostimulants as adjuvant analgesics. *J Pain Symptom Manage* 9:412–415, 1994

98. Caraceni A, Martini C, De Conno F, et al: Organic brain syndromes and opioid administration for cancer pain. *J Pain Symptom Manage* 9:527–535, 1994

99. Abel EL: Opiates and sex. *J Psychoactive Drugs* 16:205–216, 1984

100. Paice JA, Penn RD, Ryan WG: Altered sexual function and decreased testosterone in patients receiving intraspinal opioids. *J Pain Symptom Manage* 9:126–131, 1994

101. McGuire DB, Sheidler VR: Pain, in Groenwald SL, Frogge MH, Goodman M, Yarbro CH (eds): *Cancer Nursing: Principles and Practice* (ed 4). Boston: Jones & Bartlett, 1997, pp. 529–584

102. Houde RW: Systemic analgesics and related drugs: Narcotic analgesics, in Bonica JJ, Ventafridda V (eds): *Advances in Pain Research and Therapy*, vol 2. New York: Raven Press, 1979, pp. 263–272

103. Inturrisi CE: Management of cancer pain: Pharmacology and principles of management. *Cancer* 63:2308–2320, 1989

104. Walsh TD: Oral morphine in chronic cancer pain. *Pain* 18:1–11, 1984

105. Houde RW: Misinformation: Side effects and drug interactions, in Hill CS, Fields WS (eds): *Advances in Pain Research and Therapy*, vol 11. New York: Raven Press, 1989, pp. 145–161

106. Szeta HH, Inturrisi CE, Houde R, et al: Accumulation of normeperidine, an active metabolite of meperidine, in patients with renal failure or cancer. *Ann Intern Med* 86: 738–741, 1977

107. Kaiko RF, Foley KM, Grabinski PY, et al: Central nervous system excitatory effects of meperidine in cancer patients. *Ann Neurol* 13:180–185, 1983

108. Pitorak EF, Kraus JC: Pain control with sublingual morphine. *Am J Hosp Care* 4:39–41, 1987

109. Bell MDD, Murray GR, Mishra P, et al: Buccal morphine—A new route for analgesia. *Lancet* 8420:71–73, 1985

110. Fine PG, Marcus M, DeBoer AJ, et al: An open label study of oral transmucosal fentanyl citrate (OTFC) for the treatment of breakthrough cancer pain. *Pain* 45:149–153, 1991

111. Kaiko RF, Fitzmartin RD, Thomas GB, et al: The bioavailability of morphine in controlled-release 30-mg tablets per rectum compared with immediate-release 30-mg rectal suppositories and controlled-release 30-mg oral tablets. *Pharmacotherapy* 12:107–113, 1992

112. McCaffery M, Martin L, Ferrell BR: Analgesic administration via rectum or stoma. *J ET Nurs* 19:114–121, 1992

113. Breda M, Bianchi M, Ripamonti C, et al: Plasma morphine and morphine-6-glucuronide patterns in cancer patients after oral, subcutaneous, sublabial and rectal short-term administration. *Int J Clin Pharmacol Res* 11:93–97, 1991

114. Citron ML, Johnston-Early A, Fossieck BE, et al: Safety and efficacy of continuous intravenous morphine for severe cancer pain. *Am J Med* 77:199–203, 1984

115. Hill HF, Chapman CR, Kornell JA, et al: Self-administration of morphine in bone marrow transplant patients reduces drug requirement. *Pain* 40:121–129, 1990

116. Storey P, Hill HH, St. Louis RH, et al: Subcutaneous infusions for control of cancer symptoms. *J Pain Symptom Manage* 5:33–41, 1990

117. Moulin DE, Kreeft JH, Murray-Parsons N, et al: Comparison of continuous hydromorphone infusions for management of cancer pain. *Lancet* 337:465–468, 1991

118. Paice JA, Buck MM: Intraspinal devices for pain management. *Nurs Clin North Am* 28:921–935, 1993

119. Paice JA, Williams AR: Intraspinal drugs for pain, in McGuire DB, Yarbro CH, Ferrell B (eds): *Cancer Pain Management* (ed 2). Boston: Jones & Bartlett 1995, pp. 131–158

120. Payne R: Transdermal fentanyl: Suggested recommendations for clinical use. *J Pain Symptom Manage* 7(suppl): 40–44, 1992

121. Farncombe M, Chater S: Case studies outlining use of nebulized morphine for patients with end-stage chronic

lung and cardiac disease. *J Pain Symptom Manage* 8:221–225, 1993

122. Wetchler BV, Alexander CD, Uhill MA: Transnasal butorphanol tartrate for pain control following ambulatory surgery. *Curr Ther Res* 52:571–580, 1992

123. Lombard DJ, Oliver DJ: The use of opioid analgesics in the last 24 hours of life of patients with advanced cancer. *Palliat Med* 3:27–29, 1989

124. Snyder S: Recent advances in extemporaneous compounding in unusual pain medications for hospice/terminally ill patients. *Pain Digest* 4:29–42, 1994

125. Ferrell BR, Wisdom C, Wenz C, et al: Effects of controlled-release morphine on QOL for cancer pain. *Oncol Nurs Forum* 16:521–526 1989

126. Cherny NI, Portenoy RK: The management of cancer pain. *CA Cancer J Clin* 44:262–303, 1994

127. Jadad AR, Carroll D, Glynn CJ, et al: Morphine responsiveness of chronic pain: Double-blind randomised crossover study with patient-controlled analgesia. *Lancet* 339: 1367–1371, 1992

128. Watson CPN: Antidepressant drugs as adjuvant analgesics. *J Pain Symptom Manage* 9:392–405, 1994

129. Mellick GA, Mellicy LB, Mellick LB: Gabapentin in the management of reflex sympathetic dystrophy. *J Pain Symptom Manage* 10:265–267, 1995

130. Watanabe S, Bruera E: Corticosteroids as adjuvant analgesics. *J Pain Symptom Manage* 9:442–445, 1994

131. Backonja M-M: Local anesthetics as adjuvant analgesics. *J Pain Symptom Manage* 9:491–499, 1994

132. Patt RB, Proper G, Reddy S: The neuroleptics as adjuvant analgesics. *J Pain Symptom Manage* 9:446–453, 1994

133. Fromm GH: Baclofen as an adjuvant analgesic. *J Pain Symptom Manage* 9:500–509, 1994

134. Watson CPN: Topical capsaicin as an adjuvant analgesic. *J Pain Symptom Manage* 9:425–433, 1994

135. Lynn B: Capsaicin: Actions on the nociceptive C-fibres and therapeutic potential. *Pain* 41:61–69, 1990

136. Watson CPN, Evans RJ: The postmastectomy pain syndrome and topical capsaicin: A randomized trial. *Pain* 51: 375–379, 1992

137. Ellison N, Loprinzi CL, Kugler J, et al: Phase III placebo-controlled trial of capsaicin cream in the management of surgical neuropathic pain in cancer patients. *J Clin Oncol* 15:2974–2980, 1997

138. Laing AH, Ackery DM, Bayly J, et al: Strontium-89 chloride for pain palliation in prostatic skeletal malignancy. *Br J Radiol* 64:816–822, 1991

139. Graffam S, Johnson A: A comparison of two relaxation strategies for relief of pain and its distress. *J Pain Symptom Manage* 2:229–231, 1987

140. Syrjala KL, Donaldson GW, Davis MW, Kippes ME, Carr JE: Relaxation and imagery and cognitive-behavioral training reduce pain during cancer treatment: A controlled clinical trial. *Pain* 63:189–198, 1995

141. Ferrell-Torry AT, Glick OJ: The use of therapeutic massage as a nursing intervention to modify anxiety and the perception of cancer pain. *Cancer Nurs* 16:93–101, 1993

142. Eisenberg E, Carr DB, Chalmers TC: Neurolytic celiac plexus block for treatment of cancer pain: A meta-analysis. *Anesth Analg* 80:290–295, 1995

143. Sweet WH, Poletti CE, Gybels JM: Operations in the brainstem and spinal canal, with an appendix on the relationship of open to percutaneous cordotomy, in Wall PD, Melzak R (eds): *Textbook of Pain* (ed 3). Edinburgh: Churchill Livingstone, 1994, pp. 1113–1135

144. Faries JE, Mills DS, Goldsmith KW, et al: Systematic pain records and their impact on pain control: A pilot study. *Cancer Nurs* 14:306–313, 1991

145. McMillan SC, Williams FA, Chatfield R, et al: A validity and reliability study of two tools for assessing and managing cancer pain. *Oncol Nurs Forum* 15:735–741, 1988

146. American Pain Society quality assurance standards for relief of acute pain and cancer pain, in Bond MR, Charlton JE, Wolff CJ (eds): *Proceedings of the Sixth World Congress on Pain*. New York: Elsevier, 1991, pp. 185–189

147. Miaskowski C, Nichols R, Brody R, et al: Assessment of patient satisfaction utilizing the American Pain Society's quality assurance standards on acute and cancer-related pain. *J Pain Symptom Manage* 9:5–11, 1994

148. Ward SE, Gordon D: Application of the American Pain Society quality assurance standards. *Pain* 56:299–306, 1994

149. Rimer BK, Kedziera P, Levy MH: The role of patient education in cancer pain control. *Hosp J* 8:171–191, 1992

150. *Managing Cancer Pain*. AHCPR Publication No. 94-0595. Rockville, MD: Agency for Health Care Policy and Research, Public Health Service, U.S. Department of Health and Human Services, March 1994

Pain

Patient Name: _____

Symptom and Description   Pain is feared by people with cancer, but most patients can get relief with proper treatment. Cancer pain can occur due to tests, surgery, chemotherapy, radiation therapy, hormonal therapy, the tumor itself, or unrelated reasons.

Learning Needs   You should let your doctor or nurse know if you have pain. They cannot know if you are in pain unless you tell them. Patients and families often don't report pain because they don't want to bother the doctor or nurse. Patients also say they do not want to appear to be complaining. Good pain management helps you better participate in your treatment and will improve your quality of life.

Many pain medicines are available to relieve your pain. These may include nonsteroidal antiinflammatory drugs (e.g., aspirin, ibuprofen), opioids (e.g., codeine, morphine), antidepressants, anticonvulsants, corticosteroids, and others.

You will not become addicted to pain medicines. If the pain medicines do not provide as much relief as you need, the doctor or nurse can give you more. There is no maximum amount of morphine. The correct dose is the dose that works for you.

Prevention   The best method to treat pain is to prevent it from returning. You also can prevent some of the side effects to pain medicines.

- Be sure you take your pain medicines as prescribed. The best way to take pain medicines is on a schedule (e.g., every 4 hours). Waiting until the pain returns means you will have to play "catch up." You may even need to take more medicine than if you treat the pain before it becomes a problem.

- Take supplemental, or as-needed, pain medicines before any activity you know will be painful. This will allow you to be active with less pain.

- Let your doctor or nurse know if you are having side effects to the pain medicines. Most side effects can be easily treated.

- Most patients taking opioid medicines will develop constipation. Take a laxative and stool softener (either as separate pills or in combination) every day to prevent constipation. As the dose of the opioid increases, so must the dose of the laxative and stool softener.

Management   If your pain is not well relieved with the medicines ordered, let your doctor or nurse know as soon as possible. Many medicines are available and everyone responds differently to each medicine. You may need to try several medicines before finding the one most effective for you.

Also, let your doctor or nurse know if you have a new pain. They will need to evaluate the cause. Tell your doctor or nurse if you are having trouble getting your medicines or if you cannot afford them.

Self-Management

- It is very important that you talk to your doctor and nurse about your pain. They cannot know how much pain you have unless you tell them. Some patients find that a daily diary of their pain score (0 = no pain, 10 = worst pain imaginable) can be useful.

- You can use a chart like this to rate your pain and to keep a record of how well the medicine is working. Write the information in the chart. Use the pain intensity scale to rate your pain before and after you take the medicine.

Pain Intensity Scale

| 0 | 1 | 2 | 3 | 4 | 5 | 6 | 7 | 8 | 9 | 10 |

No pain   Medium pain   Worst pain

Date	Time	Pain intensity scale rating	Medicine I took	Pain intensity scale rating 1 hour after taking the medicine	What I was doing when I felt the pain
1/3/99	2:35 p.m.	6	two aspirin tablets	3	Sitting at my desk and reading

Source: Payne R: Transdermal fentanyl: Suggested recommendations for clinical use. J Pain Symptom Manage 7(suppl):40–44, 1992

- Take your medicines as ordered. If they do not relieve your pain, contact your doctor or nurse.

- Relaxation and guided-imagery exercises can be very helpful in addition to your pain medicines. Many tapes and books are available to help you learn these exercises. Ask your doctor or nurse for more information.

- Distraction can be a complement to your pain medicines. Music, a funny movie or videotape, or a computer or video game can help distract you from the pain. These can be especially useful when you have periods of increased pain.

- Massage can help reduce muscle tension and relieve pain. Ask your doctor or nurse for information about massage therapists in your area. There are books and videotapes that show massage techniques. You may want to ask your family and friends for back rubs or massage of painful muscles. They may appreciate being able to help you feel better.

- Heat, cold, vibration, and other treatments can provide relief for some patients. Ask your doctor or nurse for assistance.

- Pain can affect all parts of our lives. Many people find that talking about the pain to a trained therapist can be very helpful. Support groups can also provide the opportunity to talk with others in your situation and learn what has helped them.

- Add more fruits (including prunes) and juices to your diet, if you can tolerate these, to help prevent constipation from your pain medicines.

Follow-up   Remember to talk to your doctor and nurse about your pain. There also are many resources available regarding cancer pain, including booklets, books, videos, and the Internet. Ask your doctor or nurse for more information.

Phone Numbers

Nurse: ⎯⎯⎯⎯⎯⎯⎯⎯⎯⎯⎯⎯⎯⎯⎯ Phone: ⎯⎯⎯⎯⎯⎯

Physician: ⎯⎯⎯⎯⎯⎯⎯⎯⎯⎯⎯⎯⎯ Phone: ⎯⎯⎯⎯⎯⎯

Other: ⎯⎯⎯⎯⎯⎯⎯⎯⎯⎯⎯⎯⎯⎯⎯ Phone: ⎯⎯⎯⎯⎯⎯

Comments

Patient's Signature: ⎯⎯⎯⎯⎯⎯⎯⎯⎯⎯⎯ Date: ⎯⎯⎯⎯

Nurse's Signature: ⎯⎯⎯⎯⎯⎯⎯⎯⎯⎯⎯ Date: ⎯⎯⎯⎯

Source: Paice, JA: Pain, in Yarbro CH, Frogge MH, Goodman M (eds): *Cancer Symptom Management* (ed 2). Sudbury: Jones and Bartlett, 1999. © Jones and Bartlett Publishers.

CHAPTER 10

Pruritus

Alison M. Seiz, RN, MSN, AOCN

Connie Henke Yarbro, RN, MS, FAAN

The Problem of Pruritus in Cancer

Pruritus (itching) is an unpleasant sensation in the skin that can be tickling or tormenting. The terms pruritus and itching are often used interchangeably. Pruritus elicits the desire to scratch, which may temporarily decrease the sensation of itching. Cycles of severe scratching may damage the skin, causing erythema, papules, and excoriation. This compromises the effectiveness of the skin as a protective barrier and may obscure diagnosis of the underlying pathology. For individuals with cancer, pruritus is a frequent cause of discomfort and anxiety. Because pruritus is subjective and difficult to define, it has not been researched adequately.[1,2]

Pruritus can be generalized or localized. If restricted to one anatomic region, it may point to a specific disease (e.g., allergic contact dermatitis). Pruritus that is generalized may point to a systemic disease (e.g., Hodgkin's disease). All patients with significant pruritus should be evaluated for evidence of an underlying cause.

Incidence in Cancer

Generalized pruritus can be associated with dermatologic disorders, nonmalignant diseases, psychological stress, drug reactions, cancer, and cancer therapy. The strongest association between pruritus and a malignancy is Hodgkin's disease. Pruritus is reported as a presenting symptom in 10% to 30% of patients with Hodgkin's disease, and will occur in 20% to 30% sometime during the course of their illness.[3–7] If severe, it may be an indicator of poor prognosis.[8,9]

Other malignancies in which pruritus is the presenting symptom include oat cell carcinoma of the bronchus;[10] non-Hodgkin's lymphoma, cutaneous T-cell lymphoma (mycosis fungoides), leukemia, multiple myeloma;[11] Bowen's disease, invasive squamous cell carcinoma;[12] germ cell neoplasms;[13] and central nervous system tumors.[14] Pruritus is more common in lymphocytic leukemia than in granulocytic leukemia, and in chronic leukemia than in acute leukemia.[15] In some cases, generalized pruritus has been the presenting or only symptom of hematologic or visceral malignancy[16] and an indication of occult Hodgkin's disease.[17]

Hematologic disorders associated with pruritus include polycythemia vera and iron deficiency anemia. Pruritus has been reported in 14% to 52% of patients with polycythemia vera.[11,18] Pruritus is a frequent clinical manifestation in patients with acquired immunodeficiency syndrome (AIDS) and Kaposi's sarcoma, and in the majority of patients with AIDS-related opportunistic infections.[4,19]

Impact on Quality of Life

When compared with the other symptoms of cancer, pruritus may seem insignificant; however, it should not be minimized by those responsible for patient care. Due to the tormenting nature of pruritus, it can cause severe discomfort and distress, and reduce the quality of life by preventing sleep, interfering with concentration, and becoming a constant concern.[11] It may also promote infection by damaging the skin's protective barrier.

Etiology

The exact cause of pruritus is unknown; however, it is associated with both primary skin diseases and systemic diseases. It is common in chronic renal, hepatic, hematopoietic, and endocrine diseases. Additionally, it is seen with infection, psychosis, advanced age, and certain drugs.[11] Table 10-1 lists systemic conditions associated with pruritus.

Primary Causes of Pruritus

Dry skin

Dry skin (xerosis) is the most common cause of itching.[4,5] Dryness of the epidermis and dermis causes itching, leading to injury through scratching and formation of fissures. The skin may appear dry, cracked, and scaling, or it may appear completely normal, even when the patient is tormented by itching.[5]

Some individuals may be predisposed to dry skin such as those with fair complexion who are sensitive to the sun, extreme temperatures, and wind. In addition, factors such as a low-humidity or warm, dry environment, advanced age, improper skin care, and a family history of allergies or eczema may increase the incidence of dry skin.

Systemic causes

Pruritus secondary to systemic disease may be related to toxic circulating substances, including peptides, histamine, bradykinin, and serotonin. Such substances are thought to be associated with lymphomas, leukemias, and solid tumors. Hodgkin's disease is associated with elevated blood kininogen levels.[20] Renal failure with uremia is a well-recognized cause of persistent generalized pruritus. Biliary and hepatic obstruction due to cancer metastases or pancreatic and liver tumors can lead to increased serum levels of bile acids, resulting in pruritus. Polycythemia vera, diabetes, thyrotoxicosis, and infections are associated with pruritus in the absence of clear biochemical changes in the blood. Treatment of the primary disease often results in cessation of the pruritus.

Pruritus may result from drug reactions from antibiotic therapy or analgesic therapy and may be the initial symptom before a rash develops. For example, administration of opioids commonly causes pruritus, and it is more common with epidural or spinal administration. Ballantyne et al.[21] report that 8.5% of the patients receiving epidural opioids and 46% of patients receiving intrathecal opioids developed pruritus. The pruritus was at the level of injection or localized to the face, primarily the nose.

Pruritus related to cancer therapy

The development of pruritus is associated with cancer therapy: chemotherapy, radiation therapy, and biological response modifiers.[22-26] Pruritus may be an early sign of hypersensitivity to a specific agent. Some chemotherapeutic agents, such as doxorubicin, can cause local hypersensitivity reactions, resulting in itching, redness, inflammation, and erythema along the vein. This usually subsides within minutes after the drug is stopped. Pruritus

TABLE 10-1 Systemic Conditions Associated with Pruritus

Hematologic Disorders and Malignant Neoplasms
Hodgkin's disease
Non-Hodgkin's lymphomas
Leukemia
Mycosis fungoides
Multiple myeloma
Sarcomas
Germ cell neoplasms
Bowen's disease
Invasive squamous cell carcinoma
Central nervous system tumors
Visceral tumors
AIDS
Polycythemia vera
Iron deficiency anemia
Paraproteinemia

Renal
Chronic renal failure

Hepatic
Obstructive biliary disease
Cholestasis related to pregnancy, phenothiazines, or oral
   contraceptives
Primary biliary cirrhosis
Posthepatic obstruction

Endocrine
Hyperthyroidism
Carcinoid syndrome
Diabetes mellitus

Miscellaneous
Dry skin (xerosis)
Drug ingestion
Infectious disease
Psychosis
Parasitic infestations
Advanced age

or a skin rash may also occur with antineoplastic agents and biological response modifiers (Table 10-2). These reactions can affect the sebaceous and sweat glands, resulting in dry skin.

Pruritus is a common complaint experienced by patients receiving radiation therapy.[26] An accumulated dose of 2000 to 2800 cGy obliterates the sebaceous glands, causing dryness or pruritus.[27–29] Other skin reactions that lead to pruritus include increased pigmentation, erythema, and dry and moist desquamation. The skin must be protected from any sources of irritation, such as friction and chemicals or agents, that could cause further drying. In addition, special attention should be given to areas that are more susceptible to damage from radiation therapy such as the axilla, groin, abdomen, perineum, and perirectal area.[28]

Patients who have undergone allogeneic bone marrow transplantation may experience pruritus as a result of acute graft-versus-host disease (AGVHD) or chronic graft-versus-host disease (CGVHD).[22,30] For those patients who develop CGVHD, 95% will have skin involvement and complain of itching and burning of the skin.[30]

Pathophysiology

The exact pathophysiology of pruritus is not fully understood. Much of what we know about the pathophysiology of pruritus is a result of research on pain. It is generally accepted that pain and itch are transmitted through the same nerve pathways, even though they are two different and unique sensations.[31]

Nerve endings and networks are enmeshed in a dermis of blood vessels, mast cells, and connective nerve fibers beneath the epidermis. The pattern commonly known as the "itch-scratch-itch cycle" begins when the cutaneous nerves that form a network below the epidermis are stimulated. The itch stimuli probably disturb this balanced network. The patient then perceives this disturbance as an itch, pain, or touch. The actual sensation may depend on the spacial and temporal pattern of neural excitation rather than on the nerve receptors themselves. Itch impulses are conducted from the skin by myelinated fibers to the ipsilateral dorsal root ganglia, then cross over to the opposite anterolateral spinothalamic tract, continue to the thalamus, and travel through the internal capsule to the sensory cortex.[11] There, the perceived sensation of pruritus may be intensified by such factors as anxiety, stress, and boredom, or mitigated by mental distraction.

The perception of itching is followed by a motor response to scratch. The scratch response itself is unique in that the individual feels an irresistible urge to cause tissue destruction, experiencing pleasure while at the same time tearing at the skin. The itching sensation may finally cease only after the pain elicited by scratching becomes overpowering.[32]

There are mast cells in the fine network of nerve endings beneath the epidermis. Histamine is a chemical mediator that activates cutaneous nerves, and histamine is present in mast cells.[14,20] Scratching releases histamine, and the itching is increased.[33] Other substances that act as mediators include vasoactive peptides, trypsin, enkephalins, substance P, prostaglandins, and serotonin.[11,14,32] Pruritus results from a poorly understood combination of these chemicals and their interactions.

Assessment

Measurement Tools

At present, no measurement tools are available to measure the degree of severity of itching. A diary maintained by the patient who has had or is presently experiencing pruritus may be a useful tool to determine the patterns of itch and to assist with the diagnosis and treatment plan. The written record should include the time the itching occurs, how long it lasts, what seems to aggravate it, and relief measures taken.

History and Physical Assessment

A patient who presents with itching requires a thorough history and physical examination to determine the cause. Patients may present with no detectable primary lesions or with secondary changes (papules, excoriations) that obscure the primary lesions. Secondary changes may confuse the diagnosis; thus, the intensity of the itching and the history of skin changes are major assessment factors to consider.

History

The patient should be asked about the onset, duration, intensity, sensation, pattern, and location of itching.

TABLE 10-2 Chemotherapy Agents and Biological Response Modifiers Associated with Pruritus

Allopurinol	Hydroxyurea
Aminoglutethimide	Idarubicin
Bleomycin	Interferon (high dose)
Carmustine	Interleukin
Chlorambucil	Mechlorethamine
Cyclophosphamide	Megestrol
Cytarabine	Mitomycin
Daunorubicin	Tamoxifen
Doxorubicin	

For example, in patients with Hodgkin's disease, itching is often constant and manifests as a burning sensation on the lower legs.[5,15] Clamon et al.[13] noted that patients with Hodgkin's disease reported pruritus and painful lymph nodes after alcohol consumption. Pruritus in patients with polycythemia vera often occurs after a hot shower or bath and lasts 1 hour.[2,5,16] These patients also have pruritus on going to bed at night, and this may be due to an increase in body temperature and dilation of the blood vessels.[2,16]

Patients should also be asked about allergies, environment, travel, occupation, and skin-care practices. Their psychological state should be assessed as well by asking questions about their personality and emotions. Table 10-3 identifies questions that may be asked during the history and assessment.

Physical examination

The physical examination should include a meticulous skin examination and attention given to adenopathy and organomegaly. The color, temperature, turgor, and appearance (e.g., dryness, crusting, flaking, scaling) of any lesions should be recorded (see Table 10-3). Patients receiving radiation therapy require a baseline skin assessment of the irradiated field and skin assessments before each treatment.[29] In addition, primary cutaneous lesions must be distinguished from secondary lesions due to scratching.

Diagnostic Evaluation

When the patient with cancer presents with pruritus, the assessment outlined above should be carried out and documented. A variety of diagnostic tests to evaluate the malignancy may be ordered: complete blood count, renal and liver function studies, tumor markers, chest x-ray film, computerized tomography, and bone marrow biopsy.

Degrees of Toxicity

In some cases, grading scales are available to measure altered skin integrity. For example, the Radiation Therapy Oncology Group (RTOG) has developed a scale for acute radiation toxicity that includes pruritus. Table 10-4 summarizes two grading scales for impaired skin integrity. These scales are categorized according to four levels of impairment.

Symptom Management

Although the literature is sparse regarding pruritus in cancer patients, generalized pruritus should be taken

TABLE 10-3 Assessment of Pruritus

History
When did the itching start?
How long does the itching last?
Is the itching intense? What does it feel like? (e.g., burning, tingling)
Where on the body did the itching start?
Is the itching generalized or localized?
Is the itching gradual or sudden?
Does it occur at a certain time of the year?
Do you have other symptoms along with the itching?
Is the itching worse at night?
Does the itching increase with heat or decrease with cold?
Does the itching affect normal activities of daily living?
What makes the itching worse and what relieves it?
Do you have a family history of cancer?
Have you had any treatments for cancer, infections, or pain? (e.g., antibiotics, analgesics)
Do you drink alcohol?
What medications do you take? (including over-the-counter)
Have you had any recent dietary changes?
Do you have any allergies?
Have you recently traveled out of the country?
What is your occupation?
What are your skin-care practices?
What is your environment like? Do you live in or near a wooded area, or come in frequent contact with animals or plants?
What is the humidity level of your house? (warm and dry conditions?)
Have you recently changed laundry detergents, or worn irritating fabrics or tight clothing?
How would you describe your personality? Your emotional state?

Physical Exam: Skin Assessment
Skin turgor (assess for hydration status)
Texture of skin
Color of skin
Temperature of skin
Thickening of skin (lichen simplex chronicus) or signs of scratching
Rash or erythema present?
Chapping? (Is xerosis present?)
Signs of infection or allergic reaction (redness, dryness, skin injury secondary to scratching)
Mucous membranes (dullness, dryness, color, crusting, flaking; are fissures present?)
Physical factors (tight, constrictive clothes, irritating or harsh fabrics)

seriously. Lober[2] notes that "even if initial evaluation of a patient with generalized pruritus fails to reveal a malignancy, the patient should be periodically reevaluated because pruritus may precede all other manifestations of malignancy by years" (p. 127). Management of pruritus focuses on the following areas: prevention of dry skin and irritation, maintenance of skin integrity, treatment of the underlying disease, pharmacologic therapy, environmental interventions, and comfort and relief measures.

TABLE 10-4 Grading Scales for Impaired Skin Integrity

Reference	Grade 0	Grade 1	Grade 2	Grade 3	Grade 4
National Cancer Institute's Toxicity Criteria	None or no change	Scattered macular or papular eruption or erythema that is asymptomatic	Scattered macular or papular eruption or erythema with pruritus or other associated symptoms	Generalized symptomatic macular, papular, or vesicular eruption	Exfoliative dermatitis or ulcerating dermatitis
Radiation Therapy Oncology Group (RTOG)	No change over baseline	Follicular, faint or dull erythema/epilation/dry desquamation/decreased sweating	Tender or bright erythema, patchy moist desquamation/moderate edema	Confluent, moist desquamation other than skinfolds, pitting edema	Ulceration, hemorrhage, necrosis

Prevention

A major goal of care in patients with pruritus or those who have the potential to develop pruritus is to prevent dry skin and irritation. Skin that is nongreasy and slightly dry itches less than very dry skin.

Dryness of the skin can be decreased by bathing in moderation, for no less than 10 and no longer than 20 minutes per day, and by not taking a hot bath. Heat causes vasoconstriction of the blood vessels, which in turn can cause increased itching. Instruct the patient to use mild soaps and rinse well. A bath oil or lubricating emollient cream should be applied after the bath, followed by gently patting the skin dry. If the patient prefers to add oil to the bath water, it should be added near the end of the bath. Some patients have found that Aveeno® (Rydelle Laboratories, Racine, WI) Colloidal Oatmeal baths are soothing, and they tend to help the skin hold moisture. In addition, perfumes, cosmetics, starch-based powders, and deodorants should be avoided. Baking soda can be used instead of deodorants, to decrease the chance for irritation under the arms.[34] The use of petroleum and oil-based ointments under skinfold areas can also irritate the skin, as these are not easily removed or absorbed by the skin.[34]

Harsh materials such as wool clothing and synthetic fabrics such as polyester may irritate the skin. In addition, fabrics that have been starched or washed in harsh detergents or dried in dryers with products used to eliminate static cling may cause itching. Clothing and linens should be laundered in mild detergents and can be neutralized by rinsing in a solution of 1 teaspoon vinegar per quart of water.[34] Encourage the use of clothing that is loose fitting and the avoidance of clothing that is tight and associated with increased friction such as girdles, belts, heavy seams in denim or corduroy, pantyhose, high shirt collars, bras (especially underwires), and the groin bands on men's briefs.[28]

Heat increases cutaneous blood flow, causes the skin to lose moisture, and can intensify itching. Maintain a well-ventilated, cool environment with a humidity level of 30% to 40%. Patients should be instructed not to overdress, especially at bedtime, and to use cotton bed linens and cotton clothing that is loose, because cotton allows the exchange of air and decreases moisture. If sweating provokes itching, vigorous exercise may have to be avoided for a certain period of time.

Therapeutic Approaches

Management of pruritus should be aimed at preventing injury to the skin due to scratching and at providing comfort. To decrease the risk of injury and infection, instruct the patient to keep fingernails cut short, to maintain good handwashing techniques, and to wear soft cotton mittens on both hands and socks on the feet as needed, especially at night.[22,34] Rubbing a wide area around the itch with the open palm and applying pressure may help distract from the itching sensation. However, vigorous rubbing or massage may intensify the itch.[28] Stroking the area gently with a soft toothbrush (infant type) may provide some relief.[22]

Adequate nutrition is essential to maintain healthy skin and prevent tissue hypoxia. The diet should include a balance of vitamins, proteins, carbohydrates, fats, minerals, and fluids to promote skin integrity. If possible, daily fluid intake of at least 3000 mL per day should be maintained.

Treatment of underlying disease

The most effective relief of pruritus is obtained from the treatment of the underlying disease. Specific cases have been reported in which patients who have pruritus associated with cancer have experienced immediate relief of their pruritus on removal or treatment of the tumor.[2,17] Pruritus associated with cutaneous lymphomas is often relieved by treatment with electron beam radiotherapy.[35] The pruritus associated with Hodgkin's disease responds promptly to chemotherapy. If treatment of the underlying disease is not possible, management should focus on controlling the factors that are known to worsen or provoke itching.

Pharmacologic therapy

Various pharmacologic agents have been used to treat pruritus. A trial of different agents may be necessary to determine which provides the best relief for the patient. Table 10-5 reviews the common local and systemic medications used to treat pruritus.[36]

Topical treatments   A variety of topical agents are useful in providing temporary relief from pruritus. Many topical preparations can be found over-the-counter that include ingredients such as corticosteroids, astringents such as calamine, tannic acid, and aluminum acetate, moisturizing agents, and antihistamines.

Topical corticosteroids are available in cream, ointment, and spray forms in a variety of strengths (e.g., 0.25%, 0.5%, or 2.5%). They should be applied to the affected area not more than four times a day. Hydrocortisone cream has antiinflammatory actions and reduces itching by vasoconstriction. However, the overuse of steroids can potentially cause diffuse thinning of the skin and epidermal atrophy, leading to increased risk of skin injury.[28]

Astringents are commonly found in a variety of lotions and creams. Many calamine lotions contain menthol (0.25% to 2%), phenol (0.5% to 2%), and camphor (1% to 3%), which result in a cooling and soothing effect to localized areas.[6,11,33] Although these ingredients can cause dry skin and should be used cautiously, at the same time their drying effects are beneficial for pruritic lesions or vesicles that are inflamed, weeping, or oozing. Aveeno® anti-itch cream also contains calamine to dry up weepy rashes and promote healing. Its oatmeal-enriched formula is nongreasy and invisible when rubbed into the skin. Some Caladryl® lotions contain calamine, pramoxine HCl, camphor, and glycerin, which provide a cooling and antihistamine effect.

Benadryl cream contains diphenhydramine HCl, zinc acetate, and aloe vera. It is most effective for itching resulting from histamine release, as it stops the itch at the source by blocking the action of histamine. Benadryl cream should not be used on chickenpox, measles, or blisters or on extensive areas of the skin unless directed by a physician.

Moisturizing agents may be useful for patients with dry skin. These agents come in a variety of forms such as oil and oatmeal bath additives, ointments, lotions, and creams. Oil and oatmeal baths are safe and effective for localized pruritus. The oil is a moisturizer and the oatmeal acts as an astringent. Aveeno® bath treatment is probably the most common bath additive, and when added to water it forms a soothing milky bath that helps normalize sensitive, irritated skin.

Aquaphor® is a healing ointment for severely dry, chafed, and cracked skin. It contains a special blend of waxes and oils that help the skin to retain its moisture. Aquaphor® is often used in patients who are undergoing radiation therapy.

Prax® and Sarna® are emollient lotions that are soothing to dry, itchy, irritated skin. Prax® contains pramoxine HCl 1% in a hydrophilic lotion base, and Sarna® contains 0.5% camphor and 0.5% menthol. Both lotions can be applied to the affected area two or three times daily, or as directed by the physician. Sarna® should not be applied under compresses or bandages.

Gold Bond® medicated cream is a pain-relieving anti-itch cream with oils, lidocaine, and menthol. This product should not be used in large quantities, particularly over raw surfaces or blistered areas.

Although most of these antipruritic agents can be obtained over-the-counter, several creams and lotions, such as doxepin and Zone-A, require a prescription. Doxepin cream (5%) may provide effective short-term management of moderate pruritus in adults with atopic dermatitis and lichen simplex chronicus. Zone-A cream or lotion is a combination of hydrocortisone and the topical anesthetic pramoxine. Pramoxine provides the antiinflammatory and anesthetic effects. Doxepin and Zone-A should be applied to the affected area three to four times a day or as directed by the physician. The patient should be instructed to avoid applying occlusive dressings over the site, as they may increase dermal absorption.

Systemic treatments   In cases in which histamine is thought to be the itch mediator, antihistamines may be helpful. In addition to their effect on itching, they also provide relief due to their sedative effects. Probably the most common antihistamine that is available over-the-counter is diphenhydramine HCl. Diphenhydramine HCl is available in both liquid and capsule form. The usual adult oral dosage is 25–50 mg every 6 hours as needed, not to exceed 12 capsules in 24 hours. Another common over-the-counter antihistamine is chlorpheniramine, and a common antihistamine prescribed by physicians is hydroxyzine. A common side effect of most antihistamines is drowsiness. If the sedative effects are troublesome, methdilazine, 8 mg every 6–12 hours as needed, may be tried since its sedative effects are minimal. If one antihistamine provides inadequate relief, switching to another class of antihistamine or using a combination may improve relief.[6] Contraindications to most antihistamines include the concurrent use of MAO inhibitors, pain medications, and alcohol, which may intensify CNS depression.

Cimetidine may be used as an adjunct with an antihistamine to treat pruritus. Another agent is cholestyramine, which may relieve pruritus caused by renal or hepatic abnormalities, because it binds pruritogenic substances, such as bile salts, in the intestine to form an insoluble complex that is excreted in the feces. The drug comes in an oral suspension. Initial dose is one 5-g packet, 1 to 2 times a day. Maintenance dose is two to four packets twice a day. Preparation of the mixture is important to ensure that the full dosage is taken. Instruct the patient to mix one packet in 2 ounces of water or juice, then add another 2–4 ounces of liquid and shake the mixture vigorously; drink the mixture immediately, since the

TABLE 10-5 Medications for the Treatment of Pruritus

Pharmacologic Therapy	Mechanism of Action	Usual Adult Route/Dose	Special Considerations
Antihistamines			
Chlorpheniramine	Antagonizes effects of histamine. Most cross blood-brain barrier, producing sedative effects.	*Oral:* 4 mg q4–6h or extended release (8–12 mg) q8–12h or prn	• If one type of antihistamine provides no relief, switch to another. A combination may be helpful. • Concurrent use of MAO inhibitors, pain medications, or alcohol may intensify CNS depression.
Diphenhydramine	As above	*Oral:* 25–50 mg q6h prn *Cream or lotion:* apply to affected area tid or qid, or as directed	• Concurrent use of MAO inhibitors, pain medications, and alcohol may intensify CNS depression.
Hydroxyzine	Suppression of activity in certain areas of CNS, providing antihistamine and analgesic effects.	*Oral:* 10 mg tid–25 mg/qid	• May potentiate meperidine and barbiturates. Causes drowsiness with alcohol.
Methdilazine	Antagonizes effects of histamine.	*Oral:* 8 mg q6–12h prn	• Minimal sedative effects
Trimeprazine	Antagonizes effects of histamine.	*Oral:* 2.5 mg (base) qid prn; extended-release capsules 5 mg (base) q12h prn	• Concurrent use of MAO inhibitors, pain medications, or alcohol may intensify CNS depression. • Extrapyramidal and other adverse side effects have been reported in patients with renal disease who have taken this drug.
Tricyclic Antidepressants			
Doxepin HCl (Sinequan)	Moderate inhibitor of norepinephrine and weak inhibitor of serotonin.	*Oral:* initially, 10 mg at bedtime. May increase to 25 mg/day prn	• Administer with food to avoid GI irritation. • Can cause drowsiness and dry mouth. • Drug interactions or increased side effects can occur with concurrent use of MAO inhibitors, antidepressants, cimetidine, alcoholic beverages, or antihistamines. • Elderly patients often require lower dosages.
Doxepin HCl (Zonalon)		*Topical:* cream (5%) applied qid	• Topical application is just as potent as the oral form of doxepin. • Do not prescribe this cream while patient is taking oral cimetidine, other antidepressants, or MAO inhibitors. • Do not confuse this cream with Zone-A, a cream or lotion that is also prescribed for itching.
Miscellaneous Agents			
Cimetidine	May block the synthesis of pruritogenic substances.	*Oral:* as prescribed	• Adjunct: used in combination with an antihistamine. • Elimination of other drugs that require hepatic metabolism may be decreased with concurrent use of cimetidine.

TABLE 10-5   Medications for the Treatment of Pruritus *(continued)*

Pharmacologic Therapy	Mechanism of Action	Usual Adult Route/Dose	Special Considerations
Miscellaneous Agents (cont.)			
Cholestyramine	Binds to and removes pruritogenic substances in the gut. Reduces bile acids in the intestine to form an insoluble complex that is excreted in the feces.	*Oral suspension:* Initial dose is one packet (5 g) 1–2 times daily *Maintenance dose:* 2–4 packets bid *Preparation:* Mix packet in 2 ounces water or juice, then add another 2–4 ounces and shake vigorously; take immediately, as mixture does not dissolve	• Indicated for the relief of pruritus *only* with partial biliary obstruction. Primarily used for relieving pruritus of renal or hepatic origin. • May increase nausea, constipation, acidosis. • May delay or decrease absorption of concomitant oral medications such as tetracyclines, penicillin G, phenobarbital, digitalis, thyroxine preparations. Other medications should be administered 1 hour *before* or 4–6 hours *after* cholestyramine.
Corticosteroids (local, topical treatment)			
Hydrocortisone cream	Antiinflammatory, antipruritic. Reduces itching by vasoconstriction, reducing blood flow to the skin.	*Topical forms:* 0.25%, 0.5%, or 2.5% cream, 1–4 times per day *Rectal ointment:* 0.5–0.75%, 1–4 times per day *Lotion:* 0.25–2.5%, 1–4 times per day *Ointment:* 0.5–2.5%, 1–4 times per day	• Apply to affected area as a thin film. Do not cover skin with a dressing unless ordered by physician. • Keep away from eyes. • Local or systemic side effects are infrequent or rare. • Overuse can potentially cause diffuse thinning of skin and epidermal atrophy, leading to increased risk of skin injury.

CNS = central nervous system; MAO = monoamine oxidase.

drug does not dissolve in the liquid. Other medications should be taken 1 hour *before* or 4 to 6 hours *after* cholestyramine. This drug may increase nausea and constipation and may increase acidosis. It may also delay or decrease the absorption of concomitant oral medications such as tetracyclines, penicillin G, phenobarbital, digitalis, and thyroxine preparations.

Doxepin, a tricyclic antidepressant, may be useful in the treatment of pruritus, and pruritus related to anxiety may respond to tranquilizers such as diazepam.

Other therapies   Ultraviolet light may be useful in the treatment of pruritus associated with dermatitis, urticaria pigmentosa, and biliary, renal, and hematopoietic disease.[20] Ultraviolet light produces a response due to mild cutaneous injury that includes the thickening of the epidermis and stratum corneum. This process may also cause Langerhans cells to be destroyed or diminished and melanocytes to proliferate, with increased pigmentation of the skin.[20] Ultraviolet light may also have a psychological or placebo effect. Winkelmann[20] suggests that ultraviolet light may affect blood pressure, vitamin D and calcium metabolism, and peripheral blood lymphocyte T-cell population. The combination of these effects may account for the relief patients have reported. Care must be taken not to expose the skin to doses sufficient to cause sunburn, which in turn may cause itching.

Environmental interventions

The itch threshold seems to improve in a cool and humid environment. Dry air—humidity below 40%—causes the skin to lose moisture. In the winter months, indoor heating lowers the humidity even more. The use of a humidifier may be helpful, and open basins of water and house plants can also add humidity to a room.

Comfort and relief measures

General measures can be used to provide relief from itching. Application of heat and cold may offer some relief, and the patient may need to experiment to find which one works best. However, cool applications are often preferred because they decrease inflammation of the skin.

TABLE 10-6   Clinical Nursing Guide for the Diagnosis and Management of Pruritus

Nursing Diagnosis	Nursing Interventions	Expected Outcomes	Rationale
Alteration in skin integrity related to pruritus	Educate patient about measures to prevent dry skin and irritation. Watch for signs and symptoms of infection such as redness, swelling, pain, and drainage. Report any alterations to the physician.	• Patient and significant other will report alterations in skin integrity. Patient will state the site of pruritus, treatment, and expected outcome of the intervention.	• Alteration in skin integrity could lead to infection. The patient and significant other have a right to information regarding interventions that promote comfort.
	• Encourage oral fluid intake of 3000 mL per day (unless contraindicated). Encourage balanced diet of protein, carbohydrates, iron, and vitamins to promote skin integrity. Encourage avoidance of alcoholic beverages and smoking.	• Maintain healthy skin.	• Healthy skin requires adequate fluid intake, proper vitamins, and nutrients.
	• Maintain a cool, well-ventilated, and humidified (30–40%) environment. Encourage use of tepid baths or showers, lasting from 10–20 minutes per day. Use bath additives.	• Prevent dry skin.	• Pruritus is associated with dry skin. Frequent bathing causes dry skin. Hot water causes vasodilation, which increases pruritus. Heat causes the body to lose moisture.
	• Cut fingernails short and smooth and encourage frequent hand washing. Apply lotion to hands after washing.	• Prevent skin trauma and infection.	• These measures decrease skin damage due to scratching.
	• Encourage measures such as soft mittens on hands and soft cotton socks on feet to prevent scratching.	• Prevent skin irritation.	• Soft fabrics are less irritating to the skin, and cotton fabrics allow air exchange and decrease moisture.
	• Avoid using starch or washing clothing or bed linens in harsh detergents.		• Harsh detergents can cause skin irritation.
Alteration in comfort related to pruritus	• Educate patient about measures to decrease pruritus and provide comfort.	• Patient and significant other will report alterations in comfort level.	• An alteration in comfort could indicate progression of disease.
	• Use physical modalities to counteract itch sensation: 1. Apply cool washcloth or ice over the site. 2. Apply firm pressure at the site or contralateral to the site of itching and at acupressure points to break the neural pathway. 3. Rub area gently with a soft cloth, use mild vibration, or stroke the area with a soft, small (i.e., infant-size) brush.	• Patient and significant other will use measures to increase comfort and enhance the continuance of daily activities and valued relationships.	• Cutaneous stimulation counteracts the itch sensation. • It is important for the patient to maintain as normal a lifestyle as possible.
	• Use pharmacologic agents as prescribed by physician. Use over-the-counter agents as needed.	• Patient and significant other will use over-the-counter medications appropriately.	• Some medications provide a sedative effect that decreases anxiety and allows the patient to sleep. Some topical agents give temporary relief.

TABLE 10-6 Clinical Nursing Guide for the Diagnosis and Management of Pruritus (continued)

Nursing Diagnosis	Nursing Interventions	Expected Outcomes	Rationale
Alteration in comfort related to pruritus *(cont.)*	• Wear loose-fitting, soft, cotton clothing. Avoid harsh fabrics such as wool or synthetics. Use cotton bed linens, and change them frequently.	• Patient and significant other will select and care for clothes and linens appropriately.	• Soft fabrics are less irritating to the skin, and cotton fabrics allow air exchange and decrease moisture.
Sleep pattern disturbance related to pruritus	• Use diversional activities, distraction techniques, and relaxation techniques. • Encourage adequate rest periods, and report to physician if unable to obtain sleep due to itching at night.	• Patient will get adequate rest and sleep.	• These techniques help distract thoughts from the itch sensation and decrease anxiety. • Effective sleep management is available for most patients.

Data from references [4,22,37,38].

Many folk remedies include agents that offer fast, short-term relief and feel soothing to the skin. For example, an old, home folk remedy appealing to many patients is 2 teaspoons of olive oil and one large glass of milk added to the bath. As previously mentioned, an oatmeal bath is another remedy that can be very soothing. When the mixture is added to bath water, it produces an oatmeal-milk—like appearance.

Other relief measures include the application of over-the-counter topical preparations as discussed in the pharmacologic therapy section of this chapter. Many topical preparations provide a cooling, soothing sensation that can provide relief for minutes to hours.

Because itching is a subjective phenomenon, psychological factors must be considered, such as stress due to fear of serious illness. Stress should not be underestimated, and every effort should be made to reduce it.

Multiple approaches and combined efforts may be required to promote comfort and prevent skin injury. Offer positive suggestions rather than warnings about scratching. Encourage the patient to cut fingernails short and wear soft mittens, especially at night. The use of relaxation techniques and diversional activities may help focus thoughts on subjects other than the sensation of itching. Distraction techniques include the use of electronic games such as Nintendo or computerized game programs, playing cards, videotapes, audiotapes, music therapy, meditation, and imagery. If the patient has had a previous hobby such as sewing or working with crafts, encourage resuming this activity.

Evaluation of Therapeutic Approaches

Good documentation is important to assist in the evaluation of therapeutic approaches. Response to therapy should be documented via diary, problem-oriented check-off list, narrative notes, or flow sheet. Documentation should include important information such as frequency and intensity of itching, assessment including skin integrity, relief measures taken, and individual self-report of comfort obtained. Documentation helps the patient and caregivers to identify and manage the factors that influence comfort, clarifying the strategies that have been effective in relieving pruritus. A written record can alert the patient to seek assistance and may also document that the disease state has changed.

Educational Tools and Resources

A clinical nursing guide for the diagnosis and management of pruritus is given in Table 10-6. This guide can be used as a quick reference for nurses. The expected outcomes are goals that should be the focus when planning nursing care and interventions.

Appendix 10A presents a self-care guide for the patient to use in preventing and managing pruritus. It can also be used as a guide to assist nurses with patient education efforts.

Conclusion

Pruritus is an unpleasant cutaneous sensation that elicits the desire to scratch. Pruritus can be localized or generalized and is subjective to the person experiencing it. Generalized pruritus may be a symptom of certain types of cancer or associated with cancer treatments. Management of pruritus should focus on the prevention of dry and irritated skin, maintaining skin integrity, treatment of the underlying disease, pharmacologic therapy, environmental interventions, and comfort and relief measures.

References

1. Greaves MW: Itching—Research has barely scratched the surface. *N Engl J Med* 326:1016–1017, 1992 (editorial)
2. Lober CW: Pruritus and malignancy. *Clin Dermatol* 11:125–128, 1993
3. Rubinstein N, Weinrauch L, Matzner Y: Generalized pruritus as a presenting symptom of phenytoin-induced Hodgkin's disease. *Int J Dermatol* 24:54–55, 1985
4. Dangel RB: Pruritus and cancer. *Oncol Nurs Forum* 13:17–21, 1986
5. Rosenbaum M: Pruritus of unknown origin. *Hosp Pract* 23:19–26, 1988
6. McClean DI, Haynes HA: Cutaneous manifestations of internal malignant disease, in Fitzpatrick TB, Eisen AZ, Wolff K, Freedberg IM, Austen, FM, (eds): *Dermatology in General Medicine* (ed 4). New York: McGraw-Hill, 1993, pp. 2229–2249
7. Kantor GR: Generalized pruritus: How do you manage it? *Emerg Med* 25:18–26, 1993
8. Gobbi PG, Attardo-Parrinello G, Lattanzio G, et al: Severe pruritus should be a B-symptom in Hodgkin's disease. *Cancer* 51:1934–1936, 1983
9. Gobbi PG, Cavalli C, Gendarini A, et al: Reevaluation of prognostic significance of symptoms in Hodgkin's disease. *Cancer* 56:2874–2880, 1985
10. Thomas S, Harrington C: Intractable pruritus as the presenting symptom of carcinoma of the bronchus: A case report and review of the literature. *Clin Exp Dermatol* 8:459–461, 1983
11. Gilchrest BA: Pruritus: Pathogenesis, therapy, and significance in systemic disease states. *Arch Intern Med* 142:101–105, 1982
12. Powell FC, Perry HO: Pruritus ani: Could it be malignant? *Geriatrics* 40:89–91, 1985
13. Clamon G, Henry K, Loening S: Constitutional symptoms in patients with germ cell neoplasms. *Urology* 36:465–466, 1990
14. Phillips WG: Pruritus: What to do when the itching won't stop. *Postgrad Med* 92:34–56, 1992
15. Bernhard JD: Itching as a manifestation of noncutaneous disease. *Hosp Pract* 22:81–95, 1987
16. Lober CW: Should the patient with generalized pruritus be evaluated for malignancy? *J Am Acad Dermatol* 19:350–352, 1988
17. O'Donnell BF, Alton B, Carney D, et al: Generalized pruritus: When to investigate further. *J Am Acad Dermatol* 28:117, 1993
18. Denman ST: A review of pruritus. *J Am Acad Dermatol* 14:375–392, 1986
19. Schelsinger I, Oelrich DM, Trying SK: Crusted (Norwegian) scabies in patients with AIDS: The range of clinical presentations. *South Med J* 87:352–356, 1994
20. Winkelman RK: Pharmacy control of pruritus. *Med Clin North Am* 66:1119–1131, 1982
21. Ballantyne JC, Loach AB, Carr DB: Itching after epidural and spinal opiates. *Pain* 33:149–160, 1988
22. Couillard-Getreuer DL, Heery ML: Protective mechanisms: Skin, in Gross J, Johnson BL (eds): *Handbook of Oncology Nursing* (ed 2). Sudbury: Jones and Bartlett, 1994, pp. 421–463
23. Yasko JM: *Nursing Management of Symptoms Associated with Chemotherapy* (ed 3). Columbus, OH: Adria Laboratories, 1993
24. Moldawer NP, Figlin RA: The interferons, in Rieger PT (ed): *Biotherapy*. Sudbury: Jones and Bartlett, 1995, pp. 69–93
25. Sharp E: The interleukins, in Rieger PT (ed): *Biotherapy*. Sudbury: Jones and Bartlett, 1995, pp. 93–111
26. Fleischer AB, Michaels JR: Pruritus, in Berger AM, Portenoy RK, Weissman DE (eds): *Principles and Practice of Supportive Oncology*. Philadelphia: Lippincott-Raven, 1998, pp. 245–250.
27. Hassey KM, Rose CM: Altered skin integrity in patients receiving radiation therapy. *Oncol Nurs Forum* 9:44–50, 1982
28. McDonald A: Altered protective mechanisms, in Dow KH, Hilderley LJ (eds): *Nursing Care in Radiation Oncology*. Philadelphia: WB Saunders, 1992, pp. 96–125
29. Goodman M, Hilderley LJ, Purl S: Integumentary and mucous membrane alterations, in Groenwald SL, Frogge MH, Goodman M, Yarbro CH (eds): *Cancer Nursing: Principles and Practice* (ed 4). Sudbury: Jones & Bartlett, 1997, pp. 768–822
30. Buchsel PC: Bone marrow transplantation, in Groenwald SL, Frogge MH, Goodman M, Yarbro CH (eds): *Cancer Nursing: Principles and Practice* (ed 4). Sudbury: Jones and Bartlett, 1997, pp. 459–506
31. Greaves MW: Pathophysiology and clinical aspects of pruritus, in Fitzpatrick TB, Eisen AZ, Wolff K, Freedberg IM, Austen, FM, (eds): *Dermatology in General Medicine* (ed 4). New York: McGraw-Hill, 1993, pp. 413–421
32. Banov C, Epstein J, Grayson L: When pruritus is a diagnostic puzzle. *Patient Care* 26:41–60, 1989
33. DeWitt S: Nursing assessment of the skin and dermatologic lesions. *Nurs Clin North Am* 25:235–245, 1990
34. Bord MA, Devolder-McCray N, Shaffer S: Alteration in comfort: Pruritus, in McNally JC, Somerville ET, Miaskowski C, Rostad M (eds): *Guidelines for Oncology Nursing Practice* (ed 2). Philadelphia: WB Saunders, 1991, pp. 143–147
35. Casciato DA, Lowitz BB: *Manual of Clinical Oncology* (ed 3). Boston: Little, Brown, 1995
36. USP DI: *Drug Information for the Health Care Professional*, vol 1 (ed 18). Rockville, MD: United States Pharmacopeial Convention, 1998
37. Oncology Nursing Society and American Nurses' Association: *Outcome Standards for Cancer Nursing Practice*. Kansas City, MO: American Nurses' Association, 1979
38. Clark JC, McGee RF, Preston R: Nursing management of responses to the cancer experience, in Clark JC, McGee RF (eds): *Core Curriculum for Oncology Nursing* (ed 2). Philadelphia: WB Saunders, 1992, pp. 67–155

Pruritus (Itching)

Patient Name: _____

Symptom and Description   Pruritus (itching) can occur because of your cancer and the treatment for cancer. The itching can be in one area or all over your body. Pruritus can become so severe and annoying that it causes loss of sleep and changes your daily lifestyle. Scratching and damage of the skin can lead to an infection. Decreasing the itch sensation and keeping your skin healthy is most important.

Learning Needs   You need to be aware that pruritus may occur and learn how to prevent it and how to reduce its effects.

Prevention   Pruritus may not be prevented. However, there are many things you can do to prevent dry skin and irritation:

- Drink at least _____ glasses of fluid each day
- Keep skin moist, using moisturizing agents and Aveeno® bath treatment
- Keep a humid environment
- Report changes in pruritus to physician/nurse
- Keep fingernails cut short and wear soft mittens on hands and socks on feet, especially at night
- Avoid hot baths and heat

Management   There are things you can do to help control the urge to scratch:

- Apply cool compresses or pressure, or gently rub area
- Apply lotions, creams, or emollients as directed
- Use medications as directed by your physician
- Use distractions and relaxation techniques to decrease pruritus
- Take lukewarm baths, using Aveeno® oatmeal treatment
- Keep a diary of what helps your pruritus and what doesn't help
- Wear cotton clothes to reduce sweating

Follow-up   If you develop pruritus or your pruritus gets worse, call your physician or nurse. Be prepared to tell them the following information:

- Location of itching and how long it lasts
- Is it getting worse?
- Treatment you are using
- Any problems with daily activities, sleep, or rest

(continued) 159

Phone Numbers

Nurse: _____ Phone: _____

Physician: _____ Phone: _____

Other: _____ Phone: _____

Comments

Patient's Signature: _____ Date: _____

Nurse's Signature: _____ Date: _____

Source: Seiz AM, Yarbro CH: Pruritus, in Yarbro CH, Frogge MH, Goodman M (eds): *Cancer Symptom Management*. Sudbury: Jones and Bartlett, 1999. © Jones and Bartlett Publishers.

CHAPTER 11

Sleep Disturbances

Suzanne B. Yellen, PhD

Jane V. Dyonzak, PhD

The Problem of Sleep Disturbances in Cancer

Cancer diagnosis, treatment, and subsequent unpleasant sequelae present challenges to patients, to their families, and to the treatment team. Sleep disturbance is a common side effect of the cancer experience, though little empirical data is available. Problems in sleep often do not emerge until several weeks after diagnosis and treatment planning and may not emerge until after treatment has been initiated. Sleep problems may be transient and related to the normal responses associated with a diagnosis of cancer. For example, a patient may complain of insomnia that remits spontaneously several weeks later. Transient insomnia is a manifestation of the emotional reaction to a cancer diagnosis and of fears about treatment; it generally abates with successful psychological adaptation to illness and treatment. Insomnia does not necessarily imply that a problem exists; rather, is considered to be a part of normal psychosocial adjustment to a diagnosis of cancer.[1]

On the other hand, sleep problems may persist and become chronic, affecting overall quality of life and suggesting either high levels of prolonged stress or poor adaptation to diagnosis and treatment. Long-term sleep deprivation, which may result from chronic insomnia, is most commonly associated with a reduced ability to work, to partake in social activities, and to experience pleasure in daytime functioning. Because sleep disturbance in cancer may take the form of either *insomnia* (inability to sleep when desired) or *hypersomnia* (inability to maintain wakefulness when desired), these two most frequently encountered manifestations of sleep disturbance are addressed in this chapter.

Many factors are important in the regulation of timing and duration of sleep, including sleep need, the balance between rapid eye movement (REM) and non–rapid eye movement (NREM) sleep, and circadian factors. For any given individual, the main period of sleep tends to occur at approximately the same time in a 24-hour period. However, there is wide variability among people in terms of their internal sleep schedules (e.g., "early birds" versus "night owls"). The sleep schedule is closely associated with the circadian oscillations of body temperature that occur with sleep onset and continue throughout the sleep cycle. Disruptions to sleep are likely to reflect disruptions to circadian oscillations. This not only has deleterious effects on daytime functioning and quality of life, but it also interferes with appropriate delivery of certain treatment protocols. For example, circadian patterning of the chemotherapeutic agent, floxuridine, has been shown to reduce toxicity, allowing higher dose intensity to patients with widespread cancer.[2] Further, circadian patterning has been shown to affect the efficacy of delivery of hematopoietic growth factors.[3] Oncologists and oncology nurses can play an important role in the prevention and management of sleep-related problems that emerge as a function of cancer and cancer treatment, because there is likely an important relationship among sleep, quality of life, and possibly even immune function.[4,5]

Incidence in Cancer

It is difficult to determine the true prevalence of sleep disorders in cancer patients because of the paucity of empirical work investigating this problem.[6] Of the few reported studies conducted within the last 15 years, estimates of the prevalence of sleep disorders in cancer patients have ranged from a low of 29% in an autologous bone marrow transplant population[7] to a high of 95% in reports of transient or persistent insomnia from a sample of 300 cancer patients.[8]

The most common form of sleep disorder found both in the general population and in cancer patients is insomnia. This is not surprising, given the general prevalence of insomnia at 30% to 35%.[9] Insomnia can be primary or secondary, and can take the form of sleep onset difficulty, sleep maintenance difficulty, early morning awakening, or all three. Insomnia in cancer patients typically falls under the domain of secondary insomnia. As such, secondary insomnia has been routinely treated pharmacologically, but this approach has the potential side effect of further disrupting the sleep cycle.[10]

Less is known about the true incidence of insomnia in cancer patients, but it is suggested that the likelihood of developing insomnia may peak at several times during the illness trajectory.[11] Specifically, sleep pattern disturbance may be likely to become problematic during initial diagnosis, during chemotherapy, radiation therapy, or immunotherapy, and in end-stage disease.[12] Most often the sleep disturbance takes the form of insomnia, but hypersomnia and other fatigue syndromes may result from preexisting conditions, disease-related factors, cancer treatments, or the demands of coping with cancer.[13]

In a review of the literature, Hu and Silberfarb[6] summarize the empiric findings concerning the relationship between cancer and sleep. In general, the sleep of cancer patients has been found to be disturbed, and findings supporting this well-known clinical phenomenon are more prevalent than those reporting no differences in quality or duration of sleep. Their review reveals the following: (1) cancer patients are approximately three times more likely to have sleep maintenance problems compared to a control group;[14] (2) cancer patients have greater difficulty with both sleep onset and maintenance than the general population;[15] (3) the sleep of the cancer patient is similar to that of the suicidally depressed patient but dissimilar in depressive symptomatology;[16] and (4) the second most commonly prescribed psychotropic medications after antiemetics are those intended to assist in sleep.[17,18] In a retrospective chart review, Derogatis et al.[17] found that hypnotics accounted for 48% of total prescriptions for hospitalized cancer patients. Forty-four percent of all psychotropic prescriptions for cancer patients were written for sleep, with flurazepam accounting for 33% of the prescriptions. This suggests that sleep disturbance is a highly prevalent problem among cancer patients and that physicians commonly treat this problem symptomatically with medications (e.g., hypnotics or benzodiazepines) rather than undertaking a thorough assessment of factors underlying the sleep problem.

Other findings support the high prevalence of sleep problems in cancer patients. Nail et al.[19] found that 55% of cancer patients experience sleep difficulty 2 days after chemotherapy, and the mean severity rating of this problem was moderate to severe. Terminally ill cancer patients are often prescribed a benzodiazepine intended to promote sleep.[18] The diagnosis of lung cancer has been associated with sleep disturbance, and the incidence of insomnia increases with recurrent disease.[20] Even a positive Pap smear as a screen for cervical cancer has been associated with impairment in sleep patterns.[21] Again, the use of benzodiazepines to promote sleep or to help manage nighttime restlessness is problematic because the underlying problem may be *anxiety*, related to either impaired physical function or shortness of breath (as in lung cancer), rather than a sleep problem per se. In general, sleep problems should be treated with appropriate pharmacologic or behavioral techniques. Anxiety or other psychological syndromes associated with restlessness can be treated pharmacologically or nonpharmacologically during daytime hours.

Two recent studies conflict with traditional views concerning the association of cancer and sleep. Lamb[22] compared 15 newly diagnosed cancer patients with a control group and found no differences in either the amount of sleep or in sleep quality, despite the fact that cancer patients were found to be more depressed and anxious. The site of cancer also is relevant, affecting the amount and quality of sleep. Specifically, Silberfarb et al.[23] compared the sleep of breast cancer patients and lung cancer patients with both healthy controls and healthy insomniacs. Their results suggest that the sleep of breast cancer patients is similar to that of healthy volunteers, whereas the sleep of lung cancer patients approximates that of healthy insomniacs. Of interest is the fact that the lung cancer patients underestimate their sleep difficulty despite objective verification of this problem in the sleep laboratory.

Finally, complaints of sleep disturbance may be a secondary manifestation of an underlying malignant process. For example, hypersomnia secondary to sleep apnea from a restricted upper airway has been found in lymphocytic lymphoma,[24] and excessive lethargy secondary to renal cell cancer metastatic to the pituitary gland has been described by Weiss et al.[25] In another example, a case of cataplexy, one of the diagnostic symptoms of narcolepsy, led to a diagnosis of lymphoma, and this sleep disturbance was reported to have resolved with cancer treatment.[26]

In general, cancer diagnosis, treatment, and progressive disease are associated with sleep disturbance, primarily in the form of insomnia. By virtue of the fact that insomnia commonly produces fatigue, irritability, and depression, it may have a devastating effect on quality of life during cancer treatment.[10]

Impact on Quality of Life

There are no published data reporting the impact of sleep disturbance on overall subjective, patient-rated quality of life (QOL). This is surprising, because most QOL questionnaires include sleep disturbance among symptoms rated by patients. However, it has been suggested that insomnia has an adverse impact on QOL.[10,27] As part of an ongoing study of stage of disease, expected treatment toxicity, and QOL, assessment of the impact of subjectively rated sleep ("I am sleeping well") on overall QOL was measured by the Functional Assessment of Cancer Therapy scales (FACT-G).[28] The correlation between the sleep item and the total QOL score on the FACT-G minus the item was $r = .60$, and this relationship was highly significant in a sample of 254 patients ($p < .0001$). These findings suggest that sleep is an important component of overall QOL in cancer patients. More importantly, this relationship was independent of whether patients were in the early or later stages of the disease trajectory.

Other studies have assessed sleep disturbance as it relates to other symptomatology, such as pain or anxiety. In a sample of 84 patients with cancer-related pain, 58% reported poor quality of sleep secondary to cancer pain.[29] Cleeland[30] suggests that cancer pain and anxiety lead to poor sleep, appetite disturbance, and coping difficulties, making cancer treatment more difficult. Sleep problems persist even 1 year after treatment. Chao et al.[31] found that 5% of patients reported sleep difficulties 1 year after autologous bone marrow transplantation. These findings suggest a strong relationship between sleep and cancer-related QOL, persisting long after cancer treatment has ended. Thus, it is important to recognize and appropriately treat sleep problems of cancer patients to enhance coping and functioning during treatment and to minimize long-term treatment-related sequelae.

Pathophysiology

Sleep and Immune Function

Sleep has long been believed to have a restorative function in behavior. Sleep deprivation over long periods of time has been linked to problems ranging from disruption in mentation to psychotic states and even death.[45,46] More recently, attention has been focused on the relationship between the sleep-wake cycle and immune, neuroendocrine, and thermal systems of the body. In an article describing the relationship between sleep and the immune system, Moldofsky[47] reviews the current literature, drawing from both animal and human studies. His findings support the notion that certain cytokines and peripheral immune functions are associated with sleep, among them natural killer (NK) cell activity and plasma interleu-

kin-1 (IL-1) and interleukin-2 (IL-2), endogenous pyrogens. This is supported by his research indicating a nocturnal decline in NK cell activity and increases in plasma IL-1 and IL-2 in young adults, corresponding to stage 4 slow-wave sleep (SWS). Clinical studies of sleep deprivation also have been implicated in immunologic functions. Sleep deprivation in men over a period of 48 hours resulted in reduced lymphocyte stimulation in response to phytohemagglutinin (PHA) and depressed granulocyte phagocytosis.[48] Sleep deprivation studies by others have also suggested immunologic consequences, among them reductions in phagocytosis and increases in interferon production and plasma cortisol, with restoration of immunologic functions after several days of rest. Based on evidence from a series of studies attempting to distinguish sleep effects from circadian effects on cellular and cytokine functions, Moldofsky concludes that (1) evidence supports the notion of greater activity of plasma IL-1 during stage 4 SWS, independent of circadian changes in plasma cortisol; and (2) activities of NK cells and plasma IL-1 are related to sleep. Other studies have assessed the effects of the sleep-wake cycle on production of tumor necrosis factor (TNF)-α, with levels of TNF-α and IL-1β increasing during wakefulness.[49] Finally, insomnia has been associated with a reduction of NK activity independent of the presence of a mood disorder.[50] An obvious inference from the above studies suggests that disorganization or loss of the sleep-wake system that commonly occurs with diagnosis and treatment of neoplastic disease interferes with immunologic, neuroendocrine, and thermal systems and may contribute to pathologic processes, among them increased vulnerability to infection.

Etiology

The most common sleep-related sequela of treatment itself is either insomnia or hypersomnia. Insomnia has been associated with use of corticosteroid agents, such as those used in treatment of childhood cancers.[32,33] Specifically, Harris reports that use of prednisone at doses of 60 mg/m^2 per day is associated with increases in appetite, changes in facial appearance, increased irritability and argumentativeness, and increased nighttime awakenings. It is apparent that even very low doses of steroids can disrupt sleep in some individuals. However, there is a high degree of variability in people in terms of their susceptibility to sleep disturbance from these agents.

Treatment-related hypersomnia is another clinical phenomenon, often associated with cranial radiation. The "Somnolence Syndrome," first described as a sub-acute encephalopathy in 1929, consists of "symptoms of somnolence, ranging from mild drowsiness to marked lethargy with prolonged periods of sleep" appearing 3 to 12 weeks after treatment and resolving spontaneously in 3 to 14 days.[34] Patients describe their sleepiness as "exhausted doing nothing" and any activity as "a struggle."[35] This syndrome has also been reported after bone marrow transplantation in cases of acute nonlymphocytic leukemia,[36] and with use of teniposide at 3 to 5 times the conventional dose for children with acute lymphocytic leukemia.[37] Even noncranial radiation therapy has been associated with increased fatigue and sleep. Specifically, Greenberg et al.[38] found a fatigue syndrome in breast cancer patients treated with localized radiation therapy to the breast. Further, Greenberg et al.[38] have suggested that radiation therapy for prostate cancer increases sleep, which itself is associated with relative changes in serum interleukin-1 and may possibly serve as a biological marker for treatment-related fatigue. Complaints of fatigue have also been associated with interleukin-2 or interferon alfa-2a treatments.[39]

Treatment-related disturbances notwithstanding, there are many other causal factors associated with sleep and cancer diagnosis and treatment. One of the most common causes of sleep disturbance in cancer patients is cancer pain, and the importance of adequate pain relief has been targeted as a primary goal by the World Health Organization.[40] Portenoy et al.[41] suggest that 90% of ambulatory cancer patients experience pain more than 25% of the time, with at least half this number reporting moderate or greater pain interference in sleep, mood, and enjoyment of life. Bowdler[42] reports that quality of sleep secondary to cancer pain was poor in 54% of his sample, and Cleeland[30] suggests that cancer pain and anxiety contribute to loss of sleep and inability to cope.

Disruptions in sleep can result from a number of other factors in addition to cancer-related treatments and cancer pain, among them physical illnesses (hypoxia, urinary frequency, fever, pruritus, endocrine disorders), hot flashes, psychiatric syndromes including anxiety, medications, and a disturbing home or hospital environment (Table 11-1).[43] The diagnosis of malignancy is commonly associated with stress, anxiety, and depression, with an inverse relationship between these feelings and amount of sleep.[5] Indeed, it is often difficult to distinguish whether sleep disturbances are a function of the treatment and disease factors or are instead secondary to emotional factors; therefore, they are less helpful in making a diagnosis of depression or anxiety in the cancer patient. For example, early-morning awakening, a form of insomnia, can be an important diagnostic indicator of depression. This suggests that affective factors unrelated to the cancer cannot be ignored as etiologic factors in sleep disturbance and may need to be treated independently. Consultation and evaluation by a mental-health professional can be most useful in making this determination.

Patients themselves give many clues as to the causes of sleep problems in cancer treatment. Some problems identified by patients as contributory factors in sleep disturbance include the following: (1) decreases in physical activity, with increases in the amount of time spent in bed and napping; (2) profound daytime fatigue and a preference for sedentary activities; (3) fears of pain on awakening; (4) lack of knowledge regarding foods and beverages containing caffeine; (5) lack of knowledge of behavioral relaxation techniques; and (6) frequent and regular use of pharmacologic sleep inducers.[5]

Finally, it is important to know whether the sleep disturbance is primary or secondary. For example, disturbances in the sleep-wake cycle can be a function of organic brain syndrome, a syndrome likely to occur either in elderly patients,[44] or from organic or metabolic disturbance. Many medications are known to cause insomnia; for example, prolonged use of central nervous system (CNS) stimulants, steroids, certain antidepressants, antihypertensives, alcohol, and withdrawal from hypnotic sedatives can cause insomnia. Regular use of diuretics can contribute to insomnia due to increased awakenings with the need to void, as can withdrawal from CNS depressants and hypnotics, anxiolytics, antidepressants, antipsychotics, and recreational drugs.[43] Again, there is wide variability among individuals with respect to susceptibility to these agents.

Assessment

A thorough assessment of a patient's sleep complaint is critical to understanding the etiology of the problem and to designing an appropriate management strategy. For example, insomnia secondary to the diagnosis of cancer or specific drug therapies may be treated behaviorally, whereas other sleep disorders, such as narcolepsy (a primary sleep disorder), is likely to be treated pharmacologically. It is also important to rule out underlying physical and emotional causes of sleep disturbance.[51] These include premorbid major depressive or anxiety disorders or reactive adjustment disorders, each of which includes disturbed sleep among its symptomatology. Treatment of underlying emotional problems warrants a careful assessment to determine if behavioral treatments, pharmacologic treatments (e.g., institution of antidepressant therapy), or a combination of the two would be helpful.

TABLE 11-1 Causes of Insomnia in Cancer Patients

Physical illness (hypoxia, urinary frequency, fever, pruritus, endocrine disorders)

Pain

Psychiatric syndromes (depression, mania, delirium)

Anxiety

Medication/drugs (prolonged use and withdrawal)

Disturbing hospital and/or home environment

Massie MJ, Lesko LM: Psychopharmacological management, in Holland R, Rowland J (eds): *Handbook of Psychooncology: Psychological Care of the Patient with Cancer*. New York: Oxford U Press, 1989, p. 482.[43] Reprinted with permission.

Cancer patients typically complain of daytime sleepiness that results from poor nighttime sleep. Complaints may also take the form of fatigue or lethargy, difficulty with concentration and memory, or irritability. As with any medical or nursing history format, specifics should be obtained as to the problem, duration, and recurrence. In addition to the more traditional information obtained in a medical history, it is essential to obtain additional information specific to sleep: (1) normal (premorbid) habitual sleep schedule (bedtime and wake time); (2) amount of time to fall asleep (sleep latency); (3) number of nocturnal awakenings and the time to return to sleep with each; (4) any unusual behaviors during sleep (snoring, irregular breathing, leg jerking/kicking); (5) nonroutine daytime naps and inappropriate or abrupt sleep in the daytime; and (6) psychological stress or adjustment difficulties. In her assessment of sleep problems, Thomas[5] includes pre-sleep routines, daily activities, environmental considerations (e.g., light, noise, temperature), physiologic associations (e.g., pain), current medications (including hypnotics), caffeine and alcohol intake, and the patient's perception of the problem. Table 11-2 is a modified version of Thomas's assessment that includes her categories as well as those delineated previously. In addition to a detailed patient history, it is often very helpful to obtain the bed partner or family member's observations of or complaints about the patient's sleep. When more sleep information is needed, the treatment team may wish to use the assessment tool developed by Kaempfer and Johnson[52] as an alternative (Table 11-3).

Another good way to obtain specific information concerning sleep is the completion of a sleep diary. Appendix 11A is an example of a sleep log (diary) that includes factors other than latency and duration of sleep. Such a log can be used to identify problem areas and creative approaches to facilitating more healthy sleep habits.

When a primary sleep disorder (e.g., narcolepsy, parasomnias) or multiple etiologies of the sleep problem is suspected, referral to an accredited sleep disorders center is essential for appropriate evaluation and management. Referral to a sleep specialist is also appropriate to help manage chronic insomnia which does not readily remit with traditional interventions.[53] These specialists may determine that further evaluation via a sleep study (polysomnogram) is needed. The American Sleep Disorders Association (507-287-6006) can be very helpful in locating accredited sleep disorder centers throughout the country.

TABLE 11-2 Categories of the Sleep Assessment Tool

Pre-cancer sleep habits
  Bedtime/wake time
  Total hours slept each night
  Presence of daytime sleepiness
  Presence of daytime napping

Quality and quantity of sleep since diagnosis
  Bedtime/wake time
  Total hours slept each night
  Presence of daytime sleepiness
  Presence of daytime napping

Patterns of insomnia
  Sleep onset problems
  Wakenings in the middle of the night with return to sleep
  Early morning awakenings

Present pre-sleep routine

Present daily activities

Environmental considerations (noise, light, temperature)

Physiologic associations (pain, dyspnea, hot flashes)

Medications (including anti-anxiety and sleeping pills)

Caffeine/alcohol intake

Emotional considerations

Patient's perception of the problem. Look for:
  Patient's beliefs about the causes of sleep problems
  Patient's beliefs about the causes of nighttime awakenings

When to refer for outside consultation or evaluation:
  When sleep problem persists for longer than 3 weeks
  When there is increased dependency on sleep medications
  When there is a strong possibility of mood disturbance
  When daytime sleepiness is no longer tolerable to the patient

Modified with permission from Thomas C: Insomnia: Identification and management. *Semin Oncol Nurs* 3:263–266, 1987.[5]

Symptom Management

In the ideal world, it would be most helpful to anticipate and prevent disturbances in sleep that arise from cancer diagnosis and treatment. In reality, however, the oncology team rarely takes a prophylactic stance with respect to this issue. Discussion and problem-solving most often occur well after sleep disturbance has become a problem to the patient, with concomitant fatigue and irritability. A contributory factor is that some patients believe that they are depressed rather than sleep-deprived, and thus are reluctant to communicate about sleep problems during the course of treatment because of fears that their response is not a normal one. Perhaps a better understanding that sleep patterns may change with diagnosis and treatment or that sleep disturbance is a common response to treatment may encourage individuals to report their problems earlier.

The treatment of cancer-related insomnia has been similar to the management of insomnia in the general public.[6] In order to select the most appropriate form of treatment, all underlying physical and emotional causes of insomnia must be ruled out. For example, it is important to determine that cancer pain has been adequately treated either pharmacologically or nonpharmacologically. To minimize disruption in sleep, narcotics should be administered every 12 hours rather than every 4 hours. Findings from research suggest that quality of nighttime sleep, daytime functioning, pain, and overall QOL are improved when narcotics for pain

TABLE 11-3   Factors That Influence Sleep and Assessment of Sleep Disturbance in Cancer Patients

Factor	Assessment
General (age and developmental level)	What are the patient's age and development level (infant, school age, adolescent, young adult, middle age, elderly)? How has the patient been sleeping (describe sleep habits, usual amount of sleep)?
Time retires to bed	What time does the patient usually go to bed?
Patterns of insomnia	
Initial	How long does it take the patient to fall asleep? Does the patient fall asleep right away? How does the patient feel before falling asleep? How often does the patient have trouble falling asleep?
Intermittent	Does the patient wake up during the night? What causes awakening? How often does the patient awaken during the night? What helps the patient get back to sleep?
Terminal	What time does the patient wake up? What wakes the patient up early? How often do early awakenings occur? Is the patient depressed? What does the patient do upon awakening early?
Patient's response to quality of sleep	Does the patient feel rested after a night's sleep? How does the patient feel after getting up? Does the patient appear to be well rested? Validate patient vs. nurse perceptions.
Naps	Does the patient nap during the day? How long? Does the patient have day/night reversal (sleeps more during the day than at night)? Does the patient have excess daytime sleepiness (e.g., due to a brain tumor)?
Recreation/exercise	Does the patient exercise? What sort of activity is involved? When does the patient exercise in relation to bedtime?
Emotional factors	
Anxiety	Is the patient worried about the outcome of the illness? Is there an inability to manage normal responsibilities?
Depression	What is the patient's mood (cheerful, depressed)?
Stress	Has the patient received a recent diagnosis of cancer or recurrence? Are there any other obvious sources of stress in the patient's life (e.g., a new course of treatment)?
Sleep environment	What is the patient's usual sleep environment? What have been the previous experiences when sleeping in an unfamiliar place?
Lighting	Does having a light on at night disturb the patient?
Ventilation	Does the patient like to sleep with a door or window open?
Bedding	How many and what type of pillows does the patient use? Is any special bedding used (blankets, mattress, or pads)?
Temperature	Does the patient need the room warm or cool to sleep well?
Noise	Do noises wake the patient or keep the patient awake? Does the patient need quiet to sleep?
Positioning	What is the patient's usual sleep position? Does the patient need to be turned every 2 hours?
Social factors	Does the patient usually sleep alone, share a room, or share the bed? Does the patient have increased social stimulation before bedtime?
Presleep routine	What does the patient do immediately before going to bed?
Beverages	Does the patient like a beverage before going to bed?
Hygiene	Does bathing at bedtime help the patient sleep?
Food	Does the patient like to eat something at bedtime?
Medication	What medications is the patient receiving? Is the patient on steroids (which can produce chronic insomnia)? Does the patient take any medications (including alcohol) to produce sleep?
Personal beliefs about sleep	How much sleep does the patient think is necessary? What does the patient feel are the consequences of insufficient sleep?
Disease/treatment factors	What is the patient's diagnosis, disease status, and course of treatment?
Pain/discomfort	What is the source of any pain (e.g., recent surgery, mucositis)? Is pain control adequate? Is the patient febrile? Is pain preventing sleep or causing awakening?
Fatigue	Does the patient have a balance of activity and rest during the day? Has the patient undergone a late evening test or treatment?
Impaired nutritional status	Is the patient NPO? Is there nausea or vomiting?
Dyspnea/cough	Does the patient need oxygen or suctioning? Is coughing disrupting sleep?
Urinary frequency/incontinence	Is the patient receiving IV therapy or diuretics? Is the patient aware of the urge to void? If present, is the bladder catheter patent?

TABLE 11-3 Factors That Influence Sleep and Assessment of Sleep Disturbance in Cancer Patients (continued)

Factor	Assessment
Disease/treatment factors (*cont.*)	
Diarrhea	What are the frequency and consistency of stools?
Nighttime confusion	Does the patient's mental status undergo changes from day to night? Does the patient have an electrolyte imbalance?
Altered skin integrity	Are there pressure ulcers? Are there draining wounds or lesions that require frequent dressing changes?
Disruption in hormonal balance	Does the woman experience hot flashes at nighttime? How many a night?
Disruptive caregiver routines (tests, treatments, routine care, health team rounds)	What procedures are absolutely necessary (e.g., antibiotic administration), and which can be eliminated or postponed until the patient is awake (e.g., q2h mouth care)?

Kaempfer SH, Johnson BL: Sleep, in Gross J, Johnson BJ (eds): *Handbook of Oncology Nursing*, (ed 2). © 1994 Sudbury: Jones and Bartlett Publishers, pp. 314–316.[52] Reprinted with permission.

control are delivered in a 12-hour format.[54] It may also be important to explore different routes of administration of narcotics. For example, intrathecal delivery of morphine has been associated with significant improvements in sleep, gait, and daily activities.[55] Hypnosis, as a nonpharmacologic adjunct, has also been shown to both decrease pain and improve sleep.[56]

There are two main approaches to the management of sleep disturbance in cancer, one being pharmacotherapy management and the other being management using nonpharmacologic (behavioral or stimulus control) techniques. These approaches can be considered separately or as adjuncts to one another. In general, however, it is useful to consider nonpharmacologic or behavioral techniques first, because pharmacotherapy may lead to problems with habituation, long-term ineffectiveness, side effects, and withdrawal symptoms.[27] Patient guides for a healthy night sleep and management of insomnia and hypersonmia can be found in Appendices B–D.

Nonpharmacologic Approaches

Education about sleep hygiene

Difficulties getting to sleep and maintaining sleep may worsen over time due to sleep habits. Attending to these habits may aid in eliminating the sleep problem. Sleep hygiene consists of becoming involved in specific behaviors that promote good sleep. Not all individuals respond equally to the following suggestions, and necessary changes in lifestyle for appropriate sleep hygiene must be tailored to meet the individual's needs. The following sleep hygiene guidelines have been adapted from Hauri and Orr.[57] It is best not to overwhelm the individual with too many changes at once; therefore, it may be best to start with one or two suggestions and move on to others after the initial goals have been achieved. Table 11-4 is a summary of sleep hygiene guidelines.

1. *Set the alarm clock, but then hide it.* Eliminate all clocks from the bedroom.
2. *Stay in bed only for the hours intended for sleeping.* Most

individuals have a tendency to remain in bed "to try to get some sleep" when they are not sleeping. This is counterproductive because the association between being in bed and not sleeping is strengthened. It is better to reduce the time spent in bed by 1 to 2 hours, as remaining in bed longer typically leads to lighter sleep and an increased number of awakenings.

3. *Establish a bedtime and wake time and maintain them,* even though it may be difficult to establish these times during the first few weeks. The wake time appears to be particularly important in establishment of a sleep-wake rhythm. If there are awakenings during the night or difficulty getting to sleep, the individual should still get up at his or her chosen wake time, and not "sleep in." Those who consistently awake too early (for reasons other than depression) should go to bed later.
4. *Do not worry about getting sleep.* The more an individual tries to sleep, the less likely sleep will be achieved. Worrying, anger, and frustration all increase arousal, which in turn inhibits sleep. Sleep is achieved most easily when the body is relaxed and the mind is either not active or is focused on some mundane, unexciting subject.
5. *Try to deal with worries that may inhibit sleep before bedtime.* Frequently, bedtime is the first time of the day when

TABLE 11-4 Sleep Hygiene Guidelines

Set the alarm clock but then *hide* it. Eliminate all clocks from the bedroom.

Stay in bed only for the hours intended for sleeping.

Establish a bedtime and wake time and maintain them.

Do not worry about getting sleep.

Deal with worries that may inhibit sleep before bedtime.

Avoid stimulants.

Avoid CNS depressants.

Exercise on a consistent basis, 4–7 hours before bedtime.

Individualize the sleep environment.

Adapted from Hauri PJ, Orr WC: *Current Concepts: The Sleep Disorders.* Kalamazoo, MI: Upjohn, 1982.[57]

one can step aside from his or her busy schedule and have time to focus on some other concerns or tasks to be completed. One option is to set aside 30 minutes to think about concerns and perhaps even write them down. This helps clear the mind but maintains these items in memory.

6. *Avoid stimulants.* Caffeine and other stimulants interfere with the quality of sleep, even in those who fall asleep quickly after drinking coffee.[58] Caffeine is found in its highest potency in coffee, but is also found in many soft drinks (colas, Mountain Dew), tea, and chocolate. Reducing or eliminating caffeine consumed after late afternoon helps reduce its effects on sleep. Nicotine, found in tobacco products, also is a stimulant and disruptive to sleep.[59] Reduction of smoking, or at least elimination of nighttime consumption of tobacco, will help improve sleep quality. Reducing nicotine consumption may need to be accomplished gradually so as not to experience withdrawal. Finally, many medications (e.g., steroids, methylphenidate) contain CNS stimulants that interfere with sleep. It may be possible to change the timing of such medications to a time well before sleep onset.

7. *CNS depressants,* such as alcohol, may help sleep onset but can be very disruptive to sleep quality.[60] Typically, alcohol leads to frequent awakenings after the initial 1 to 2 hours of sleep. Insomnia is frequently given as a reason for beginning to drink or for relapse from recovery. Knowledge of past alcohol use is important because it can affect sleep long after discontinuation. It has been suggested that heavy drinkers show significantly disrupted sleep patterns for months and years past abstinence.[61]

8. *Exercise on a consistent basis* tends to improve sleep and promote deeper sleep.[62] Intense exercise raises the body temperature during exercise and for approximately 6 hours after exercise. For this reason, it is important to exercise at least 6 hours before bedtime. For those who cannot exercise, a hot bath for 20 minutes taken 2 hours before bedtime produces a similar effect.[63]

9. *The perfect sleep environment should be individualized.* Most find a dark, slightly cooler room to be comfortable. Many need a quiet environment, whereas others respond best to a steady noise (e.g., fan) that masks other noises in the environment.

Stimulus control technique (SCT)

The SCT has been shown to be one of the most effective behavioral treatments for insomnia.[64] The goal of this technique is to change the behavioral conditioning regarding the bed (bedroom) and sleeping that eventually develops among many individuals who have had extended periods of sleepless nights. In these cases, the bed (a stimulus) signals frustration, tension, and arousal due to spending time in bed while tossing, turning, and hoping for sleep to come. The goal of the SCT is to associate the bed with relaxation and falling asleep quickly. SCT has been used extensively with individuals who present to sleep disorders centers with complaints of insomnia arising from multiple etiologies.

There are five basic tenets: (1) go to bed only when sleepy and intending to sleep; (2) use the bed only for sleeping, not watching television, reading, or eating; (3) if unable to fall asleep quickly, get out of bed and move to another room, staying there until sleepy and only then returning to the bed to fall asleep; (4) set an alarm and get up at the same time every day regardless of the amount of nighttime sleep; and (5) do not nap. On average, SCT takes between 3 to 6 weeks to master. The initial weeks of SCT are difficult, and often patients will need a tremendous amount of encouragement to persevere.

Behavioral relaxation techniques

Anxiety reduction by means of behavioral relaxation techniques has also been useful in the treatment of insomnia. There are myriads of training procedures to induce behavioral relaxation, all having four common features but each unique in the manner in which relaxation is achieved. Features common to all relaxation techniques include (1) instruction to attend to some low-intensity event (e.g., breathing or trainer's voice); (2) instructions to ignore distractions and to avoid self-evaluation; (3) promotion of decreased muscle tonus; and (4) decreased environmental stimuli.[65] Despite these common features, relaxation training methods may differ tremendously in that they emphasize or ignore specific response modalities.[66] Six major relaxation training methods specified in Table 11-5 are elaborated below:

1. *Progressive muscle relaxation training*[67–69] gives instructions to systematically tense and relax muscle groups. The goal is to teach observational skills and localiza-

TABLE 11-5 Cognitive-Behavioral Techniques to Facilitate Sleep

Behavioral Relaxation Techniques
Progressive muscle relaxation training
Passive muscle relaxation training
Meditation
Autogenic training
Hypnosis
Guided imagery
Cognitive Control Techniques
Counting/distraction
Cognitive refocusing
Transcendental meditation
Guided imagery
Ocular relaxation

tion of tension so as to allow for rapid reduction of tension.

2. *Passive muscle relaxation training* differs from progressive muscle relaxation in that patients are instructed to observe tension in specific muscle groups and to use covert statements (e.g., letting the muscles become limp, loose, and comfortably heavy) to promote tension reduction. Often passive relaxation techniques are more appropriate for the medically ill patient than are progressive techniques, which may lead to increased levels of pain.

3. *Meditation* targets verbal, visceral (breathing), and observational behavior.[70] In meditation, a sonorous syllable is repeated on each exhalation, and patients passively observe their verbal and breathing activity. The focus is on observation of passive behavior rather than on an active goal.

4. *Autogenic training* involves verbal and observational behavior in which a series of statements is made to suggest heaviness, warmth, and calmness in various parts of the body.[71] The patient repeats the phrase and observes the described sensation.

5. *Hypnosis* involves a narrowing of consciousness, inertia, and passivity.[72] Relaxation is induced by providing verbal descriptions of motoric and observational behavior, and the patient is instructed to engage in the behavior (e.g., "your hand and arm feel heavy as if something were pressing down").[66]

6. *Guided imagery* involves descriptions of scenes and actions in which the patient imagines himself or herself. During guided imagery, patients are instructed to observe the scene in terms of its sensory modalities, such as sight, sound, temperature, touch, and smell.[65]

Cognitive control techniques

Cognitive techniques focus on managing the cognitive arousal that often accompanies poor sleep. In the clinical interview, cognitively aroused patients attribute sleep problems to "worrying too much in bed" or "racing thoughts." Cognitive control techniques are described in detail by Lacks.[73] The goal of the following techniques is to reduce cognitive arousal and augment cognitive control (see Table 11-5).

1. *Counting* is one of the most common control techniques, such as lying in bed and counting sheep. Despite the emergence of this technique from folk remedies, research has supported its effectiveness, and a number of other techniques have developed from it.[74]

2. *Cognitive refocusing* is based on the concept of competing behaviors. This treatment involves learning the techniques of visual imagery, distraction, and attention-focusing that disrupt sleep-incompatible thoughts. For example, patients may be asked to focus on things external to themselves, such as the sound of a ticking clock or the smell of a scented candle. The goal is concentration on these strategies rather than on sleep-incompatible thoughts and behaviors.

3. *Transcendental meditation* is similar to cognitive refocusing in that attention is paid to a particular syllable or "mantra." It has been theoretically linked both to anxiety reduction and cognitive control.

4. *Guided imagery* is another technique that fosters cognitive control by means of distraction and anxiety reduction. Individuals who utilize this technique are guided through a preconstructed visualized scene by a therapist, and the individual is instructed to focus all his or her attention on the images.

5. *Ocular relaxation* is a technique first developed by Jacobson[67] and later modified. The modified procedure involves having individuals move their eyes in various directions and then holding the position for 7 seconds. In between movements, individuals are instructed to focus for 40 seconds on relaxing sensations.

If techniques of good sleep hygiene, SCT, behavioral relaxation, and cognitive control have been followed rigorously without success, then psychotherapy should be considered to (1) help the patient cope with daily life stressors and (2) identify and manage interpersonal problems that are not dealt with adequately during the day and are intruding into sleep.

Pharmacologic Approaches

Treatment of hypersomnia

Medication prophylaxis can be a helpful tool in averting the somnolence syndrome associated with cranial radiation. Specifically, steroid coverage (prednisone) at a dose of 15 mg/m^2 or greater can be useful in reducing the incidence of acute radiation reactions and somnolence in children.[40] Other medications are used to treat hypersomnia. Methylphenidate, a psychostimulant recently prescribed to treat vegetative depressive symptoms in the elderly, has also been used to counter the sedating effects of strong narcotics in cancer patients.[74] Methylphenidate is a mild central nervous system stimulant presumed to activate the brain-stem arousal system and cortex. It has a rapid onset of action, and beneficial effects can be seen within a matter of days.

Treatment of insomnia

More often, however, medications are prescribed to promote rather than inhibit sleep. Typically these are the benzodiazepines, which are widely available and effective in fostering sleep (see Table 11-6 for a listing of hypnotics). Most sedative-hypnotics (e.g., alprazolam) display similar effects on sleep—among them, shorter time to achieve sleep, reduced number of awakenings during

TABLE 11-6   Sleep Promoters: Hypnotics

Generic	Trade	Half-Life Hours	Dose (mg)
Benzohypnotics			
Estazolam	Prosom (Abbott)	10–24	1, 2
Flurazepam	Dalmane (Roche)	47–100	15, 30
Quazepam	Doral (Baker-Cummins)	39–70	7.5, 15.0
Temazepam	Testorial (Sandoz)	10–20	7.5, 15, 30
Triazolam	Halcion (Upjohn)	1.6–5.4	0.125, 0.25
Imidazopyridine			
Zolpidem tartrate	Ambien (Searle)	1.4–3.8	5, 10
Other Benzodiazepines			
Alprazolam	Xanax (Upjohn)	12–15	0.25, 1.0
Chlordiazepoxide	Librium, Libritabs (Roche)	5–30	5, 10
Clonazepam	Klonopin (Roche)	18–50	0.5, 1.5
Clorazepate	Tranxene (Abbott)	3–300	3.75, 15
Diazepam	Valium (Roche)	20–50	2, 10
Lorazepam	Ativan (Wyeth-Ayerst)	10–20	0.5, 2.0
Oxazepam	Serax (Wyeth-Ayerst)	3–21	10, 30
Prazepam	Centrax (Parke-Davis)	30–200	20, 60

Used with permission from the National Sleep Foundation, 1994.

the night, and suppression of delta (deep) sleep and sometimes a reduction in REM sleep. The ideal bedtime sleep aid should have a half-life equivalent to an average night's sleep, immediate effectiveness, no active metabolites, minimal disruption of sleep architecture, and limited potential for abuse.[75]

Two newer benzodiazepines, quazepam (Doral) and estazolam (Prosom), have been developed to be more specific in their pharmacokinetic and pharmacodynamic properties. The newer hypnotic on the market in the United States, zolpidem (Ambien), is not a benzodiazepine but appears to act similarly to them without suppressing delta sleep, the stage of sleep during which physiologic restoration is thought to be the greatest. The shorter half-life agents reduce the experience of sedation or "hangover" effects in the morning. While these drugs have good effects on promoting the occurrence of sleep, they may not sustain sleep throughout the night depending on the length of their action. A non-benzodiazepine agent under development possesses an even shorter half-life and could be taken later in the course of the night, if an individual awakens and cannot return to sleep prior to their final morning wake time.

Caution is advised in prescribing either benzodiazepines or other hypnotics for sleep. While the intent is to inhibit insomnia, the long-term effects include persistent insomnia, physiologic and psychological tolerance, and rebound insomnia with increased symptomatology following withdrawal.

A guiding principle in pharmacologic management of insomnia is that sleeping pills treat only the symptom, not the cause of the complaint. Prior to administration of pharmacotherapy, the etiology of the sleep complaint should be sought, and behavioral or other nonpharmacologic interventions, oriented to the correction of the originating cause of the problem, should be attempted.

If pharmacologic interventions are used, the following considerations are important. First, hypnotic medications should be cautiously prescribed and their use closely supervised.[76,77] Second, tolerance to short-acting hypnotics can be acquired in as little as 2 weeks.[78] To delay or avoid tolerance or dependence, hypnotics should be used on an intermittent basis for the shortest duration possible. Third, discontinuation of many hypnotics may result in the recurrence or worsening of symptoms of insomnia. To minimize this possibility, the dose should be tapered before discontinuation. This is particularly relevant for short-acting agents.[79,80] Fourth, use of hypnotics may lead to impairment of daytime performance due to oversedation caused by a lengthy half-life of the medication.[81] Daytime sedation can be minimized by selecting a drug with the shortest half-life possible.

Avoidance of adverse effects is best achieved by the careful selection of medication, dose, and frequency based on the individual's age, body mass, current medications, medical status, psychological status, and the type of insomnia. Because most medications used as hypnotics are CNS depressants, attention should be directed to possible interactions with other medications having CNS effects. Clear contraindications exist in the following situations: sleep apnea syndrome or other sleep-related breathing problems, excessive alcohol consumption, pregnancy, and for those who must perform complex activities during either the night or day.

Other medications have been used in the treatment of insomnia. These include the sedating antidepressants, sedating anxiolytics, chloral hydrate, antihistamines, and aspirin. While some of these medications have been effective, their role and impact on sleep and sleep stages is not well defined and may be limited. For example, antidepressants are the appropriate treatment for insomnia secondary to depression. Use of antidepressants for their hypnotic effects when there is no underlying depression, however, may be less effective than use of other medications due to the slow onset of action and long half-life. Another effective hypnotic is chloral hydrate; however, its efficacy is limited to short-term use.[51] Finally, the age of the patient and comorbid medical conditions must be taken into account when prescribing medications for sleep. For example, the use of a benzodiazepine that has an active metabolite and a long half-life (e.g., flurazepam) may potentially contribute to oversedation, particularly in the elderly cancer patient or the patient with hepatic impairment.[82]

Nonprescription agents

Nonprescription agents have come into popular use as a means of promoting sleep. In the past 5 years, melatonin has become a highly used hypnotic. Melatonin (*N*-acetyl-5-methoxytryptamine) is a hormone produced during dark hours by the pineal gland, a neuroendocrine transducer.[83,84] In humans, endogenous melatonin secretions increase soon after darkness, peak in the middle of the night, gradually tapering during the second half of the night. Importantly, age appears to be related to serum melatonin levels, with declining levels in the elderly. Doses of orally administered melatonin vary widely, typically ranging from 1 to 5 mg. These doses result in serum melatonin concentrations 10 to 100 times the usual nighttime peak within 1 hour, followed by a decline to baseline values within 4 to 8 hours. Exogenously administered (oral) melatonin has a half-life of 35 to 50 minutes, is rapidly metabolized by the liver and excreted in the urine, and does not appear to be associated with any serious side effects or risks.[83,84] It has been suggested that exogenous melatonin administration is efficacious in terms of its sedative-hypnotic effects only in people with low levels of endogenous circulating melatonin plasma.[83] In the elderly, a sustained-release preparation (2 mg) can extend melatonin plasma levels for 5 to 7 hours, reducing sleep maintenance disturbance, a common complaint of the elderly occurring independent of disease or treatment processes.

An important aspect of melatonin is that it does not appear to have carcinogenic properties. In fact, it has been suggested that melatonin, when properly administered, has stimulatory effects on immune function. Tamarkin et al.[85] report that pinealectomies enhance tumor growth in rats, with this effect being reversed or inhibited by melatonin administration. Although the mechanism by which melatonin may inhibit tumor growth is still largely unknown, it has been suggested that melatonin may have (1) antimitotic activity; (2) immunomodulatory activity; and (3) may act as a "potent radical scavenger" (p. 193), shielding DNA molecules from oxidative damage, especially at high concentrations.[84] In several small studies, the effects of extraordinarily high doses of melatonin (20–700 mg/day) have been explored in patients with advanced cancers.[86–88] When given in combination with radiation therapy or chemotherapy, melatonin has

been associated with increased survival in patients with glioblastomas,[86] slowed the progression of disease in women with metastatic breast cancer,[87] and decreased tumor size in patients with malignant melanomas.[88] It has even been suggested that melatonin may minimize treatment-related damage to blood cells.[89]

Valerian root extract, an herbal remedy sold in many health and drug stores, has also seen increasing use as a sleep aid. It is available as either a pill or an extract (liquid). Similar to melatonin, no undesirable side effects are reported. Only a few studies have investigated the efficacy of this herbal remedy on subjective and objective measures of sleep. These studies show that when subjective measures are used to evaluate the effects of valerian on sleep, sleep latency and the number of awakenings are reduced, and sleep quality is improved.[90–93] However, objective measure of sleep (EEG laboratory studies) have indicated inconsistent results. Confirmation of subjective evaluation has been found only in one study,[90] with others failing to support subjective effects with objective findings.[93,94]

It is important that consumers of over-the-counter herbal remedies recognize that these preparations are not under the control of the FDA, and therefore purity of the remedies and the doses needed to achieve results may vary greatly between brands.

Conclusion

Given the potential adverse effects of pharmacologic interventions, nonpharmacologic interventions to treat sleep problems should be attempted before prescribing medication. Patient-related factors, such as patient willingness to be actively involved in their treatment and the absence of obvious organic impairment, predict whether pharmacologic or nonpharmacologic techniques should be considered in successful treatment planning.

Cancer patients are at significant risk to develop a sleep disturbance during their disease or treatment trajectory.[5] Evidence suggests that patient-related QOL is closely intertwined with adequate sleep. It is essential that all members of the healthcare team be familiar with the evaluation of sleep-related complaints and creative management strategies.

References

1. Massie MJ, Holland JC: Overview of normal reactions and prevalence of psychiatric disorders, in Holland R, Rowland J (eds): *Handbook of Psychooncology: Psychological Care of the Patient with Cancer.* New York: Oxford U Press, 1989, pp. 273–282
2. von Roemeling R, Hurshesky W: Circadian patterning of

continuous floxuridine infusion reduces toxicity and allows higher dose intensity in patients with widespread cancer. *J Clin Oncol* 7:1710–1719, 1989

3. Wood P, Vyzula R, Hurshesky W: Circadian hematopoietic growth factor chromotherapy. *J Infusional Chemotherapy* 3: 89–95, 1993

4. Blakeslee S: Mysteries of sleep yield as studies reveal immune ties. *New York Times,* August 3, 1993

5. Thomas C: Insomnia: Identification and management. *Semin Oncol Nurs* 3:263–266, 1987

6. Hu D, Silberfarb PM: Management of sleep problems in cancer patients. *Oncology* 5:23–27, 1991

7. Andrykowski M, Henslee P: Assessment of current adaptation and functioning of adult survivors of allogeneic bone marrow transplantation (BMT). *Proc Am Soc Clin Oncol* 7: A1041, 1988 (abstract)

8. Thomas C: Insomnia among individuals with cancer. *Proc Oncol Nurs Soc* 13:63, 1986 (abstract)

9. Kales A, Kales JD, Soldatos CR: Insomnia and other sleep disorders. *Med Clin North Am* 66:971–988, 1982

10. Cannici J, Malcolm R, Peek L: Treatment of insomnia in cancer patients using muscle relaxation training. *J Behav Ther Exp Psychiatry* 14:251–256, 1983

11. Page M: Sleep pattern disturbance, in McNally J, Stair J, Somerville E (eds): *Guidelines for Cancer Nursing Practice.* Orlando, FL: Grune & Stratton, 1985, pp. 89–95

12. Hodgson L: Why do we need sleep? Relating theory to nursing practice. *J Adv Nurs* 16:1503–1510, 1991

13. Winningham ML, Nail LM, Barton-Burke M, et al: Fatigue and the cancer experience: The state of the knowledge. *Oncol Nurs Forum* 21:23–36, 1994

14. Kaye J, Kaye K, Madow L: Sleep patterns in patients with cancer and patients with cardiac disease *J Psychol* 114: 107–113, 1983

15. Beszterczey A, Lipowski Z: Insomnia in cancer patients. *Can Med Assoc J* 116:355, 1977

16. Holland J, Plumb M: A comparative study of depressive symptoms in patients with advanced cancer. *Proc Am Assoc Cancer Res* 18:201, 1977 (abstract)

17. Derogatis LR, Feldstein M, Morrow G, et al: A survey of psychotropic drug prescriptions in an oncology population. *Cancer* 44:1919, 1979

18. Goldberg R, Mor V: A survey of psychotropic use in terminal cancer patients. *Psychosomatics* 26:745–751, 1985

19. Nail L, Lones L, Greene D, et al: Use and perceived efficacy of self-care activities in patients receiving chemotherapy. *Oncol Nurs Forum* 18:883–887, 1991

20. Sarna L: Correlates of symptom distress in women with lung cancer. *Cancer Pract* 1:21–28, 1993

21. Lerman C, Miller S, Scarborough R, et al: Adverse psychologic consequences of positive cytologic cervical screening. *Am J Obstet Gynecol* 165:658–662, 1992

22. Lamb MA: The sleeping patterns of patients with malignant and nonmalignant diseases. *Cancer Nurs* 5:389–396, 1982

23. Silberfarb P, Hauri P, Oxman T, et al: Assessment of sleep in patients with lung cancer and breast cancer. *J Clin Oncol* 11:997–1004, 1993

24. Zorick F, Roth T, Kramer M, et al: Exacerbation of upper-airway sleep apnea by lymphocytic lymphoma. *Chest* 77: 689–691, 1980

25. Weiss R, Corvalan A, Dillon R: Metastatic renal cell carcinoma presenting as impotence. *J Urol* 149:821–822, 1993

26. Onofrj M, Curatola L, Ferracci F, et al: Narcolepsy associated with primary temporal lobe B-cell lymphoma in an HLA DR2 negative subject. *J Neurol Neurosurg Psychiatry* 55: 852–853, 1992

27. Stam H, Bultz B: The treatment of severe insomnia in a cancer patient. *J Behav Ther Exp Psychiatry* 17:33–37, 1986

28. Cella D, Tulsky D, Gray G, et al: The Functional Assessment of Cancer Therapy Scale: Development and validation of the general measure. *J Clin Oncol* 11:570–579, 1993

29. Strang P, Ovarner H: Cancer-related pain and its influence on quality of life. *Anticancer Res* 10:109–112, 1990

30. Cleeland C: Psychological aspects of pain due to cancer. *Curr Manag & Pain* 3:33–48, 1989

31. Chao N, Tierney D, Bloom J, et al: Dynamic assessment of quality of life after autologous bone marrow transplantation. *Blood* 80:825–830, 1992

32. Harris J, Cynthia C, Rosenberg L, et al: Intermittent high-dose corticosteroid treatment in childhood cancer: Behavioral and emotional consequences. *J Am Acad Child Psychiatry* 25:120–124, 1986

33. Drigan R, Spirito A, Sallan S, et al: Behavioral effects of corticosteroids in children with acute lymphoblastic leukemia (ALL). *Proc Am Soc Clin Oncol* 6:A1010, 1987 (abstract)

34. Mandell LR, Walker R, Steinherz P, et al: Reduced incidence of the somnolence syndrome in leukemic children with steroid coverage during prophylactic cranial radiation therapy: Results of a pilot study. *Cancer* 63:1975–1978, 1989

35. Faithfull S: Patients' experiences following cranial radiotherapy: A study of the somnolence syndrome. *J Adv Nurs* 16:939–946, 1991

36. Goldberg S, Tefferi A, Rummans T, et al: Post-irradiation somnolence syndrome in an adult patient following allogeneic bone marrow transplantation. *Bone Marrow Transplant* 9:499–501, 1992

37. McLeod H, Baker D, Pui C, et al: Somnolence, hypotension, and metabolic acidosis following high-dose teniposide treatment in children with leukemia. *Cancer Chemother Pharmacol* 29:150–154, 1991

38. Greenberg D, Gray J, Shipley W, et al: Treatment-related fatigue: Prostate radiation and interleukin-1 (IL-1). *Proc Am Soc Clin Oncol* 11:A1311, 1992 (abstract)

39. Janisch L. Nursing management of side effects of interleukin-2 and interferon alfa-2a administered as subcutaneous injections. *Oncol Nurs Forum* 17(suppl):163, 1990

40. World Health Organization: *Cancer Pain Relief.* Geneva: World Health Organization, 1986

41. Portenoy R, Miransky J, Thaler H, et al: Pain in ambulatory patients with lung or colon cancer: Prevalence, characteristics, and effect. *Cancer* 70:1616–1624, 1992

42. Bowdler I: The use of a standardized questionnaire for the routine assessment of pain in cancer patients. Workshop: Goals of Palliative Cancer Therapies, March 23–26, 1992

43. Massie MJ, Lesko LM: Psychopharmacological management, in Holland R, Rowland J (eds): *Handbook of Psychooncology: Psychological Care of the Patient with Cancer.* New York: Oxford U Press, 1989, pp. 470–491

44. Welch-McCaffrey D, Dodge J. Acute confusional states in elderly cancer patients. *Semin Oncol Nurs* 4:208–216, 1988

45. Tinuper T, Montagna P, Medori R, et al: The thalamus participates in the regulation of the sleep-wake cycle. A clinico-pathological study in fatal familial thalamic degeneration. *Electroencephalogr Clin Neurophysiol* 73:117–123, 1989

46. Medori R, Montagna P, Tritschler HJ, et al: Fatal familial insomnia: A second kindred with mutation of prion protein gene at codon 178. *Neurology* 41:669–670, 1992

47. Moldofsky H: Sleep and the immune system. *Int J Immunopharmacol* 17:649–654, 1995

48. Plambad J, Petrini B, Wasserman J, et al: Lymphocyte and granulocyte reactions during sleep deprivation. *Psychosom Med* 41:273–278, 1979

49. Uthganannt D, Schoolmann D, Pietowski R, et al: Effects of sleep on the production of cytokines in humans. *Psychosom Med* 57:97–104, 1995

50. Irwin M, Smith TL, Gillin JC: Electroencephalographic sleep and natural killer activity in depressed patients and control subjects. *Psychosom Med* 54:10–21, 1992

51. Levine S, Jones L, Sack D: Evaluation and treatment of depression, anxiety, and insomnia in patients with cancer. *Oncology* (suppl):119–125, 1993

52. Kaempfer SH, Johnson BL: Sleep, in Gross J, Johnson BJ (eds): *Handbook of Oncology Nursing* (ed 2). Sudbury: Jones and Bartlett, 1994, pp. 310–327

53. Moran M, Stoudemire A: Sleep disorders in the medically ill patient. *J Clin Psychiatry* 53:(suppl)29–36, 1992

54. Lazarus H, Fitzmartin R, Goldenheim P: A multi-investigator clinical evaluation of oral controlled-release morphine administered to cancer patients. *Hospice J* 6:1–15, 1990

55. Sjoberg M, Appelgren L, Einarsson S, et al: Long-term intrathecal morphine and bupivacaine in "refractory" cancer pain: I. Results from the first series of 52 patients. *Acta Anaesthesiol Scand* 35:30–43, 1991

56. LaClave L, Blix S: Hypnosis in the management of symptoms in a young girl with malignant astrocytoma: A challenge to the therapist. *Int J Clin Exp Hypn* 37:6–14, 1989

57. Hauri PJ, Orr WC: *Current Concepts: The Sleep Disorders.* Kalamazoo, MI: Upjohn, 1982

58. Nicholson AN, Stone BM: Heterocyclic amphetamine derivatives and caffeine of sleep in man. *Br J Clin Pharmacol* 9:195–203, 1980

59. Bale P, White M: The effects of smoking on the health and sleep of sportswomen. *Br J Sports Med* 12:149–153, 1980

60. Rundell OH, Lester BK, Griffiths WJ, et al: Alcohol and sleep in young adults. *Psychopharmacologia* 26:201–218, 1972

61. Adamson J, Burdick JA: Sleep of dry alcoholics. *Arch Gen Psychiatry* 28:146–149, 1973

62. Shapiro CM, Warren PM, Trindler J, et al: Fitness facilitates sleep. *Eur J Appl Physiol* 53:1–4, 1984

63. Horne JA, Reid AJ: Night-time sleep EEG changes following body heating in a warm bath. *Electroencephalogr Clin Neurophysiol* 60:154–157, 1985

64. Bootzin RR, Nicassio PM: Behavioral treatments for insomnia, in Hersen M, Eisler RM, Miller PM (eds): *Progress in Behavioral Modification,* vol 6. New York: Academic Press, 1978, pp. 1–45

65. Benson H, Beary JF, Carol MP: The relaxation response. *Psychiatry* 37:37–46, 1974

66. Poppen R: *Behavioral Relaxation Training and Assessment.* New York: Pergamon, 1988

67. Jacobson E: *Progressive Relaxation* (ed 2). Chicago: U of Chicago Press, 1938

68. Wolpe J: *Psychotherapy by Reciprocal Inhibition.* Stanford, CA: Stanford U Press, 1958

69. Bernstein DA, Borkovec TD: *Progressive Relaxation Training.* Champaign, IL: Research Press, 1973

70. Benson H: *The Relaxation Response.* New York: William Morrow, 1975

71. Schultz J, Lothe W: *Autogenic Training,* vol. 1. New York: Grune & Stratton, 1969

72. Davis M, Eshelman E, McKay M (eds): *The Relaxation and Stress Reduction Workbook* (ed 2). Oakland, CA: New Harbinger Publications, 1982

73. Lacks P: *Behavioral Treatment for Persistent Insomnia.* New York: Pergamon, 1987

74. Wilwerding M, Loprinzi C, Mailliard J, et al: A randomized crossover evaluation of methylphenidate in cancer patients receiving strong narcotics. *Proc Annu Meet Am Soc Clin Oncol* 12:A1615, 1993 (abstract)

75. Hollister LE: *Clinical Pharmacology of Psychotherapeutic Drugs* (ed 2). New York: Churchill-Livingstone, 1983

76. Lader M: A practical guide to prescribing hypnotic benzodiazepines. *BMJ* 293:1048–1049, 1986

77. Consensus conference on drugs and insomnia: The use of medications to promote sleep. *JAMA* 251:2410–2414, 1984

78. Kales A, Kales JD: Sleep laboratory studies of hypnotic drugs: Efficacy and withdrawal effects. *J Clin Psychopharmacol* 3:140–150, 1983

79. Kales A, Soladtos CR, Bixler EO, et al: Early morning insomnia with rapidly eliminated benzodiazepines. *Science* 220:95–97, 1983

80. Greenblat DJ, Harmatz JS, Zinny MA, et al: Effect of gradual withdrawal on the rebound sleep disorder after discontinuation of triazolam. *N Engl J Med* 317:772–778, 1987

81. Church MW, Johnson LC: Mood and performance of poor sleepers during repeated use of flurazepam. *Psychopharmacology* 61:309–316, 1979

82. Goldberg R, Cullen L: Use of psychotropics in cancer patients. *Psychosomatics* 27:687–700, 1986

83. Brezezinski A: Melatonin in humans. *N Engl J Med* 36:186–195, 1997

84. Haimov I, Shochat T, Lavie P: Melatonin—a possible link between sleep and the immune system. *Isr J Med Sci* 33:246–250, 1997

85. Tamarkin L, Cohen M, Roselle D, et al: Melatonin inhibition and pinealectomy enhancement of 7,12-demethyl-benz (a)anthracene-induced mammory tumors in the rat. *Cancer Res* 41:4432–4436, 1981

86. Lissoni P, Meregalli S, Nosetto L, et al: Increased survival time in brain glioblastomas by a radioneuroendocrine strategy with radiotherapy plus melatonin compared to radiotherapy alone. *Oncology* 53:43–46, 1996

87. Lissoni P, Barni S, Meregalli S, et al: Modulation of cancer endocrine therapy by melatonin: A phase II study of tamoxifen alone. *Br J Cancer* 71:854–856, 1995

88. Gonzalez R, Sanchez A, Ferguson JA, et al: Melatonin therapy of advanced human malignant melanoma. *Melanoma Res* 1:237–243, 1991

89. Lissoni P, Barni S, Ardizzoia A, et al: A randomized study with the pineal hormone melatonin versus supportive care alone in patients with brain metastases due to solid neoplasms. *Cancer* 73:699–701, 1994

90. Leathwood PD, Chauffard F: Quantifying the effects of mild sedatives. *J Psychiatr Res* 17:115–122, 1982

91. Lindahl O, Lindwall L: Double blind study of a valerian preparation. *Pharmacol Biochem Behav* 32:1065–1066, 1989

92. Leathwood PD, Chauffard F, Heck E, et al: Aqueous extract of valerian root (Valeriana officinalis L.) improves sleep quality in man. *Pharmacol Biochem Behav* 17:65–71, 1982

93. Balderer G, Borbely AA: Effect of valerian on human sleep. *Psychopharmacol* 87:406–409, 1985

94. Schulz H, Stolz C, Muller J: The effect of valerian extract on sleep polygraphy in poor sleepers: A pilot study. *Pharmacopsychiatry* 27:147–151, 1994

Daily Sleep Log

Patient Name: _____

	Monday	Tuesday	Wednesday	Thursday	Friday	Saturday	Sunday
Day's events (record any naps)							
Medication							
Bedtime mood*							
Time in bed							
Lights out							
No. of minutes (or hours) to sleep							
No. of wakings							
Total time awake							
Wake-up time							
Get-up time							
Wake-up mood*							

*Rank moods from 1 = very upset to 10 = very good.
Source: Yellen SB, Dyonzak JV: Sleep disturbances, in Yarbro CH, Frogge MH, Goodman M (eds): *Cancer Symptom Management* (ed 2). Sudbury: Jones and Bartlett, 1999. © Jones and Bartlett Publishers.

Insomnia

Patient Name: _____

Symptom and Description   Seven to eight hours of sleep a night is important for your functioning and well-being. Cancer and cancer treatment can lead to a lack of sleep.

Insomnia is a problem in either falling asleep or staying asleep. Insomnia may occur when you first learn you have cancer. You may have problems with sleep throughout your treatment and for several weeks after treatment is finished.

Learning Needs   You will need to learn the symptoms of insomnia, how to describe them, and when to report them to your doctor. During a 3-week period, you may notice the following symptoms:

- It takes 30 minutes or longer to fall asleep, or
- You wake up frequently during the night, or
- It takes 30 minutes or longer to return to sleep after you wake up during the night.

Prevention   Please refer to the Guide to Healthy Sleep (Appendix 11C) to learn more about preventing insomnia.

Management   One common problem in insomnia is that the bed has become connected with things other than sleep. This makes it hard to use the bed for sleep when you want. These guidelines may help you:

- Go to bed only when you are sleepy and planning to sleep.
- Use the bed only for sleeping, *not* for watching TV, reading, or eating.
- Don't stay in bed for longer than 15 minutes if you can't fall asleep. Move to another room and stay there until sleepy, and then return to your bed. Do this as many times as needed until you fall asleep.
- Set an alarm and get up at the same time every day even if you have not had a good night's sleep. Get up at the same time even on days that you are not working.
- Do not nap during the day, even if you are very tired.
- Tell your physician or nurse of any other medications (e.g., melatonin, valerian) you use for sleep.
- If sleep medications are prescribed, follow directions carefully.

Evaluation   If the above guidelines do not help your sleep, you may need to discuss this problem with your doctor. Let your doctor know if you are experiencing any of the following:

- Your sleep problem lasts longer than 3 weeks.
- If you take a sleep aid and you need more of it to get to sleep or to stay asleep.

- If you are unable to sleep because of sadness or personal problems.
- There is too much stress in your life.
- It is hard to do things during the day because you are sleepy.

Follow-up

Medications:

Referrals:

Phone Numbers

Nurse: _____ Phone: _____

Physician: _____ Phone: _____

Other: _____ Phone: _____

Comments

Patient's Signature: _____ Date: _____

Nurse's Signature: _____ Date: _____

Source: Yellen SB, Dyonzak JV: Sleep disturbances, in Yarbro CH, Frogge MH, Goodman M (eds): *Cancer Symptom Management* (ed 2). Sudbury: Jones and Bartlett, 1999. © Jones and Bartlett Publishers.

A Guide to Healthy Sleep

Patient Name: _____

Symptom and Description   Seven to eight hours of sleep a night is important to healthy daytime functioning and general well-being. Cancer and cancer treatment can lead to a lack of sleep or too much sleep. There are things that you can do to help your sleep remain healthy (or even make your sleep better) during cancer treatment. This guide contains rules for healthy sleep during your treatment.

Management

- Stay in bed only for the hours you plan to sleep.
- Set a bedtime and wake time and follow them.
- Try not to worry about either getting to sleep or getting enough sleep.
- Try to deal with your problems or worries during the day, before bedtime.
- Avoid foods and liquids that have caffeine in them (for example, coffee or soda) and nicotine (cigarettes).
- Avoid alcohol.
- Try to get exercise on a regular basis, even if it is only a small amount.
- Learn what things help your sleep (for example, no noise, dark room, cool room), and use them in planning your sleep.

Follow-up

Medications:

Referrals:

Phone Numbers

Nurse: _____   Phone: _____

Physician: _____   Phone: _____

Other: _____   Phone: _____

Comments

Patient's Signature: _____   Date: _____

Nurse's Signature: _____   Date: _____

Source: Yellen SB, Dyonzak JV: Sleep disturbances, in Yarbro CH, Frogge MH, Goodman M (eds): *Cancer Symptom Management* (ed 2). Sudbury: Jones and Bartlett, 1999. © Jones and Bartlett Publishers.

Hypersomnia

Patient Name: _____

Symptom and Description   A good night's sleep is important for your functioning and well-being. Too much sleep can be a problem. One side effect of cancer
and cancer treatment is sleeping too much. This is called hypersomnia, meaning
"too much sleep."

   Hypersomnia is a problem in staying awake when you want to and try to. You
may sleep 10 hours at night and still be unable to stay awake during the day.
Hypersomnia is different from fatigue. Fatigue is the feeling of being tired, but
you are able to stay awake if you try. You may have hypersomnia when you are
sleeping more than 10 hours at night or when you are unable to keep from falling
asleep during the day after a full night of sleep. The most common causes of
hypersomnia are your treatment or your mood.

Learning Needs   You will need to learn the symptoms of hypersomnia, how to
describe them, and when to report them to your doctor. During a 3-week period,
you may notice the following symptoms:

- Ten hours or more of sleep at night
- Problems in staying awake during the day

Prevention   This sleep problem is hard to prevent if it is due to your treatment.

Management   If your sleep problem is due to your treatment, then your doctor
may want to prescribe medication to help you stay awake. If your sleep problem is
due to sadness or personal problems, your doctor may either prescribe medicine
or refer you to a counselor.

Evaluation

Follow-up

Medications:

Referrals:

Phone Numbers

Nurse: _____ Phone: _____

Physician: _____ Phone: _____

Other: _____ Phone: _____

Comments

Patient's Signature: _____ Date: _____

Nurse's Signature: _____ Date: _____

Source: Yellen SB, Dyonzak JV: Sleep disturbances, in Yarbro CH, Frogge MH, Goodman M (eds): *Cancer Symptom Management* (ed 2). Sudbury: Jones and Bartlett, 1999. © Jones and Bartlett Publishers.

PART III

SYMPTOMS OF ALTERATIONS IN NUTRITION

CHAPTER 12

Anorexia-Cachexia Syndrome

Nancy S. Tait, RN, BSN, OCN®

The Problem of Anorexia-Cachexia Syndrome in Cancer

Anorexia-cachexia is a complex problem for patients and their families, as well as for the physicians and nurses who care for them. As many as 31% to 87% of all cancer patients[1] and 62% to 78% of AIDS patients[2,3] are affected by this syndrome, in which *anorexia* (lack of appetite) and *cachexia* (physical wasting) interact in a complex but vicious cycle. Those at greatest risk are the elderly, whose digestive and absorptive functions are already compromised by the aging process. Children and adolescents, people who are anorectic for long periods, and those whose malignancies, chemotherapy, and radiation therapy interfere with ingestion, digestion, or absorption are also at risk for cachexia.[4,5]

Cachexia may be the earliest manifestation of a tumor-host interaction and, in patients with cancer and AIDS, is the most common cause of death, solely from progressive weakness and wasting of host tissue.[6–8] Anorexia-cachexia is a debilitating syndrome characterized by loss of appetite, early satiety, weight loss, muscle wasting, protein depletion, and other metabolic abnormalities.[6,7,9–11] This is manifested in the patient as weakness, muscle atrophy, easy fatigability, impairment of immune function, decrease in motor or mental skills, and decline in attention span or concentration abilities.[1,12] Anorexia contributes to weight loss, which leads to weakness and a decrease in performance status. Performance status is the ability to do the physical and mental tasks of daily living.

Weight loss and performance status have been used to predict patient response to therapy, toxicity, and survival.[13,14] In an analysis of more than 3000 patients enrolled in various cancer research trials, DeWys et al.[15] found a positive correlation between a decrease in weight and a decrease in performance status. Patients with at least 5% weight loss had a shorter median survival and a lower chemotherapy response rate. This factor of weight loss is also a predictor of survival in AIDS. An estimated 20% of HIV patients have at least 10% involuntary weight loss, which leads to early death.[8,16]

The catabolic processes of anorexia-cachexia lead to progressive deterioration of nutrition, compromise of other bodily functions, lower resistance to infection, slow healing, and aggravate the toxicities of many treatments. The weakness and fatigue related to muscle wasting and changes in metabolism affect physical appearance, leading to a loss of self-esteem. As food intake decreases, weakness and fatigue continue, leading to a decrease in activity levels in the patient. It becomes difficult to perform even simple tasks such as eating and breathing.[5,12] Unless reversed, this vicious cycle continues, having a significant impact on every aspect of daily life, until death occurs.

Etiology

Although the exact etiology of cachexia still remains enigmatic, it appears to be a multifactorial problem resulting in or caused by an imbalance between caloric intake and metabolic needs.[17,18] Factors that may influence this negative balance include anorexia, nausea, alterations in gastrointestinal function, chronic blood loss, proteinuria, and gastrointestinal loss of albumin.[19]

Anorexia

Anorexia is defined as a loss of appetite. Many factors influence a person's desire to eat, such as alterations in taste, alterations in gastrointestinal function, influences of metabolism or behavior, and effects from the tumor itself.[19]

Alterations in taste

Taste changes affect appetite. Alterations in taste perception may result from a direct effect of the tumor itself, oral infections such as *Candida*, or from the effect of various treatments such as chemotherapy, radiation therapy, surgery, or antibiotics.[2,20] Commonly reported taste sensations include a decreased threshold for bitter taste, causing a dislike or aversion to beef, pork, chocolate, coffee, or tomatoes. An increased threshold for sweet taste leads the patient to add sugar to food, whereas a decreased threshold for sweet taste causes an aversion to sweet foods. Other reported taste changes include an increased need for salt on foods, an avoidance of sour foods, and a metallic or medicinal taste that may be related to zinc deficiency or to an increase in calcium or lactate.[1,6,20,21] Taste abnormalities may lead to decreases in digestive enzymes, which may yield a delay in digestion.[7]

Alterations in the gastrointestinal function

Alterations in gastrointestinal function may also influence appetite. Ulceration of the mucous membranes—a complication of chemotherapy, radiation therapy, or opportunistic infections (such as herpes simplex, *Candida*, or cytomegalovirus)—may produce mucositis or diarrhea, which interferes with ingestion, digestion, or absorption. HIV patients are especially prone to diarrhea due to the many opportunistic infections they encounter. HIV itself may cause intestinal virus atrophy, which can lead to carbohydrate malabsorption. Fifty percent of all HIV patients have no etiologic factor for malabsorption or diarrhea. Nausea and vomiting may decrease appetite and create food aversions.[1–3,8,11,22,23] Antibiotics and analgesics such as morphine may promote anorexia.[24]

Early satiety is frequently reported by patients with cancer or AIDS. It may be related to gastrointestinal tumors, ascites, hepatomegaly, or splenomegaly. Organ enlargement may be due to progressive tumor or infiltration by infection.[2,3,11,25] Chronic nausea is often associated with autonomic failure, which results in prolonged or delayed gastric emptying.[7,26]

Metabolic abnormalities

Other possible physiologic factors that may "lead to" anorexia include abnormalities in glucose metabolism,

increases in circulating amino acids or lactic acid, and increases in free fatty acids, all of which may cause early satiety. Glucose intolerance leads to prolonged elevations in blood glucose levels, which may suppress appetite. Also noted have been increases in brain levels of serotonin or tryptophan, which affect central nervous system control over appetite.[25,27,28]

Psychological abnormalities

Psychological factors such as depression, grief, or anxiety resulting from the disease or cancer treatment also may lead to poor appetite, abnormal eating behaviors, and learned food aversions, thus diminishing food intake.[29] Social or cultural factors that influence food preferences or dining behaviors may be altered by physical or psychological factors, adding to the problem of anorexia.[27] Other psychophysical factors such as pain or fatigue also may decrease appetite.[11]

Effects of the tumor

Recent studies have demonstrated the release of *cytokines* (substances released by macrophages and lymphocytes in response to inflammation) such as interleukin-1 (IL-1), tumor necrosis factor (TNF or cachectin), interleukin-2 (IL-2), gamma interferon (IFN-γ), and interleukin-6 (IL-6) as possible mediators of cachexia.[30,31] Under normal conditions, cytokines respond to injury or infection to promote wound healing and protein synthesis, and to eradicate microorganisms.[32,33] Plasma levels of these cytokines are elevated in cancer and AIDS.[2,34] Anorexia can be produced by TNF and IL-1, as demonstrated in clinical studies utilizing these cytokines for treatment. It is also presumed that TNF and IL-1 decrease gastric emptying, which delays digestion and causes satiety.[17,31,34]

These cytokines may raise the metabolic rate and increase protein catabolism and skeletal muscle protein metabolism as demonstrated by involuntary weight loss in many malignancies and in AIDS.[2,35] Patients with AIDS exhibit an episodic weight loss with partial recovery during each bout of infection that differs from the continuous weight loss in cancer.[3]

Tumors, such as in small-cell lung cancer, produce peptides such as bombesin that cause anorexia.[36,37] Gibbs and Smith systemically administered bombesin-like peptides and monitored effects on food intake. A satiety action was produced in both animals and humans.

Cachexia

Cachexia can be divided into two categories, primary and secondary. *Primary cachexia* includes anorexia, decrease in nutrients, and changes in metabolic pathways. In *secondary cachexia*, weight loss is due to mechanical factors limiting intake.[8,13]

Increased nutrient needs

Cachectic patients may have increased nutrient needs due to changes in metabolic rate or metabolic demands. The basal metabolic rate may be increased as an initial response to infection or malignancy.[2] Metabolic rate can be affected by other influences such as age, nutritional status, temperature, hormones, trauma, or alterations in resting metabolic rate.[39] In a healthy person, the adaptation to a decrease in food intake is a lowered metabolic rate.[30] This does not occur in the anorexia-cachexia syndrome. As appetite decreases, nutritional demands result in weight loss and muscle wasting. Cytokines not only promote anorexia, they also promote cachexia through an increase in resting energy expenditure and skeletal muscle wasting.[34]

As nutrition is impaired, nutrients such as zinc, selenium, and iron, which help to maintain immune function, are eliminated. The resulting decreased immunocompetence potentiates the patient's risk for infection and influences response to therapy and survival.[3,5,39]

Alterations in gastrointestinal function

Dysfunction of the GI tract may be the result of malignancy, infection, or malnutrition. Tumors of the GI tract invade the esophagus, stomach, or bowel, causing compression or obstruction that limits or inhibits food intake. Surgery to eradicate these malignancies removes necessary portions of organs, decreasing organ function and production of needed digestive enzymes. This results in inadequate digestion or absorption of fats, carbohydrates, and proteins. Damage from chemotherapy, therapy, radiation, or infection may shorten the intestinal villi, reducing the absorptive surface of the bowel.[40–42] The resulting maldigestion may alter the body's utilization of protein, carbohydrates, and fats, promoting weight loss and decreasing immune competence.

Pathophysiology

As the anorexia-cachexia syndrome continues, disruptions in normal metabolic function occur that result in further muscle wasting, immune dysfunction, and fatigue. These metabolic changes include increased energy expenditure and alterations in carbohydrate, protein, or fat metabolism. As a result of energy expenditure, oxygen consumption and carbon dioxide production may be increased, which leads to increased work of the respiratory muscles.[43] The metabolic alterations result in weight loss and muscle wasting, which may diminish cellular and humoral immunity, allowing for a decrease in resistance to infection.[39] Muscle wasting also promotes weakness and fatigue, which lead to further anorexia, weight loss, asthenia, and eventually death (Figure 12-1).

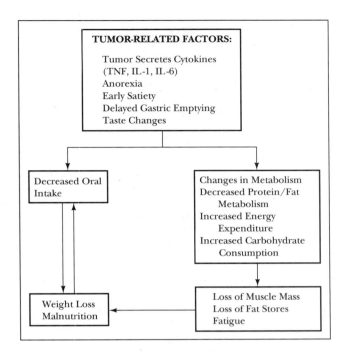

FIGURE 12-1   Anorexia-cachexia syndrome.

Carbohydrate Metabolism

Carbohydrates provide the major source of energy for the body. Glucose is synthesized from lactic acid or glucogenic amino acids, in response to hormonal signals, to meet the energy needs of glucose-dependent tissue.[14] This allows glucose to be converted to lactic acid in tissues and then reconverted to glucose in the liver in an energy-consuming process known as the Cori cycle.[45] In cachexia, this cycle is increased so that glucose usage is greater than glucose conversion. To keep up with the increased demand, additional amino acids are needed along with lactic acid to continue the cycle[27,29] Amino acids are less energy efficient, as additional energy is required to eliminate the protein by-product of nitrogen.[5] In patients with weight loss, accelerated glucose turnover or recycling can be seen.[44]

A second problem seen is impairment of insulin sensitivity or glucose intolerance. Insulin normally stimulates appetite and promotes fat and protein synthesis in response to a rise in glucose levels.[45] Insulin inhibits amino acid release from muscle. It can also inhibit gluconeogenesis, reducing amino acid degradation and conserving muscle mass.[10] In cachexia, a slower clearance in blood glucose levels is seen due to insensitivity of insulin to tissue, which results in a lower insulin response to hyperglycemia or lack of exogenous glucose production in response to hypoglycemia. This lack of response may decrease appetite and thus food intake.[46] Insulin resistance is also seen. To meet the energy needs for glucose, synthesis of glucose from glycerol or lactic acid occurs rather than the lipid oxidation that usually takes place.

This promotes a wasteful energy cycle, resulting in anorexia, decreased fat and protein synthesis, and increased energy expenditure.[45] Thus weight loss and wasting are seen.

Protein Metabolism

Protein is used as an energy source when glycogen stores are decreased. Amino acids are mobilized from the muscle to continue this energy cycle. In the noncachectic host, the body compensates for this muscle breakdown by eventually using fat and fatty acids for energy, yielding a decrease in glucose utilization and muscle sparing. This compensatory mechanism is not apparent in patients with cachexia.[10]

Also seen in cachexia is a decrease in protein synthesis that may be due, in part, to inadequate intake of protein or a decrease in albumin production by the liver. This decrease in synthesis causes a loss of muscle mass and hypoalbuminemia as the muscle protein stores are utilized to keep up with energy needs. The clinical result is a patient with impaired wound healing, susceptibility to infection, asthenia, and decreased performance status.[45,47]

Fat Metabolism

The oxidation of fatty acids is the major source of fuel for energy needs in humans.[48] As muscle wasting continues, fat stores are eventually mobilized to keep up with the increasing energy needs produced by the tumor. Fat loss may account for most of the weight loss seen in patients with anorexia-cachexia.[45,48] In addition, there may be an abnormal metabolism of fat, stimulated by insulin resistance, which results in hyperlipidemia and further decreased fat stores. The continued depletion of body stores causes further weakness, further anorexia, progressive weight loss or wasting, and a perpetuation of the cachexia cycle.

Assessment

The key to potentially altering the spiral of cachexia is to improve or maintain the nutritional status of the patient. A nutritional assessment is the first step (Figure 12-2). Assessment of various physical and psychosocial parameters allows for a baseline collection of information from which to build a plan of care. This includes a diet history, physical assessment of the patient for signs of malnutrition, and evaluation of somatic and visceral protein stores through various anthropometric or laboratory indices. The assessment is meant to screen for potential or existing problems in nutrition status; to evaluate the

patient for potential deficits of knowledge about nutrition, nutritional support, disease symptoms, or treatment side effects; and to determine response to treatment or dietary intervention.[49] The nurse may do the initial assessment with other health team members, such as a dietitian, a nutrition team, or the physician.

Diet History

A diet history is the first stage of a nutritional assessment. A complete history will elicit information about an individual's usual dietary habits, current disease symptoms, and possible side effects of treatment. Other parameters of focus include food preferences, food intolerances, food aversions, psychological factors such as family support, ability to obtain or prepare meals, and education needs on diet and nutrition.[50]

Another important way to assess individual food intake is with a food diary. This is usually done over three consecutive 24-hour periods but may be done weekly. The nurse or dietitian should review the food diary with the patient to ensure accuracy of intake during the period monitored. (See Appendix 12A for a sample food diary.)

A physical assessment of the patient should also be done to evaluate potential sites for complication from treatment (such as oral or gastrointestinal mucosa) that may influence appetite and eating, and to evaluate for potential signs of malnutrition. Some signs of malnutrition include dry, flaky skin; muscle wasting; pale skin or sclera; unhealed wounds; sparse, dry hair; and cheilitis.[51]

Anthropometric Measurements

Weight is an important measure of nutritional status. A comparison is done between a patient's current weight and a usual or ideal body weight. A recent history (3 months or less) of weight loss of 10% of the usual body weight may signal nutritional depletion.[52] Weight loss of 20% or greater is associated with an increase in morbidity and mortality.[8,51] As a result of such extreme changes in weight, the patient may appear haggard and emaciated.

Weights should be obtained and entered in the patient record each visit, using the same scale and same conditions if possible. Fluctuations in weight are influenced by the presence of edema, ascites, or dehydration.[49] Rapid weight loss may be an indication of depletion of visceral protein stores. This depletion of protein causes muscle wasting, not only of skeletal muscle but also of cardiac and respiratory muscle. The latter muscle wasting may contribute to the symptoms of easy fatigability and dyspnea seen in many cancer patients.[5,53]

Other anthropometric measurements used by the dietitian or nutritional support team to assess muscle and fat stores are skinfold measurements of the triceps, biceps, and subscapular area (Table 12-1). These measurements are done to determine subcutaneous fat stores.

Nutrition Assessment and Plan

Patient Name: _____   Phone: _____   Date: _____

Height: _____cm/in   Usual weight: _____kg/lb   Current weight: _____kg/lb

Age: _____   BSA: _____   Percent of Usual Weight: _____

Medical History/Risk Factors: _____

_____

_____

_____

Physical Assessment: _____

_____

_____

_____

Symptoms: _____

_____

_____

Food Preferences: _____

_____

_____

Food Intolerances: _____

_____

Food Aversions: _____

_____

Meal Preparation Requirements: _____

_____

_____

Educational Needs: _____

_____

_____

Treatment Regimen: _____

_____

_____

Nutrition Plan: _____

_____

_____

_____

Referrals: _____

_____

Follow-up: _____

FIGURE 12-2   Nutrition assessment and plan.

TABLE 12-1 Anthropometric Measurements

Measurement	Description	Normal Value	Significance
Midpoint of arm	Halfway point from acromion process of scapula to tip of olecranon process of ulna. Used to help measure TSF/MAC.	Individual	—
Triceps skinfold thickness (TSF)	Grasp fold of skin on posterior surface of upper arm 1 cm above midpoint and pull away from underlying muscle mass. Measure tissue with calipers. Measures subcutaneous fat.	Male: 18 mm Female: 22 mm	Severe depletion Male: ≤ 11 mm Female: ≤ 17 mm May need nutritional intervention.
Mid-arm circumference (MAC)	Measure circumference of upper arm at midpoint with an insertion tape measure. Used to calculate MAMC.	Individual	—
Mid-arm muscle circumference (MAMC)	Computed with the following formula: MAMC = MAC − (TSF × 0.314). Used to measure muscle mass.	Male: 31.7 mm Female: 28.7 mm	Severe depletion Male: ≤ 29.6 mm Female: ≤ 26.2 mm May need nutritional intervention.
Subscapular skinfold	Grasp fold of skin below border of scapula. Skinfold is angled 45 degrees upward and medial from horizontal plane. Apply calipers 1 cm from fold. Measures subcutaneous fat.	Male: 14 mm Female: 16 mm	Severe depletion Male: ≤ 10 mm Female: ≤ 10.5 mm May need nutritional intervention

TABLE 12-2 Biochemical Measures of Nutrition

Lab Index	Normal Value	Moderate Risk Malnutrition	Severe Risk Malnutrition	Interpretation of Findings/Significance
Albumin	3.8–4.5 g/dL	2.1–2.7 g/dL	<2.1 g/dL	Indicates protein depletion; may be used as an individual indicator of nutritional repletion
Transferrin	250–450 mg/dL	100–150 mg/dL	<100 mg/dL	May reflect acute changes in visceral protein. May be used as an individual indicator of nutritional repletion
Prealbumin	17–40 mg/dL	5–10 mg/dL	<5 mg/dL	Indicates protein depletion
Urinary creatinine	1.2 g/24h	960 mg/24h	720 mg/24h	Represents protein depletion
Total lymphocyte count	≥2000/mm³	800–1199/mm³	<800/mm³	Indicates cellular immune status
Nitrogen balance	Positive	Negative	Negative	Positive nitrogen balance is an indication of nutritional repletion
Anergy panel	≥5 mm induration is positive skin test	Negative	Negative	Negative anergy panel may be reversed with nutritional repletion

Additionally, estimates of muscle mass and protein stores are determined by mid-arm muscle circumference (MAMC). A tape measure is placed around the midpoint of the upper arm to measure mid-arm circumference (MAC). This measurement is coupled with triceps skinfold measurements to calculate muscle mass, which gives an estimate of somatic protein stores. These values—MAC and MAMC—are then compared with standard values.[54]

Laboratory Evaluation

A variety of laboratory tests are done to estimate somatic and visceral protein stores as well as immune function, all of which are influenced by malnutrition. These tests include serum evaluation of transport proteins, such as albumin, transferrin, prealbumin, or lymphocyte count; urinary evaluation of creatinine and nitrogen; and anergy testing (Tables 12-2, 12-3, 12-4). Most of these tests are expensive and not necessarily helpful in cachexia.[55,56]

TABLE 12-3 Significance of Creatinine-Height Index (CHI)*

Value	Degree of Protein Depletion	Implications
100%	None	None
80–99%	Mild	Encourage protein intake
60–80%	Moderate	May need assistance to increase protein intake
<60%	Severe	Needs assistance to increase protein intake

*CHI = Actual urinary creatinine excretion divided by ideal urinary creatinine excretion × 100.

Ideal creatinine for males: 23 mg/kg (based on ideal body weight).

Ideal creatinine for females: 18 mg/kg (based on ideal body weight).

Albumin levels may be influenced by body stresses such as trauma or infection, changes in hydration status, and alteration in liver and renal function. Because of the effect of nutrition on immune response, albumin has been used by some investigators as an indicator for increased risk of compromise. Albumin can be easily followed with a routine chemistry panel.[55,57]

Symptom Management

The goal in managing cachexia is to increase nutritional intake, thus improving nutritional status. Increasing the appetite may potentially reverse some of the deleterious effects of cachexia. Repletion of protein stores will increase muscle mass, which may lead to a decrease in fatigue and weakness and an increase in self-esteem. As weight is gained, the patient may experience a reduction in complications from therapy or surgery and an improvement in immune function with an increase in host resistance to infection. The patient may also experience an increase in well-being that permits administration of more intensive therapy. This may alter response to therapy and improve survival and quality of life.

Treating and controlling the cancer or infection may reverse the cachectic spiral, improving the nutritional status of the patient with cancer.[58–61] Appetite improvement and body mass repletion have been seen with the treatment of HIV infections.[41] Not all tumors or infections, however, respond to treatment, and relapse may occur despite effective treatment. Other methods that may reverse the cachexia should be tried, such as increasing intake through supplements or enteral and parenteral support, or using methods of appetite stimulation.

TABLE 12-4 Significance of Albumin, Transferrin, Prealbumin Depletion

Degree of Protein Depletion	Serum Albumin (half-life 20 days)	Serum Transferrin (half-life 8 days)	Prealbumin (half-life 2 days)
Mild	2.8–3.5 g/dL	150–200 mg/dL	10–15 mg/dL
Moderate	2.1–2.7 g/dL	100–150 mg/dL	5–10 mg/dL
Severe	<2.1 g/dL	<100 mg/dL	<5 mg/dL

Nutritional Support

Nutritional support is aimed at replenishing the body with proteins, carbohydrates, fats, vitamins, and minerals being lost through the anorexia-cachexia syndrome. Increasing the calorie-protein intake may be accomplished through oral supplementation, enteral feeding, or parenteral nutrition.

Enteral and parenteral support in the treatment of cachexia is an area of controversy in the treatment of cachexia. Animal models clearly demonstrate stimulation of tumor-cell proliferation with the use of oral or parenteral nutrition. However, similar studies in humans have not shown conclusively that parenteral nutrition may affect tumor growth or tumor protein synthesis.[62]

Nutritional support does improve nitrogen balance and may prevent further nutritional deterioration.[63] Copeland[64,65] found that cell-mediated immunity was restored with nutrition repletion. This may result in fewer infectious complications from therapy. In addition, when given parenteral support preoperatively, patients experience fewer surgical complications.[17,66] However, in spite of the potential benefits of nutritional support, no improvement in survival, tumor response, or tolerance of therapy has been shown.[61,63,67]

Enteral feeding utilizes the GI tract for digestion and absorption of nutrients.

- Nasogastric: Tube placed through nose to stomach
- Esophagostomy: Tube placed in esophagus to stomach via neck incision
- Gastrostomy: Tube either surgically or percutaneously placed into stomach
- Jejunostomy: Tube either surgically or percutaneously placed beyond pylorus of stomach into jejunum

Some of the complications of enteral nutrition and their causes are listed in Table 12-5. Nasogastric feeding is contraindicated in the presence of oral or esophageal ulcers. Further irritation of already painful ulcers is seen if a nasogastric tube is used.[22,68] If local comfort measures, such as popsicles, analgesics, or viscous Xylocaine (lidocaine hydrochloride), are inadequate to promote oral intake, alternative methods of nutrition support need to be considered. Feeding schedules and formulas are prescribed for individual tolerance and caloric needs. Teaching the patient and family to maintain the tube and feeding schedule is important in allowing the patient to remain at home, thus promoting self-esteem and potentially improving quality of life. (See Appendix 12B, Self-Care Guide: Enteral Feeding.) Patients with gastrostomies or jejunostomies can even be taught to blenderize table foods, which may cut down on expense, promote more normal digestion, and psychologically provide satiety. In general, enteral alimentation is safer than total parenteral nutrition (TPN), is less expensive, does not require sterile equipment or a trained maintenance team, is closer to a physiologic method of nutritional repletion, and may be perceived by the patient as an improvement in daily living.[56,69,70] Nursing care is aimed at assessing the patient, maintaining safety and comfort, and minimizing potential complications.

Unlike enteral support, which uses the GI tract, parenteral nutrition provides nutrients via the intravascular route. Because of the hyperosmotic solution used and the method of administration, parenteral support has many potential complications, which include venous thrombosis, air embolism, infection, hypoglycemia, and hyperglycemia. Nursing care and management of these complications are discussed in Table 12-6. As with enteral alimentation, schedules are designed for individual tolerance, caloric needs, and potential for home care. (See Appendix 12C, Self-Care Guide: Parenteral Feeding.)

The American Society for Parenteral and Enteral Nutrition has set up general guidelines for the diagnosis and treatment of malnutrition.[71,72] These guidelines take into consideration the anticipation of lack of oral intake, the use of the GI tract as the preferred route of feeding, the need for gradual refeeding without overfeeding to minimize organ or metabolic complications, and the use of solutions that meet patient needs with minimal side effects. All patients should be observed for actual or potential malnutrition. Patients should be considered at risk for malnutrition if they have had inadequate intake for 7 days or more, have had unintentional weight loss of 10% of pre-illness weight, and demonstrate a decrease in serum albumin. All patients should be given nutrition counseling early. If causes of nutrition depletion are identified, these should be corrected whenever possible. Unless the GI tract is dysfunctional, enteral feeding should be utilized rather than parenteral support. Keep in mind that parenteral support is unlikely to benefit patients with advanced cancer or those patients for whom adequate intake is anticipated. Nutritional support may provide

TABLE 12-5 Complications of Enteral Support

Complication	Presentation	Cause	Prevention/Management
Aspiration of gastric contents	• Coughing • Fever	• Excessive residual feeding • Large-bore feeding tube	• Aspirate gastric contents prior to beginning feeding. If >50 mL aspirated, wait 1 hour and try again • Patient should be in sitting position during feeding and 1 hour after feeding • Consider placing tube in jejunum to bypass pylorus • May administer metoclopramide tid to increase gastric emptying
Dumping syndrome	• Dizziness • Nausea • Abdominal cramps • Diarrhea • Skin feels cold, clammy	• High volume, hyperosmotic solution pulls fluid from upper GI tract and rapidly empties into lower GI tract	• Initiate and advance formula rate and concentration gradually • Administer feeding at room temperature • Continuous feeding may be necessary • Reduce rate/concentration temporarily
Diarrhea	• Watery stool with each feeding	• Hyperosmotic solution • Rapid rate infusion • Lactose intolerance • Contaminated equipment	• Initiate and advance formula rate and concentration gradually • Reduce rate/concentration temporarily • Continuous feeding may be necessary • Use lactose-free formula • Administer diphenoxylate hydrochloride (Lomotil)/loperamide (Imodium) after each stool • Prepare liquid meal using table food to promote more normal digestion/elimination • Change solutions and equipment daily
Constipation	• Hard, infrequent stools	• Inadequate fluid intake • Reduced gastric motility • Inadequate fiber intake • Analgesia or other drug therapy	• Increase fluid intake to two L/day • Increase activity as allowed • Administer stool softeners/laxatives • Encourage increased fiber intake • Administer prune juice as tolerated
Skin irritation	• Redness, pain, bleeding around tube	• Friction on tissue at opening • Spillage of gastric contents	• Reposition or replace tube if leaking • Keep skin around tube site clean/dry • Cleanse area daily with warm water/mild soap • Maintain gauze dressing or clear dressing • Keep catheter secured to prevent dislodgement • May require skin barrier
Clogging of feeding tube	• Unable to infuse food or air	• Inadequate flush following meals • Incompletely dissolved meds or food	• Flush tube following each meal with 80–100 mL water • Flush tube with 30–50 mL water following administration of meds • Inject 20 cc ¼ strength Hydrogen peroxide • Inject 20–30 cc air to dislodge clog • Allow 50 mL cola or cranberry juice to dwell in catheter for 20 minutes

benefit to a select group of patients but not to all cachectic patients. Other mechanisms of increasing oral intake have, therefore, been investigated.

Pharmacologic methods of appetite stimulation in cachexia

Over the past decade, many investigators have been studying possible alternatives to stimulate appetite and increase oral intake. Pharmacologic enhancement has included such drugs as hydrazine sulfate, cyproheptadine, insulin, tetrahydrocannabinol, metoclopramide, and steroids.[17,26,45,73–75] Each method has shown possible

improvement in appetite, but toxicities or insufficient data or clinical experience have limited use. One drug that has received much attention and study is megestrol acetate (MA). It produces weight gain, increased appetite, and an increased sense of well-being

Megestrol acetate Megestrol acetate is a synthetic progesterone most commonly used in the treatment of breast cancer. In a study using escalating doses of MA in stage IV breast cancer, Tchekmedyian and his group found that nearly all patients gain weight regardless of tumor response or site of disease.[76] Even patients who are anorectic or cachectic demonstrate a rapid increase

TABLE 12-6 Complications of Parenteral Support

Complication	Presentation	Cause	Prevention/Management
Venous thrombosis	• Patient complains of shoulder, neck, back, or arm pain • Swelling at base of neck or arm	• Venous irritation by catheter • Hypercoagulable states • Bed rest • Dehydration • Venous stasis • Malignancy	• Removal of catheter • Local site care to prevent infection • Local application of heat • Administration of anticoagulants
Air embolism	• Sudden-onset chest pain, apprehension, tachycardia, hypotension • Can progress to loss of consciousness and cardiac arrest	• Occlusion of small vessel by air • Insufficient hydration • Improper position • Lack of appropriate clamping	• Maintain patient in supine or Trendelenburg position when exposing catheter to atmosphere • Encourage patient to do Valsalva maneuver during tubing changes • Keep all connections taped securely • Inspect infusion system for leaks or cracks • Administer oxygen as needed
Infection/sepsis	• Fever, chills • Leukocytosis • Positive blood culture and sensitivity • Erythema, tenderness along catheter • May progress to sepsis/shock	• Inadequate aseptic care of catheter • Decreased immunocompetence	• Remove catheter • Administer appropriate antibiotic/antifungal therapy • Maintain adequate peripheral access • Administer TPN under aseptic conditions • Maintain aseptic care of catheter • Monitor for signs of infection
Hyperglycemia	• Dry, hot, flushed skin • Thirst • Fatigue • Polyuria • Nausea/emesis	• Excess carbohydrate administration • Lack of insulin	• Add insulin to TPN titrated to blood sugars • Monitor urine or blood glucose levels every 6 hours during initiation period of TPN • TPN solution may be changed based on glucose
Hypoglycemia	• Diaphoresis • Nervousness • Hunger • Weakness • Irritability, tremors • Numbness of tongue or lips • Headache • Palpitations	• Sudden withdrawal of glucose • Excessive insulin	• Administer 5% dextrose and water or 10% dextrose and water at same infusion rate if TPN interrupted • Gradually increase and decrease infusion rate for cyclic infusions • Adjust insulin • Monitor blood glucose levels

in appetite and weight gain.[77] Although the exact mechanism for this weight gain is not clearly understood, laboratory studies have been conducted that demonstrate that MA may have a role in adipose differentiation and fat synthesis.[78] These findings led to a series of clinical trials in people with cachexia resulting from cancer and AIDS.

Tchekmedyian's group conducted a randomized, double-blind, placebo-controlled trial of high-dose MA (1600 mg/day) in advanced hormone-insensitive cancer patients. Eighty-nine patients receiving MA for a least 1 month were evaluated. The results demonstrated improvement in appetite and food intake with MA. Also noted were an increase in weight and an improvement in loss of taste and aversion to sweets.[79,80] Side effects were reported as tolerable.

Loprinzi et al.[81] conducted several studies using MA as an appetite stimulant. In a randomized, double-blind, placebo-controlled trial of MA (800 mg/day), Loprinzi noted an increase in appetite and food intake, with 16%

of patients with cancer-associated anorexia and cachexia gaining 15 pounds or more over baseline.[81] In a subsequent dose-comparison study (range MA 160–1280 mg/day), a positive dose-response effect for MA on appetite stimulation was seen. Of patients receiving MA 800 mg/day, 85% had significantly more appetite stimulation when compared with those who received MA 160 mg/day. Nonfluid weight gain was seen in the higher drug doses.[82] Again, toxicities were minimal. Because of cost, Loprinzi has recommended that a lower dose of MA be used.

Other investigators have found that higher doses of MA are related to weight gain.[83–88] Von Roenn[89] has studied appetite stimulation and weight gain in AIDS cachexia. In a preliminary trial using MA (320 mg/day) in AIDS patients, weight gain of 6.3 kg was seen at a rate of 0.5 kg/wk. As in the cancer population, a marked improvement in sense of well-being was noted.[89] Additional studies in patients with AIDS demonstrated an improvement in well-being, an increase in appetite, and a significant weight gain when MA 800 mg/day was used.[90,91] Although the toxicity of MA was tolerable in all studies, doses above 800 mg/day are associated with a higher incidence of toxicity. In a quality-of-life study conducted in conjunction with a dose-response trial of MA in advanced breast cancer, women treated with 160 mg/day reported less severe side effects, better physical functioning, less psychological distress, and improvement in quality of life as compared with those women receiving 1600 mg/day.[92]

Because of the positive benefit these studies have demonstrated in potentially increasing appetite and caloric intake, promoting an increase in body mass and fat stores, and improving the patient's perception of self-image and well-being MA has now been approved as a treatment in anorexia-cachexia or weight loss associated with AIDS. It is recommended as a possible treatment of cancer cachexia. The dose recommended by the manufacturer is 800 mg/day, as it results in the greatest percent weight change. Lower doses have also shown positive results and can be used if the higher dose is not tolerated, or as a maintenance dose once the desired weight gain is achieved.[93,94] The 800 mg dose of MA requires that the patient take twenty (40 mg each) tablets per day at a cost of approximately $20 per day. To ease administration and ensure compliance, an oral suspension has been released at a cost less than the tablets.[55]

Patients receiving MA should be counseled on the potential side effects, such as hypertension, hyperglycemia, constipation, edema, gastrointestinal upset, phlebitis or deep vein thrombosis, impotence, fatigue, and bloating, which increase in frequency with increased dosing. An increase in appetite may be seen within the first week, whereas weight gain may take more than a month. Follow-up, to date, has been monthly, which may be too long an interval to accurately assess changes in appetite, as patients may accommodate to the changes.[95] Assessment may need to take place by phone and records kept in the chart in order to accurately document trends in appetite stimulation.

Growth hormone   Because it is believed that cytokines mediate cachexia, investigators have theorized that utilizing these cytokines may reverse the anorexic effects produced. During the last few years, recombinant growth hormone (rhGH) has been studied in patients with HIV. Multiple placebo-controlled or open-label studies have been conducted that demonstrate an increase in lean body mass and stabilization or increase in weight with the use of rhGH.[96–102] At a dose of 0.1 mg/kg/day, side effects include joint stiffness, puffiness, paresthesias, nausea, headache, and allergy.[16] As a result of these data and lobbying by activist groups, the U.S. Food and Drug Administration (FDA) has approved (Serostim) for the treatment of AIDS-related wasting.[103]

Other pharmacologic approaches   HIV may affect testicular function, causing lower testosterone levels. These low levels have been linked to the wasting syndrome in AIDS.[104] Replacement of testosterone in HIV-infected men with hypogonadism may improve energy, appetite, mood, and weight.[3] The FDA has approved the marketing of the synthetic anabolic steroid (Oxandrin) for treatment of AIDS-related wasting.[105]

To manage the anorexia-cachexia syndrome, marinol has also been used as an appetite stimulant.[94] Beal et al.[106] continued the use of marinol for up to 12 months in a group of patients included in a double-blind trial. Side effects included anxiety, confusion, dizziness, and euphoria.

A variety of medications have demonstrated a positive benefit in many cachexic patients. Not all patients, however, achieve weight gain or an increase in appetite. This has prompted investigation of combination drug studies in appetite enhancement to manage the debilitating axorexia-cachexia syndrome.[107,108]

Other methods of appetite stimulation

The literature supports the use of nonpharmacologic methods, such as exercise, to stimulate appetite. Relaxation exercises before meals or light exercise approximately 30 minutes before meals may reduce tension, thus improving appetite.[3,7,109] Winningham and others have conducted a number of studies that demonstrate the benefit of exercise in reducing side effects of cancer therapy such as fatigue and nausea/vomiting.[110–113] In animal models, physical exercise has been shown to have a detrimental effect on tumor metabolism.[114]

When planning an exercise regimen, assessment of the patient for disease-related or cancer therapy–related problems is necessary in ensuring individual physical readiness for exercise. Keep in mind that one of the side-effects of exercise is fatigue, which if exacerbated may cause the patient psychological and physical distress.[7,115]

Nursing Interventions to Manage Cachexia

Nursing care of the cancer patient centers around prevention and management of those symptoms related to the disease and its treatment that may adversely affect appetite and nutrition status. Interventions to alleviate unwanted symptoms should be employed as early as possible to promote an increase in appetite and nutrient intake. Patients may require additional assistance through mechanical nutrition support or appetite stimulation. Education is important to ensure understanding and promote compliance of these various interventions. (See Appendix 12D, Self-Care Guide: Appetite Stimulation.)

Nursing interventions to counteract cachexia should aim at minimizing the negative effects of nausea, vomiting, diarrhea, pain, fatigue, changes in taste, or food preferences that may influence appetite. Promoting comfort by providing antiemetics or analgesics, encouraging oral care, or encouraging rest periods may influence appetite.

Encouraging patient and family interaction and providing emotional and educational support are often helpful. When family members can provide the patient's favorite foods, food intake usually improves and family bonds are strengthened. A clean uncluttered environment can promote relaxation and result in an unhurried meal.

High-protein foods should be consumed at the most tolerated time of the day. The patient should be encouraged to participate in meal planning and to choose appealing foods high in proteins. Small, frequent meals are often better tolerated than larger, infrequent ones. Pleasant food aromas and light exercise may stimulate appetite. To conserve energy and decrease the negative impact of odors on appetite, the patient should be encouraged to allow others to cook, not coming to the table until after the meal is prepared. Using small amounts of seasonings or flavorings may enhance taste. The patient may require more seasoning than previously noted for food to have a pleasant taste. (See Appendix 12E, Self-Care Guide: Taste Changes.) The use of wine or beer before meals, if allowed, is also relaxing and may stimulate appetite.[109]

Monitoring the patient for signs of malnutrition or for potential interferences in intake is an important responsibility of the oncology nurse. Encouraging the patient to adequately complete calorie diaries and accurately report symptoms that may influence intake is helpful in planning and evaluating nutrition plans. The nurse can assess the patient for the potential need for support and suggest the use of appetite stimulation or mechanical support. Communicating with the physician or other healthcare members ensures the patient of a multidisciplinary approach to care. The patient record is an excellent resource to document a plan of care and patient response.

Conclusion

Anorexia-cachexia is a complex problem encountered by many patients. Knowledge about nutrition and cachexia has increased over the last several decades, holding promise for the future. Further research is needed to understand the mechanisms of cachexia and to find possible inhibitions to the wasteful metabolic cycles. Early assessment and intervention are essential in improving symptom control and, ultimately, quality of life. For a few patients, controlling disease-related or therapy-related symptoms may be all that is necessary. However, for most patients some pharmacologic intervention may be required. Increasing appetite and oral intake is necessary to replete protein stores, thus restoring nutrition status. Reversing the cachectic spiral decreases weight loss, mus-

cle weakness, and fatigue, improves immune function, increases tolerance of therapy, and may increase survival.

References

1. Puccio M Nathanson L: The cancer cachexia syndrome. *Semin Oncol* 24:277–287, 1997
2. *Wasting in AIDS and Cancer.* Princeton, NJ: Bristol-Myers, Squibb CO., 1995
3. Von Roenn J, Knopf K: Anorexia-cachexia in patients with HIV: Lessons for the oncologist. *Oncology* 10:1049–1056, 1996
4. Tait NS, Aisner J: Nutritional concerns in cancer patients. *Semin Oncol Nurs* 5(suppl):58–62, 1989
5. Lindsey AM: Cancer cachexia: Effects of the disease and its treatment. *Semin Oncol Nurs* 2:19–29, 1986
6. Foltz A: Nutritional disturbances, in Groenwald SL, Frogge MH, Goodman M, Yarbro CH, (eds): *Cancer Nursing: Principles and Practices* (ed 4). Sudbury: Jones and Bartlett, 1997, pp. 655–683
7. Bruera E, Higginson I (eds): *Cachexia-Anorexia in Cancer Patients.* New York: Oxford University Press, 1996, pp. 1–197
8. Ottery F: *Integrating Nutrition Into Cancer and AIDS Care.* Princeton, NJ: Bristol-Myers, Squibb CO., 1995
9. Hellerstein MK, Kahn J, Maudie H, et al: Current approach to the treatment of human immunodeficiency virus—Associated weight loss: Pathophysiologic considerations and emerging management strategies. *Semin Oncol* 17 (suppl):17–33, 1990
10. Langstein HN, Norton JA: Mechanisms of cancer cachexia. *Hematol Oncol Clin North Am* 5:103–123, 1991
11. Cunningham R: *The Anorexia-Cachexia Syndrome in Cancer.* Princeton, NJ: Bristol-Myers, Squibb CO., 1997
12. Reilly H: Nutritional Assessment. *Br J Nurs* 5:18–24, 1996
13. Ottery F: Supportive nutrition to prevent cachexia and improve quality of life. *Semin Oncol* 22(suppl):98–111, 1995
14. Ottery F: Rethinking nutritional support of the cancer patient: The new field of nutritional oncology. *Semin Oncol* 21:770–778, 1994
15. DeWys WD, Begg C, Lavin PT, et al: Prognostic effect of weight loss prior to chemotherapy in cancer patients. *Am J Med* 69:491–497, 1980
16. Kocurek K: Primary care of the HIV patient. *Med Clin North Am* 80:375–410, 1996
17. Parnes HL, Aisner J: Protein-calorie malnutrition and cancer therapy. *Drug Safety* 7:404-416, 1992
18. Chlebowski RT: Nutritional support of the medical oncology patient. *Hematol Oncol Clin North Am* 5:147–159, 1991
19. Buhle EL: Nutritional support. *Oncolink,* Sept 1997, http://cancer.med.upehn.edu/Specia Hymed.orc/nutri-support.html
20. Bender CM: Taste alterations, in Yasko JM (ed): *Nursing Management of Symptoms Associated with Chemotherapy* (ed 3). Columbus: Adria Laboratories, 1993, pp. 67–74
21. Strohl R: Nursing management of the patient with cancer experiencing taste changes. *Cancer Nurs* 5:353–359, 1983
22. Sharpstene D, Gazzard B: Gastrointestinal manifestations of HIV infection. *Lancet* 348:379–383, 1996

23. Herber D, Tchekmedyian NS, Galvin M, et al: Metabolic and nutritional disorders in the HIV-positive and AIDS patient, in Torosian M (ed): *Nutrition for the Hospitalized Patient.* New York: Marcel, Dekker, 1995, pp. 551–565

24. Keithly JK, Kohn CL: Managing nutritional problems in people with AIDS. *Oncol Nurs Forum* 17:23–27, 1990

25. Pearlstone DB, Pisters PW, Brennan MF: Nutrition and cancer, in Torosian M (ed): *Nutrition for the Hospitalized Patient.* New York: Marcel Dekker, 1995, pp. 393–424.

26. Strong P: The effect of megestrol acetate on anorexia, weight loss and cachexia in cancer and AIDS patients. *Anticancer Res* 17:657–662, 1997

27. Grant M, Ropka ME: Alterations in nutrition, in Baird S, McCorkle R, Grant M. (eds): *Cancer Nursing: A Comprehensive Textbook.* Philadelphia: WB Saunders, 1991, pp. 717–741

28. Meguid MM, Muscaritoli M, Beverly JL, et al: The early cancer anorexia paradigm: Changes in plasma free tryptophan and feeding indexes. *J Parenter Enter Nutr* 16(suppl): 56S–59S, 1992

29. Daly JM, Shinkwin M: Nutrition and the cancer patient, in Holleb AI, Fink DJ, Murphy GP (eds): *American Cancer Society Textbook of Clinical Oncology.* Atlanta: American Cancer Society, 1991, pp. 498–512

30. Keush GT, Thea DM: Malnutrition in AIDS. *Med Clin North Am* 77:795–811, 1993

31. Lowry SF, Moldawer LL: Tumor necrosis factor and other cytokines in the pathogenesis of cancer cachexia. *Principles Practices Oncol Update* 4:1–12, 1990

32. Thompson WA, Coyle SM, Loury SF: Nutrition and cytokines, in Torosian M (ed): *Nutrition for the Hospitalized Patient.* New York: Marcel Dekker, 1995, pp. 97–117.

33. Laviano A, Renvyle T, Yang ZJ: From laboratory to bedside: New strategies in the treatment of malnutrition in cancer patients. *Nutrition* 12:112–122, 1996

34. Moldawer LL, Rogy MA, Lowry SF: The role of cytokines in cancer cachexia. *J Paren Enter Nutr* 16(suppl):43S–49S, 1992

35. Cooney RN, Kimball SR, Vary TC: Regulation of skeletal muscle protein turnover during sepsis: Mechanisms and mediators. *Shock* 7:1–16, 1997

36. LaCivita C: Nutrition support, in Finley R (ed): *Concepts in Oncology Therapeutics.* Bethesda, MD: American Society of Hospital Pharmacists, 1991, pp. 361–386

37. McNamara MJ, Alexander HR, Norton JA: Cytokines and their role in the pathophysiology of cancer cachexia. *J Parenter Enter Nutr* 16(suppl):50S–55S, 1992

38. Gibbs J, Smith GP: The actions of Bombesin-like peptides on food intake. *Ann NY Acad Sci* 547:210–216, 1988

39. Krenitsky J: Nutrition and the immune system. *AACN* 7: 359–369, 1996

40. Crocker KS: Gastrointestinal manifestations of acquired immunodeficiency syndrome. *Nurs Clin North Am* 24: 395–406, 1989

41. Von Roenn JH, Roth EL, Craig R: HIV-related cachexia: Potential mechanisms and treatment. *Oncology* 49(suppl): 50–54, 1992

42. Szeluga DJ: Nutritional disturbances, in Groenwald SL, Frogge MH, Goodman M, Yarbro CH (eds): *Cancer Nursing: Principles and Practices* (ed 2). Sudbury: Jones and Bartlett, 1992, pp. 495–519

43. DeWys WD: Pathophysiology of cancer cachexia: Current understanding and areas for future research. *Cancer Res* 42(suppl):721S–726S, 1982

44. Chlebowski RT, Herber D: Metabolic abnormalities in cancer patients: Carbohydrate metabolism. *Surg Clin North Am* 66:957–963, 1986

45. Nelson KA, Walsh D, Sheehan F: The cancer anorexia-cachexia syndrome. *J Clin Oncol* 12:213–225, 1994

46. Chen MK, Souba WW, Copeland EM: Nutritional support in the surgical oncology patient. *Hematol Oncol Clin North Am* 5:125–142, 1991

47. Iwamoto R: Cancers of the head and neck, in Hassey-Dow K, Bucholtz J Iwamoto R, et al (eds): *Nursing Care in Radiation Oncology.* Philadelphia: Saunders 1997, pp. 239–260

48. McAndrew PF: Fat metabolism and cancer. *Surg Clin North Am* 66:1003–1011, 1986

49. Schulmeister L: Nutrition, in Otto S (ed): *Cancer Nursing.* St. Louis: Mosby–Year Book, 1991, pp. 373–387

50. Iwamoto RR: Altered nutrition, in Hassey-Dow KM, Hilderley LJ (eds): *Nursing Care in Radiation Oncology.* Philadelphia: Saunders, 1992, pp. 69–94

51. Bernard M, Jacobs D, Rombeau J (eds): Nutrient requirements, in *Nutritional and Metabolic Support of Hospitalized Patients.* Philadelphia: Saunders, 1986, pp. 11–45

52. Driscoll DF, Bistrian BR: Clinical issues in the therapeutic monitoring of total parenteral nutrition. *Clin Lab Med* 7: 699–714, 1987

53. DeWys WD: Management of cancer cachexia. *Semin Oncol* 12:452–460, 1986

54. Edelstein S: Nutritional assessment in cancer cachexia. *Pediatric Nurs* 17:237–240, 1991

55. Tchekmedyian NS: Costs and benefits of nutrition support in cancer. *Oncology* 9(suppl):79–84, 1995

56. Lin EM: Nutrition support making the difficult decisions. *Cancer Nurs* 14:261–269, 1991

57. Bistrian BR: Some practical and theoretic concepts in the nutritional assessment of the cancer patient. *Cancer* 58: 1863–1866, 1986

58. Feron KC, Carter DC: What's new in general surgery: Cancer cachexia. *Ann Surg* 208:1–5, 1988

59. Bonneterre J, Beaucaire J, Vennin P, et al: Cancer cachexia. *Ad Clin Oncol* 3:391–405, 1988

60. Tchekmedyian NS, Tait N, Moody M, et al: Appetite stimulation with megestrol acetate in cachectic cancer patients. *Semin Oncol* 13(suppl):37–43, 1986

61. Ng EH, Lowry SF: Nutritional support in cancer cachexia. *Hematol Oncol Clin North Am* 5:161–180, 1991

62. Torosian MH: Stimulation of tumor growth by nutrition support. *J Parenter Enter Nutr* 16:725–755, 1992

63. De Cicco M, Panarello G, Fantin D, et al: Parenteral nutrition in cancer patients receiving chemotherapy: Effects of toxicity and nutrition status. *J Parenter Enter Nutr* 17: 513–518, 1993

64. Copeland EM: Intravenous hyperalimentation and cancer: A historical perspective. *J Parenter Enter Nutr* 10:337–342, 1986

65. Copeland EM, MacFadyen BV, Dudrick SJ: Effects of intravenous hyperalimentation on established delayed hypersensitivity in the cancer patient. *Ann Surg* 184:60–64, 1976

66. Sclafani LM, Brennan MF: Nutritional support in the cancer patient, in Fischer JE (ed): *Total Parenteral Nutrition* (ed 2). Boston: Little, Brown, 1991, pp. 323–345

67. Sax HC, Souba WW: Enteral and parenteral feedings. *Med Clin North Am* 77:863–880, 1993

68. Zibell-Fisk D: Tube feeding: Practical suggestions, in Bloch

AS (ed): *Nutrition Management of the Cancer Patient*. Rockville, MD: Aspen Publishers, 1990, pp. 277–284

69. Stuart S, Stuart M, Unger L: Enteral and parenteral nutrition support, in Morrison G, Hank L (eds): *Medical Nutrition in Disease*. Boston: Blackwell Science, 1996, pp. 339–368

70. Page C, Hardin T, Melnik G (eds): *Nutritional Assessment and Support* (ed 2). Baltimore: Williams & Wilkins, 1994, pp. 1–230

71. American Society for Enteral and Parenteral Nutrition: Guidelines for the use of parenteral and enteral nutrition in adult and pediatric patients. *J Parenter Enter Nutr* 17 (suppl):1SA–15SA, 1993

72. Klein S, Kinney J, Jujcebhey K, et al: Nutritional support in clinical practice: Review of published data and recommendations for future research directions. Summary of a conference sponsored by the NIH, ASPEN, and ASCN. *Am J Clin Nutr* 66:683–706, 1997

73. Chlebowski RT, Bulcavage L, Grosvenor M, et al: Hydrazine sulfate in cancer patients with weight loss: A placebo-controlled clinical experience. *Cancer* 59:406–410, 1987

74. Kardinal CG, Loprinzi CL, Schaid DJ, et al: A controlled trial of cyproheptadine in cancer patients with anorexia and/or cachexia. *Proc Am Soc Clin Oncol* 9:325, 1990 (abstract)

75. Beal JE, Olson R, Laubenstein L, et al: Dronabinol as a treatment for anorexia associated with weight loss in patients with AIDS. *J Pain Symptom Manage* 2:89–97, 1995

76. Tchekmedyian NS, Tait N, Aisner J: High-dose megestrol acetate in the treatment of postmenopausal women with advanced breast cancer. *Semin Oncol* 13(suppl):20–75, 1986

77. Aisner J, Tchekmedyian NS, Tait N, et al: Studies of high-dose megestrol acetate: Potential applications in cachexia. *Semin Oncol* 15(suppl):68–75, 1988

78. Hamburger AW, Parnes H, Gordon GB, et al: Megestrol acetate-induced differentiation of 3T3-L1 adipocyte in vitro. *Semin Oncol* 15(suppl):76–78, 1988

79. Tchekmedyian NS, Hariri L, Siau J, et al: Megestrol acetate in cancer anorexia and weight loss. *Proc ASCO* 9(suppl): 336, 1990

80. Tchekmedyian NS, Hickman M, Siau J, et al: Megestrol acetate in cancer anorexia and weight loss. *Cancer* 69: 1268–1274, 1992

81. Loprinzi CL, Ellison NM, Schaid DJ, et al: Controlled trial of megestrol acetate for the treatment of cancer anorexia and cachexia. *J Natl Cancer Inst* 82:1127–1132, 1990

82. Loprinzi CL, Michale JC, Schaid DJ, et al: Phase III evaluation of four doses of megestrol acetate as therapy for patients with anorexia and/or cachexia. *J Clin Oncol* 11: 762–767, 1993

83. Bruera E, MacMillian K, Kuelyn N, et al: A controlled trial of megestrol acetate on appetite, caloric intake, nutritional status and other symptoms in patients with advanced cancer. *Cancer* 66:1279–1282, 1990

84. Bruera E, MacMillian K, Kuelyn N, et al: A double-blind trial of megestrol acetate on appetite, calorie intake, nutritional status and other symptoms in patients with advanced cancer. *Proc Am Soc Clin Oncol* 8:327, 1989 (abstract)

85. Schmoll E, Wilke H, Thole R, et al: Megestrol acetate in cancer cachexia. *Semin Oncol* 18(suppl 2):32–34, 1991

86. Schmoll E: Risks and benefits of various therapy for cancer anorexia. *Oncology* 49(suppl):43–45, 1992

87. Gebbia V, Testa A, Gebbia N: Prospective randomized trial of two dose levels of megestrol acetate in the management of anorexia-cachexia syndrome in patients with metastatic cancer. *Br J Cancer* 73:1576–1580, 1996

88. Heckmayer M, Gatzemeier U: Treatment of cancer weight loss in patients with advanced lung cancer. *Oncology* 49 (suppl):32–34, 1992

89. Von Roenn JH, Murphy RL, Weber KM, et al: Megestrol acetate for the treatment of cachexia associated with human immunodeficiency virus (HIV) infection. *Ann Intern Med* 109:840–841, 1988

90. Von Roenn J, Armstrong D, Kotler D, et al: Megestrol acetate in patients with AIDS-related cachexia. *Ann Intern Med* 121:393–399, 1994

91. Oster M, Enders S, Samuels S, et al: Megestrol acetate in patients with AIDS and cachexia. *Ann Intern Med* 121: 400–408, 1994

92. Kornblith AB, Hallis DR, Zuckerman E, et al: Effect of megestrol acetate on quality of life in a dose-response trial in women with advanced breast cancer. *J Clin Oncol* 11: 2081–2089, 1993

93. Tchekmedyian NS, Hickman M, Herber D: Treatment of anorexia and weight loss with megestrol acetate in patients with cancer or acquired immunodeficiency syndrome. *Semin Oncol* 18(suppl 2):35–42, 1991

94. Tchekmedyian NS, Halpert C, Ashley J, et al: Nutrition in advanced cancer: Anorexia as an outcome variable and target of therapy. *J Parenter Enter Nutr* 16(suppl): 88S–92S, 1992

95. Tchekmedyian NS, Hickman M, Siau J, et al: Treatment of cancer anorexia with megestrol acetate: Improved quality of life. *Oncology* 4:185–192, 1990

96. Daar ES, LaMarca A, Schambelan M, et al: Effect of continuous growth hormone therapy on lean body mass (LBM) and AIDS-defining events in HIV-associated wasting (HIV-W) *3rd Conf Retro Opportun Infect*, p. 125, 1996

97. Klaude S, Fruhauf L, Michels B, et al: HIV-associated wasting syndrome—Therapy with mammalian cell-derived human growth hormone (rhGH). *Intern Conf AIDS* 11:121, 1996

98. Berger DS, LaMarca A, Landy H, et al: A Phase III study of recombinant human growth hormone (mammalian (cell-derived) in patients with AIDS wasting. *Intern Conf AIDS* 11:26, 1996

99. Tai VW, Mulligan K: Culp J, et al: The effects of chronic growth hormone therapy on dietary intake in patients with HIV-associated weight loss. *Intern Conf AIDS* 11:122, 1996

100. Schambelin M, Mulligan K. Hormonal anabolic agents and cytokine inhibitors in the treatment of HIV-associated wasting. *3rd Conf Retro Opportun Infect*, p. 171, 1996

101. Luna-Castanos G, Osornio L, Gomez DM, et al: Growth hormone in the treatment of weight AIDS-related. *Intern Conf AIDS* 11:122, 1996

102. Pierson R, Wang J, Landy H, et al: Clinical relevance of DEXA-determined lean body mass in patients with AIDS wasting. *Intern Conf AIDS* 11:123, 1996

103. James JS: Human growth hormone approved for wasting. *AIDS Treat News* 254:1–4, 1996

104. Hernandez-Lopez G, Feregrino-Goyos M, Eid-Lidt G, et al: Low levels of testosterone in AIDS wasting syndrome: The effect of anabolic steroids on muscular body mass and better nutritional support. *Intern Conf AIDS* 11:454, 1996

105. Anonymous: Anabolic steroid available again. *Posit Aware* 7:5, 1996

106. Beal JE, Olson R, Laubenstein L, et al: Long-term efficacy

and safety of dronabinol for acquired immunodeficiency syndrome-associated anorexia. *J Pain Symptom Manage* 14: 7–14, 1997

107. Timpone JG, Wright D, Li N, et al: The safety and pharmacokinetics of single agent and combination therapy with megestrol acetate and dronabinol for the treatment of HIV-wasting syndrome. *3rd Conf Retro and Opportun Infect,* p. 125, 1996

108. McMillian DC, O'Gorman P, Fearon KC, et al: A pilot study of megestrol acetate and ibuprofen in the treatment of cachexia in gastrointestinal cancer patients. *Br J Cancer* 76: 788–790, 1997

109. Rosenbaum EH, Stitt CA, Drasin H, et al: Daily nutritional care for cancer patients, in Newell GR, Ellison NW (eds): *Nutrition and Cancer: Etiology and Treatment.* New York: Raven Press, 1981, pp. 339–354

110. Winningham ML, MacVicar MG: The effect of aerobic exercise on patient reports of nausea. *Oncol Nurs Forum* 15:447–450, 1988

111. Winningham ML, Nail LM, Burke MB, et al: Fatigue and the cancer experience: The state of knowledge. *Oncol Nurs Forum* 21:23–36, 1994

112. Friendenreich CM, Courneya KS: Exercise as rehabilitation for cancer patients. *Clin J Sport Med* 6:237–244, 1996

113. Dimeo FC, Tilmann MH, Bertz H, et al: Aerobic exercise in the rehabilitation of cancer patients after high dose chemotherapy and autologous peripheral stem cell transplantation. *Cancer* 79:1717–1722, 1997

114. Department of Surgery, Sahlgrens Hospital: Effects of spontaneous physical exercise on experimental cancer anorexia and cachexia. *Eur J Cancer* 26:1083–1088, 1990

115. St. Pierre BA, Dasper CE, Lindsey AM: Fatigue mechanisms in patients with cancer: Effects of tumor necrosis factor and exercise on skeletal muscle. *Oncol Nurs Forum* 19:419–425, 1992

Weekly Food Diary

Patient Name: _____

Meal Preparation: Self _____ Spouse _____ Other _____

Meal Supplement: Yes _____ No _____ Type: _____

Community Assistance Program: Yes _____ No _____ Phone: _____

Appetite Stimulant: Yes _____ No _____ Type: _____

	Amt Food/Fluid	Comments	Value/Calories
Date:			
Breakfast			
Lunch			
Dinner			
Snack			
Supplement			

Instructions for a Food Diary

You will be asked to keep a record of all foods eaten for the next 7 days. Accurately write down what you eat immediately after eating.

Amount of Food   Use measuring spoons and cups and a ssmall diet scale if possible, to accurately record amounts. Describe food as "plain, baked, broiled, fried, breaded, sweetened, whole, half, sliced," etc. Record all beverages at meals and between meals. remember to record all food items, including fats (margarine, butter, etc.), sauces, gravies, cream, sugar, ketchup, mustard, pickles, and other added foods. The following abbreviations may be used.

Cup	c.	Medium	med.
Teaspoon	tsp.	Large	lg.
Tablespoon	T.	Inches	in.
Ounce	oz.	Slices	sl.
Small	sm.	Sweetened	sw.

Also include any vitamin and mineral supplements taken. Please keep the food record as accurately as possible. Remember to bring the record back on follow-up visits.

(continued) 199

Phone Numbers

Nurse: _____ Phone: _____

Physician: _____ Phone: _____

Other: _____ Phone: _____

Comments

Patient's Signature: _____ Date: _____

Nurse's Signature:Patient's Signature: _____ Date: _____

Source: Tait NS: Anorexia-cachexia syndrome, in Yarbro CH, Grogge MH, Goodman M (eds): *Cancer Symptom Management* (ed 2). Sudbury: Jones and Bartlett, 1999. © Jones and Bartlett Publishers.

Enteral Feeding

Patient Name: _____

Symptom and Description   When weight loss or lack of appetite become severe, nutrition supplements can be given. These supplements provide protein, vitamins, and other nutrients your body needs for energy. If you are unable to take these supplements by mouth, special tubes can be placed that allow you to receive the necessary nutrients without eating or drinking. The types of special tubes are:

- Nasogastric tube: A tube that goes from the nose down the esophagus to the stomach.
- Gastrostomy tube: A tube that is placed by the surgeon into the stomach through a small hole outside the stomach wall.
- Jejunostomy tube: A tube that is placed into the upper part of the intestine (jejunum), just beyond the stomach. The tube is placed by the surgeon through a small hole in the abdomen.

Learning Needs   You will need to learn to care for the nutrition tube and learn to give yourself the nutrients. You will also need to learn about some of the problems that can occur with tube feedings and what to report to your doctor.

Preventing Problems   Tube feeding is important in giving you the nutrients you need. When care is taken to give the tube feeding safely, many problems can be avoided.

1. Aspiration:
   - Sit up to take feeding and for 1 hour after feeding.
   - If feeding is continuous, keep your head elevated on two or three pillows.
   - Check for residual food before giving feeding. If more than 50 mL or 2 ounces of residual food, do not take a feeding at that time. Try again in 1 hour.
   - Check placement of tube before beginning.
   - Do not begin feeding if you feel full or bloated.
2. Diarrhea:
   - Allow feeding solution to warm to room temperature before giving.
   - Do not use feeding solution that has been opened and out for more than 6 to 8 hours.
   - Do not use feeding solution left open in refrigerator longer than 24 hours.
   - Wash hands before handling tube or feeding solution.
   - Keep feeding container clean.
3. Constipation:
   - Take additional water.
   - Ask about adding fiber to diet.
   - Consider a stool softener/laxative.
   - Increase your physical activity as allowed.

4. Skin irritation:
   - Keep skin around tube clean and dry.
   - Check for leakage around tube and report this immediately to your caregiver.
   - Tape tube securely to prevent pulling.
   - Change dressing daily.
   - Apply skin protectant as needed.

5. Dehydration (loss of body fluids):
   - Increase amount of water given in the tube between feedings.
   - Observe for increased urination.
   - Observe for signs of thirst, fever.
   - Check with physician about changing formula.

6. Tube clogging:
   - Make sure there are no kinks in tube.
   - Flush tube with 3 to 4 ounces water after meals.
   - Dissolve all medications placed in the tube in at least 1 ounce water.
   - Rinse your tube with water before and after medications.
   - Rinse tube with cola or 1 part hydrogen peroxide in 3 parts water, if tube becomes sluggish.

Management Your tube feeding will be given on a schedule that best fits your needs for care and amount of calories required. The doctor, dietitian, or nurse will explain the schedule that is best for you. The choices of schedules are as follows:

- Intermittent or bolus: The amount of tube feeding for the day will be divided up into smaller portions to be given at set times during the day over short periods. May be done by gravity or syringe.
- Continuous tube feeding: The amount of tube feeding for the day will be given slowly over the 24-hour period. It is usually given by a pump to keep the rate steady.

It is important to make sure the tube is in the right place before starting each feeding.

1. Nasogastric tube:
   - Wash your hands.
   - Draw up 10 to 20 cc air into a syringe.
   - Insert the tip of the syringe into the end of the feeding tube.
   - Unclamp the tube.
   - Put stethoscope into ears and place bell over abdominal area.
   - Quickly push air into feeding tube. You should hear a "whoosh," a bubbling, or a quick high-pitched gurgling sound.
   - Do not give your feeding if you cannot hear this sound. Contact the doctor, nurse, or dietitian.

2. Gastrostomy or jejunostomy tube:
   - Wash your hands.
   - Measure the number of inches from the stomach wall to the end of the tube.
   - If more than _____ inches, do not give feeding.
   - Contact the doctor, nurse, or dietitian.

Report any of the following symptoms to your doctor:

- Tube feeding into lungs (aspiration): Coughing or gagging, especially associated with fever.
- Diarrhea: Loose, watery stools can occur alone or associated with other symptoms such as cramping, upset stomach, or dizziness.
- Constipation: Hard, infrequent stools.
- Skin irritation: Pain, redness, or bleeding around the tube.
- Dehydration: Thirst, weight loss, dry mouth, lack of energy, extreme tiredness.
- Tube clogging: Difficulty flushing tube with water or air.

Follow-up   Should any of these problems happen, call your doctor:

1. If you feel your feedings are not working well for you, check with your doctor or dietitian about changing rate of feeding or method of feeding.
2. If the tube becomes dislodged or falls out, apply a dressing over the opening if the tube is in your stomach, and call your caregiver immediately.
3. Notify your caregiver if you have any of the following:
   - temperature of 100.4°F (38°C) or more
   - diarrhea
   - nausea or vomiting
   - constipation
   - abdominal distention
   - tube dislodgement
   - clogging of the tube

Phone Numbers

Nurse: _____ Phone: _____

Physician: _____ Phone: _____

Dietitian: _____ Phone: _____

Comments

Patient's Signature: _____ Date: _____

Nurse's Signature: _____ Date: _____

Source: Tait NS: Anorexia-cachexia syndrome, in Yarbro CH, Frogge MH, Goodman M (eds): *Cancer Symptom Management* (ed 2). Sudbury: Jones and Bartlett, 1999. © Jones and Bartlett Publishers.

Parenteral Feeding

Patient Name: _____

Symptom and Description   When weight loss or lack of appetite becomes severe, nutrition can be given by vein. This allows you to get the protein, vitamins, and other nutrients your body needs for energy. This special nutrition solution can be given into an implanted port, a tunneled catheter, or any other long-term catheter placed in a large vein.

Learning Needs   You will need to learn to care for the catheter and learn to give yourself the nutrients. Your nutrition solution will be given on a schedule that best fits your needs for care and amount of calories required. The doctor, nurse, or dietitian will explain the schedule that is best for you. The choices of schedules are:

- Continuous: The amount of solution for the day will be given slowly over the 24-hour period.
- Cyclic: The amount of solution for the day will be given over a 12-hour period. You will also need to learn about some of the problems that can occur with nutrition solutions and what to report to your doctor.

Preventing Problems   The parental feeding is important in giving you the nutrients you need. When care is taken to give the solution safely, many problems can be avoided. Such as:

1. High blood sugar: Your blood sugar level may become high as a result of the amount of sugar in the solution. You will need to have blood tests to monitor this level as often as the doctor thinks is necessary, usually two to three times per week.
   - Special medication called insulin may be added to your nutrition solution.
   - The type of solution may need to be changed.
2. Low blood sugar: Your blood sugar will become low if there is an interruption in the infusion of the nutrient solution.
   - Infuse the solution with the rate as you have been instructed to use.
   - Do not stop or interrupt the solution without calling the doctor first.
   - Blood tests will be done to measure your blood sugar levels.
3. Infection: Clean the catheter daily as follows.
   - Use only sterile technique when changing the dressing of the catheter or hooking up the solution.
   - Wash hands.
   - Remove old dressing, being careful not to pull tube or dislodge needle.
   - Begin cleaning next to catheter with hydrogen peroxide, working outward to push bacteria away from catheter.

- Clean same area a second time with povodine iodine (Betadine), working outward to push bacteria away from catheter.
- Clean catheter with povodine iodine where it exits from your body.
- Check for redness, soreness, or drainage.
- Put antibacterial ointment around catheter or needle.
- Place new gauze to cover catheter or needle, and tape.
- Do not use the nutrient solution if it looks cloudy or has particles in it. Call the doctor or pharmacist for instructions.

Management

- Have blood tests for sugar level drawn as directed.
- Should low blood sugar occur, drink 1 or 2 glasses of juice or eat several pieces of hard candy. Symptoms should resolve quickly. The symptoms are sweating; nervousness; shaking of hands; hunger; weakness; irritability; numbness of tongue or lips; headache.
- Self-administer insulin as you have been instructed or call doctor immediately if symptoms of high blood sugar occur: dry, hot flushed skin; thirst; fatigue; frequent urination; upset stomach.
- Call doctor for any temperature of 100.4°F (38°C) or higher.
- Do not adjust rate of nutrition solution without talking with your doctor.

Follow-up

1. Discuss any difficulties with solution infusion with your doctor, nurse, or dietitian.
2. Notify your caregiver if any of the following occur:
   - Temperature of 100.4°F or higher
   - Chills
   - Tenderness, redness at catheter site
   - Swelling of neck or arm
   - High blood sugar: dry, hot, flushed skin; thirst; fatigue; frequent urination; upset stomach
   - Low blood sugar: sweating; nervousness; shaking of hands; hunger; weakness; irritability; numbness of tongue or lips; headache

Phone Numbers

Nurse: _____ Phone: _____

Physician: _____ Phone: _____

Dietitian: _____ Phone: _____

Comments

Patient's Signature: _____ Date: _____

Nurse's Signature: _____ Date: _____

Source: Tait NS: Anorexia-cachexia syndrome, in Yarbro CH, Frogge MH, Goodman M (eds): *Cancer Symptom Management* (ed 2). Sudbury: Jones and Bartlett, 1999. © Jones and Bartlett Publishers.

Appetite Stimulation

Patient Name: _____

Symptom and Description   Loss of appetite is a loss of the desire to eat. Not eating can lead to weight loss. Weight loss can cause weakness and fatigue, which affect your ability to perform normal activities. Proper nutrition also helps your body prevent and fight infection. Weight loss or lack of appetite may be due to the cancer or sometimes to treatments for the cancer.

Learning Needs   You will need to learn the possible causes for loss of appetite and inform your doctor of the signs. You should report the following causes for loss of appetite.

- Tiredness
- Pain
- Taste changes such as with sugar, salt, caffeine, meats
- Side effects from medications

Prevention/Management   Increasing food intake is important in maintaining your weight. Maintaining your weight will help you perform your daily activities.

1. Stimulate appetite: Eat small meals five to six times a day.
   - Limit liquids around mealtime to avoid feeling full quickly. Take liquids at least 30 minutes before meals.
   - Eat high-protein foods such as cheeses, milk, yogurt, eggs, beans or meats, nuts, puddings.
   - Help family members plan meals you would like to eat.
   - Eat high-protein, high-carbohydrate snacks between meals.
   - Drink juices or milk shakes between meals.
   - Eat in pleasant surroundings in the company of friends/family.
   - Allow others to prepare foods to your liking.
   - Avoid the area where food is being prepared if aromas bother you.
   - Serve cold foods if odors bother you.
   - Plan light exercise before meals.
   - Try new recipes.
   - Drink a glass of wine or juice before meals.
   - Avoid cigarette smoke or smoking, which can affect your sense of smell, thus changing sense of taste.
2. Feeling of fullness:
   - Avoid high-fat foods.
   - Take liquids 30 minutes before meals.
   - Chew food slowly.
   - Avoid gas-forming foods such as cabbage or broccoli and carbonated liquids such as beer or soda.

3. Safety considerations:
   - Cook all raw protein foods, such as eggs, meats, poultry, fish.
   - Thaw frozen foods in refrigerator or microwave, not at room temperature.
   - Wash all fruits and vegetables.
   - Use only pasteurized dairy products.
   - Wash hands well with soap and water when preparing or serving foods.
   - Use strict cleaning procedures for all utensils and cooking/storage containers.
   - Refrigerate all foods in need of refrigeration after shopping or meal completion.
   - Serve hot foods hot and cold foods cold. Avoid leaving foods at room temperature.
   - Do not use foods beyond expiration dates.

4. Other methods of appetite stimulation may include the use of medications approved as appetite stimulants. The medications are Megace (megesteral acetate), Marinol (drenabinol), Seroshin (recombinant human growth horemone).
   - Megestrol acetate (Megace) is a hormone that has been shown to help increase appetite and weight. Some of the common side effects are high blood pressure, a rise in blood sugar, fluid retention, bloating, constipation, fatigue, gastrointestinal upset, and blood clots.
   - Marinol is an antinausea medication that increases appetite and improve mood. Common side effects include dizziness, confusion, and sleepiness.
   - Serostim is a growth hormone that to increases weight and reverses muscle wasting. It is usually well tolerated, but side effects include headache, fluid retention, nausea, and allergy.

5. Managing side effects:
   - Report any side effects to your doctor or nurse.
   - Ask if your medication needs changing.
   - Keep a log or diary of changes in mood, appetite, or other feelings you experience while on any of these.

6. Evaluation: Management of weight loss or lack of appetite is aimed at increasing food intake. To monitor your success:
   - You may be asked to keep a food diary.
   - Your weight should be recorded regularly.

Follow-up   Notify your nurse and/or physician if any of the following occur:
   - Unable to drink fluids.
   - Feeling dizzy when standing.
   - Unable to take solid food.
   - Change in diet habits.

Phone Numbers

Nurse: _____   Phone: _____

Physician: _____   Phone: _____

Dietitian: _____   Phone: _____

Comments

Patient's Signature: _____   Date: _____

Nurse's Signature: _____   Date: _____

Source: Tait NS: Anorexia-cachexia syndrome, in Yarbro CH, Frogge MH, Goodman M (eds): *Cancer Symptom Managenent* (ed 2). Sudbury: Jones and Bartlett, 1999. © Jones and Bartlett Publishers.

Taste Changes

Patient Name: _____

Symptom and Description   Change in taste can be a change in the sensation of sweet, salty, sour, or bitter. A change in the way foods taste may cause a dislike for foods, which may lead to lack of appetite or weight loss. The taste buds are affected by the cancer or its treatment.

Learning Needs   You will need to learn the possible changes in taste sensation and inform your doctor if a lack of appetite occurs. The following are possible changes in taste you could experience.

- Foods are not sweet enough.
- Foods taste too sweet.
- Foods taste too salty.
- Foods are not salty enough.
- Foods taste spoiled or very bitter.
- Foods taste metallic.

Prevention/Management

- Add small amounts of seasonings to food, such as oregano, basil, cinnamon, ginger.
- Avoid food found to be unpleasant.
- Brush teeth before and after meals to keep mouth clean.
- Use gravies or sauces on foods.
- Marinate meats to enhance or disguise flavor.
- Avoid unpleasant odors.
- Serve cold foods if aromas bother you.
- Use other high-protein foods, such as cheese, milk, eggs, beans, nuts, yogurt, puddings, or wheat germ, in place of meat.
- Avoid cigarette smoke or smoking, which can affect your sense of smell, thus changing sense of taste.

Follow-up   Notify your nurse or doctor if taste changes affect your appetite.

- Ask to talk with a dietician if you experience weight loss or loss of appetite.

Phone Numbers

Nurse: _____   Phone: _____

Physician: _____   Phone: _____

Dietician: _____   Phone: _____

Comments

Patient's Signature: _____   Date: _____

Nurse's Signature: _____   Date: _____

Source: Tait NS: Anorexia-cachexia syndrome, in Yarbro CH, Frogge MH, Goodman M (eds): *Cancer Symptom Management* (ed 2). Sudbury: Jones and Bartlett, 1999. © Jones and Bartlett Publishers.

CHAPTER 13

Dysphagia

Laurel A. Barbour, RN, MSN, AOCN

The Problem of Dysphagia in Cancer

The term *dysphagia* is derived from the Greek *dys* (with difficulty) and *phagia* (eating); it is used to describe difficulty in swallowing. Dysphagia disrupts peoples' lives not only by hindering their ability to take in food and nutrients, but also by inhibiting their ability to dine out and socialize comfortably. Dysphagia can be manifested as a structural or neurologic abnormality in the oral cavity, oropharynx, or esophagus.[1]

Manifestations

Dysphagia occurs during the act of swallowing, which consists of four phases: (1) the oral preparatory phase, (2) the oral phase, (3) the pharyngeal phase, and (4) the esophageal phase.[1] Individuals with dysphagia may complain of difficulty swallowing a solid or liquid during any of the four phases of swallowing. Manifestations of dysphagia include difficulty initiating the swallow, packing of food into the cheeks, the presence of drooling, intermittent coughing, or liquid leaking from the nose after swallowing.[2] Interestingly, persons with dysphagia can usually tell at what phase of swallowing the problem exists.[1]

Knowledge of anatomy, physiology, nutrition, and dysphagia, combined with the many observations and assessments of the dysphagic person, make the oncology nurse a vital member of the treatment team. For successful rehabilitation, the recommended approach is interdisci-plinary collaboration among physicians, speech pathologists, nurses, and dietitians. Figure 13-1 outlines the usual pattern of care for persons with dysphagia.

Incidence and Impact on Quality of Life

Dysphagia, whether temporary or permanent, has a significant impact on the quality of life and functional status of individuals with cancer. Though dysphagia can occur with many types of cancer and treatment, the head and neck cancer population is affected most frequently. Persons with head and neck cancer may experience significant and persistent swallowing disturbances for as long as 5 years posttreatment.[2] Reports indicate that 37% to 46% of individuals in this population are unable to return to a solid diet,[4] and 79% have significant eating problems. In addition, many experience an increase in eating time that interferes with dining in the company of others.[4] Thus, the quality of life for most persons with head and neck cancer changes dramatically. Maximum rehabilitation offers the greatest hope of minimizing the impact on quality of life.

Etiology

Dysphagia resulting from cancer can occur due to a tumor and the effects of cancer treatment: chemotherapy, radiation therapy, or surgery. Difficult and painful swallowing can develop due to radiation therapy to the head and

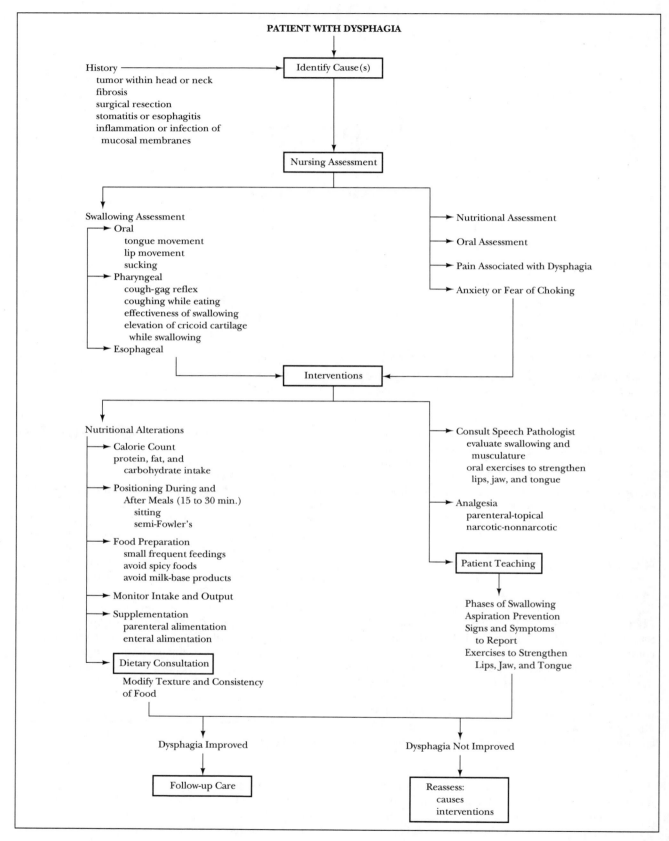

FIGURE 13-1 Dysphagia decision tree. (Source: Donoghue M: Dysphagia, in Baird S (ed): *Decision Making in Oncology Nursing.* Philadelphia: BC Decker, 1988, p. 97.[3]) Reprinted with permission.

neck. Radiation may cause long-term xerostomia, recurrent fungal infections, tissue fibrosis, or inflammation of the mucous membranes. The cytotoxic effects of chemotherapy may cause stomatitis or esophagitis. Also, tumor obstruction (oral, pharyngeal, or esophageal) may cause dysphagia. Chemoradiotherapy combination treatment regimens result in more swallowing difficulties; however, benefits include a decrease in the extent of surgical resection and subsequent impairment.[5]

Dysphagia may result from manipulation or interruption of cranial nerves V, VII, IX, X, XI, or XII, either by cancer or by surgical resection. Table 13-1 describes the function of these cranial nerves in chewing and swallowing and describes the effect of their loss. Dysphagia may also result from temporary weakness and permanent paralysis of the muscles innervated by these cranial nerves.[7]

Pathophysiology

This discussion will be limited to the oral preparatory, oral, and pharyngeal stages of the swallow, which are most affected by dysphagia. These stages are also most responsive to therapy. Esophageal swallowing disorders are not responsive to swallowing interventions.

Swallowing is critical to adequate nutrition. A constant concern for the individual with swallowing difficulties is aspiration, which is the entry of material into the airway below the true vocal cords. Though there are no clear guidelines as to the amount of aspiration that can be tolerated before pneumonia develops, aspiration should always be kept to a minimum. Usually, aspiration of food or fluid is signaled by coughing; however, silent aspiration can occur.[7,8] Silent aspiration is usually diagnosed only after pneumonia develops.

Phases of Swallowing and Dysphagia

Dysphagia may occur during any of the four phases of swallowing: oral preparatory, oral, pharyngeal, or esophageal. Figure 13-2 illustrates the phases of swallowing.

The oral preparatory phase

This phase consists of repeated coordinated movements of the mandible, tongue, and teeth. The amount of time needed to form a food or liquid bolus varies with each individual. Liquids require minimal oral preparation, whereas meats and vegetables need considerable chewing and lubricating before swallowing. Poor dentition will also lengthen the time of the oral preparatory stage. Mastication involves a rotating lateral movement of the tongue and mandible. The bolus is positioned in the middle or back of the mouth, with the posterior tongue elevating against and dropping from the hard palate. Once the swallow begins, the anterior tongue elevates first, then the body of the tongue elevates, pushing the bolus posteriorly. This entire sequence can take 1 second, and any residue should be cleared by tongue sweeps and repeated swallowing.

The individual who has undergone a partial or total glossectomy will experience difficulty transporting and controlling a bolus of food or liquid to the oropharynx. The number of oral structures resected will directly influence the extent of swallowing impairment. Specifically affected are the mastication process, bolus control, and the anteroposterior propulsion processes. Generally, if tongue resection is less than 50%, the oral preparatory phase will be functional. If more than 50% of the tongue is resected, lingual peristalsis and control of the food are severely reduced.[9] Reconstruction of the mandibular region may cause scarring, muscle contracture, and temporomandibular joint pain, which interfere with mastication.[10]

TABLE 13-1 Cranial Nerve Function and Loss as Related to Chewing and Swallowing

Cranial Nerve	Function	Loss
V: Trigeminal	Controls muscles of mastication; provides sensation to face, teeth, gums, and tongue	Sensation loss; inability to move mandible
VII: Facial	Provides sense of taste; controls the muscles of the face	Increased salivation; pouching of food in cheeks
IX: Glossopharyngeal	Transmits sensations to the tongue, pharynx, and soft palate; influences sense of taste, production of saliva, and swallowing	Decreased taste and salivation; diminishes or inhibits the gag reflex
X: Vagus	Sensation (touch, pressure, and pain) in pharynx and ability to swallow	Loss of sensation in pharynx and gag reflex
XI: Spinal accessory	Controls vocal cords and head/shoulder movement	Paralysis of vocal cord and loss of shoulder shrug
XII: Hypoglossal	Controls the extrinsic and intrinsic muscles of the tongue	Difficulty positioning food for chewing, resulting in pouching, choking, drooling

Data from Gabe-Skabowski M, Archini S, Bedinger K, et al: The home care team approach to dysphagia. *Caring* 9:66–69, 1990.[6]

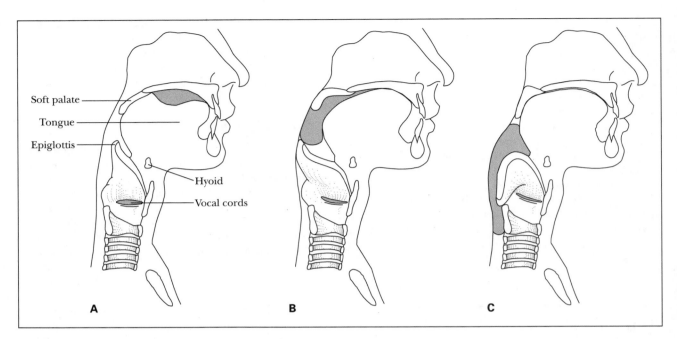

Soft palate

Tongue

Epiglottis

Hyoid

Vocal cords

A   B   C

FIGURE 13-2   Phases of swallowing: Views from three of the four phases of swallowing of food bolus: oral (A), pharyngeal (B), and esophageal (C). (Artist: Camille Rea.)

The oral phase

The oral phase of the swallow is initiated when the tongue begins posterior movement of the bolus. During this phase, the tongue squeezes the bolus posteriorly against the hard palate. When the bolus passes the anterior faucial arches, the oral phase is concluded, and the swallowing reflex is triggered.

The pharyngeal phase

The pharyngeal phase begins with the swallowing reflex. This complex process involves closure of the velopharyngeal port. The purpose of closure is to prevent reflux of food into the nose and to transport the bolus backward over the posterior tongue and into the pharynx. These structures are innervated by cranial nerves IX, X, and XI. The brain stem acts as a neuronal pool to organize impulses to perform the swallow reflex. Individuals cannot swallow unless something is in their mouth: be it food, liquid, or saliva.[1]

Surgery of the oropharynx that results in loss of the soft palate and tonsillar pillars usually involves reconstructive flaps. These flaps interfere with food bolus transport because of sensory loss. The tissue flaps also lack the normal propulsive action usually provided by the pharyngeal constrictor musculature. Individuals may experience nasal regurgitation, decreased bolus transit, aspiration, and dysfunction of the pharyngoesophageal segment.[11]

The esophageal phase

The esophageal phase of swallowing comprises the point from when the bolus enters the esophagus at the cricopharyngeal juncture until it passes into the stomach at the gastroesophageal juncture. The peristaltic wave begins in the pharynx when the swallowing reflex is triggered and continues in a sequential fashion through the esophagus.

Effects of Specific Surgical Procedures on Swallowing

Surgical procedures of the head and neck area can result in significant alterations of structure and function. Each procedure results in a specific set of rehabilitation needs.

Oral and oropharyngeal cancers

The two most important pieces of information needed for swallowing therapy are the exact structures removed and the reconstruction techniques used. An intraoral prosthesis may be used in palatal resections.

Supraglottic laryngectomy

Following supraglottic laryngectomy, swallowing rehabilitation will be necessary. The surgery involves the removal of the sphincters that provide airway protection (the epiglottis and aryepiglottic folds) and the false vocal cords. The true vocal cords are the only remaining protective mechanism (Figures 13-3A and 13-3B for anatomy of the larynx). If surgery extends into the base of the tongue, food tends to fall onto the closed true vocal cords. Aspiration is likely if closure of the larynx at the level of the true vocal cords is not strong.[1]

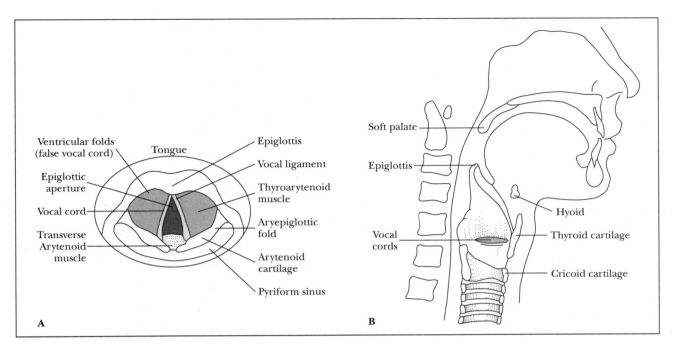

FIGURE 13-3   View of normal larynx as seen through fiberoptic laryngoscope (A). Normal larynx anatomy: the true vocal cords protect the airway (B). (Artist: Camille Rea.)

Hemilaryngectomy

Hemilaryngectomy is a vertical laryngectomy that removes half of the larynx. Most hemilaryngectomy patients will swallow well, provided they assume a flexed head posture. If arytenoid cartilage is removed, normal swallowing without aspiration is unlikely.[8]

Individuals will remain asymptomatic for a long period of time, then develop pulmonary complications (i.e., minimal basilar pneumonia, fibrosis, aspiration pneumonia, and lung abscess).[10]

Laryngectomy

Aspiration of food is not a problem with total laryngectomy because of the physical separation of the respiratory and GI tracts. However, some swallowing complications may occur. The most common cause of problems is the development of a band of scar tissue at the base of the tongue, necessitating ingestion of a liquid diet. Treatment for this is typically resection of the scar tissue. Fortunately, most persons who have a total laryngectomy can tolerate both liquid and solid food.[2]

Tracheotomy

The presence of a tracheotomy tube can contribute to difficulty in swallowing and increase the incidence of dysphagia. The tracheotomy tube impedes laryngeal elevation and results in poor clearance of the larynx. Management of the tracheotomy cuff may vary with clinician preferences. Some clinicians keep the cuff inflated, while others prefer it deflated so they can

evaluate the amount of aspiration. In general, advantages of any tracheotomy tube outweigh any disadvantages, because aspiration of food is readily visible and easily detectable.[7]

Assessment

Risk Factors

The following factors will predispose one to dysphagia:

- tumor invasion or obstruction
- radiation fibrosis
- recurrent fungal infection of the pharynx
- surgical resection
- neuropathy secondary to therapy
- stomatitis
- esophagitis

Aspiration is a significant indicator that a person is experiencing dysphagia. Additionally, the following may indicate risk of aspiration:[12]

- intermittent or frequent choking
- difficulty swallowing
- fever
- abnormal lung sounds
- oral changes

History and Physical Examination

A complete history and physical examination will provide information about the individual's respiratory status, history of tracheotomy tube placement, current symptoms, and proposed or accomplished cancer treatment. Nutritional status may be determined according to the standard methods. Information about the swallowing disorder is obtained, including the person's description of the problem.

Assessment of the oral cavity includes the lips, tongue, and jaw. Evaluation of the range of motion of these structures includes checking for lateralization, protrusion, and elevation of the tongue; observing the lips for protrusion, retraction, and closure; and determining the ability of the jaw to close and to produce rotary movement.[1] Strength and symmetry of the jaw and facial muscles may be evaluated by palpating the lower facial area while the individual clenches the jaw. To evaluate cranial nerves V, VII, IX, X, XI, and XII, ask the person to frown, smile, blow a whistle, pucker, raise eyebrows, wrinkle the forehead, tightly close the eyes, and attempt to resist opening the eyes.[6]

Determine the level of alertness and discuss any fear or anxiety the individual may have about choking. If a prosthetic device is present, evaluate the fit. Inspect the dentition and secretions in the oral cavity. Oral sensations may be tested by evaluating temperature, ability to feel, or presence of taste. Observe the individual during eating for choking, drooling, regurgitation of fluid in the nose, and retention of food in the oral cavity; note foods that are not well tolerated.[9]

Specialized Assessments

The cough reflex, whether voluntary or involuntary, prevents food and fluid from entering the upper respiratory tract. To initiate an involuntary cough reflex, a substance would have to enter the airway and touch the vocal cords, thus triggering forceful expulsion of the substance. It is safer to elicit a voluntary cough for clinical assessment. Ask the person to cough at least twice in rapid succession. As this is done, estimate the person's ability to protect the airway by evaluating the amount of coughing and choking. An intact voluntary cough reflex will be strong and brisk, but this does not imply a strong involuntary cough reflex. Presence of the gag reflex may also be evaluated by tickling the back of the throat with a wet cotton swab.[10]

If the nursing assessment has identified a real or potential swallowing dysfunction, the speech/swallowing pathologist is consulted to collaborate with the medical rehabilitation team and further assess the degree of dysphagia.

Radiologic Assessment

Further assessment of the impact of dysphagia on swallowing can be performed through radiologic studies.

The radiographic swallowing evaluation called *videofluoroscopy* visualizes the timing of the swallowing phases and extent of aspiration in the form of a videoesophagram. Initially, oral pharyngeal, laryngeal, and upper esophagus tissues and structures are viewed. The videofluoroscope enables visualization while the person ingests various food consistencies in a barium or barium food form. Additional observations made during the study evaluate feeding posture and technique. If a tracheotomy tube is in place during the videofluoroscopy, occlusion of the tracheotomy will allow for more normal swallowing pressure.[1]

Nutritional Assessment

Persons with dysphagia are at a great risk of nutritional debilitation. A comprehensive nutritional assessment will provide necessary baseline measures. Observe for physical signs of malnutrition. Evaluate laboratory and physical indicators. Assess the individual's knowledge of nutrition, calorie intake, and protein, carbohydrate, and fat intakes. Initially, ask the patient to record nutritional/fluid intake for 24 hours, including a calorie count and fluid intake. In addition to typical nutritional assessments, determine on a weekly or monthly basis anthropometric measurements and laboratory values (albumin, total protein, total iron-binding capacity, serum transferrin, electrolytes, glucose, lymphocyte count).

Explore the resources available to the patient, such as financial means, stores in area, food preparation facilities, and community supports. For more information on nutritional assessment and management, see Chapter 12, Anorexia-Cachexia Syndrome.

Pain Assessment

Pain in swallowing (*odynophagia*) is commonly related to infection, inflammation, or tumor infiltration in the oropharyngeal region.[10] Qualitative and quantitative pain assessments are performed by the nurse using appropriate tools. Odynophagia may occur in combination with stomatitis and xerostomia as a result of radiation therapy or chemotherapy. Initially, there will be pain eating solid foods, with eventual regression to liquids.

Symptom Management

Prevention

Prevention of dysphagia for the cancer patient is difficult, because dysphagia usually results from standard treatment efforts to control or eliminate the cancer. However, pretreatment counseling is essential to prepare the person physically and psychologically for anticipated swallowing difficulty. Soliciting the cooperation of the individual and significant other in the rehabilitation process may result in a more satisfactory and realistic outcome. Furthermore, anticipation of potential nutritional deficits with dysphagia will facilitate the early implementation of supplemental or alternative feeding methods.

Therapeutic Approaches

Early measures

Pain management Treatment of painful oral lesions, xerostomia, and candidiasis will improve swallowing. Management of early painful lesions may be achieved by topical anesthetic, systemic nonnarcotic analgesic, or nonsteroidal antiinflammatory agents. Artificial saliva and systemic pilocarpine may decrease the pain of swallowing by increasing oral lubrication.

Swallowing therapy After the assessment of oral functioning and a videofluoroscopic examination, swallowing therapy can begin for those persons diagnosed with dysphagia. Adequate movement of oral structures is essential, especially for persons who have undergone surgical rehabilitation. Treatment measures include exercises designed to strengthen musculature, increase range of motion, and develop compensatory strategies.[10]

Direct swallowing exercises Oromotor exercises are required to improve muscle control for swallowing. Exercises can begin simultaneously with radiation treatment or begin 10 to 14 days postoperatively when wound healing is complete. Areas to exercise include the lips, tongue, jaw, and palate.[13]

Incomplete lip closure and decreased labial strength will improve with oromotor exercises. To reduce the deficit and improve muscle tone, stretch the lips widely during production of the sound *ee* and pucker the lips as if kissing. Each of these movements should be performed fifteen times for 1 second each, five times per day, until improvement is identified.

Range-of-motion exercises for the tongue are designed to increase lateralization and elevation in an attempt to improve oral transit time. (See Appendix 13A for a teaching guide and flow sheet on how to perform the exercises and a method for recording performance.) With the mouth opened as wide as possible, the individual elevates the tongue tip, elevates the posterior tongue, moves the tongue laterally, and extends the tongue out of the mouth. In each position, the individual's tongue is moved as far as possible and the position held for 1 second in each position, then released.[2]

Coordination of tongue movements may be improved through manipulation of objects, such as a licorice whip tied to a string and placed in the mouth. The licorice is grasped between the tongue and palate, then moved side to side and front to back. When the person masters this technique, the motion is replaced with a circular movement from the middle of the mouth to the teeth and back again, as if chewing. With progress, the licorice can be replaced with a piece of O-shaped candy tied to a string and later with a cloth soaked in juice. In each case, the nurse holds one end of the string to prevent choking.[13]

Once the ability to manipulate material in the mouth has been established, the focus of exercises shifts to holding and moving a bolus. A ¼-teaspoon paste-consistency bolus is placed in the mouth and moved with the tongue. The amount of bolus allowed to fall into the buccal gutters is minimal. When the exercise is complete, the bolus should be expectorated. As progress in manipulating the bolus is identified, the size and consistency of the bolus should vary.

Practicing backward propulsion of the bolus may be accomplished by instructing the individual to squeeze juice from a long, thin cloth placed in the mouth. Anterior to posterior glossal-palatal contact should occur. The amount of juice in the cloth is varied according to the individual's ability to swallow. These exercises are designed to increase the strength and range of motion of the structures of the oral and pharyngeal cavities. Well-sequenced movement of these structures is crucial to swallowing. The individual in swallowing therapy requires frequent and consistent reinforcement of these strategies to accomplish swallowing.[13] Rehabilitation professionals provide support and encouragement to minimize frustration, fear, and isolation.

Anticipatory/compensatory strategies Preventive strategies provide the individual with alternative techniques in addition to those previously mentioned in order to reduce the chance of aspiration and increase the efficiency of the swallow. The two main compensatory strategies are postural changes and food consistency modifications. The following postural changes are recommended to improve the safety and efficiency of the swallow:[14]

1. Tilt the chin backward to facilitate oral movement or decrease oral transmit time.

2. Tilt the head forward to widen the vallecular space in the larynx and reduce the chance of aspiration in an individual with a delayed pharyngeal swallow. This posture assists the epiglottis in protecting the airway during the swallow.

3. Turn the head to the weaker side of the pharynx in order to close the weaker side and use the stronger pharyngeal wall. This position improves vocal-cord adduction, making it useful for individuals with unilateral vocal-cord paralysis.

4. Tilt the head toward the stronger side of the oral cavity and pharynx to allow gravity to keep food on the stronger side of the oral cavity and pharynx during

swallowing. This helps persons with posterior oral cavity resections.

5. Tilt the head downward while putting food in the mouth, then tip the head backward when swallowing; hold breath during the swallow to protect the airway.

Because eating is also considered a social activity, efforts are made to make eating pleasant and leisurely, with attractively prepared and good-smelling food. Preferably, the individual is out of bed, with oral care performed before eating. To be conducive to eating, the environment should have limited distractions and environmental noise. Additionally, you will want to talk with the individual if you are present during eating; but do not ask the person to speak until a few seconds after swallowing. This decreases the risk of aspiration.

Determine the best feeding position to promote swallowing. If the potential or fear of aspiration exists, have suction equipment readily available. Begin feeding with ¼ to ½ teaspoon of a thickened liquid. Avoid thin liquids, such as water and juice, because they are difficult to control during the swallow. Observe for up/down laryngeal movement following each ¼ teaspoon of food.[2]

Following the swallows, ask the individual to speak. If the voice is wet and gurgles, request a cough to clear the oropharynx. Inspect the oral cavity for residual food or saliva. If there is difficulty propelling food to the posterior tongue, it may help to use a long-handled spoon or syringe to place food on the posterior of the tongue. The finger-sweep maneuver may be used to clear food that was not swallowed. A reminder to swallow twice will complete clearance of the pharyngeal tract. In addition, using an oral suction catheter to remove accumulated oral/pharyngeal fluids is often helpful. Halt feeding if difficulties arise, such as coughing, choking, or extreme fatigue. Maintain the patient in an upright position for 30 minutes after eating to minimize regurgitation that could result in aspiration.[6]

Frequently, dysphagia may be controlled and oral feeding attempted if the head is in the recommended position or a diet of a particular consistency is used. It is often necessary to alter food consistency to decrease the chance of aspiration. Table 13-2 describes the range of food consistencies and representative foods.[15] (See Appendix 13B for a patient education tool on suggested food modifications.) Simultaneously, swallowing therapy may be used to strengthen musculature or to learn a new swallowing technique.

The time needed to swallow a single bolus of a particular consistency of food appears to be an important parameter in nutritional management. If the videoesophagram indicates that more than 10 seconds are required for swallowing all consistencies of food, the individual may require a tube feeding, either nasogastric or gastrostomy.[2]

Persons with a tracheotomy tube who require mechanical ventilation may still eat. The inflated tube cuff will prevent aspiration but may also make swallowing more difficult. The individual with a tracheotomy tube not on a ventilator may require the cuff to be inflated during feeding to prevent aspiration. When eating is complete, the mouth and throat secretions should be suctioned before deflating the cuff. Stop the feeding if food appears in or around the tracheotomy tube.[8]

Late or advanced dysphagia measures

Advanced symptomatology management Weekly oropharyngeal assessment is indicated to identify the development of fungal infections that may impede the swallowing process. For individuals experiencing severe pain while swallowing, progression to narcotic analgesics will be indicated.

Individuals who experience continued drooling may benefit from continued attempts to close the lips and change the head position to encourage posterior movement of saliva. Interventions may include atropine to decrease secretions, and holding gauze in the mouth to absorb secretions.

Individuals who experience an obstruction at the esophageal level will have increased secretions. Usually, constant expectoration is required to manage this symptom. A container to collect secretions will be needed at all times.

Odor from the oral cavity may be managed by frequent oral care, approximately four to six times a day, especially following meals. A suggested oral care guideline follows.

- Dentulous
    Brush teeth with soft brush, fluoridated toothpaste
    Brush tongue
    Floss with dental floss (avoid injuring gums)
- Edentulous
    Cleanse mouth with gauze and a very soft brush
    Massage gums
    Clean dentures with denture cleaner/baking soda
        and water
- Rinse mouth several times per day with baking soda flavored with peppermint

Psychological support should be ongoing by all professionals involved in the dysphagic individual's care. Often, the interventions described are not satisfactory for the frustrating symptoms experienced.

Alternative feeding methods For a person with cancer, the goal of nutritional support is to achieve and maintain desirable weight and to prevent or correct nutritional deficiencies.[16] Nonoral feeding is recommended if the individual has demonstrated consistent aspiration or severe pain with swallowing. If either swallowing exercise or oral gratification is still desired, nonoral supplementation is recommended if it is determined that oral intake is calorically insufficient.[17]

In some cases, nonoral feeding is initiated prior to medical intervention that will likely disrupt swallowing

TABLE 13-2 Food Consistencies

Consistency	Examples
Semisolid, traditionally prepared foods that are cohesive	Baked egg dishes (e.g., soufflés, quiches, custards) Salads with mayonnaise or other binding agents (e.g., egg, tuna, macaroni, or meat salad) Cheese that is soft (cream cheese) or melted Pasta or rice casseroles with thick binders (eggs) Aspic, pudding, cheesecake, mousse, and gelatin Thick hot cereals
Soft foods that tend to fall apart or separate and may be difficult to control	Whole-grain breads Foods that separate into liquid and pulp (e.g., thin puréed fruits and vegetables) Dry cottage cheese Plain rice, ground meats Thin hot cereals Foods of two or more consistencies (e.g., canned fruits in juice or syrup, soups with whole vegetables, pasta, or grains)
Dense foods that are sticky and bulky	Moist white bread Peanut butter Plain mashed potatoes Bananas Refried beans
Thin liquids	Apple, cranberry, citrus, and grape juices Broth and thin cream soups Coffee, tea, and hot chocolate Frozen pops, fruit ices* Water, soda, and alcohol Most 1.0 kcal/mL oral supplements
Thin to medium liquids	Vegetable juice; fruit nectars
Thick liquids	Blenderized or cream soups Eggnog, buttermilk Ice cream, sherbet* Milk shakes, malts, and yogurt shakes* Most 1.5–2.0 kcal/mL oral supplements
Spoon-thick liquids	Yogurt drink (kefir) Gelatin

* Unstable liquids (e.g., milk shakes, ice cream, sherbets, ice slushes, and frozen pops) separate into a combination of thin liquid and food mass or melt completely when allowed to stand at room temperature or when placed in the mouth. For a patient with delayed swallow, these foods should be stabilized with thickening agents.

© 1995, The American Dietetic Association. *Manual of Clinical Dietetics.* 5th ed. Used by permission.[15]

abilities. Intermittent nonoral feeding may be required following chemotherapy administration or during radiation therapy.[13]

The options for enteral access are transnasal intubation, percutaneous endoscopic gastronomy or jejunostomy, and surgical gastrostomy or jejunostomy. The enteral access route is adapted to individual needs.

Selection of nutritional products involves consideration of characteristics such as osmolality, viscosity, nutrient adequacy, cost, and convenience. Once enteral feeding is chosen, the method of formula administration is considered. The bolus feeding method involves the rapid administration by gravity or pump infusion of 250–500 mL of solution several times per day, for approximately 30 minutes each time. Individuals at home may be able to tolerate cyclic nighttime feeding over an 8- to 10-hour period. The feeding delivery technique and nutritional product selected for an individual determines the guidelines for initiation of enteral therapy.[12] (For specific guidelines on self-administration of tube feedings, refer to Appendix 13C.)

Evaluation of Therapeutic Approaches

The information outlined in this chapter provides those interventions we believe will improve the quality of life for the individual with dysphagia. This text does not convey the constant, almost hourly, assessment and evaluation performed by the individual experiencing dysphagia and his or her caregivers, family, or other professionals.

The symptom of dysphagia usually does not follow a progressive desirable outcome. The multimodal therapy approach used for cancer treatment will cause the severity of dysphagia to wax and wane over the course of treatment and prolonged rehabilitation intervals. The assessment flowsheet (Figure 13-4) will help nurses plot the dysphagic individual's status; however, narrative documentation may be necessary. Items to be noted in the nursing assessment include weight, caloric intake, methods of feeding, supplements, and emotional response to swallowing status.

Conclusion

The oncology nurse, as a member of a multidisciplinary team, evaluates and treats individuals who exhibit oral and pharyngeal dysphagia. The nurse can use knowledge of normal swallowing to characterize and assess the dysphagia. Furthermore, identifying food consistencies, posi-

---

NUTRITION ASSESSMENT

Patient Name _____

Date _____   Weight _____

Albumin _____   Protein _____

Symptoms (describe degree)

    Pain _____

    Cough _____

    Choking _____

Nasal regurgitation _____

    Other _____

    Other _____

Nutrition

    Soft diet _____

Supplement PO _____

Tube feeding _____

    Other _____

Food Intake

    Adequate _____

    Good _____

    Poor _____

    Other _____

Swallowing Therapy: Yes _____   No _____

Comments:

FIGURE 13-4   Nutrition/dysphagia assessment.

tions, and procedures that facilitate safe eating will minimize the risk of aspiration. The nurse, physician, dietitian, and speech pathologist together design a highly individualized treatment plan and approach to follow-up and re-evaluation. This approach ensures the best management for the individual who has swallowing problems.

References

1. Perlman A: Videofluoroscopic predictors of aspiration in patients with oropharyngeal dysphagia. *Dysphagia* 9:90–95, 1994

2. Logemann J, Bytell DE: Swallowing disorders in three types of head and neck surgical patients. *Cancer* 44:1095–1105, 1979

3. Donoghue M: Dysphagia, in Baird S (ed): *Decision Making in Oncology Nursing.* Philadelphia: BC Decker, 1988, pp. 96–97

4. Lansky S, List M, Ritter-Sterr C: Quality of life in head and neck cancer survivors. *Proc Am Soc Clin Oncol* 8:A656, 1989 (abstract)

5. Price M, DiIorio C: Swallowing: A practice guide. *Am J Nurs* 90(7):42–44, 1990

6. Gabe-Skabowski M, Archini S, Bedinger K, et al: The home care team approach to dysphagia. *Caring* 9:66–69, 1990

7. LaBlanc GR, Kraus K, Steckol K: Rehabilitation of swallowing and communication following glossectomy. *Rehabil Nurs* 16:266–270, 1991

8. Logemann J: Aspiration in head and neck surgical patients. *Ann Otol Rhinol Laryngol* 94:373–376, 1985

9. DiIorio C, Price M: Swallowing: An assessment guide. *Am J Nurs* 90(7):38–41, 1990

10. Groher M: *Dysphagia* (ed 3). Stoneham, MA: Butterworth-Heinemann, 1997

11. Gelfand DW: *Dysphagia Diagnosis and Treatment.* New York: Igka-Shoin, 1989

12. Cole-Arvin C, Notich L, Underhill A: Identifying and managing dysphagia. *Nurs* 24:48–49, 1994

13. Logemann J: Swallowing and communication rehabilitation. *Semin Oncol Nurs* 5:205–212, 1989

14. Meehan M: Nursing diagnosis: Potential for aspiration. *RN* 55:30–34, 1992

15. Chicago Dietetic Association and South Suburban Dietetic Association: *Manual of Clinical Dietetics.* Chicago: American Dietetic Association, 1993

16. Grady R, Farnen J, Asheman P: Nutrition alteration in less than body requirements related to dysphagia, in McNally JC, Somerville ET, Miaskowski C, et al (eds): *Guidelines for Cancer Nursing Practice* (ed 2). Philadelphia: Saunders, 1991, pp. 179–184

17. Urade M, Igarashi T, Sugi M, et al: Functional recovery of swallowing, speech, and taste in an oral cancer patient with subtotal glossectomy. *J Oral Maxillofac Surg* 45:282–285, 1987

Difficulty Swallowing:
Exercises for the Tongue

Patient Name: _____

Symptom and Description   Your surgery or treatment may make it difficult for you to swallow or to control food in your mouth. These exercises will improve your ability to move your tongue well. Your tongue is important for eating, speaking, and swallowing.

Learning Needs   You will learn exercises to make your tongue stronger. You also need to know when to call your doctor or nurse.

Prevention   It is not likely you can prevent this problem from occurring, but these techniques can make it easier for you to swallow:

- Do these exercises five to ten times a day.
- Keep a record of the exercises.
- Note any changes you feel while eating or swallowing.
- Call your doctor or nurse if it becomes more difficult to swallow or eat.

Management/Procedure

1. General exercises: Do these five to ten times a day.
   - Open mouth as wide as possible.
   - Lift tongue as high as possible; hold 1 second; repeat five times.
   - Lift back of tongue as far as possible; hold 1 second; repeat five times.
2. Tongue exercises (Figure 13A-1). Do these five to ten times a day.
   - Push tongue forward against a tongue blade or your fingers; hold for 1 second.
   - Then push tongue to one side and forward again.
   - Then push tongue to the other side and forward again; hold for 1 second.
   - Repeat these exercises five times.
3. Measure progress.
   - Keep a chart of exercises done and the response (such as more movement and strength).
   - These exercises will become easier to perform.
   - It will become easier to move foods in your mouth.
   - Share this information with your nurse and swallowing therapist.
   - Talk with your nurse and swallowing therapist if you believe that the exercises are not helping your tongue strength.

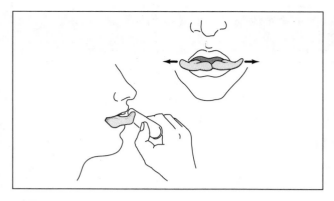

FIGURE 13A-1 Tongue exercises. (Artist: Camille Rea.)

Log of Tongue Exercises

Patient Name: _____

Date	Times Done	Response (How is tongue working)

Phone Numbers

Nurse: _____ Phone: _____

Physician: _____ Phone: _____

Other: _____ Phone: _____

Comments

Patient's Signature: _____ Date: _____

Nurse's Signature: _____ Date: _____

Source: Barbour LA: Dysphagia, in Yarbro CH, Frogge MH, Goodman M (eds): *Cancer Symptom Management* (ed 2). Sudbury: Jones and Bartlett, 1999. © Jones and Bartlett Publishers.

Food Suggestions for the Person with Difficulty Swallowing

Patient Name: _____

Symptom and Description   Your surgery or treatments may make it difficult for you to swallow. Certain foods are easier to swallow. It is important to eat enough calories and have a balanced diet.

Learning Needs   You will learn to change your food choices to keep a balanced diet with enough calories. You will learn when to call your doctor or nurse for more advice.

Management

- *Eat small meals or snacks.* It is sometimes easier to eat a small amount of food at one time. Remember to eat many times a day to get enough calories.
- *Add calories to your food.* Gravies, sauces, and protein shakes can add calories. Sauces and gravies can also make the food easier to swallow.
- *Choose high-protein foods.* These include cheese, poultry, meat, fish, and beans. You may need to cut, blend, or shred the food to make it easier to swallow. Gravies and sauces may help.
- *Try milkshakes or puddings.* These are easy to swallow. The cool, smooth texture can be soothing.
- *Try cold foods or bland foods.* Cold or cool foods are soothing. Spicy foods may need to be avoided.
- *Freeze nutritional shakes.* The texture and taste of this is like ice cream, but it is more nutritious.

Follow-up   Call your doctor or nurse if you have:

- more difficulty swallowing
- a feeling of choking
- coughing while swallowing or drinking
- a decrease in your weight

Phone Numbers

Nurse: _____ Phone: _____

Physician: _____ Phone: _____

Other: _____ Phone: _____

Comments

Patient's Signature: _____ Date: _____

Nurse's Signature: _____ Date: _____

Source: Barbour LA: Dysphagia, in Yarbro CH, Frogge MH, Goodman M (eds): *Cancer Symptom Management* (ed 2). Sudbury: Jones and Bartlett, 1999. © Jones and Bartlett Publishers.

(continued)

Tube Feeding

Patient Name: _____

Symptom and Description   Tube feedings are given if you have difficulty swallowing. The difficulty swallowing is usually caused by your cancer treatment. The tube feeding is needed to prevent weight loss and to provide calories and nutrition.

Learning Needs   You will learn to feed yourself with the tube. You will also learn to care for and clean the tube. You need to know when to call your doctor or nurse.

Management   A feeding tube will be inserted into your nose or stomach to deliver liquid food, water, and medication. (Figures 13C-1 and 13C-2).

To get ready to feed yourself:

1. Follow the doctor's order for the type, amount, and time of feeding.
2. Wash hands to prevent infection.
3. Gather the supplies. Formula may be given by syringe or feeding bag:
   - Feeding bag or large (60-cc) syringe
   - Small (10-cc) syringe
   - Two ounces of water
   - Tube feeding formula (type and amount): _____

     _____

   - Disposable gloves, if desired
   - Optional: a feeding pump (a pump can control flow of liquid)

To begin feeding:

1. Sit upright (45- to 90-degree angle).
2. Remove clamp, and pinch tubing at the end away from nose or abdomen. This prevents leakage.
3. Using the small (10-cc) syringe, push 10 cc of air into the tube. If no choking, coughing, or pain occurs, please proceed. If choking, coughing, or pain occurs, stop now and clamp the tube. Call your doctor or nurse for advice.
4. For syringe feeding:
   - Attach syringe to end of tube. Raise syringe 18 inches above head (if tube is through nose) or 18 inches above stomach (if tube is through stomach).
   - Fill large syringe with 2 ounces of water and run through tubing.
   - Fill syringe with formula; allow flow to empty gradually. Slower feeding will prevent cramping and diarrhea.

- Refill syringe and feed until proper amount of feeding formula has been given.

5. For feeding bag:
   - Fill bag with 2 ounces of water and run through tubing.
   - Fill bag with the feeding formula amount prescribed.
   - Let formula flow through bag tubing to remove air from tube.
   - Then clamp the tube of the feeding bag.
   - Connect feeding bag to feeding tube.
   - Raise bag 18 inches above head or abdomen to start flow of formula.
   - Change the rate of feeding flow by loosening or tightening the clamp.
   - Feeding will flow in within _____ hours. Slower feeding will prevent cramping.

6. At end of feeding, clear the tube by running 2 ounces of water through the tube.

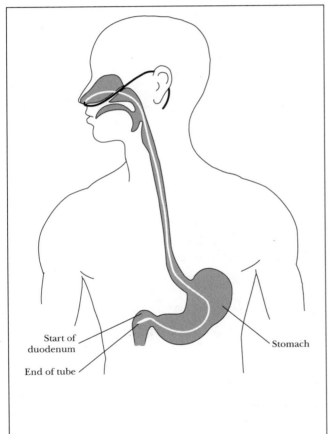

FIGURE 13C-1   Nasal feeding tube is placed through nose into stomach. (Artist: Camille Rea.)

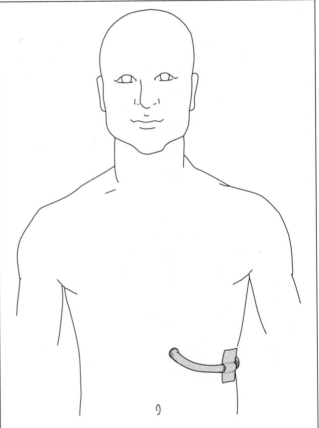

FIGURE 13C-2   Gastrostomy feeding tube is placed through skin into stomach. (Artist: Camille Rea.)

To give medicine:

1. Use the large (60-cc) syringe. Remove the plunger from the syringe. Connect syringe to tube.

2. Clear the tube by first pushing 2 ounces of water into the tube.

3. Then pour liquid medication into the syringe.

4. If tablets are to be given:

   - Crush the tablet with the back of a spoon.

   - Put crushed tablet into 1 ounce of water.

   - Pour water and tablet into syringe.

5. Push syringe plunger to advance medication into feeding tube.

6. Keep rinsing medication from cup with water until all medicine is given.

7. Finally, rinse tube by giving 2 ounces of water.

8. Clamp feeding tube and disconnect syringe.

9. Call nurse if tube is clogged.

10. Record how much feeding is given and how much water is taken.

Call medical personnel if any of the following occur:

1. Coughing or choking

2. Feeding coming from tracheotomy (if present), mouth, or nose

3. Nausea, vomiting, diarrhea, or stomach cramps

4. Continued weight loss

5. Tube becomes clogged

Evaluation:

- To be sure that the tube feeding procedure is correct, you and/or a family member will be asked to perform the tube feeding procedure for your nurse.

Follow-up

- Keep a daily record of your weight.

- Record the amount of feeding taken each time.

- Bring the record of your feedings and your weights to your next appointment.

- The physician, nurse, and dietitian may be able to see where more help is needed.

- Call your doctor or nurse if you experience any of the following: diarrhea, constipation, continued weight loss, or indigestion.

- If you are unsure of any of the instructions, be sure to ask for help.

- Be sure you understand what to expect, what to do about it, and when to call your doctor or nurse.

- Have emergency phone numbers available.

Log of Tube Feedings

Patient Name: _____

Date	Weight	Bowel Movement	Amount of Water	Amount of Feeding	Comments

Phone Numbers

Nurse: _____ Phone: _____

Physician: _____ Phone: _____

Other: _____ Phone: _____

Comments

Patient's Signature: _____ Date: _____

Nurse's Signature: _____ Date: _____

Source: Barbour LA: Dysphagia, in Yarbro CH, Frogge MH, Goodman M (eds): *Cancer Symptom Management* (ed 2). Sudbury: Jones and Bartlett, 1999. © Jones and Bartlett Publishers.

CHAPTER 14

Nausea and Vomiting

Rita Wickham, RN, PhD, AOCN

The Problem of Nausea and Vomiting in Cancer

Incidence in Cancer

Nausea and vomiting (N&V) are major problems during cancer, with as many as 50% of patients experiencing N&V secondary to cancer treatment (despite antiemetics), and more than 50% having N&V related to progressive disease or other therapies.[1–4] Nausea alone probably occurs more frequently, but because it is a subjective symptom, it is often underappreciated and thus underassessed.

Impact on Quality of Life

Among patients, the same level of nausea and vomiting may vary in the degree to which it affects quality of life (QOL). For instance, nausea or vomiting can result in negative emotional responses or altered roles, leading to major disruptions for one person but having little effect on another.[5] Negative QOL effects are greatest when N&V are severe or long-lasting, or when these symptoms interfere with important activities of daily living, enhance other toxicities of treatment (e.g., increased nephrotoxicity with cisplatin; bladder toxicity with cyclophosphamide because of poor oral intake of fluids secondary to vomiting), and when associated with terminal disease.

Research has confirmed that chemotherapy-related N&V negatively affect QOL.[6–8] For instance, Lindley et al.[9] found that nausea, as well as vomiting after chemotherapy, affected activities and enjoyment of daily living, including maintaining leisure activities, doing usual household tasks, eating and drinking, spending time with family and friends, and maintaining other daily activities. It is difficult to substantiate the degree of this effect, but it has been shown that despite the use of serotonin-antagonist antiemetics, patients still rank nausea as their most bothersome chemotherapy side effect, while vomiting is ranked as third to fifth most bothersome.[10,11]

Etiology

The causes of nausea and vomiting in persons with cancer can be broadly differentiated as being therapy related (chemotherapy and radiation therapy) or related to disease or other factors (visceral, chemical, drug, CNS, vestibular, and other). An individual may endure one or multiple causes for their N&V.

Chemotherapy-Induced Nausea and Vomiting

Postchemotherapy N&V have been characterized as acute, delayed, persistent, and anticipatory, but there are no standard definitions for these categories. The first 24 hours after chemotherapy administration is generally considered to be the period of acute N&V, and this arbitrary definition assumes that N&V from most antineoplastic agents resolve within that time. This is not true for many agents, however. The actual period of acute N&V may be 16 to 20 hours, because serotonin-receptor antagonists will typically delay symptoms for that long after cisplatin is administered.[12] This time frame may vary for other agents. On the other hand, du Bois et al.[13] proposed that serotonin antagonists delay vomiting and extend the period of acute N&V to 48 hours, which includes "late-onset peak emesis." A third hypothesis is that delayed N&V occur in those individuals who did not experience acute N&V, while persistent N&V extend from the day of chemotherapy administration to subsequent days. These conflicting definitions underscore our incomplete understanding of the pathogenesis and time course of chemotherapy-induced N&V.[14] For the purposes of this chapter, delayed and persistent N&V will be discussed as a single entity.

Cisplatin and other moderately to highly emetogenic chemotherapy can induce N&V that persist for several days in almost all patients who do not receive adequate antiemetics, and delayed or persistent N&V also may occur after administration of agents considered to be mildly to moderately emetogenic (i.e., cyclophosphamide, doxorubicin, carboplatin, and mitomycin).[15,16] Anticipatory nausea and vomiting (ANV) usually develop within three or four cycles of chemotherapy, when acute (and perhaps delayed and persistent) N&V are not adequately controlled. Other risk factors include being less than 50 years old; feeling warm or hot after chemotherapy; having nausea or vomiting rated as moderate, severe, or intolerable; feeling generalized weakness after chemotherapy; or a history of motion sickness.[17] ANV is considered to be a case of classical conditioning, in which the events and cues surrounding chemotherapy (e.g., odors, tastes of drugs, visual cues) or other precipitating causes become linked to N&V, and the cues themselves induce N&V. ANV is difficult to control, and may persist for years after therapy is complete.[18]

The risks for chemotherapy-induced N&V are related to the antineoplastic drug(s) administered and to patient-related factors. Both the drugs themselves and the doses administered affect emetogenic potential, as shown in Table 14-1.[19,20] Emetogenicity, latency (time to onset of vomiting), and duration of N&V are highly variable among various agents, but drugs with the shortest latency tend to be the most emetogenic. Other factors may also alter emetogenicity: alternate schedules (i.e., lower doses given over several days or continuous infusions) often change the pattern (i.e., decreased vomiting and increased nausea), while multiple drug regimens increase the intensity and perhaps the duration of N&V. The effect of multiple chemotherapy agents is taken into account and is used to estimate the emetogenic potential of particular combination chemotherapy regimens and to plan antiemetic management accordingly.[20] (See footnote to Table 14-1.) A regimen such as cyclophosphamide (<750 mg/m²), methotrexate (≤ 50 mg/m²), fluorouracil (<1000 mg/m²) (CMF), which has typically been considered to be moderately emetogenic, is reclassified as level 4, or moderately highly emetogenic (60%–90% of individuals treated will have emesis). It is important to gauge emetogenicity accurately to plan antiemetic interventions, because the administration of highly emetogenic chemotherapy, particularly cisplatin, and poor control of acute N&V are the most important predictors for delayed N&V.[21]

Gender is the most important patient-related risk factor for chemotherapy-induced N&V. Age and a history

TABLE 14-1 Emetogenicity of Antineoplastic Agents

Emetic Potential	Agent/Dose (mg/m²)	Latency (hrs)	Reported Duration (hrs)
Level 5 Very high (>90%)	Carmustine ≥ 250 mg	2–6	4–24
	Cisplatin ≥ 50 mg	1–6	48–72⁺
	Cyclophosphamide > 1500 mg	4–12	12–24⁺
	Dacarbazine	0.5–6	6–24
	Lomustine ≥ 60 mg	4–6	12–24
	Mechlorethamine	0.5–2	6–24
	Melphalan, high dose	0.3–6	6–12
	Streptozocin	1–6	12–24
Level 4 Moderately high (60–90%)	Carboplatin	4–9	12–48
	Carmustine < 200 mg	2–6	4–24
	Cisplatin < 50 mg	1–6	48–72
	Cyclophosphamide > 750 ≤ 1500	4–12	12–24⁺
	Cytarabine > 1 g	2–4	12–24
	Doxorubicin > 60 mg	4–6	6–24⁺
	Lomustine < 60 mg	4–6	12–24
	Methotrexate > 1000 mg	4–12	3–12 days
	Procarbazine (oral)	24–72	variable

(continued)

TABLE 14-1 Emetogenicity of Antineoplastic Agents (continued)

Emetic Potential	Agent/Dose (mg/m²)	Latency (hrs)	Reported Duration (hrs)
Level 3 Moderate (30–60%)	Asparaginase	4–12	—
	Cyclophosphamide ≤ 750 mg	—	12–24+
	Cyclophosphamide (oral)	2–6	—
	Daunorubicin	4–6	24
	Doxorubicin 20–60 mg	—	6–24+
	Epirubicin ≤ 90 mg	—	—
	Fluorouracil ≥ 1000 mg	—	24+
	Hexamethylmelamine (oral)	—	—
	Idarubicin	—	—
	Ifosfamide	4–12	—
	Methotrexate 250–1000 mg	4–6	3–12 days
	Mitoxantrone < 15 mg	—	6+
	Paclitaxel	—	—
	Teniposide	1–6	2–12
Level 2 Moderately low (10–30%)	Docetaxel	—	—
	Doxorubicin ≤ 20 mg	—	—
	Etoposide	3–8	6–12
	5-fluorouracil < 1000 mg	—	—
	Cytarabine ≤ 20 mg	3–12	—
	Gemcitabine	—	—
	Irinotecan	—	—
	Melphalan	6–12	—
	Mercaptopurine	4–8	—
	Mitomycin	1–4	48–72
	Paclitaxel	—	—
	Topotecan	—	—
	Taxotere	—	—
	Vinblastine	4–8	—
Level 1 low (<10%)	Bleomycin	3–6	—
	Busulfan	—	—
	Chlorambucil	8–12	—
	2-Chlorodeoxyadenosine	—	—
	Fludarabine	—	—
	Hydroxyurea	—	—
	Methotrexate < 50 mg	4–12	—
	L-phenylalanine mustard (oral)	—	—
	Thioguanine (oral)	—	—
	Vinblastine	—	—
	Vincristine	4–8	—
	Vinorelbine	—	—

Dash = no data reported.

Follow these steps (1 through 5) to identify the level of emetogenicity of single agent and combination chemotherapy.

1. Identify the most emetogenic agent in the combination.
2. Assess the relative contribution of other agents to the emetogenicity of the combination.
3. Level 1 agents do not contribute to the emetogenicity of the combination.
4. Adding one or more level 2 agents increases the emetogenicity of the combination by one level greater than the most emetogenic agent in the combination.
5. Adding level 3 or 4 agents increases the emetogenicity by one level per agent.

Adapted from Ettinger DS: Preventing chemotherapy-induced nausea and vomiting: An Update and Review of Emesis. *Semin Oncol* 23(suppl 10):6–18, 1995[19]; and from Hesketh PJ, Kris MG, Grunberg SM, et al: Proposal for classifying the acute emetogenicity of cancer chemotherapy. *J Clin Oncol* 15:103–109, 1997.[20]

of chronic alcohol use are implicated less often. Overall, women who are of menstrual age are more likely to experience more severe N&V from therapy or disease and, correspondingly, to attain poorer antiemetic control than are men or older women.[21–24] The gender effect may be hormonally influenced[25] and may also be interrelated with age, because persons younger than 45 to 55 years report more intense acute N&V and are more likely to develop ANV than older persons.[17,26] Furthermore, people younger than 30 years are more likely to experience extrapyramidal symptoms (EPS) with dopamine antagonist drugs. Conversely, patients who have a history of chronic, high alcohol intake (definitions vary from one to five drinks per day) have been found to be more likely to experience complete antiemetic control than nondrinkers in some studies[27] but not in others.[28] In addition, there may be a small number of individuals who are at greater risk for N&V with chemotherapy because of previous life events, such as motion sickness or hyperemesis of pregnancy.[29]

Radiation Therapy

Radiation therapy (RT)–related N&V is dependent on the site and volume irradiated and the fractionation schedule. RT fields that include a large percentage of the epigastric tissue—which includes the enterochromaffin cells—are most likely to induce N&V (Figure 14-1).[30,31] The role of the enterochromaffin cells is illustrated in hemibody irradiation: as many as 88% of those treated to the upper and mid-hemibody experience vomiting, while as few as 15% to 17% of those treated to the lower hemibody do so.[32] Approximately 50% of those receiving conventional doses of 180 to 200 centiGray [cGY]/fraction to the upper abdomen experience N&V. The latency period between radiation administration and onset of N&V is typically 1 to 2 hours, and N&V may last for several hours after radiotherapy.[33]

Large field size has an impact on latency, and 85% to 100% of individuals who receive total body irradiation (TBI) or hemibody radiation in large fractions (i.e., >500 cGy) vomit 10 to 15 minutes after therapy.[34] Patients treated with TBI in preparation for stem cell or bone marrow transplantation are also likely to be receiving high doses of emetogenic chemotherapy, which also increases the risk for N&V.

Nausea and Vomiting of Terminal Disease

Intermittent or constant N&V are common symptoms in terminal cancer (pain and dyspnea may occur more frequently) and are experienced by as many as 60% of patients.[3,4,35] In most instances, intractable vomiting occurs only during the last few days of life. N&V are at least moderately severe for most terminally ill persons, but small numbers report their N&V to be "horrible"[3] or "unendurable."[36] Gender is also predictive of N&V of terminal disease, which are more frequent problems for women.[3,37,38] N&V are most often related to advanced stomach or breast cancers but can occur with almost any malignancy.[3] N&V in these instances are often multicausal and include visceral, biochemical/metabolic, drug-induced, CNS, vestibular, and others causes, which may increase the difficulty of selecting treatment (Figure 14-2).

Pathophysiology

The pathogenesis of N&V is complex and not totally understood. Neural structures in the fourth ventricle and brain stem comprise the final common pathway, and sev-

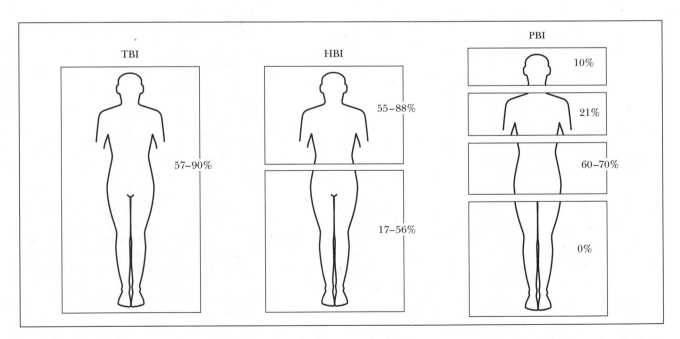

FIGURE 14-1   Percentage of patients with vomiting following radiation therapy. TBI = total body irradiation; HBI = hemibody irradiation, divided at the umbilicus into upper and lower hemibody irradiation; PBI = partial body irradiation. (Reprinted with permission from King GL, Makale MT: Postirradiation emesis, in Kucharcyzk J, Stewart DJ, Miller AD (eds): *Nausea and Vomiting: Recent Research and Clinical Advances.* Boca Raton, FL: CRC Press, 1991, p. 106.[30] © CRC Press, Boca Raton, FL.)

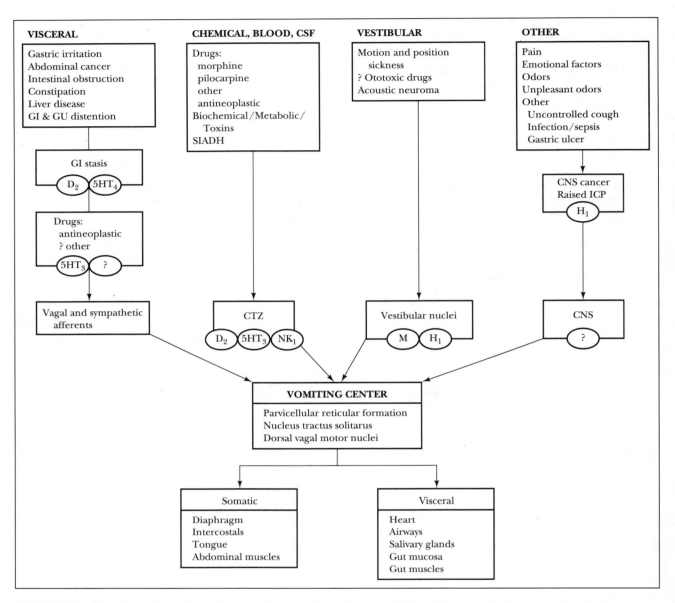

FIGURE 14-2 Vomiting reflex pathways. Neurotransmitters: D_2 = dopamine D_2; H_1 = histamine H_1; M = muscarinic cholinergic; $5HT_3$ = serotonin subgroup-3; $5HT_4$ = serotonin subgroup-4; NK_1 = neurokinin, CTZ = chemoreceptor trigger zone; SIADH = syndrome of inappropriate antidiuretic hormone; LCP = intracranial pressure; GI = gastrointestinal; GU = geniburinary. (Source: Adapted from Lichter I: Which antiemetic? *J Palliat Care* 9:42–50, 1993.[37])

eral putative neurotransmitters and afferents to this area have been identified. During the last 25 years, a large body of research regarding N&V has focused on chemotherapy-related emesis. However, much less is known about emesis from other causes, the pathogenesis of nausea, and about potential physiological differences in children. Current hypotheses of the vomiting reflex pathways, as well as the causes that theoretically fall within these pathways, are summarized in Figure 14-2.[37,39] N&V are different entities and may be mediated in different ways or may exist on a continuum. Vomiting, and possibly nausea, is a highly conserved reflex, and occurs in many lower animals and in humans. Emesis is a mechanism

meant to protect the organism from ingested substances that are interpreted as being poisonous or toxic.[40]

Nausea is a recognized feeling of the need to vomit and thus involves the cerebral cortex.[41] Nausea is mediated by the autonomic nervous system and is accompanied by symptoms such as pallor, tachycardia, and cold sweat. It corresponds to the pre-ejection phase, in which the stomach relaxes and gastric acid secretion is inhibited. Then a single retrograde giant contraction (RGC) of the small intestine occurs, and the alkaline small bowel contents are propelled back into the stomach, decreasing the acidity of the stomach contents. Thus, ingested toxins are alkalinized and confined to the stomach. Retching and vomiting do not occur until RGC reaches the stomach.[41]

The first event in this ejection phase is *retching*, during which the intrathoracic pressure is negative and the intraabdominal pressure is positive. When the contractions of the abdominal muscles and the diaphragm become coordinated, and the pressure in the thorax and abdomen become positive, they compress the stomach, and its contents are forced upward through the mouth and nose in the act of vomiting.

Neural Structures and Transmitters Involved in Emesis

Several neural structures are involved in emesis, including the vomiting center (VC), the vagus and other abdominal visceral nerves, the chemoreceptor trigger zone, the vestibular apparatus, and the higher cortical centers. It is the VC that receives input from the other structures and that ultimately sends impulses to the motor nuclei that bring about vomiting.

The VC is not a discrete anatomical entity; rather, it is a central integrating complex within the reticular formation of the brain stem. Within the VC is a network of neuroanatomical connections of several brain-stem nuclei, including the parvicellular reticular formation (PCRF), the nucleus tractus solitarus (NTS), and the somatic motor nuclei involved with emesis (the dorsal motor vagal nucleus innervating the abdominal viscera, as well as the dorsal and ventral respiratory groups).[39,41,42]

The vagus nerve plays a key role in acute emesis caused by chemotherapy, by radiation therapy to the epigastrium, and by abdominal distention or obstruction. Antineoplastic drugs and radiation to the gut damage or somehow stimulate enterochromaffin cells, causing them to release serotonin (5HT; 5-hydroxytryptamine), which then binds to serotonin subtype-3 (5HT$_3$) chemoreceptors on the vagus nerve that lie in close proximity in the proximal gut wall (Figure 14-3).[43] The result is an impulse to vomit, which is transmitted to the nucleus tractus solitarus and the chemoreceptor trigger zone (CTZ) in the CNS. Other neurochemicals found in the upper GI tract may also play a role in emesis and include dopamine, neurotensin, vasoactive intestinal peptide (VIP), and polypeptide PYY.[37,41] Mechanoreceptors within the gut wall respond to contraction and overdistension, and stimulate the vagal and splanchnic nerves.

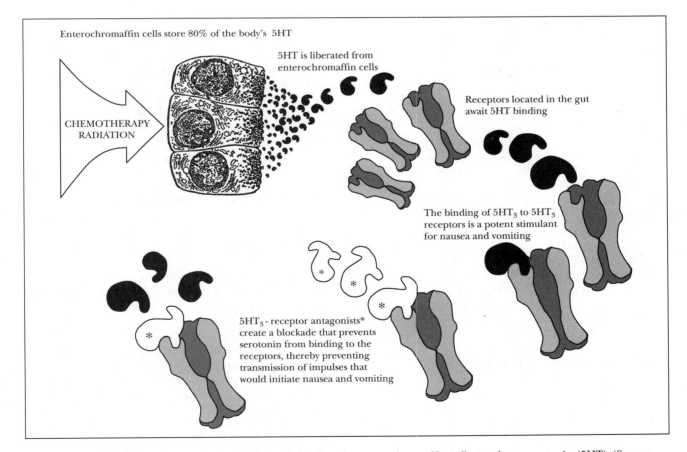

Enterochromaffin cells store 80% of the body's 5HT

CHEMOTHERAPY RADIATION

5HT is liberated from enterochromaffin cells

Receptors located in the gut await 5HT binding

The binding of 5HT$_3$ to 5HT$_3$ receptors is a potent stimulant for nausea and vomiting

5HT$_3$ - receptor antagonists* create a blockade that prevents serotonin from binding to the receptors, thereby preventing transmission of impulses that would initiate nausea and vomiting

FIGURE 14-3 Chemotherapy and radiation therapy stimulate the enterochromaffin cells to release serotonin (5HT) (Source: Cunningham RS: 5HT$_3$-receptor antagonists: A review of Pharmacology and Clinical efficiency *Oncol Nurs Forum* 24(suppl 7):35, 1997.) Reprinted with permission.

The amount of 5HT released is measured by its urinary metabolite, 5-hydroxyindoleacetic acid (5-HIAA), and may be related to emetogenic potential of the chemotherapy administered. This, in turn, is reflected in the onset, severity, and duration of emesis. For instance, after dacarbazine or high-dose cisplatin administration, 5-HIAA excretion increases rapidly to a high level; low-dose cisplatin causes a lower increase in 5-HIAA excretion. Cyclophosphamide causes a later and lower but more persistently elevated level of 5-HIAA excretion, which corresponds with late-onset and persistent emesis.[16,44] Fractionated high-dose total body irradiation (i.e., 1.2 Gy/fraction in 11 fractions over 4 days) also leads to elevated urinary 5-HIAA each day radiation is given and is associated with recurrent emesis. Greater elevations in 5-HIAA are documented with radiation to the upper and midabdomen than to the lower abdomen.[32]

The CTZ, a highly vascular organ, lies in the area postrema of the fourth ventricle, in close proximity to the nucleus tractus solitarus. The CTZ is not confined within the blood-brain barrier, and thus can detect chemical stimuli (e.g., drug, biochemical product, toxins) in the cerebrospinal fluid and in blood. The CTZ plays a general role as a chemoreceptor and is also implicated in food intake and conditioned taste aversion,[41] and plays a role in GI tract motility.[39] There are many neurotransmitters in or about the CTZ, including dopamine (D), noradrenaline, somatostatin, substance P, serotonin (5HT) histamine (H), noradrenaline, enkephalins, and acetylcholine, and corresponding receptors.[39] Thus, the CTZ plays a role in chemotherapy N&V, as well as in emesis from other causes.[40]

Motion sickness and labyrinthitis are the most common stimuli to the vestibular apparatus (VA) of the inner ear that induce N&V, whereas tumor involvement (i.e., acoustic neuroma or metastases to the base of the skull) is a rare cause. The VA may play a minor role in chemotherapy-related N&V, as people who have experienced motion sickness may be at greater risk to develop ANV.[17] Furthermore, drugs that are ototoxic, such as cisplatin, may secondarily induce N&V via the VA.[41]

Higher cortical centers also play a part in modulating vomiting, nausea, taste aversions, and ANV, but the neural connections between the cortex and the VC, as well as the neurotransmitters involved, have not yet been identified. Input seems to come from several areas in this region.[39]

Other Potential Structures and Mechanisms

Other unidentified structures or chemoreceptors in the brain or visceral organs (e.g., the liver) may play a role in the initiation of N&V.[42] Several levels of neurologic control probably come into play, and second or third messengers for emesis may exist. The neurological systems for N&V have plasticity—that is, if the message to

vomit is blocked in one neural route, it can be rerouted via another.[40] Other neurotransmitters and hormones that may be involved in the onset of emesis include serotonin subtype-4 (5HT$_4$) receptors in the gut and CNS, which may play a role in gastrointestinal motility and in emesis.[42] In addition, endogenous cortisol may be a factor in the onset of N&V. In one study, individuals with low urinary cortisol levels had more intense N&V than did those with high urinary cortisol levels, and dexamethasone administration enhanced antiemetic efficacy only in patients with low urinary cortisol excretion.[45]

Current research is focusing on a new class of antiemetics, the neurokinin$_1$ (NK$_1$) receptor antagonists. Substance P, which can induce vomiting, is found in the area postrema. NK$_1$-receptor antagonists have been shown to decrease the incidence of acute and delayed N&V from chemotherapy, as well as N&V from other causes.[46] These agents act centrally and are thus likely to be widely effective in controlling N&V deriving from a variety of causes. In one initial human study, a NK$_1$ receptor antagonist (CP-122,721) was highly effective alone and increased the efficacy of a 5HT$_3$-receptor antagonist plus dexamethasone to control both acute and delayed N&V.[47] With both agents, 100% of patients had control of acute emesis, and 80% had no delayed emesis after highly emetogenic chemotherapy.

Vasopressin (antidiuretic hormone [ADH]) may also be an endogenous mediator of N&V. Serum levels of ADH may rise 20- to 50-fold in animals and humans in response to emetogenic stimuli (e.g., chemotherapy, apomorphine, and motion sickness).[41] In humans, ADH increases only in those who experience nausea and may thus either mediate N&V or be a response to promote water conservation when confronted with losses from vomiting. Vasopressin plays a role in memory, and so may be instrumental in the onset of ANV.

Delayed Nausea and Vomiting

Serotonin plays a diminished role in delayed and persistent N&V after chemotherapy. Evidence for this is that second elevations of 5-HIAA do not occur in persons who develop delayed N&V.[48] Andrews and Davis's[41] model for cisplatin-induced N&V (Figure 14-4) assumes that the role for 5HT progressively diminishes after 24 hours, and proposes phases of N&V in which different antiemetic agents might be effective. During the acute phase, steroids might affect the permeability of the CTZ to emetic stimuli. During delayed N&V, prokinetic agents might be effective because cisplatin causes a dose-related inhibition of gastric emptying and gastroparesis in animals and humans that may last for several days. In addition, chemotherapy and radiation therapy to the GI tract damage the rapidly dividing cells of the gut, leading to breaches in gut wall integrity. Such damage could allow potentially emetogenic toxins (e.g., lipopolysaccharides, hormones such as polypeptide PYY) to leak into the bloodstream.

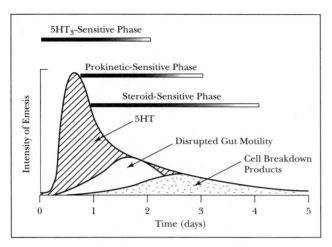

FIGURE 14-4 Conceptual model of mechanisms that may be involved in acute and delayed vomiting from cisplatin. The model is intended to illustrate that there are multiple mechanisms of N&V, and the predominant cause of emesis may be different for each phase, which accounts for the changing efficacy of various antiemetic agents with time. (Source: Andrews PLR, Davis CJ: The mechanisms of emesis induced by anti-cancer therapies, in Andrews PLR, Sanger GJ (eds): *Emesis in Anti-Cancer Therapy: Mechanisms and Treatment*. London: Arnold, 1993, p. 147.[41] Reprinted with permission.)

Steroids might be effective at this point, essentially to mend these breaches.

Assessment

Baseline and ongoing assessment and documentation are critical to optimal management of N&V. Nausea and vomiting should each be assessed by patient self-report, because physicians' and nurses' ratings of symptom severity often do not agree with patients' ratings.[49,50] Furthermore, patients often deem control of nausea as most important, while physicians may think control of vomiting and retching is more important. Nurses spend a great deal of time with patients who are receiving chemotherapy and may be the best care providers to gain an accurate understanding of the severity and duration of N&V, the side effects of antiemetics that the patient finds objectionable, and the effects of both on patients' QOL and activities of daily living (ADLs).

Estimating the Potential for Therapy-Induced Nausea and Vomiting

The ultimate antiemetic management goals are that persons undergoing chemotherapy or radiation therapy will not experience acute, delayed, or anticipatory N&V. Un-

fortunately, these goals are not attainable in all instances. A baseline assessment considers the risk factors for N&V. (See Appendix 14A for an example.) This information helps the nurse to identify individuals who may have better antiemetic control (men, older persons including postmenopausal women, and those with a history of chronic alcohol use), or worse N&V (premenopausal women, younger men, and persons who drink little or no alcohol). The nurse should also ask the patients about pharmacologic and nonpharmacologic management strategies that they have tried in the past that have or have not been helpful.

After chemotherapy, patient self-assessment can again be used to evaluate the antiemetic plan. One method is a short, easily understood daily diary (see Appendix 14B). The diary should record important information regarding the control of N&V, including estimates of intensity of N&V, assessment of the effect that N&V have on activities important to the individual, and of their effect on QOL.[29] These factors are critical in helping the nurse and physician to gauge the efficacy of previous antiemetics and the need to change the antiemetic management plan.

The nurse should telephone the patient on the day after first cycle of chemotherapy is received to assess whether or not the patient has nausea *or* vomiting, if the antiemetic has caused any objectionable side effects, and to change antiemetic interventions as necessary. The nurse can also remind patients to complete the diary for 3 to 5 days. A diary can be used for four to six cycles of chemotherapy, which is the usual time frame in which ANV develops. The diary could be adapted for use with persons receiving radiation therapy, to cue the patient to report N&V to the nurse or physician.

Nausea and Vomiting as an Actual Problem

Many patients experience N&V despite taking antiemetics, so the nurse must continue to assess for their occurrence. Symptom assessment includes whether the individual is experiencing nausea, vomiting, or both; and the onset, duration, frequency, intensity, aggravating and ameliorating factors; and effects on QOL and ADLs. Assessment cues are given in Figure 14-5. Because many events can precipitate N&V, the nurse should consider that chemotherapy, radiation therapy to the epigastrium, new opioid therapy, or other drugs may be contributing factors. In other instances, the person may be experiencing another problem that can lead to N&V (e.g., constipation, intermittent bowel obstruction, hypercalcemia, infection, uncontrolled cough).

Physical Assessment

In addition to considering multiple etiologies, the nurse must correlate other system problems that may exacer-

---

ASSESSMENT OF VOMITING

Client: _____

Age: _____ (under 50 increases risk)

Gender: _____ (female increases risk)

Chief complaint:
"What brought you to the clinic/hospital?"
"Why are you telephoning?"

Clarification/amplification:
"Tell me what you mean by . . . . ?"
"Tell me more about . . . . ?"
(Make sure you use words the client understands.)

Establish possible cause:
"What do you think your nausea and/or vomiting are due to?"

Onset/duration:
"When did the nausea and/or vomiting begin?"

Frequency:
"Do you have the nausea and/or vomiting all the time, or do they come and go?"
(If intermittent, ask when they occur.)

Intensity: Assess nausea and vomiting separately.
"On a scale of 0 to 10, with 0 being no nausea/vomiting and 10 being the worst nausea/vomiting you can imagine, rate your nausea/vomiting: 1) now; 2) at its worst."
"Rate your nausea/vomiting: none, slight, moderate, severe: 1) now; 2) at its worst."

Quality of vomitus:
"What does the material you vomit look like? Smell like?"

Effects on quality of life and daily living:
"Does your nausea/vomiting affect:
Your eating?
Your sleep?
Things you like to do?
Your work?
Your relationships with family and friends?"

Aggravating and ameliorating factors:

"What makes your nausea/vomiting worse?"

"What makes your nausea/vomiting better?"

"What medicines for nausea and vomiting did your doctor prescribe?"

"How often do you take them?"

"How much of your nausea/vomiting does the medicine take away?"

"For how long does the medicine work?"

"Does the medicine give you any side effects that you do not like?"

"How satisfied are you with your antiemetic medicine(s)?"

FIGURE 14-5 Cues to assess the patient who is vomiting.

---

bate or cause N&V with physical findings and laboratory values. For instance, assessment of the mouth may confirm candidiasis; palpation of the abdomen may confirm hepatomegaly; examination of urine for cloudiness and odor increase suspicion for infection; and rectal examination confirms constipation.

Significant vomiting can result in fluid volume deficit (FVD), which includes water and electrolyte losses. Several liters of electrolyte-rich gastrointestinal secretions are normally produced each day, and all but 150 to 200 mL of the water and all electrolytes are resorbed in the small and large bowel before stool is passed. Prolonged vomiting (or gastric suctioning) leads to losses of hydrogen (H^+), chloride (Cl^-), potassium (K^+), and large amounts of water (Figure 14-6). Metabolic alkalosis and hypokalemia result, so the lungs (rapidly) and the kidneys

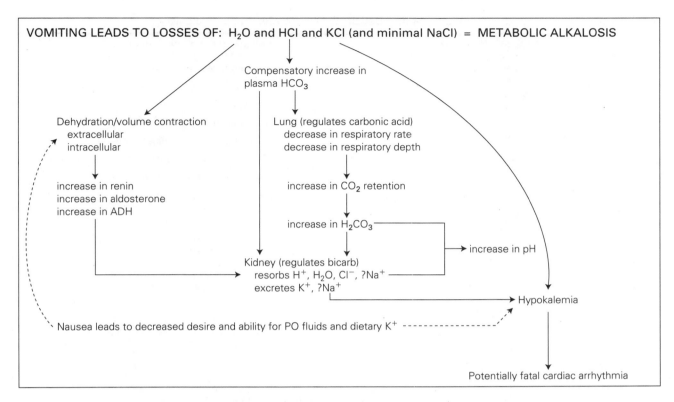

FIGURE 14-6   Effect of nausea and vomiting on fluid volume and acid-base balance.

(more slowly) attempt to return pH toward normal. The action of the kidneys initially actually worsens hypokalemia, as H^+ and Cl^- are preferentially resorbed and K^+ is excreted in urine. In the face of water loss, the pituitary secretes ADH and the kidneys secrete renin, which further induces the adrenal glands to secrete aldosterone. The result is the conservation of water loss in urine.[51,52] Persistent nausea exacerbates the problems to the extent that the individual is not able to drink or eat.

Assessment parameters may vary somewhat depending on whether the patient is in the hospital, in the clinic, or at home. Parameters to assess include the estimated volume of vomitus, the patient's ability to drink fluids, level of thirst, the color of urine (dilute versus concentrated), and if they have experienced any rapid weight loss (Table 14-2). It is important to identify the character of vomitus to determine whether it is stomach contents or regurgitated from further along the GI tract, which could indicate obstruction or obstipation. Stomach contents may look like food, medication, or greenish, bilelike fluid, whereas contents from the distal ileum would be brown and have a fecal odor. Blood from the stomach resembles coffee grounds.

In the hospital or clinic, the nurse can also assess the patient's skin and tongue turgor, oral cavity moisture, vital signs, and cardiac rhythm to estimate FVD. Intake-and-output measurements (I&O) are initiated in hospitalized patients. I&Os are notoriously inaccurate and provide

more accurate information when combined with daily weights. A 2% weight loss is considered to be mild FVD, 5% is moderate FVD, and 8% is severe FVD.[51] When fluid losses are significant, the homeostatic response is increased thirst. The amount of rapid water loss can be calculated easily because 1 liter of water weighs 2.2 pounds.

Skin turgor and oral moisture may be useful measures of FVD. Skin turgor is assessed by pinching the skin over the sternum, forehead, inner thigh, or the abdomen (of children). The skin springs back immediately when turgor is normal, but the pinched skin may stay elevated (tented) for several seconds with FVD. Skin turgor reflects skin elasticity as well as interstitial fluid, so it may not accurately reflect the hydration status of persons older than 55 to 60 years.[51] Assessing tongue turgor is more accurate: Well-hydrated individuals have one longitudinal furrow, whereas those with FVD have additional furrows, their tongues become smaller, and they have little oral cavity moisture. To differentiate this from dryness caused by mouth breathing, the nurse should assess the patient's mouth for moisture or dryness between the gingiva and buccal mucosa.

Altered vital signs may occur with moderate to severe FVD. For instance, temperature may decrease, but this is often not a reliable indicator in persons with cancer who are at high risk for infection. Respirations become slower and more shallow as the lungs try to conserve CO_2, and the heart rate increases to compensate for decreased

TABLE 14-2 Physical Findings of Fluid Volume Deficit (FVD) with Metabolic Alkalosis

Indicator	Signs and Symptoms	Assessment and Intervention
I&O	PO intake down with N&V Variable volume emesis Decreased urine volume Urine concentrated	Accurate measurement of: • PO fluids (foods/beverages) • IV fluids • Vomitus (loss of electrolytes) • Urine (estimate incontinent urine) • Diarrhea stools (increased loss of electrolytes) • Wound and fistula drainage
Rapid weight loss	1 lb rapid loss ≈ 500 mL fluid loss	Daily weights using same scale Weigh in A.M. after voiding and before breakfast Wear same type clothes
Oral moisture	Dry oral cavity	Oral assessment: differentiate between dryness secondary to FVD and mouth breathing

Turgor
  Skin
  Tongue
	Tenting of pinched skin
	More than 1 longitudinal furrow
	Decreased tongue size
		Not reliable in older adults

Vital signs	Temperature may be low RR down HR up Postural hypotension	Not reliable with infection, neutropenia Check orthostatic BPs
Cardiac functioning	Arrhythmias may occur Flattened T waves and ST depression may be seen Increased sensitivity to digitalis	Place person on cardiac monitor if they have ≥ moderate FVD Check pulse

I&O = intake and output; RR = respiratory rate; HR = heart rate; BP = blood pressure.

intravascular volume. Postural hypotension is also likely to occur. A decrease of at least 15 mm Hg in systolic BP or an increase of 15 heartbeats per minute from lying to sitting suggests intravascular volume deficit.[51] Electrocardiogram (ECG) may reveal flattened T waves and ST segment depression.

Laboratory tests are used in conjunction with physical findings to confirm the severity of FVD and alkalosis (Table 14-3). Tests of urine concentration, including specific gravity (SG) and osmolality, as well as urinary chloride may be done. Decreased urine chloride is the most reliable way to confirm metabolic alkalosis from excessive vomiting or gastrointestinal suction. Serum tests are done to determine electrolyte imbalances and their severity, the degree of dehydration (blood urea nitrogen [BUN]: creatinine ratio) and serum osmolality, and the degree of alkalosis. Other laboratory values that may assist in identifying other underlying causes of N&V include serum calcium, liver function values, BUN, and urinalysis or urine culture.

Degrees of Toxicity

Little has been done to substantiate the degree of toxicity from N&V from the patients' perspective. The Common Toxicity Criteria is used by several oncology study groups in the United States,, e.g., Eastern Cooperative Oncology Group (ECOG), Southwest Oncology Group (SWOG), and evaluates N&V separately (Table 14-4). These type of criteria may reflect subjective judgment on the part of the physician or nurse rater, and may not capture the patients' view of their experiences. For instance, one study found that nurses' and physicians' ratings of the patients' nausea agreed with patient ratings 52% and 37% of instances, respectively, and with their vomiting ratings 78% and 59%, respectively.[53]

In antiemetic trials, control of emesis (vomiting plus retching) is the primary outcome variable of interest, but there is no accepted standard for response rates. Complete response/protection certainly means the patient does not vomit or retch, but definitions of lesser responses vary. For example, in some studies a major response is 1 to 2 emeses in 24 hours, a minor response refers to 3 to 5 emeses, and failure is more than 5 emeses. Some studies also include the assessment of nausea, and others evaluate antiemetics as effective if both N&V are controlled. Studies that include patients' subjective evaluations provide additional important information on which to base antiemetic selection decisions. Because criteria for antiemetic control differ from study to study, comparison of studies is difficult.

TABLE 14-3 Laboratory Values

Laboratory Value	Normal/Alteration	Comment
Urine		
Specific gravity	Normal = 1.008–1.035 Increases in FVD	
Urine osmolality	Normal = 500–800 mOsm/kg Increases in FVD	
Chloride	Normal = 110–250 mEq/24 hours <10–15 mEq/L when metabolic alkalosis is due to vomiting	Varies with salt intake
Serum		
Potassium	Normal = 3.4–5.3 mEq/L Hypokalemia < 3.4	When pH increases, K^+ decreases Average .1 increase in pH = .5 decrease in K^+
Chloride	Normal = 94–108 mEq/L Hypochloremia < 94 mEq/L	Associated with hypokalemia and metabolic alkalosis
Osmolality	280–295 mOsm/kg Increases with dehydration	Review both serum and urine osmolality
BUN: creatinine ratio	Normal = 10:1 (approximate) FVD > 10:1	Seen with hypovolemia and dehydration
Carbon dioxide (CO_2)	Normal = 22–28 Alkalosis < 22	

Source: Metheny NM: *Fluid and Electrolyte Balance: Nursing Considerations* (ed 3). Philadelphia: Lippincott, 1996, pp. 34–40.[51]

TABLE 14-4 Common Toxicity Criteria for N&V

	0	1	2	3	4
Nausea	None	Able to eat reasonable intake	Intake significantly decreased but can eat	No significant intake	—
Vomiting	None	One episode in 24 hours	Two to five episodes in 24 hours	Six to ten episodes in 24 hours	Greater than 10 episodes in 24 hours requiring parenteral support

Symptom Management

Optimal antiemetic management includes the prevention of N&V and the minimization of antiemetic side effects. If N&V occur, ongoing assessment will lead to prompt recognition of the problem(s), and new interventions will be implemented and reevaluated on a timely basis. Appropriate interventions (type and duration of use) require knowledge of the probable etiologies, as well as evidence-based and empirically reported intervention strategies. Antiemetics are almost always necessary, whether N&V are related to disease, cancer therapy, or other factors. Nonpharmacologic measures may be useful adjuncts in some cases.

Pharmacologic Management

Several classifications of drugs have antiemetic activity. These include serotonin antagonists, dopamine antago-

nists, corticosteroids, cannabinoids, benzodiazepines, and others. No agent in any of these classes controls N&V 100% of the time, illustrating the complex nature of N&V and the difficulties of management. Each class of agents is discussed separately, and for each mechanisms of action, indications, adverse effects, and administration considerations (doses, routes, and schedules) are given. Antiemetics indicated for therapy (chemotherapy, radiation therapy, and for postanesthesia) are included in Table 14-5, and those for other indications are given in Table 14-6. Selection of the appropriate antiemetic requires careful assessment and evaluation of efficacy (Figure 14-7).

Serotonin antagonists

Ondansetron (Zofran), granisetron (Kytril), and dolasetron (Anzemet) are the 5HT$_3$-receptor antagonists available in the United States. These highly effective antiemetics were developed to be selective for 5HT$_3$ receptors and have little activity at other receptors. These antiemetics bind tightly to 5HT$_3$ receptors on the afferent vagus

TABLE 14-5 Antiemetics for Cancer Therapy

Antiemetic	Indications: Dose/Schedule	Comments
Serotonin Antagonists		
Ondansetron (Zofran)	Acute N&V (level 3–5 chemotherapy): 8–32 mg IV Acute N&V (level 3–4 chemotherapy); delayed N&V; radiation therapy–induced N&V: 8 mg PO qd or bid Postanesthesia N&V: 4–8 mg IV PO	All are administered once before therapy unless otherwise indicated 5HT$_3$ regimens for moderate to highly emetogenic chemotherapy should include dexamethasone (see below) Some clinicians advocate adding lorazepam or other benzodiazepine to a 5HT$_3$ regimen; may decrease anxiety but increases sedation
Granisetron (Kytril)	Acute N&V (level 3–5 chemotherapy): 10 μg/kg IV or 2 mg PO	Some evidence that addition of a small dose of phenothiazine (i.e., prochlorperazine) increases efficacy
Dolasetron (Anzemet)	Acute N&V (level 3–5 chemotherapy): 100 mg IV Acute N&V (level 3–4 chemotherapy): 100 mg PO Postanesthesia N&V: 12.5–100 mg IV	Granisetron and dolasetron can be administered over 30–60 sec; ondansetron over 15 min or more Dolasetron will precipitate with dexamethasone in D5W
Dopamine Antagonists		
Metoclopramide (Reglan)	Acute N&V (level 4 chemotherapy): 1–3 mg/kg q2h × 3–5 doses Delayed N&V: 10–20 mg PO tid/qid × 3–5 days	Metoclopramide has minor 5HT$_3$ antagonist activity; emesis typically starts at approximately 5 hours, is more severe, and persists longer than after a 5HT$_3$ antagonist regimen
Prochlorperazine (Compazine)	Acute N&V (level 2 chemotherapy); add to 5HT$_3$ antagonist regimen; delayed N&V; postanesthesia N&V: 10 mg IV/PO q4–6h, or 15–30 mg timed release (i.e., compazine spansules) q8–12h	Add dexamethasone to dopamine antagonist regimens used for delayed N&V Haloperidol less sedating than prochlorperazine and high-dose metoclopramide
Haloperidol (Haldol)	Acute N&V (level 3–4 chemotherapy): 0.5–2 mg IV/IM q 4–8 hr Acute N&V (level 2–3 chemotherapy), delayed N&V: 2–5 mg PO q4h	Dystonic reactions (i.e., EPS) are not allergies; premedicate to prevent, or treat reaction with a benzodiazepine (lorazepam) or diphenhydramine. Does not preclude retreatment
Corticosteroids		
Dexamethasone (Decadron)	Acute N&V: add to 5HT$_3$ antagonist regimen: 10–20 mg IV, or 8–20 mg PO Delayed N&V: varying doses, i.e., 4 mg PO bid/tid × 2 to 4 days, sometimes tapered	Addition of a corticosteroid will increase efficacy of antiemetic regimens by about 15%–25% Rapid IV administration of dexamethasone may cause perineal burning or itching May cause anxiety or insomnia
Methylprednisolone	250–500 mg IV	
Benzodiazepines		
Lorazepam (Ativan)	Add to other regimens for level 3–5 chemotherapy: 1–1.5 mg/m² IV (maximum 3 mg) or 1 mg IV or sublingual	Higher doses may be extremely sedating; use in caution with ambulatory individuals and those taking other sedating drugs More efficacious in younger adults, who may experience fewer side effects
Cannabinoid		
Dronabinol (Marinol)	Acute N&V (level 2 chemotherapy): 2.5–10 mg bid/tid	Second- or third-line antiemetic, or adjuvant agent Monitor dosing carefully because of adverse effects

D5W = 5% dextrose in water; EPS = extrapyramidal symptoms.

and splanchnic nerves in the GI tract and CTZ for approximately 24 hours, which blocks the message to vomit from being transmitted to the VC. This occurs because 5HT released from the enterochromaffin cells in response to emetogenic stimuli (chemotherapy or radiation therapy to the GI tract) cannot bind with the 5HT$_3$ receptors.

Indications The major indication for intravenous and oral 5HT$_3$ antagonists is to prevent N&V (or to stop emesis after onset) caused by moderately to highly emetogenic chemotherapy.[54,55] These agents are not standard first-line therapy for less emetogenic chemotherapy, but can be used as second-line antiemetic therapy for patients

TABLE 14-6   Antiemetics in Palliative Cancer Care

Class/Drug	Site of action/ receptor	Doses	Indications	Comments/adverse effects
Phenothiazines				

Thiethylperazine	CTZ/D_2	10 mg PO, PR, IM q4–8h	1st line:
			    opioids
			    other drugs
			    bowel obstruction
			    radiation therapy
				• Side effects do not correlate with dose

Prochlorperazine		5–20 mg PO q4–6h, 25 mg PR q6–8h, 5–15 mg IM/IV q4–6h		• Oral dose: poor bioavailability • IM painful, IV desirable • Irritating, cannot be given CSQI

Perphenazine		2–8 mg PO q6–8h, 5–10 mg IM q4–8h	$\geq$ 2nd line:
			    vestibular
			    chronic unexplained
			        nausea of cancer
				• Hypotension (with IV) greater in patients with dehydration, cardiac disease

Chlorpromazine	CTZ/D_2
	$alpha_1$
		10–50 mg PO q4–6h, 25–100 mg PR q6–8h, 25–50 mg IM/IV q2–4h	chlorpromazine:
			    hiccups
			    uremia
			    hypercalcemia
			    hyponatremia
				• Most sedation with chlorpromazine and methotrimeprazine; use when sedation is desirable or only at night

Methotrimeprazine		? doses		
Benzamides				

Metoclopramide*	CTZ/D_2
	$GI/5HT_3$, $5HT_4$
		Begin dosing at 10 mg PO tid or ac and hs, increase to 10–40 q4–6h; 10 IV q2–4h	Primary indications:
			    opioids
			    hepatomegaly leading to
			        gastric compression
			        with nausea and
			        anorexia
			    radiation therapy
			    chronic unexplained
			        hiccups
			    gastric stasis
				• Can administer CSQI, used for chronic unexplained nausea of cancer: start 10 mg/day and increase prn
				• Compatible with MSO_4
				• Side effects may limit high doses

Cisapride	$GI/5HT_4$	? doses		• Can combine with phenothiazine/haloperidol for increased effect; EPS rare • Contraindicated if bowel obstruction • Hypotension greater if patient dehydrated • EPS increases with multiple-day use, younger, and female patients • Cisapride does not cross into CNS, so no D_2 side effects
Butyrophenone				
Haloperidol*	CTZ/D_2	0.5–2 q4–8h	Same as phenothiazines	• See phenothiazines • Less sedating than most phenothiazines • Can administer CSQI for chronic unexplained nausea of cancer: start 20 mg/day and increase prn • Compatible with MSO_4 • Effectiveness may vary with dose; titrate up or down prn

(continued)

TABLE 14-6 Antiemetics in Palliative Cancer Care (continued)

Class/Drug	Site of action/ receptor	Doses	Indications	Comments/adverse effects
Antimuscarinic/Anticholinergic				
Hyoscine*	vestibular/H_1 VC/M_1	0.3–1.2 mg IM q6h (usual 0.6), transdermal q72h	1st line: position/motion ≧2nd line: bowel obstruction abdominal cancer liver disease opioids	• Can administer CSQI: start at 5 mg/day • Compatible with MSO_4 • Both are sedating, so start one at a time
Antihistamines				
Promethazine*	? H_1, D_2, M_1	25–50 mg PO, PR, or IM q4–6h	1st line: position/motion ≥ 2nd line: ↑ICP opioids hepatomegaly gastric compression with nausea and anorexia biliary obstruction	• Promethazine has a higher rate of anticholinergic side effects than other phenothiazines; EPS rare
Cyclizine	H_1	50 mg PO, IM q4–6h, 100 mg PR q4–6h		
Diphenhydramine	H_1	25–100 mg PO q4–6h, 10–50 mg IV, IM q4–8h		
Corticosteroids				
Dexamethasone	CNS/GABA	4–20 mg IV, PO q4–6h	1st line: ↑ICP meningeal metastases hepatomegaly gastric compression with nausea and anorexia stomach cancer 2nd line: GI obstruction (pylorus; small, large bowel) hypercalcemia opioids	• Rapid IV may cause transient perineal, perioral, or abdominal burning, itching • Do not cause classical steroid side effects, even in high doses, over short periods • Can cause increase in sense of well-being, anxiety, or insomnia • If not effective in 3–4 days, discontinue
Anxiolytics				
Lorazepam*	CNS/benzodi-azepine receptor	PO, SL, IV	Emotional factors Amnesia desired N&V accompanied by agitation	• Antiemetic effect may be related to sedative effects • Do not give diazepam IM
Diazepam		PO, IV		
Serotonin Antagonists				
Ondansetron	GI, CNS/5HT_3	IV, PO	No clear indications ? postoperative ? delayed (day 2)	• Use when trials of escalated doses of other antiemetics are ineffective • No established doses • Constipation increased with chronic use
Granisetron				
Other				
Benzquinamide	unknown	50 mg (or .5–1 mg/kg) IM, repeat in 1h, then q3–4h	≧2nd line: bowel obstruction opioid, other drug chronic unexplained nausea of cancer	• Use when other antiemetics have been ineffective or caused excessive side effects

*Drugs of choice (Lichter, 1993).[37]

CSQI = continuous subcutaneous infusion; EPS = extrapyramidal symptoms; ↑ICP = increased intracranial pressure; MSO_4 = morphine sulfate; PO = oral; PR = rectal; SL = sublingual.

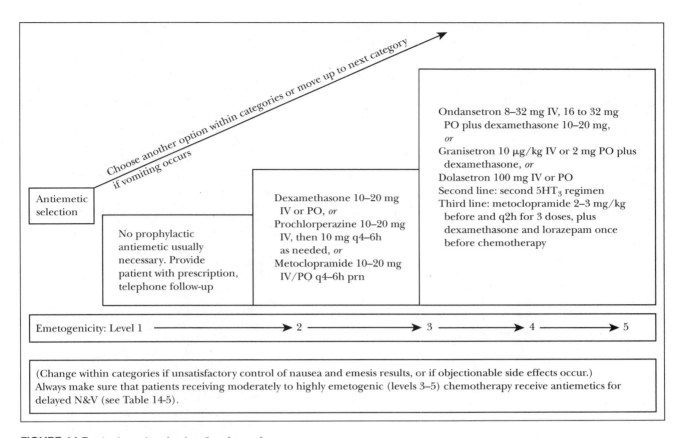

FIGURE 14-7 Antiemetic selection for chemotherapy.

who experienced N&V or had objectionable side effects after receiving a non-5HT$_3$ antagonist regimen. In addition, 5HT$_3$ antagonists are indicated to prevent N&V from radiation therapy to the epigastric area, abdomen, and pelvis, for TBI,[56] and for postanesthesia N&V in some instances.[57] However, there are limited indications for delayed/persistent N&V from chemotherapy, for N&V from other drugs, and for N&V related to terminal cancer. When N&V are caused by mechanisms that are not related to 5HT release, such as opioid-related N&V and motion sickness, 5HT$_3$ antagonists will probably not be effective.

After chemotherapy, ondansetron, granisetron, or dolasetron are similarly efficacious in adults, and reported rates of complete control of emesis range from about 40% to 80%.[16,28,58–66] Differences in response rates in these studies were influenced by highly emetogenic chemotherapy (decreased control), gender (poorer in women), and age (poor control in younger individuals). Furthermore, in all studies control of nausea was inferior to control of vomiting. In studies that defined complete control as "no emesis and no greater than mild nausea," complete control therefore reflected the number of individuals who had little or no nausea.

The 5HT$_3$ antagonists are also safe and effective for children. Nausea and vomiting are prevented in approximately 75% of children after standard-dose chemotherapy, and in 50% after high-dose chemotherapy plus TBI

who have received 5HT$_3$ antagonists.[67–69] There is little research to substantiate optimal doses and schedules of 5HT$_3$ antagonists for children, who may require larger doses than adults. Evidence for this is that children who received 10 µg/kg of granisetron experienced breakthrough vomiting after chemotherapy sooner than those who received higher doses (20 and 40 µg/kg).[70]

Oral and intravenous 5HT$_3$ antagonists are more effective than other antiemetics (i.e., oral metoclopramide 10 mg tid or prochlorperazine 10 mg tid) to prevent radiation therapy–induced N&V. For example, 58 to 92% of persons who took oral ondansetron (8 mg tid) for fractionated radiation therapy to the upper epigastric area had no vomiting during their entire treatment.[31,71,72] Granisetron was also shown to be superior to metoclopramide, dexamethasone, and lorazepam for TBI, and rates of complete control (no vomiting and no or mild nausea) were 53.3% and only 13.3%, respectively.[73]

Many individuals who have cancer undergo surgery, which may or may not be related to their malignancy. Risk factors for postoperative N&V include female gender (women are three times more likely to vomit than men), younger age (including children), obesity, a history of motion sickness, highly anxious persons, and a past history of postoperative N&V.[57,74] 5HT$_3$ antagonists effectively reduce the risk for postanesthesia N&V in these individuals.[75–78] Ondansetron (4 mg IV before or during anesthesia) and dolasetron (100 mg within 2 hours before surgery) are FDA-approved for postoperative N&V. In one study, ondansetron 8 mg was superior to 4 mg,[76] so a higher dose may be indicated for some individuals. In addition, lower doses of dolasetron (12.5 mg, 25 mg, and 50 mg) are as effective as 100 mg,[77] so the optimal dose of dolasetron may be much lower than the dose recommended by the manufacturer.

Other potential uses Because of high cost, 5HT$_3$ antagonists should not routinely be used for delayed and persistent N&V from chemotherapy, as they are usually no more effective than other antiemetics (such as metoclopramide) after cisplatin or other chemotherapy, or for the second and subsequent days of fractionated chemotherapy.[26,79,80] These findings support the hypothesis that delayed N&V are mediated by other than 5HT$_3$ mechanisms. On the other hand, the number of women who required rescue antiemetics or who experienced multiple, delayed emeses after chemotherapy for breast cancer was lower after oral ondansetron than after placebo.[81] Clinical experience also demonstrates that oral ondansetron (8 mg bid or tid) sometimes controls delayed N&V when other antiemetics have failed. The recommended dose of ondansetron for delayed N&V is 8 mg PO bid, but in one study of 297 patients, both 4 mg and 8 mg tid prevented emesis (over 3 days) in approximately 65% of patients.[16] 5HT$_3$ antagonists are most effective on day 1 of fractionated chemotherapy, and control of vomiting decreases substantially on subsequent days.[82] Nonetheless, most clinicians would administer a low dose of 5HT$_3$ antagonist, such as ondansetron 8 mg once a day or bid, on each day of fractionated chemotherapy.

There is little evidence to substantiate that 5HT$_3$ antagonists are effective for N&V of terminal disease. However, a few case reports illustrate that they may be useful in combination with other antiemetics (e.g., haloperidol, dexamethasone) for patients in whom conventional antiemetics have failed to control N&V.[83–85] Indications may include intractable vomiting for which a cause cannot be determined, failure to respond to all other standard antiemetics (e.g., metoclopramide, cyclizine, haloperidol, dexamethasone), and clear indication that the 5HT$_3$ is beneficial (vomiting resumes if the 5HT$_3$ antagonist is discontinued) and that control can be achieved with conversion to an oral 5HT$_3$ antagonist. There is no standard dose for these indications, but it would seem prudent to use the lowest effective doses. Thus, if a high intravenous dose is initially administered and results in control of N&V, subsequent doses might be reduced and/or converted to a single oral dose each day. This would reduce not only costs, but also the risk for side effects, particularly constipation.

Side effects 5HT$_3$ antagonists have a similar and relatively tolerable adverse effect profile. The most common side effects are headache, constipation, lightheadedness, and sedation.[16,63–65] Headache occurs in as many as 40% of patients after receiving a 5HT$_3$ antagonist and

seems to be more prevalent with rapid administration (<10 minutes) of ondansetron. Constipation occurs in 3% to 20% of patients, because 5HT$_3$ antagonists slow colonic transit time; it is more common when these agents are administered for several days. A lightheaded feeling has been documented in up to 21% of patients, and sedation may occur in 10% to 40% of patients. Sedation is less severe with 5HT$_3$ antagonists than with other antiemetics such as metoclopramide, and more than half of patients treated with ondansetron specifically commented that the lack of sedation, when compared to a previous antiemetic, was a desirable feature.[86] Low sedation may not only be important in terms of patient comfort (and potentially QOL), but also in terms of safety (e.g., decreased falls, fractures). 5HT$_3$ antagonists are more likely to be associated with normal appetite after chemotherapy than other antiemetics.

Infrequent side effects include dizziness, diarrhea (which may have been related to cisplatin), tremor, anxiety, and cardiovascular effects.[16,87] Only the dolasetron package insert has a warning about potential ECG changes, but this may not reflect true differences in the potential for cardiovascular effects among 5HT$_3$ antagonists. These effects were not documented before approval of ondansetron and granisetron, and cardiovascular effects of intravenous 5HT$_3$ antagonists have since been examined. One study compared granisetron and ondansetron, and two subjects (one in each group) experienced transient elevations in systolic blood pressure.[88] Mean corrected QT intervals (QT$_c$) after ondansetron were significantly longer than those after granisetron, but differences in pre- and post-QT$_c$ intervals were approximately 7 msec and were not clinically significant. Similar findings were documented in another study that compared IV dolasetron (1.2, 1.8, and 2.4 mg/kg) with ondansetron 32 mg.[89] There were statistically significant postantiemetic differences in PR, QRS, and QT$_c$ intervals after dolasetron but not after ondansetron. Again, changes were transient and not clinically significant. Because nonspecific serotonin antagonists, including tricyclic antidepressants, can lead to delayed cardiac repolarization and ventricular arrhythmias,[88] the nurse should consider that patients who have a cardiac history *might* be at risk for arrhythmias with any 5HT$_3$ antagonist.

Administration considerations Important administration considerations for 5HT$_3$ antagonists are schedule, dose, and cost. Dose-finding studies of ondansetron demonstrated that three doses (administered every 2, 4, or 8 hours) were similarly effective in preventing emesis.[58,90] It is now agreed that because there is no relationship between serum levels of drug and antiemetic control, repeated doses of 5HT$_3$ antagonists are not necessary.[54,55] Two recent studies clearly demonstrated the superiority of a single large dose over divided doses: When dolasetron 1.8 mg/kg was administered as a single dose, 48% of patients did not vomit, while only 23% of those who received the same total dose but in three divided doses did not vomit.[91] Furthermore, patients who received the divided doses vomited earlier (median time to emesis 10 hours versus >24 hours). In a second study, patients received either one or two doses of oral dolasetron 200 mg plus dexamethasone.[92] The same percentage of patients (76%) did not vomit whether they received one dose before chemotherapy or a second dose 12 hours later. Thus, the most important factor in achieving optimal antiemetic control is to administer a sufficiently high dose to block a maximal number of receptors before therapy is given. Multiple or as-needed doses or continuous infusions of $5HT_3$ antagonists are not indicated.

While there is no compelling evidence for the overall superiority of any $5HT_3$ antagonist, this does not necessarily mean that a single, least expensive drug should be used in a treatment setting. Ondansetron, granisetron, and dolasetron are not structurally identical, and recommended doses of each depend on relative binding affinity for the $5HT_3$ receptor. Structural differences may result in differences in therapeutic efficacy and side effects in particular patients. Ondansetron, for example, has some agonist activity at the $5HT_4$ receptor and thus increases gastric motility, while granisetron and dolasetron do not.[54] Furthermore, crossover studies have shown that patients who do not attain adequate antiemetic control with a first $5HT_3$ antagonist may achieve satisfactory control with a second $5HT_3$ antagonist.[59,61,93,94]

Cost of $5HT_3$ antagonists can be lowered by using lower doses of IV ondansetron, or by using oral formulations of ondansetron, granisetron, or dolasetron. Some studies have shown that IV doses of ondansetron 8 to 24 mg (with or without dexamethasone) are as effective for moderately to moderately high emetogenic chemotherapy as 32 mg is for highly emetogenic chemotherapy,[27,95,96] while other studies have found lower doses to be less effective than 32 mg.[58] Based on this evidence, some institutions have implemented antiemetic guidelines that include lower doses of ondansetron for moderately emetogenic chemotherapy,[97] and one consensus paper recommends a single intravenous dose of ondansetron 8 mg (or granisetron 10 μg/kg IV, or granisetron 2 mg PO, or dolasetron 1.8 mg/kg IV) for highly emetogenic chemotherapy.[55] Doses of intravenous granisetron or intravenous dolasetron cannot be down-dosed, because they are marketed at their optimal doses. Thus, a single dose of IV granisetron 10 μg/kg before moderately to highly emetogenic chemotherapy is used in the United States, which is as effective as the higher dose used in Europe.[63] Dolasetron is most effective at doses of 1.8 mg/kg or 100 mg.[55,98]

Not only are single oral doses of $5HT_3$ antagonists as effective as multiple oral doses, but they are also as effective as single or multiple intravenous doses. For instance, granisetron 2 mg PO once before chemotherapy was equivalent to ondansetron 32 mg IV to prevent emesis from cyclophosphamide- or carboplatin-based chemotherapy,[99] and from cisplatin-based chemotherapy.[100] In both studies, complete prevention of emesis was approximately 60 to 65% for all patients. In addition, another large study found that oral dolasetron 100 and 200 mg were equivalent for moderately high emetogenic chemotherapy.[101] Single large doses of oral ondansetron have not been compared to another intravenous $5HT_3$ antagonist, but 86% of patients who had received cisplatin 40 to 80 mg/m² and 57% of those who received moderately emetogenic chemotherapy had no emesis after receiving ondansetron 8 mg PO for three doses (plus dexamethasone).[102,103] Oral $5HT_3$ antagonists (to be used within 48 hours of chemotherapy) are now paid for by Medicare as full replacement for intravenous $5HT_3$ antagonists if the oral antiemetic is dispensed by the physician.

Dopamine antagonists

Several classes of drugs, including metoclopramide, phenothiazines, and butyrophenones, bind to dopamine (D_2) receptors in the area postrema and block impulses to vomit from being transmitted to the VC. D_2 antagonists are useful for N&V induced from a variety of causes such as low to moderate emetogenic chemotherapy, delayed N&V, radiation therapy, and N&V from other causes. D_2 antagonists bind with other receptors (sometimes with equivalent or greater affinity), which may enhance their antiemetic effect as well as increase adverse effects.[39,104,105] For example, binding at $5HT_3$, $5HT_4$, muscarinic cholinergic receptors may enhance the antiemetic effect, whereas binding at the alpha$_1$ adrenergic receptors causes sedation, dizziness, and orthostasis.[37] In addition, binding histamine (H_1) receptors may result in sedation and anticholinergic effects (e.g., dry mouth, constipation, nasal congestion).

The major disadvantages for all D_2 antagonist antiemetics are that they may cause EPS and are often administered in complex regimens. The most common manifestation of EPS is akathisia, sometimes called "dancing legs." Akathisia may range from a feeling of inner disquiet to an inability to sit still at all. Less commonly, dystonia occurs and is manifested as torticollis or spasm of the lower jaw. This can be very frightening, and patients feel like they cannot breathe. EPS is preventable or reversible in most people. Diphenhydramine (Benadryl) 25 to 50 mg PO or IV, or benztropine (Cogentin) 1–2 mg IV, will reverse dystonia, while a benzodiazepine (lorazepam [Ativan] or diazepam [Valium]) is more useful to reverse akathisia.[21]

Metoclopramide Metoclopramide (Reglan), a substituted benzamide, exerts a direct antiemetic effect on D_2 receptors in the CTZ, and indirectly decreases vomiting by accelerating gastric emptying and increasing small bowel transit (via prokinetic activity at the $5HT_4$ receptor).[54] Metoclopramide also has weak $5HT_3$-antagonist activity, which is confirmed by the finding that cisplatin-treated patients vomit sooner after receiving metoclopramide than after receiving a $5HT_3$ antagonist.[21]

Indications Metoclopramide is a valuable drug and may be useful in controlling acute and delayed N&V,

as well as N&V of terminal illness. Metoclopramide is indicated for the prevention of acute N&V caused by mild to moderately emetogenic chemotherapy but is inferior to 5HT$_3$ antagonists for highly emetogenic chemotherapy such as high-dose cisplatin.[26,106,107]

Oral metoclopramide 10 to 20 mg tid or qid for 4 or 5 days (in combination with a corticosteroid) is recommended for delayed N&V. It is equally or more efficacious than a 5HT$_3$ antagonist for delayed N&V from cisplatin and other chemotherapy[27,94] and for day 2 through day 5 of fractionated cisplatin-based chemotherapy.[83] A related drug, cisapride (Propulsid), does not cross into the blood-brain barrier and thus does not cause EPS; it may be useful for some patients.[37] However, because cisapride is more expensive than metoclopramide, it would be used as second-line therapy. These agents may be advantageous during delayed nausea because they have 5HT$_4$ agonist activity, which might decrease gastroparesis during the prokinetic-sensitive phase after chemotherapy.[41]

Other potential uses Metoclopramide is also useful for N&V from other causes, including gastric stasis or irritation, incomplete or high gastrointestinal obstruction, or unexplained chronic nausea.[38,108–110] In addition to its broad antiemetic spectrum, metoclopramide has a short half-life and a reasonable oral and rectal bioavailability (about 60%–80% of oral and rectal doses are bioavailable).[111] Thus, oral administration is used to prevent N&V, while parenteral or rectal administration can be used when the patient cannot take oral medications or when they have severe N&V. When N&V are intractable, metoclopramide can be administered as a continuous subcutaneous infusion (CSQI).[4]

Metoclopramide is not useful for N&V from labyrinthine disorders such as motion sickness, intestinal obstruction, and radiation therapy. Metoclopramide and cisapride are contraindicated when complete internal obstruction and obstipation are suspected or documented, because they accelerate gastric emptying and may increase the colicky pain associated with obstruction.[110] In addition, there is no published evidence that demonstrates that metoclopramide is useful to control radiation therapy–induced N&V.

Adverse effects EPS from metoclopramide occurs more often in children and younger adults than in older persons, and in women more often than men.[105,111] Diphenhydramine or lorazepam are administered to decrease the risk for EPS, but these drugs increase sedation and anticholinergic effects. The sedation may be profound, so the patient must have a caregiver/driver accompany them to the clinic, and safety will be a continuing concern after the patient returns home. Other adverse effects of metoclopramide may include hiccups, facial flushing, headache, and restlessness.[112]

Administration considerations Recommended doses of metoclopramide vary depending on the emetogenicity of the chemotherapy and whether it is being used for acute, delayed, or N&V related to other causes. Because they are complex to administer and are likely to cause side effects, high-dose metoclopramide-based regimens (2 mg/kg IV for three to five doses or 3 mg/kg IV for two doses) are indicated only for second- or third-line antiemetic therapy in patients receiving moderately high to highly emetogenic chemotherapy.[21] Administration takes several hours and thus requires more nursing resources and intravenous supplies; it also requires the patient to stay in the clinic longer.

A corticosteroid and either lorazepam (or other benzodiazepine) or diphenhydramine would be included in a high-dose metoclopramide regimen to decrease the risk for EPS and increase efficacy. The combination is almost as effective as a 5HT$_3$ antagonist alone.[107] The gender effect also occurs with metoclopramide, and approximately twice as many men as women do *not* have nausea (63% versus 38%, respectively) or vomiting (93% versus 54%, respectively).[112] Efficacy is offset by the antiemetic side effects, including sedation, decreased appetite, and perhaps EPS. There is no advantage to administering metoclopramide by continuous infusion, because this method is no more effective than bolus doses[112] but is more time consuming and technology dependent.

Phenothiazines Phenothiazines (single agent) are useful for acute N&V caused by mildly emetogenic chemotherapy, for delayed and persistent N&V, for radiation therapy–related N&V, and for N&V in terminal disease. Prochlorperazine (Compazine) is the phenothiazine most often studied, but other drugs in this class, including thiethylperazine (Torecan) and perphenazine (Trilafon), are useful. Prochlorperazine exerts a dose-related antiemetic effect, and higher-than-standard doses (20–40 mg IV) completely control vomiting in about 54% of those receiving moderately severe emetogenic chemotherapy.[21,113]

Indications Although phenothiazines are not useful as a single agent for highly emetogenic chemotherapy, there is evidence that adding one of these agents to a 5HT$_3$ antagonist–containing regimen increases antiemetic control from moderately to highly emetogenic chemotherapy.[114–116] A small dose (i.e., prochlorperazine, 15 mg, 60 minutes before and 12 hours after chemotherapy) enhances therapeutic effect without causing objectionable side effects.[116] Phenothiazines are useful to control delayed N&V. Sustained-release prochlorperazine (Compazine spansules 15–30 mg bid or tid) are taken on day 2 and day 3, and then 15-mg spansules bid for another 2 or 3 days.

Phenothiazines have been termed "all-purpose antiemetics" for N&V of terminal illness because they have affinity for alpha$_1$, M$_1$, and H$_1$, as well as D$_2$ receptors.[37] Multiple receptor effects may enhance the usefulness of phenothiazines, because the CTZ is assumed to play a primary role in N&V from opioids and other drugs, metabolic abnormalities, bowel obstruction, and postoperative N&V.[38,105,110] Efforts should be made to determine the cause(s), even when N&V are suspected to be multicausal. In this way, the most potent antiemetic for each recognized or probable cause can be administered, rather than selecting a multipurpose but less effective antiemetic.[37] Agents with high affinity for D_2 receptors and low affinities for other receptors (thiethylperazine, fluphenazine, and prochlorperazine) should be selected for most patients, because these agents are the least sedating. Conversely, when sedation is desirable, chlorpromazine—which has a higher affinity for alpha$_1$ than for D_2 receptors—is the drug of choice.[109] Another phenothiazine, methotrimeprazine (Levoprome) has analgesic as well as antiemetic properties. It is extremely sedating and can cause orthostasis. Thus, it is reserved as a drug of choice in hospice patients in whom N&V are severe and in whom sedation is also desirable (i.e., terminal restlessness or intractable N&V).[117] When a phenothiazine is initiated for N&V in terminal care, it is started at a relatively low dose, particularly if the patient is elderly.[105] If the original dose is inadequate, it may be carefully escalated until the patient experiences adequate control of N&V or until intolerable side effects occur.[37]

Administration considerations   Intravenous administration of prochlorperazine is safe and rarely causes postural hypotension. The risk can be minimized by making certain that the patient is adequately hydrated and by administering prochlorperazine to the recumbent patient. Higher intravenous doses increase the risk for sedation and perhaps EPS. Parenteral administration (IM and SQ) is painful, and phenothiazines cannot be administered by CSQI because they are irritating.[118] The oral and rectal bioavailability of prochlorperazine is lower than that of similar parenteral doses.[111]

Butyrophenones   Butyrophenones are structurally similar to phenothiazines and are generally used for the same indications. Intravenous droperidol (Inapsine) is useful to control cisplatin-induced N&V, but it causes a high level of sedation. Haloperidol (Haldol) is a wide spectrum antiemetic that is less sedating than droperidol and most phenothiazines. Haloperidol may be useful not only when other antiemetics fail, but in combination with other antiemetics for chemotherapy-induced N&V, for postoperative N&V, and for the management of N&V in the terminally ill individual.[21,105,110] It is an ideal drug for persons in whom sedation could be problematic; for example, the elderly and in opioid-naive individuals who experience N&V with escalations of opioid doses.[107,108] Another advantage of haloperidol is that it can be infused by CSQI, which is generally used when N&V are unrelieved by oral medications.[117]

Corticosteroids

Corticosteroids are extremely useful in controlling N&V from a wide variety of causes, including acute and delayed N&V, postoperative N&V, and N&V of terminal cancer.[38,119–121] How corticosteroids work as antiemetics is not known, but they may have central and peripheral effects. Proposed actions include that they decrease capillary permeability in CNS (specifically the CTZ) to emetic stimuli, deplete the precursor of serotonin (tryptophan) in neural tissue, and prevent release of $5HT_3$ from enterochromaffin cells and activation of $5HT_3$ receptors.[122] These might all be important during the phase of acute N&V. During the delayed phase, corticosteroids might decrease the permeability of the damaged mucosal crypt cells and thereby minimize the escape of emetogens from the gut to the bloodstream and CTZ.[41]

Indications   Corticosteroids may also be used (alone or in combination) to control N&V from other causes. Dexamethasone (Decadron) is the most common corticosteroid used as an antiemetic, but prednisolone and prednisone also effectively decrease N&V. Dexamethasone (oral or IV) is superior to standard-dose prochlorperazine and is as effective as a $5HT_3$ antagonist for moderately emetogenic chemotherapy.[62,123] Single-agent dexamethasone is now considered to be standard antiemetic therapy for such chemotherapy.[57,80] Furthermore, the addition of dexamethasone to other antiemetic regimens increases complete control of acute N&V from moderately to highly emetogenic chemotherapy by approximately 15% to 25%.[119,124]

Oral dexamethasone is equally or more effective than oral ondansetron for delayed N&V[123] and so is used alone or in combination. In addition, corticosteroids decrease N&V associated with TBI. Indications for palliative use include N&V from increased intracranial pressure, gastrointestinal obstruction, and biochemical problems (e.g., hypercalcemia, uremia).[37,109,110] Doses in such instances range from 8 to 60 mg/day.

Administration considerations   Dexamethasone is compatible with metoclopramide, ondansetron, and granisetron in IV solutions. There is no agreement regarding the minimally effective or optimal dose and schedule of dexamethasone.[125] Doses typically range from 8 to 20 mg IV or PO. Single or multiple doses are similarly effective.[109] No major adverse effects have been substantiated with short-term use of corticosteroids as antiemetics, and there is no evidence that using corticosteroids causes immunosuppression or enhances tumor progression.

Adverse effects   Rapid IV administration of dexamethasone may cause the patient to experience perineal or perioral burning, tingling, or itching, which may be decreased by administering dexamethasone over several minutes. A major advantage of corticosteroids is that they are nonsedating and in fact may cause insomnia. They may increase appetite and enhance the sense of well-being (or conversely cause dysphoria).

Benzodiazepines

Benzodiazepines have modest antiemetic effects and thus are usually used in combination with other antiemetics. Lorazepam (Ativan) is most commonly used. The exact mechanism of benzodiazepines is not known, but they do bind with gamma-aminobutyric acid$_2$ (GABA$_2$) receptors that are widely distributed throughout the CNS (cortex, reticular formation, and limbic region).[105]

Indications   Lorazepam decreases anxiety and agitation and may alter the recollection of N&V, which may be the reason that lorazepam is useful to minimize ANV.[125] Benzodiazepines are occasionally recommended for N&V of terminal illness that is exacerbated by anxiety related to progressive physical disease.[4] There are no clear dose recommendations for terminally ill persons, but an initial dose of lorazepam might be 1 to 2 mg PO or IV every 6 to 8 hours, and the dose titrated as necessary.[38] Lorazepam may be administered orally, but to achieve a rapid and similar effect to intravenous administration, it should be given sublingually.

Adverse effects   Intravenous administration may cause some persons to experience adverse effects, including perceptual disturbances, urinary incontinence, hypotension, and sedation. Benzodiazepines can cause respiratory depression and so should be administered carefully to patients receiving other CNS depressant drugs.

Cannabinoids

There are two cannabinoids, but only dronabinol (Marinol) is available commercially in the United States. Cannabinoids are equivalent to or slightly more efficacious than standard doses (10 mg PO or IV) of prochlorperazine[125] and are generally used as second- or third-line agents for moderately emetogenic chemotherapy. In rare instances, cannabinoids may be used for N&V of terminal illness. There is no evidence for their use to prevent N&V from radiation. The mechanism of antiemetic action of cannabinoids is not clear, and it is possible that they act at specific cannabinoid receptors in the cortex, hippocampus, and hypothalamus to inhibit cyclic adenosine monophosphate (cAMP), or at opioid receptors.[105]

Indications   Cannabinoids have been useful to control intractable N&V from gastrointestinal mucosal metastases.[126] Low doses are recommended for progressively or terminally ill persons. For example, dronabinol 5 mg before meals and at bedtime completely controlled previously intractable vomiting in individuals with HIV. Cannabinoids also have an appetite stimulant effect, and so may be used for this purpose.

Adverse effects   There are several reasons why cannabinoids are not widely used. Dronabinol is formulated for oral administration, which limits use in the vomiting person (the gel caps can be broken and the drug instilled on the buccal space). In addition, dronabinol is a class II drug and thus requires a triplicate prescription in some states. At the recommended dose for chemotherapy (5–10 mg/m^2 qid), adverse effects including depersonalization, drowsiness, dizziness, euphoria or dysphoria, loss of coor-

dination, dry mouth, and postural hypotension may be dose limiting.[106,127] Therefore, it may be more prudent to start dronabinol at 5 mg/m^2 and carefully titrate upward to maximal effect (or adverse effects).

Other antiemetics

Agents that act at histamine (H$_1$) receptors (dimenhydrinate, diphenhydramine, hydroxyzine, and promethazine) or muscarinic cholinergic (M) receptors (scopolamine) are most commonly used for palliative management and for postoperative N&V. These drugs are useful for N&V from vestibular and motion/position disorders, for N&V secondary to liver disease, for opioid-related N&V, and for N&V from gastrointestinal obstruction.[37,108,110] H$_1$- and M-receptor antagonists have minimal activity for N&V from chemotherapy, but H$_1$ agents are used to minimize EPS. Scopolamine is occasionally used as late-line treatment for chemotherapy-related N&V.[111] One other antiemetic, benzquinamide (Emete-con), is occasionally used to manage N&V. Although there is no research to support its use for chemotherapy, it is unrelated to phenothiazines and thus may be useful as second-line treatment for persons who experience EPS with D$_2$ antagonists.[109] Trimethobenzamide (Tigan), on the other hand, is considered to be a relatively ineffective antiemetic. The adverse effects of antihistamines and anticholinergics are similar and include sedation, dry mouth, and constipation. Dry mouth may be alleviated by oral fluids or ice chips.

Nonpharmacologic Interventions

Antiemetics are the cornerstone for managing N&V, but nonpharmacologic interventions often enhance the patients' sense of self-control as well as antiemetic effect. The interventions that have been advocated include behavioral interventions, acupressure, and dietary modifications.

Behavioral interventions

Behavioral interventions have been used to successfully treat a variety of cancer-related symptoms, most commonly ANV from chemotherapy.[128,129] The three types of interventions are relaxation with guided imagery (includes hypnosis, passive relaxation, active relaxation, and EMG biofeedback), systematic desensitization, and attentional distraction. The last two specifically require a trained therapist, usually a psychologist. Relaxation techniques may be taught by a nurse, physician, social worker, psychologist, or another individual, and are thus used more frequently. These techniques may be useful adjuncts with antiemetics to prevent acute and delayed N&V, but they have not been systematically tested. Even if nurses wish to use behavioral interventions, there are no clinical guidelines for patient selection or means by which to decide which interventions might be combined.[128]

Acupressure

There is a small but growing body of research that suggests acupressure (transcutaneous electrical and manual) is effective alone or with an antiemetic in enhancing the antiemetic effects of ondansetron, metoclopramide, and phenothiazines for chemotherapy, bone marrow transplantation, and surgery.[130–132] Control of acute and delayed N&V is better with the combination of ondansetron and acupressure than with ondansetron alone. Acupressure is useful to decrease postoperative N&V and N&V from chemotherapy.

Nurses can inform their patients about acupressure, which involves stimulation of the P6, or Neiguan point, of the dominant arm. The P6 point is located on the inner wrist about three fingerbreadths above the skin crease of the wrist, between the tendons of the palmaris longus and flexor carpi radialis. Acupressure bands are commercially available. They are adjustable elastic wrist bands equipped with a stud that is placed over the P6 point (on one or both wrists).

Dietary interventions

Nurses often recommend dietary modifications to patients receiving chemotherapy.[133] Dietary modifications are useful adjuncts to antiemetics and must be individualized for each patient. Examples include capitalizing on interventions the patients used for past episodes of N&V (such as with pregnancy, illness, or during stressful periods). Suggestions regarding food intake include eating cold or room-temperature foods, as these give off fewer odors than do hot foods. Related suggestions are that patients cook meals between chemotherapy regimens when they are not nauseated and freeze them for later use, or that they have another family member cook meals. The types of foods eaten during periods of nausea may decrease or increase symptoms. High fat content in foods delays gastric emptying, which may increase nausea. Sour foods may increase comfort, whereas spicy, salty, or sweet foods may exacerbate N&V.[133] Favorite foods should be avoided on the day of chemotherapy and while N&V persist, so that food aversions to them do not develop.

Another dietary suggestion is ginger, which is known in folk medicine to decrease N&V. One study found that ginger capsules (1 g), which are available in health food stores or in vitamin sections of other stores, were more likely than placebo—to a statistically significant degree—to prevent postoperative N&V.[134]

Education Tools

Appendix 14A provides a baseline assessment tool for patients receiving chemotherapy that is completed by the nurse and the patient. Appendix 14B is a chemotherapy treatment diary that can be given to the patient.

Self-care guides are included for patients experiencing N&V from chemotherapy (Appendix 14C), radiation therapy (Appendix 14D), and from cancer (Appendix 14E).

Conclusion

Optimal control of N&V in the person with cancer requires that caregivers use a wide variety of drugs, depending on the etiology of N&V. Adjunctive nonpharmacologic measures may increase control of N&V with few or no added adverse effects. Management must be, to a great extent, individualized. Strategies to manage acute N&V from chemotherapy and N&V of terminal disease may differ widely. For the patient receiving chemotherapy, the nurse and physician consider emetogenicity and the possibility of delayed N&V, and plan regimens accordingly. Patients who receive level 2 chemotherapy or higher should receive prophylactic antiemetics (see Table 14-5). For palliative management of N&V, the etiology must be established whenever possible so that appropriate antiemetics are used. Concepts regarding optimal antiemetic management include:

- Baseline assessment for risk of N&V is critical. No matter what the cause, menstruating women are likely to have N&V that is poorly controlled. Age younger than 60 years may also increase risk.

- Treat prophylactically. Administer antiemetics around the clock or at a schedule considering mechanisms of action (i.e., once a day for $5HT_3$ antagonists).

- Reassess frequently for degree of control of both N&V, adverse effects of antiemetics, and satisfaction with regimen.

- In palliative care, establish the cause of N&V; if unable to establish cause, start with a nonsedating phenothiazine or butyrophenone.

- Nausea and vomiting from any cause are likely mediated by more than one mechanism; thus, combination antiemetic therapy will be more effective than single-agent therapy.

- Consider the bioavailability of the dosage form used. Oral and rectal bioavailability may be high or low, requiring dose adjustments when drugs are administered by these routes.

- Select the "best" agent from each class in combination therapy; that is, choose the drugs that are most likely to result in the control of N&V ($\pm$ sedation) without excessive adverse effects.

- Escalate doses of selected antiemetic before switching to an alternate drug within a class or to another class of antiemetics.

- Although classified by major action at one receptor, antiemetics typically act at more than one receptor, which produces other effects (therapeutic and adverse).

- The oral route is easy and the least expensive; it is used for mild N&V and for prophylaxis.
- Use parenteral antiemetics for patients unable to take oral antiemetics (e.g., because of uncontrolled N&V, gastrointestinal obstruction, altered mental status).
- Avoid repeated SQ/IM injections, as they are painful.
- Rectal or vaginal administration of suppositories or oral tablets is better for terminally ill persons.
- Continuous SQ infusion of metoclopramide or haloperidol is useful for terminally ill patients who have intractable N&V.
- Explore the addition of nonpharmacologic measures with the patient.

References

1. Martin M: Myths and realities of antiemetic treatment. *Br J Cancer* 19:S46–S50, 1992
2. Lindley CM, Hirsch JD: Nausea and vomiting and cancer patients' quality of life: A discussion of Professor Selby's paper. *Br J Cancer* 66(suppl 19):S26–S29, 1992
3. Reuben DB, Mor V: Nausea and vomiting in terminal cancer patients. *Arch Intern Med* 146:2021–2023, 1986
4. Baines M: Nausea and vomiting in the patient with advanced cancer. *J Pain Symptom Manage* 3:81–85, 1988
5. Cella DF: Quality of life. Concepts and definitions. *J Pain Symptom Manage* 9:186–192, 1994
6. Cooper S, Georgiou V: The impact of cytotoxic chemotherapy—Perspectives from patients, specialists and nurses. *Eur J Cancer* 28A(suppl 1):S36–S38, 1992
7. Johansson S, Steineck G, Hursti T, et al: Aspects of patient care: Interviews with relapse-free testicular patients in Stockholm. *Cancer Nurs* 15:54–60, 1992
8. O'Brien BJ, Rusthoven J, Rocchi A, et al: Impact of chemotherapy-associated nausea and vomiting on patients, functional status and on costs: Survey of five Canadian centres. *Can Med Assoc J* 149:296–302, 1993
9. Lindley CM, Hirsch JD, O'Neill CV, et al: Quality of life consequences of chemotherapy-induced emesis. *Qual Life Res* 1:331–338, 1992
10. Griffen AM, Butow PN, Coates AS, et al: On the receiving end. V. Patient perceptions of the side effects of cancer chemotherapy in 1993. *Ann Oncol* 7:189–195, 1996
11. De Boer-Dennert M, de Wit R, Schmitz PI, et al: Patient perceptions of the side effects of chemotherapy: The influence of 5HT3 antagonists. *Br J Cancer* 76:1055–1061, 1997
12. Gralla RJ: Current issues in the management of nausea and vomiting. *Ann Oncol* 4(suppl 3):S3–S7, 1993
13. du Bois A, Meerpohl HG, Vach W, et al: Course, patterns, and risk factors for chemotherapy-induced emesis in cisplatin-pretreated patients: A study with ondansetron. *Eur J Cancer* 28:450–457, 1992
14. Cubeddu LX: Serotonin mechanisms in chemotherapy-induced emesis in cancer patients. *Oncology* 53(suppl 1):18–25, 1996
15. Fraschini G, Ciociola A, Esparza L, et al: Evaluation of three oral doses of ondansetron in the prevention of nausea and emesis associated with cyclophosphamide-doxorubicin chemotherapy. *J Clin Oncol* 9:1268–1274, 1991
16. Cubeddu LX, Pendergrass K, Ryan T, et al: Efficacy of oral ondansetron, a selective antagonist of 5-HT$_3$ receptors in the treatment of nausea and vomiting associated with cyclophosphamide-based chemotherapy. *Am J Clin Oncol* 17:137–146, 1994
17. Morrow G, Rosenthal SN: Models, mechanisms and management of anticipatory nausea and emesis. *Oncology* 53 (suppl 1):4–7, 1996
18. Cella DF, Pratt A, Holland JC: Persistent anticipatory nausea, vomiting, and anxiety in cured Hodgkin's disease patients after completion of chemotherapy. *Am J Psychiatry* 143:641–643, 1986
19. Ettinger DS: Preventing chemotherapy-induced nausea and vomiting: An update and review of emesis. *Semin Oncol* (suppl 10):6–18, 1995
20. Hesketh PJ, Kris MG, Grunberg SM, et al: Proposal for classifying the acute emetogenicity of cancer chemotherapy. *J Clin Oncol* 15:103–109, 1997
21. Pisters KMS, Kris MG: Treatment-related nausea and vomiting, in Berger A, Portenoy RK, Weissman D (eds): *Principles and Practice of Supportive Oncology.* Philadelphia: Lippincott Raven, 1998, pp. 165–177
22. Navari R, Gandara D, Hesketh P, et al: Comparative clinical trial of granisetron and ondansetron in the prophylaxis of cisplatin-induced emesis. *J Clin Oncol* 13:1242–1248, 1995
23. Latreille J, Stewart D, Laberge F, et al: Dexamethasone improves the efficacy of granisetron in the first 24 h following high-dose cisplatin chemotherapy. *Support Care Cancer* 3:307–312, 1995
24. Ettinger DS, Eisenberg PD, Fitts D, et al: A double-blind comparison of the efficacy of two dose regimens of oral granisetron in preventing acute emesis in patients receiving moderately emetogenic chemotherapy. *Cancer* 78:144–151, 1996
25. Anonymous: Discussion of Dr. Martin's paper. *Br J Cancer* 19:S50–S51, 1992
26. Heron JF, Goedhaes L, Jordaan JP, et al: Oral granisetron alone and in combination with dexamethasone: A double blind randomized comparison against high-dose metoclopramide plus dexamethasone in the prevention of cisplatin induced emesis. *Ann Oncol* 5:579–584, 1994
27. Kaizer L, Warr D, Hoskins P, et al: Effect of schedule and maintenance on the antiemetic efficacy of ondansetron combined with dexamethasone in acute and delayed nausea and emesis in patients receiving moderately emetogenic chemotherapy: A phase III trial by the National Cancer Institute of Canada Clinical Trials Group. *J Clin Oncol* 12:1050–1057, 1994
28. Brown GW, Paes D, Bryson J, et al: The effectiveness of a single intravenous dose of ondansetron. *Oncology* 49:273–278, 1992
29. Goodman M: Risk factors and antiemetic management of chemotherapy-induced nausea and vomiting. *Oncol Nurs Forum* 24(suppl):20–32, 1997
30. King GL, Makale MT: Postirradiation emesis, in Kucharczyk J, Stewart DJ, Miller AD (eds): *Nausea and Vomiting: Recent Research and Clinical Advances.* Boca Raton, FL: CRC Press, 1991, pp. 103–142
31. Robert JT, Priestman TJ: A review of ondansetron in the management of radiotherapy-induced emesis. *Oncology* 50:173–179, 1993

32. Scarantino CW, Ornitz RD, Hoffman LG, et al: On the mechanism of radiation-induced emesis: The role of serotonin. *Int J Radiat Biol Phys* 3:825–830, 1994

33. Harding RK, Young RW, Anno GH: 1993. Radiotherapy-induced emesis, in Andrews PLR, Sanger GJ (eds): *Emesis in Anti-cancer Therapy: Mechanisms and Treatment*. London: Chapman & Hall Medical, 1994, pp. 163–178

34. Scarantino CW, Ornitz RD, Hoffman LG, et al: Radiation-induced emesis: Effect of ondansetron. *Semin Oncol* 19 (suppl 15):38–43, 1992

35. Fainsminger R, Miller MJ, Bruera E: Symptom control during the last week of life on a palliative care unit. *J Palliat Care* 7:3–11, 1991

36. Ventafridda V, Ripamonti C, DeConno F, et al: Symptom prevalence and control during cancer patients' last days of life. *J Palliat Care* 6:7–11, 1990

37. Lichter I: Which antiemetic? *J Palliat Care* 9:42–50, 1993

38. Enck RE: General symptoms in dying patients. Nausea and vomiting, in Enck RE (ed): *The Medical Care of Terminally Ill Patients*. Baltimore: The Johns Hopkins University Press, 1993, pp. 11–17

39. Seynaeve C, DeMulder PHM, Verweij J: Pathophysiology of cytotoxic drug-induced emesis: Far from crystal-clear. *Pharm Weekbl Sci* 13:1–6, 1990

40. Andrews PLR, Davis CJ: The physiology of emesis induced by anti-cancer therapy, in Reynolds DJM, Andrews PLR, Davis CJ (eds): *Serotonin and the Scientific Basis of Anti-emetic Therapy*. London: Oxford Clinical Communications, 1995, pp. 25–49

41. Andrews PLR, Davis CJ: The mechanisms of emesis induced by anti-cancer therapies, in Andrews PLR, Sanger GJ (eds): *Emesis in Anti-cancer Therapy: Mechanisms and Treatment*. London: Chapman & Hall Medical, 1993, pp. 113–155

42. Leslie RA, Reynolds DJM: Neurotransmitters and receptors in the emetic pathway, in Andrews PLR, Sanger GJ (eds): *Emesis in Anti-cancer Treatment: Mechanisms and Treatment*. London: Chapman & Hall Medical: 1993, pp. 91–112

43. Cunningham RS: 5-HT_3-receptor antagonists: A review of pharmacology and clinical efficacy. *Oncol Nurs Forum* 24 (suppl):33–40, 1997

44. du Bois A, Vach W, Holy R, et al: 5-hydroxyindoleacetic acid excretion following combination chemotherapy with cyclophosphamide, epirubicin, and 5-fluorouracil plus ondansetron compared to ondansetron alone. *Support Care Cancer* 4:384–389, 1996

45. Fredrikson M, Hursti T, Furst T, et al: Nausea in cancer chemotherapy is inversely related to urinary cortisol excretion. *Br J Cancer* 65:779–780, 1992

46. Watson JW, Nagahisa A, Lucot JB, et al: The tachykinins and emesis: Toward complete control?, in Reynolds DJM, Andrews PLR, Davis CJ (eds): *Serotonin and the Scientific Basis of Anti-emetic Therapy*. London: Oxford Clinical Communications, 1995, pp. 233–238

47. Kris MJ, Radford JE, Pizzo BA, et al: Use of an NK_1 receptor antagonist to prevent delayed emesis after cisplatin (correspondence). *J Natl Cancer Inst* 89:817–818, 1997

48. Wilder-Smith OHG, Borgeat A, Chappuis P, et al: Urinary serotonin metabolite excretion during cisplatin chemotherapy. *Cancer* 72:2239–2241, 1993

49. Bonneterre J, Hecquet B, Adenis A, et al: How do patients and physicians decide which anti-emetic is best in a cross-over study? *Proc Am Soc Clin Oncol* 10:323, 1991 (abstr)

50. Olver IN, Mattews JP, Bishop JF, et al: The roles of patient and observer assessments in anti-emetic trials. *Eur J Cancer* 30A:1223–1227, 1994

51. Metheny NM: *Fluid and Electrolyte Balance: Nursing Considerations* (ed 3). Philadelphia: Lippincott, 1996

52. Sabatini S, Kurtzman NA: Metabolic alkalosis, in Narins RG (ed): *Maxwell & Kleeman's Clinical Disorders of Fluid and Electrolyte Metabolism*. New York: McGraw-Hill, 1993, pp. 933–956

53. Franklin HR, Simonetti GPC, Dubbleman AC, et al: Toxicity grading systems: A comparison between the WHO scoring system and the Common Toxicity Criteria when used for nausea and vomiting. *Ann Oncol* 5:113–117, 1994

54. Perez EA: A risk-benefit assessment of serotonin 5-HT_3-receptor antagonists in antineoplastic therapy-induced emesis. *Drug Safety* 18:43–56, 1998

55. Gandara DR, Roila F, Warr D, et al: Consensus proposal for $5HT_3$ antagonists in the prevention of acute emesis related to highly emetogenic chemotherapy. *Support Care Cancer* 6:237–243, 1998

56. Feyer PC, Stewart AL, Titlbach OJ: Aetiology and prevention of emesis induced by radiotherapy. *Support Care Cancer* 6:253–260, 1998

57. Cohen M, Duncan PG, BeBoer DP, et al: The postoperative interview: Assessing risk factors for nausea and vomiting. *Anesth Analg* 78:7–16, 1994

58. Beck TM, Hesketh PJ, Madajewicz S, et al: Stratified, randomized, double-blind comparison of intravenous ondansetron administered as a multiple-dose regimen versus two single-dose regimens in the prevention of cisplatin-induced nausea and vomiting. *J Clin Oncol* 10:1969–1975, 1992

59. Noble A, Bremer K, Goedhals L, et al: A double-blind, randomized, crossover comparison of granisetron and ondansetron in 5-day fractionated chemotherapy: Assessment of efficacy, safety, and patient preference. *Eur J Cancer* 30A: 1083–1088, 1994

60. Ruff P, Paska W, Goedhals L, et al: Ondansetron compared with granisetron in the prophylaxis of cisplatin-induced acute emesis: A multicentre double-blind, randomized, parallel group study. *Oncology* 51:113–118, 1994

61. Bonneterre J, Hecquet B: Granisetron (IV) compared with ondansetron (IV plus oral) in the prevention of nausea and vomiting induced by moderately-emetogenic chemotherapy: A cross-over study. *Bull Cancer* 82:1038–1043, 1995

62. Italian Group for Antiemetic Research: Ondansetron versus granisetron, both combined with dexamethasone, in the prevention of cisplatin-induced emesis. *Ann Oncol* 6: 805–810, 1995

63. Navari RM, Kaplan HG, Gralla RJ, et al: Efficacy and safety of granisetron, a selective 5-hydroxytryptamine-3 receptor antagonist, in the prevention of nausea and vomiting induced by high-dose cisplatin. *J Clin Oncol* 12:2204–2210, 1994

64. Chevallier B, Cappelaere P, Splinter T, et al: A double-blind, multicentre comparison of intravenous dolasetron mesilate and metoclopramide in the prevention of nausea and vomiting in cancer patients receiving high-dose cisplatin chemotherapy. *Support Care Cancer* 5:22–30, 1997

65. Hesketh P, Navari R, Grote T, et al: Double-blind, randomized comparison of the antiemetic efficacy of intravenous dolasetron mesilate and intravenous ondansetron in the prevention of acute cisplatin-induced emesis in patients with cancer. *J Clin Oncol* 14:2242–2249, 1996

66. Audhay B, Cappelaere P, Martin M, et al: A double-blind, randomised comparison of the anti-emetic efficacy of two intravenous doses of dolasetron mesilate and granisetron in patients receiving high dose cisplatin chemotherapy. *Eur J Cancer* 32A:807–813, 1996

67. Matera MG, Di Tullio M, Lucarelli C, et al: Ondansetron, an antagonist of 5-HT$_3$ receptors, in the treatment of antineoplastic drug-induced nausea and vomiting in children. *J Med* 24:161–170, 1993

68. Stevens RF: The role of ondansetron in paediatric patients: A review of three studies. *Eur J Cancer* 27(suppl 1): S20–S22, 1991

69. Jurgens H, McQuade B: Ondansetron as prophylaxis for chemotherapy and radiotherapy-induced emesis in children. *Oncology* 49:279–285, 1992

70. Lemerle J, Amaral D, Southall DP, et al: Efficacy and safety of granisetron in the prevention of chemotherapy-induced emesis in paediatric patients. *Eur J Cancer* 27:1081–1083, 1991

71. Henriksson R, Lomberg H, Israelsson G, et al: The effect of ondansetron on radiation-induced emesis and diarrhea. *Acta Oncol* 31:767–769, 1992

72. Collis CE, Priestman TJ, Lucraft H, et al: The final assessment of a randomized double-blind comparative study of ondansetron versus metoclopramide in the prevention of nausea and vomiting following high-dose upper abdominal irradiation. *Clin Oncol* 3:241–243, 1991

73. Prentice HG: Efficacy and safety of granisetron in the treatment of emesis induced by total body irradiation: A comparison with standard antiemetic therapy. *Proc Am Soc Clin Oncol* 12:1547, 1993

74. Markham A, Sorkin EM: Ondansetron: An update of its therapeutic use in chemotherapy-induced and postoperative nausea and vomiting. *Drugs* 45:931–952, 1993

75. Naguib M, El Bakry AK, Khoshim MHB, et al: Prophylactic antiemetic therapy with ondansetron, tropisetron, granisetron and metoclopramide in patients undergoing laparoscopic cholecystectomy: A randomized, double-blind comparison with placebo. *Can J Anaesth* 43:226–231, 1996

76. Claybon L: Single dose intravenous ondansetron for the 24-hour treatment of postoperative nausea and vomiting. *Anaesthesia* 49(suppl):24–29, 1994

77. Graczyk SG, McKenzie R, Kallar S, et al: Intravenous dolasetron for the prevention of postoperative nausea and vomiting after outpatient laparoscopic gynecologic surgery. *Anesth Analg* 84:325–330, 1997

78. Wrench IJ, Ward JE, Walder AD, et al: The prevention of postoperative nausea and vomiting using a combination of ondansetron and droperidol. *Anaesthesia* 51:776–778, 1996

79. Latreille J, Pater J, Johnston D, et al: Use of dexamethasone and granisetron in the control of delayed emesis for patients who receive highly emetogenic chemotherapy. *J Clin Oncol* 16:1174–1178, 1998

80. Gandara DR, Harvey WH, Monoghan GG, et al: Delayed emesis following high-dose cisplatin: A double-blind randomised comparative trial of ondansetron (GR 38032F) versus placebo. *Eur J Cancer* 29A (suppl 1):S35–S38, 1993

81. Stewart A, McQuade B, Cronje JDE, et al: Ondansetron compared with granisetron in the prophylaxis of cyclosphosphamide-induced emesis in out-patients: A multicentre, double-blind, double-dummy, parallel group study. *Oncology* 52:202–210, 1995

82. Granisetron Study Group: The antiemetic efficacy and safety of granisetron compared with metoclopramide plus dexamethasone in patients receiving fractionated chemotherapy over 5 days. *J Cancer Res Clin Oncol* 119:555–559, 1993

83. Cole RM, Robinson F, Harvey L, et al: Successful control of intractable nausea and vomiting requiring combined ondansetron and haloperidol in a patient with advanced cancer. *J Pain Symptom Manage* 9:48–50, 1994

84. Nicholson S, Evans C, Mansi J: Ondansetron in intractable nausea and vomiting (letter). *Lancet* 339:490, 1992

85. Vohra S, Juricic J: High-dose and long-term use of ondansetron (letter). *Ann Pharmacother* 26:128–129, 1992

86. Harvey VJ, Evans BD, Mitchell PLR, et al: Reduction of carboplatin induced emesis by ondansetron. *Br J Cancer* 63:942–944, 1991

87. Cook CE, Mehra IV: Oral ondansetron for preventing nausea and vomiting. *Am J Hosp Pharm* 51:762–771, 1994

88. Boike SC, Ilson B, Zariffa N, et al: Cardiovascular effects of i.v. granisetron at two administration rates and of ondansetron in healthy adults. *Am J Health Syst Pharm* 54:1172–1176, 1997

89. Benedict CR, Arbogast R, Martin L, et al: Single-blind study of the effects of intravenous dolasetron mesylate versus ondansetron on electrocardiographic parameters in normal volunteers. *J Cardiovasc Pharmacol* 28:53–59, 1996

90. Hesketh PJ, Murphy WK, Lester EP, et al: GR38032F (GR-507/75): A novel compound effective in the prevention of acute cisplatine-induced emesis. *J Clin Oncol* 7:700–705, 1989

91. Harman GS, Omura GA, Ryan K: A randomised, double-blind comparison of single-dose and divided multiple-dose dolasetron for cisplatin-induced emesis. *Cancer Chemother Pharmacol* 38:323–328, 1996

92. Kris MG, Radford JE, Pizzo BA, et al: Use of an NK$_1$ receptor antagonist to prevent delayed emesis after cisplatin (correspondence). *J Natl Cancer Inst* 89:817–818, 1997

93. Martoni A, Angelelli B, Guaraldi M, et al: An open randomised cross-over study of granisetron versus ondansetron in the prevention of acute emesis induced by moderate dose cisplatin-containing regimens. *Eur J Cancer* 26(suppl 1): S28–S32, 1996

94. Jantunen IT, Flander MK, Heikkinen MJ, et al: Comparison of ondansetron with customary treatment in the prophylaxis of nausea and vomiting induced by non-cisplatin containing chemotherapy. *Acta Oncol* 32:413–415, 1993

95. Seynaeve C, Schuller J, Buser K, et al: Comparison of the anti-emetic efficacy of different doses of ondansetron, given as either a continuous infusion or a single intravenous dose, in acute cisplatin-induced emesis: A multicentre, double-blind, randomised, parallel group study. *Br J Cancer* 66:192–197, 1992

96. Tyson LB, Kris MG, Baltzek, et al: Randomized phase II trial comparing two versus three doses of ondansetron when used in combination with dexamethasone in patients receiving cisplatin ≥100 mg/m². *Am J Clin Oncol* 17:269–272, 1994

97. Nolte MJ, Berkery R, Pizzo B, et al: Assuring the optimal use of serotonin antagonist antiemetics: The process for development and implementation of institutional antiemetic guidelines at Memorial Sloan-Kettering Cancer Center. *J Clin Oncol* 16:771–778, 1998

98. Audhay B, Whitmore J, Cramer J, et al: Optimal IV dolasetron dose for prevention of nausea and vomiting (NV) after cisplatin (CDDP) chemotherapy: Analysis of mg doses from 14 pooled trials (abstract). *Support Care Cancer* 4:249, 1996

99. Perez EA, Hesketh P, Sandbach J, et al: Comparison of single-dose oral granisetron versus intravenous ondansetron in the prevention of N&V induced by moderately emetogenic chemotherapy: A multicenter, double-blind, randomized parallel study. *J Clin Oncol* 16:754–760, 1998

100. Gralla RJ, Navari RM, Hesketh PJ, et al: Single-dose oral granisetron has equivalent antiemetic efficacy to intravenous ondansetron for highly emetogenic cisplatin-based chemotherapy. *J Clin Oncol* 16:1568–1573, 1998

101. Rubenstein EB, Gralla RJ, Hainsworth JD, et al: Randomized, double-blind, dose-response trial across four oral doses of dolasetron for the prevention of acute emesis after moderately emetogenic chemotherapy. *Cancer* 79:1216–1224, 1997

102. Franchi M, Donadella N, Zanaboni F, et al: Oral ondansetron and intravenous dexamethasone in the prevention of cisplatin-induced emesis. *Oncology* 52:509–512, 1995

103. Clavel M, Bonneterre J, d'Allens H, et al: Oral ondansetron in the prevention of chemotherapy-induced emesis in breast cancer patients. *Eur J Cancer* 31A:15–19, 1995

104. Hamik A, Peroutka SJ: Differential interactions of traditional and novel antiemetics with dopamine D_2 and 5-hydroxytryptamine$_3$ receptors. *Cancer Chemother Pharmacol* 24:307–310, 1989

105. Mitchelson F: Pharmacological agents affecting emesis: A review (part I). *Drugs* 43:295–315, 1992

106. Hainsworth J, Harvey W, Pendergrass K, et al: A single-blind comparison of intravenous ondansetron, a selective serotonin antagonist, with IV metoclopramide in the prevention of nausea and vomiting associated with high-dose cisplatin chemotherapy. *J Clin Oncol* 9:721–728, 1991

107. Chevallier B: The control of acute cisplatin-induced emesis—a comparative study of granisetron and a combination regimen of high-dose metoclopramide and dexamethasone. *Br J Cancer* 68:176–180, 1993

108. Tonnessen TI: *Control of Pain and Other Symptoms in Cancer Patients.* New York: Hemisphere Publishing Corporation, 1990

109. Billings JA: *Outpatient Management of Advanced Cancer.* Philadelphia: Lippincott, 1985, pp. 46–57

110. Ventafridda V, Ripamonti C, Caraceni A, et al: The management of inoperable gastrointestinal obstruction in terminal cancer patients. *Tumori* 76:389–393, 1990

111. Campbell M, Bateman DN: Pharmacokinetic optimisation of antiemetic therapy. *Clin Pharmacokinet* 23:147–160, 1992

112. Saito H, Shimokata K, Yamori S, et al: Continuous infusion versus intermittent short infusion of metoclopramide for cislatin-induced acute emesis. *Am J Clin Oncol* 17:422–426, 1994

113. Olver JN, Wolf M, Laidlaw C, et al: A randomized double-blind study of high-dose intravenous prochloperazine versus high-dose metoclopramide as antiemetics for cancer chemotherapy. *Eur J Cancer* 28A:1798–1802, 1992

114. Herrstedt J, Sigsgaard T, Boesgaard M, et al: Ondansetron plus metopimazine compared with ondansetron alone in patients receiving moderately emetogenic chemotherapy. *N Engl J Med* 328:1076–1080, 1993

115. Grunberg SM: Potential for combination therapy with the new antiserotonergic agents. *Eur J Cancer* 29A:S39–S41, 1993

116. Hesketh PJ, Gandara DR, Hesketh AM, et al: Improved control of high-dose cisplatin-induced acute emesis with the addition of prochlorperazine to granisetron/dexamethasone. *Cancer J Sci Am* 3:180–183, 1997

117. Storey P: Medical management of nonchemotherapy-induced nausea and vomiting in advanced cancer patients. *Cancer Bull* 43:433–436, 1991

118. Trinkle R: Compatibility of hydromorphone and prochlorperazine, and irritation due to subcutaneous prochlorperazine infusion (letter). *Ann Pharmacother* 31:789–790, 1997

119. Bishop JF, Matthews JP, Wold MM, et al: A randomised trial of dexamethasone, lorazepam and prochlorperazine for emesis in patients receiving chemotherapy. *Eur J Cancer* 28:47–50, 1992

120. Moreno I, Rosell R, Abad A, et al: Comparison of three protracted antiemetic regimens for the control of delayed emesis in cisplatin-treated patients. *Eur J Cancer* 28A:1344–1347, 1992

121. Mataruski MR, Keis NA, Smouse DJ, et al: Effects of steroids on postoperative nausea and vomiting. *Nurse Anesthes* 1:183–188, 1990

122. Hursti TJ, Frederickson M, Steineck G, et al: Endogenous cortisol exerts antiemetic effect similar to that of exogenous corticosteroids. *Br J Cancer* 68:112–114, 1993

123. Jones AL, Hill AS, Soukop M, et al: Comparison of dexamethasone and ondansetron in the prophylaxis of emesis induced by moderately emetogenic chemotherapy. *Lancet* 338:483–487, 1991

124. Roila F: Ondansetron plus dexamethasone compared to 'standard' metoclopramide combination. *Oncology* 50:163–167, 1993

125. Herrstedt J, Aapro MS, Smyth JF, et al: Corticosteroids, dopamine antagonists and other drugs. *Support Care Cancer* 6:204–214, 1998

126. Gonzales-Rosales F, Walsh D: Intractable nausea and vomiting due to gastrointestinal mucosal metastases relieved by tetrahydrocannabinol (dronabinol). *J Pain Symptom Manage* 14:311–314, 1997

127. Beal JE, Olson R, Lefkowitz, et al: Long-term efficacy and safety of dronabinol for acquired immunodeficiency syndrome-associated anorexia. *J Pain Symptom Manage* 14:7–14, 1997

128. Redd WH: Behavioral intervention for cancer treatment side effects. *Acta Oncologica* 33:113–116, 1994

129. Burish TG, Jenkins RA: Effectiveness of biofeedback and relaxation training in reducing the side effects of cancer chemotherapy. *Health Psychol* 11:17–23, 1992

130. McMillan C, Dundee JW, Abram WP: Enhancement of the antiemetic action of ondansetron by transcutaneous electrical stimulation of the P6 antiemetic point, in patients having highly emetic cytotoxic drugs. *Br J Cancer* 64:971–972, 1991

131. Shen J, Wenget NS, Glaspy JA, et al: Adjunct antiemesis electroacupuncture in stem cell transplantation (abstract). *Proc Annu Meet Am Soc Clin Oncol* 16:A148, 1997

132. Vickers AJ: Can acupuncture have specific effects on health? A systematic review of acupuncture antiemesis trials. *J R Soc Med* 89:303–311, 1996

133. Hogan CM: Nausea and vomiting. In J Yasko (ed): *Nursing management of symptoms associated with chemotherapy* (ed 3). Philadelphia: Meniscus, pp. 89–108, 1993

134. Phillips S, Ruggier R, Hutchinson SE: Zingiber officinale (ginger)—an antiemetic for day case surgery. *Anaesthesia* 48:715–717, 1993

Baseline Assessment, Chemotherapy

(Nurse Completes)

Client: _____ Risk

Age: _____   _____

_____ <50 increases risk (1)   _____ >50 decreases risk (0)

Gender: _____

_____ male decreases risk (0)   _____ female increases risk (1–2)

Alcohol use/drinks per week: _____
(1 drink = 1 glass wine, 1 12-oz beer, 1 oz hard liquor)

_____ 0 to <7/week increases risk (1)   _____ >7/week decreases risk (0)

Chemotherapy regimen (see Table 14-1 for risk: 1–5): _____ _____

N and/or V with previous chemotherapy?   _____

_____ no, may decrease risk (0)   _____ yes, may increase risk (.5)

History of motion sickness?   _____

_____ no, may decrease risk (0)   _____ yes, may increase risk (.5)

Have you had nausea and vomiting with past chemotherapy?   _____

_____ no, may decrease risk (0)   _____ yes, may increase risk (.5)

Total risk score _____

ESTIMATED RISK:

LOWER   HIGHER

1	2	3	4	5	6	7	8	9

(Patient Completes)

What medicines have you used for nausea and vomiting in the past?

_____

Which were:
  not helpful?   *helpful?*

What, if any, bothersome side effects from the medicine did you have?

_____

How satisfied were you with the medicine?

_____ Not at all   _____ A little   _____ Moderately   _____ Totally

Have you tried any nondrug measures for nausea and vomiting in the past that were helpful (examples: sleeping, ginger ale, peppermint)?

_____

Would you like to use these again?   _____ Yes   _____ No

Source: Wickham R: Nausea and vomiting, in Yarbro CH, Frogge MH, Goodman M (eds): *Cancer Symptom Management* (ed 2). Sudbury: Jones and Bartlett, 1999. © Jones and Bartlett Publishers.

Chemotherapy Treatment Diary

Patient: _____

Medicines to Take for Nausea and Vomiting		
Day	Medicines	Directions: When and how to take

Special Instructions: What Else to Do If You Have Nausea and Vomiting	
Medicine	When and how to take
Other	

Phone Numbers

Record When You Took Your Medicines and How You Felt			
Day and Time	Medicines Taken	Degree of Nausea*	Number of Times You Vomited

* 0 = No nausea
  1 = Slight nausea
  2 = Moderately severe nausea, interferes with your activities and eating
  3 = Severe nausea, intolerable

Check the box that best describes how you are able to eat and how you are feeling each day after chemotherapy for _____ days			
Day	I throw up most everything and stay in bed most of the day	I feel some nausea and have some difficulty eating, but am drinking and out of bed	I am able to eat and go about my day as usual

How well do you feel your medicines worked to prevent nausea and vomiting?

_____ Very effective _____ Moderately effective _____ Not effective

Adapted from Goodman M: Management of nausea and vomiting induced by outpatient cisplatin (Platinol) treatment. *Semin Oncol Nurs* 3:23–35, 1987.

Source: Wickham R: Nausea and vomiting, in Yarbro CH, Frogge MH, Goodman M (eds): *Cancer Symptom Management* (ed 2). Sudbury: Jones and Bartlett, 1999. © Jones and Bartlett Publishers.

Nausea and Vomiting from Chemotherapy

Patient Name: _____

Symptom and Description　Nausea (feeling queasy or sick to your stomach) and/or vomiting (throwing up) may happen from your chemotherapy. Nausea and vomiting (if they happen) are usually worst on the day of your treatment. Sometimes nausea and vomiting can last for 3 or more days after chemotherapy.

Learning Needs　Nausea and vomiting are very unpleasant. Either or both may be barely noticeable or may be severe and cause you to be unable to do things that are important to you. In addition, if you vomit a lot you can get dehydrated and have other problems from losing body salts. If you are vomiting and cannot drink fluids, you may have even worse side effects of chemotherapy to your kidneys or bladder.

　You should call your doctor or nurse if:

- You have nausea that lasts for more than a few days, or if nausea keeps you from doing things that are important to you.
- You vomit more than once or twice a day for 2 days.
- You cannot keep any liquids (such as water, juices, soda) or food down.
- You are vomiting and you lose more than 2 pounds in a day (this is from losing water). You will usually feel thirsty and your mouth will seem dry when you are losing a lot of water.
- You are vomiting many times and your urine is dark yellow and you are not going to the bathroom as often as you normally do.
- You are vomiting and feel lightheaded or dizzy, or confused (mixed up).
- The stuff you throw up looks like coffee grounds (this could be blood).

Prevention　We have many medicines to control nausea and vomiting (antiemetics). If nausea and vomiting might happen after your chemotherapy, your doctor will prescribe one or more of them for you.

- Make sure you get your antiemetics. Let your doctor or nurse know if your drugstore does not have them or if you cannot afford to pay for them.
- If you are not sure how to take your antiemetics, call your doctor or nurse.
- Take the antiemetic(s) as your doctor has ordered. If you have vomiting and cannot take them, call your doctor or nurse.
- If your antiemetics help lessen your nausea and vomiting but not as much as you would like, call your doctor or nurse. The dose of the antiemetic may have to be changed, or the doctor may change you to a different antiemetic.

Management　When nausea and vomiting are very bad, you may need to come to the office for antiemetics, and possibly for fluids, through a vein (an IV). Sometimes your doctor will also order blood tests and x-ray films to find out why you are vomiting. Most of the time, your doctor and nurse will be able to get your vomiting under control so that you can take pills to control it.

Self-Management

In addition to taking your antiemetics, you can try one or more things that other people have found helpful:

- Try eating foods and drinking beverages that were easy for you to take or have made you feel better when you had the flu, had morning sickness, or were nauseated from stress. These might be bland foods, sour candy, pickles, dry crackers, ginger ale, flat soda, or others.
- Do not eat your favorite foods when you are nauseated.
- Do not eat fatty or fried foods, very spicy foods, or very sweet foods when you are nauseated.
- If possible, have somebody else make the meals when you are nauseated.
- If you have nausea and vomiting only for a few days after chemotherapy, cook and freeze several meals that you can reheat during times you are nauseated.
- Eat foods that are at room temperature or cold. The smells from hot foods may make your nausea worse.
- Keep your mouth clean; brush at least twice a day.
- Ask your doctor or nurse if they can help you learn a relaxation exercise. This might make you feel less anxious and more in control, and decrease your nausea.
- Ask you doctor or nurse about using acupressure bands on your wrists, which may help to decrease your nausea.

Follow-up   Call your nurse and/or doctor if any of the following happen:

- You have nausea and vomiting that are not controlled with the antiemetics ordered.
- You have side effects that you do not like from your antiemetics.
- You start to have a lot of nausea and vomiting and cannot keep liquids down and are losing weight.
- You are dizzy and/or confused.

Phone Numbers

Nurse: _____ Phone: _____

Physician: _____ Phone: _____

Other: _____ Phone: _____

Comments

Patient's Signature: _____ Date: _____

Nurse's Signature: _____ Date: _____

Source: Wickham R: Nausea and vomiting, in Yarbro CH, Frogge MH, Goodman M (eds): *Cancer Symptom Management* (ed 2). Sudbury: Jones and Bartlett, 1999. © Jones and Bartlett Publishers.

Nausea and Vomiting from Radiation Therapy

Patient Name: _____

Symptom and Description   Nausea (feeling queasy or sick to your stomach) and/or vomiting (throwing up) may happen from radiation therapy. It is most likely if you get radiation to your chest, stomach, abdomen, or spine. Nausea and vomiting are rare when other parts of your body are treated. Nausea and vomiting may start within 1 to 2 hours after your radiation treatment and may last for several hours.

Learning Needs   Nausea and vomiting are very unpleasant. Either or both may be barely noticeable or may be severe and may cause you to be unable to do things that are important to you. If you vomit a lot you can get dehydrated and have other problems from losing body salts.

You should call your doctor or nurse if:

- You have nausea that lasts for more than a few days, or if nausea keeps you from doing things that are important to you.

- You vomit more than once or twice a day for 2 days.

- You cannot keep any liquids (such as water, juices, soda) or food down.

- You are vomiting and you lose more than 2 pounds in a day (this is from losing water). You will usually feel thirsty and your mouth will seem dry when you are losing a lot of water.

- You are vomiting many times and your urine is dark yellow and you are not going to the bathroom as often as you normally do.

- You are vomiting and feel lightheaded or dizzy, or confused (mixed up).

- The stuff you throw up looks like coffee grounds (this could be blood).

Prevention   We have many medicines to control nausea and vomiting (antiemetics). If you are likely to have nausea and vomiting, your doctor may prescribe one or more of them for you.

- Make sure you get your antiemetics. Let your doctor or nurse know if your drugstore does not have them or if you cannot afford to pay for them.

- If you are not sure how to take your antiemetics, call your doctor or nurse.

- Take the antiemetic(s) as your doctor has ordered. If you have vomiting and cannot take them, call your doctor or nurse.

- If your antiemetics help lessen your nausea and vomiting but not as much as you would like, call your doctor or nurse. The dose of the antiemetic may have to be changed, or the doctor may change you to a different antiemetic.

Management   When nausea and vomiting are very bad, you may need to come to the office for antiemetics, and possibly for fluids, through a vein (an IV). Most of the time, your doctor and nurse will be able to get your vomiting under control so that you can take pills to control it. In a very small number of people this is not possible. Then you may need to take antiemetics into your rectum by suppository or through your vein.

Self-Management

In addition to taking your antiemetics, you can try one or more things that other people have found helpful:

- Try eating foods and drinking beverages that were easy for you to take or have made you feel better when you had the flu, had morning sickness, or were nauseated from stress. These might be bland foods, sour candy, pickles, dry crackers, ginger ale, flat soda, or others.
- Do not eat your favorite foods when you are nauseated.
- Do not eat fatty or fried foods, very spicy foods, or very sweet foods when you are nauseated.
- If possible, have somebody else make the meals when you are nauseated.
- If you have nausea and vomiting only for a few days after chemotherapy, cook and freeze several meals that you can reheat during times you are nauseated.
- Eat foods that are at room temperature or cold. The smells from hot foods may make your nausea worse.
- Keep your mouth clean; brush at least twice a day.
- Ask your doctor or nurse if they can help you learn a relaxation exercise. This might make you feel less anxious and more in control, and decrease your nausea.
- Ask you doctor or nurse about using acupressure bands on your wrists, which may help to decrease your nausea.

Follow-up   Call your nurse and/or doctor if any of the following happen:

- You have nausea and vomiting that are not controlled with the antiemetics ordered.
- You have side effects that you do not like from your antiemetics.
- You start to have a lot of nausea and vomiting and cannot keep liquids down and are losing weight.
- You are dizzy and/or confused.

Phone Numbers

Nurse: _____ Phone: _____

Physician: _____ Phone: _____

Other: _____ Phone: _____

Comments

Patient's Signature: _____ Date: _____

Nurse's Signature: _____ Date: _____

Source: Wickham R: Nausea and vomiting, in Yarbro CH, Frogge MH, Goodman M (eds): *Cancer Symptom Management* (ed 2). Sudbury: Jones and Bartlett, 1999. © Jones and Bartlett Publishers.

Nausea and Vomiting from Cancer

Patient Name: _____

Symptom and Description   Nausea (feeling queasy or sick to your stomach) and/or vomiting (throwing up) can happen from many causes with cancer, and may be worse if you are getting chemotherapy and radiation therapy. Nausea and vomiting may come on slowly or very quickly with cancer-related problems. Your doctor will treat the problem causing the nausea and vomiting, and treat the nausea and vomiting, too.

Learning Needs   Nausea and vomiting are very unpleasant. Either or both may be barely noticeable or may be severe and may cause you to be unable to do things that are important to you. If you vomit a lot, you can get dehydrated and have other problems from losing body salts.

   You should call your doctor or nurse if:

- You have nausea that lasts for more than a few days, or if nausea keeps you from doing things that are important to you.
- You vomit more than once or twice a day for 2 days.
- You cannot keep any liquids (such as water, juices, soda) or food down.
- You are vomiting and you lose more than 2 pounds in a day (this is from losing water). You will usually feel thirsty and your mouth will seem dry when you are losing a lot of water.
- You are vomiting many times, your urine is dark yellow, and you are not going to the bathroom as often as you normally do.
- You are vomiting and feel lightheaded or dizzy, or confused (mixed up).
- The stuff you throw up looks like coffee grounds (this could be blood).

Prevention   We have many medicines to control nausea and vomiting (antiemetics). Your doctor will prescribe one or more of them for you.

- Make sure you get your antiemetics. Let your doctor or nurse know if your drugstore does not have them or if you cannot afford to pay for them.
- If you are not sure how to take your antiemetics, call your doctor or nurse.
- Take the antiemetic(s) as your doctor has ordered. If you have vomiting and cannot take them, call your doctor or nurse.
- If your antiemetics help lessen your nausea and vomiting but not as much as you would like, call your doctor or nurse. The dose of the antiemetic may have to be changed, or the doctor may change you to a different antiemetic.

Management   When nausea and vomiting are very bad, you may need to come to the office for antiemetics, and possibly for fluids, through a vein (an IV). Sometimes your doctor will also order blood tests and x-ray films to find out why you are vomiting. Most of the time, your doctor and nurse will be able to get your vomiting under control so that you can take pills to control it. In a very small number of people, this is not possible. Then you may need to take antiemetics into your rectum by suppository or through your vein.

Self-Management

In addition to taking your antiemetics, you can try one or more things that other people have found helpful:

- Try eating foods and drinking beverages that were easy for you to take or have made you feel better when you had the flu, had morning sickness, or were nauseated from stress. These might be bland foods, sour candy, pickles, dry crackers, ginger ale, flat soda, or others.
- Do not eat your favorite foods when you are nauseated.
- Do not eat fatty or fried foods, very spicy foods, or very sweet foods when you are nauseated.
- If possible, have somebody else make the meals when you are nauseated.
- If you have nausea and vomiting only for a few days after chemotherapy, cook and freeze several meals that you can reheat during times you are nauseated.
- Eat foods that are at room temperature or cold. The smells from hot foods may make your nausea worse.
- Keep your mouth clean; brush at least twice a day.
- Ask your doctor or nurse if they can help you learn a relaxation exercise. This might make you feel less anxious and more in control, and decrease your nausea.
- Ask you doctor or nurse about using acupressure bands on your wrists, which may help to decrease your nausea.

Follow-up   Call your nurse and/or doctor if any of the following happen:

- You have nausea and vomiting that are not controlled with the antiemetics ordered.
- You have side effects that you do not like from your antiemetics.
- You start to have a lot of nausea and vomiting and cannot keep liquids down and are losing weight.
- You are dizzy and/or confused.

Phone Numbers

Nurse: _____ Phone: _____

Physician: _____ Phone: _____

Other: _____ Phone: _____

Comments

Patient's Signature: _____ Date: _____

Nurse's Signature: _____ Date: _____

Source: Wickham R: Nausea and vomiting, in Yarbro CH, Frogge MH, Goodman M (eds): *Cancer Symptom Management* (ed 2). Sudbury: Jones and Bartlett, 1999. © Jones and Bartlett Publishers.

CHAPTER 15

Xerostomia

Ryan R. Iwamoto, MN, ARNP, AOCN

The Problem of Xerostomia in Cancer

Xerostomia is the term used for a condition characterized by abnormal dryness of the mouth. The dryness can range in degree from mild to severe.

Incidence in Cancer

Xerostomia occurs in the cancer patient population for many reasons.[1-6] Radiation therapy to the head and neck area is a major cause of xerostomia. Other causes include certain chemotherapeutic agents, surgery of the head and neck region involving removal of the salivary glands, and other diseases such as Sjögren's syndrome. Oral infections can also cause dryness of the mouth.

Impact on Quality of Life

The impact of xerostomia on the quality of a cancer patient's life varies with the severity of the dryness. Activities of daily living can be profoundly affected by the dryness and altered saliva.[7] These activities include eating, sleeping, speaking, and physical exercise. The patient may need to expectorate frequently or manually remove the thick saliva.

Xerostomia causes difficulty eating dry or thick foods. Meals are interrupted by frequent sips of fluids. Patients may avoid eating in the presence of others because of embarrassment. With xerostomia, wearing dentures can be difficult and uncomfortable. Saliva is important for the retention and stability of dentures. Because of denture instability, chewing food is difficult. With xerostomia, the taste of food also changes. All these symptoms can have a negative impact on the patient's nutritional status.

Sleep is interrupted because of the need to take sips of water throughout the night. These patients will frequently awaken with their tongue adhered to the roof of the mouth.

Social activities can also be affected. Patients may need to alter the way they normally conduct business, finding that telephone conversations are limited because their speech is affected. Public speaking, such as teaching a class, is difficult because of the mouth dryness and the need for frequent sips of water. Other activities such as attendance at educational lectures or recreational events are commonly curtailed because of the person's inability to be comfortable through the program. The patient may feel inhibited about participating in social activities because of the difficulty with speech and the need to frequently moisten the mouth. Travel by air is particularly difficult because of the decreased humidity in the passenger compartment of a plane.

Etiology

Xerostomia occurs as a result of cancer treatments and certain diseases. Radiation therapy to the head and neck region frequently results in xerostomia. Chemotherapeutic agents, such as doxorubicin hydrochloride, have been reported to cause a transient dryness of the mouth.[3] Xerostomia is exacerbated if the patient is taking medications that typically cause dryness of mouth, such as anticholinergics, phenothiazines, tricyclic antidepressants, antihistamines, and antispasmodics.[1,8] Climate and environmental changes can also increase the symptoms associated with xerostomia. Areas of low humidity or areas where furnaces or heaters are used during cold weather can further increase mouth dryness.

Surgical excisions within the head and neck area that include the salivary glands will cause xerostomia. These surgeries include resections of salivary gland tumors and wide resections of head and neck cancers. If one salivary gland is removed, the intact salivary glands can compensate for the decreased saliva to some extent. However, if adjuvant radiation therapy to the area is used, chronic xerostomia usually occurs.

Sjögren's syndrome is an autoimmune disease in which the salivary and lacrimal glands become nonfunctional.[1] Tissue biopsy demonstrates clusters of lymphocytes around the salivary and lacrimal ducts. Sjögren's syndrome can occur in conjunction with certain cancers, rheumatoid arthritis, systemic lupus erythematosus, primary biliary cirrhosis, chronic graft-versus-host disease, and scleroderma.[9] Xerostomia resulting from Sjögren's syndrome is usually severe and requires extensive management.

Oral infections of the mouth (e.g., candidiasis) can cause a sensation of dryness in the mouth. Infections of the mouth and esophagus ocur as a result of alteration in the normal balance of oral flora due to disease, medications, or altered mucosal integrity.[10] Chronic xerostomia has also been associated with increased esophageal acidity, gastroesophageal reflux, and esophagitis. Researchers have evaluated the effects of chronic xerostomia related to esophageal reflux and esophagitis.[11] Esophageal motility was similar in patients with xerostomia and controls. However, patients with radiation-induced xerostomia demonstrated a decreased ability to clear esophageal acid as compared with control subjects, and they experienced a higher incidence of esophagitis.

Pathophysiology

Saliva is produced by the major and minor salivary glands. Saliva is a natural lubricant that helps with chewing, formation of a bolus of food, and swallowing. Enzymes contained in saliva begin the digestive process. Saliva keeps the mouth cleansed and free of debris and bacteria, aids in taste sensation, and is also important for speech.

Saliva production is more significantly decreased if the major salivary glands are affected by treatment or disease than if the minor glands are affected. When saliva changes from a thin to a thick consistency, the saliva is unable to perform its usual function of cleansing the teeth. Thick saliva causes food and bacteria to adhere to the teeth and can result in plaque formation and periodontal disease. Caries eventually form as a result of increased acidity of saliva and growth of cariogenic bacteria within the altered mouth environment.[12]

If radiation therapy is given to the head and neck region, the salivary glands within the treatment field will be adversely affected.[1,2,5,12] The parotid salivary glands are very radiosensitive. Once the cumulative dose of radiation reaches 1000 cGy, the patient may begin to experience mild to moderate dryness of the mouth. Radiation causes salivary gland atrophy and fibrosis. The acinar cells, which contribute to the serous component of saliva, degenerate. As a result, the saliva changes from a thin and watery consistency to a thick and ropey consistency,[12,13] becoming thick and tenacious in character.

The dryness can progress through the radiation therapy and persist for more than six months after treatment is completed. If the radiation dose exceeds 4000 cGy, xerostomia usually becomes a chronic problem of progressive and permanent dryness. Some regression of dryness and return of salivary function occurs following cessation of radiation therapy, but this happens gradually and over several months' time. With xerostomia, the patient is at increased risk for developing oral stomatitis.

Assessment

Assessment for the presence of xerostomia should be done prior to the initiation of cancer treatment. In addition to the presence and quality of saliva, the patient's eating, chewing, swallowing, mouth care practices, and oral comfort should be evaluated.

Measurement Tools

Sialometry, or the objective measurement of saliva production, can be performed in a number of ways. Collection of saliva can be facilitated by the use of devices such as Carlson-Crittenden cups (Stone Machine Co., Colton, CA). These cups are placed over the salivary papillae, and measurements are taken of the amount and flow rate of saliva (Figure 15-1). More precise measurements of saliva can be achieved with cannulation of the salivary ducts. A simple technique to measure saliva production involves having the patient allow saliva to collect in the mouth for 1 minute and then spit the accumulated saliva into a preweighed container. The container is then

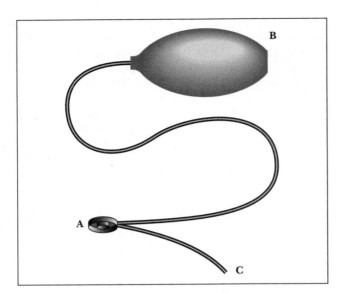

FIGURE 15-1 Carlson-Crittenden cup (Stone Machine Co., Colton, CA). Carlson-Crittenden cup is placed over salivary gland duct (A). Suction is applied by compressing bulb (B). Saliva is collected from drain tube (C). (Courtesy of MGI Pharma, Inc., Minnetonka, MN.)

weighed to determine the amount of saliva the patient produced in 1 minute. The saliva can also be analyzed for electrolytes and enzymes.

In some cases, although patients experience mouth dryness, they are able to produce some saliva with salivary gland stimulation. To determine this ability, a substance such as dilute acetic acid is placed within the mouth in measured amounts and the stimulated saliva is collected by any of the above measures.

Physical Assessment

Patients may report mouth dryness at any point in their illness trajectory. The dryness may be mild to severe depending on individual risk factors and responses to treatment. Patients may complain of pain in the mouth ranging from mild irritation to severe burning sensations.

The clinician should inspect the oral cavity for signs of xerostomia. In the presence of xerostomia, the mouth appears dry with furrowing of the tongue. Debris may adhere to the mucosa, gingiva, teeth, or tongue. The oral secretions will appear thick and ropey. Inspection of the oral cavity may reveal signs of an infection such as candidiasis or erythema.

If the patient wears dentures, the patient's comfort with the prosthesis while eating and at rest is assessed. After the dentures are removed, the oral cavity is inspected for signs of gingival irritation such as erythema, tissue breakdown, or bleeding.

Diagnostic Evaluation

A thorough periodontal and mouth evaluation by a dentist prior to the start of therapy is important, particularly if the head and neck area is being irradiated.[1,5,14] The dentist should treat any dental problems and initiate a prophylactic dental program to minimize dental complications during and after therapy.

Degrees of Toxicity

Rating scales can be used to describe the degree of xerostomia. The Radiation Therapy Oncology Group (RTOG) utilizes two scales for researchers to describe the extent of xerostomia. One scale is used for acute reactions and the other for late effects (Table 15-1). These rating scales can be used to document the degree of xerostomia as well as to monitor the effectiveness of the interventions.

Symptom Management

Interventions for xerostomia aim to provide comfort; to prevent and minimize stomatitis, oral infections, and periodontal disease; and to maintain the nutritional status of the patient.

Prevention

Xerostomia may be impossible to prevent depending on the situation, such as with definitive irradiation for head

TABLE 15-1 Radiation Therapy Oncology Group Radiation Morbidity Scoring Criteria: Salivary Gland

Acute Reactions
0: No change over baseline
1: Mild mouth dryness / slightly thickened saliva / may have slightly altered taste such as metallic taste / these changes not reflected in alteration in baseline feeding behavior, such as increased use of liquids with meals
2: Moderate to complete dryness / thick, sticky saliva / markedly altered taste
3: (Not used)
4: Acute salivary gland necrosis

Late Reactions
0: None
1: Slight dryness of mouth / good response on stimulation
2: Moderate dryness of mouth / poor response on stimulation
3: Complete dryness of mouth / no response on stimulation
4: Fibrosis

Radiation Therapy Oncology Group (RTOG), American College of Radiology, Philadelphia, PA.[15]

and neck cancer or the removal of a salivary gland tumor. However, minimizing or preventing the complications of xerostomia is possible and thus is an important nursing measure.

Preventing complications associated with xerostomia is accomplished by instructing the patient to perform consistent and meticulous mouth care (see Appendix 15A). Mouth care should be done before and after each meal and at bedtime. Brushing with a soft-bristle toothbrush and flossing, if tolerated, will clean the tooth and periodontal surfaces and prevent plaque development. Mouth care in itself will stimulate salivary flow. Frequent oral saline rinses, every 2 hours or as needed, can help cleanse and provide hydration to the oral tissues. The oral rinses will help liquefy the thick oral secretions. Commercial mouthwashes that contain alcohol, detergents, or flavorings should be avoided, because they can cause more dryness and further irritate the oral cavity.

Use of fluoride gels in dental trays or brushed on the teeth at bedtime will help strengthen the tooth enamel and minimize cavity formation. The fluoride is applied after mouth care is performed. If a dental carrier tray is used, the fluoride is placed in the carrier tray, which is then placed on the teeth for a maximum of 5 minutes. After the application of fluoride, the patient expectorates the excess fluoride and must not rinse the mouth or eat or drink for 30 minutes. The application of fluoride may be increased to twice a day if dental caries occur despite once-daily treatments.[16]

Researchers have evaluated the use of topical fluoride application in combination with a low-sugar diet to minimize cavity formation.[17] They found that the group of patients who maintained a strict low-sugar diet but did not use fluoride developed cavities more readily than the group who used fluoride but did not follow a low-sugar diet. The investigators also found that once fluoride use was initiated, the tendency to develop cavities was reversed.

Chlorhexidine mouth rinses contain antimicrobial agents and have been used to decrease the cariogenic bacteria in the mouth and reduce plaque formation.[18] However, the alcohol content of these mouth rinses can cause oral discomfort, and the solution can leave brown stains on the teeth.

Therapeutic Approaches

Early

The sensation of dryness of the mouth is best alleviated with frequent oral rinses and sips of water or juice. Performing mouth care before and after meals and at bedtime can help refresh the mouth and make eating more comfortable.

Changes in how foods are prepared and eaten will help to make eating more pleasurable and maintain nutri-

tional status. Soft, moist foods are easier to consume. Using gravies and sauces on food can help moisten the food and make it easier to chew and swallow. Instruct patients to avoid dry, sticky foods such as bread or peanut butter.

Liberal intake of fluids during meals is also helpful. Alcoholic and carbonated beverages, however, can be painful to inflamed mucosa. In addition, alcohol can further dry the oral tissues. Tobacco products should also be avoided, as they can further dry and irritate the oral mucosa.

Instruct patients to increase intake of noncarbonated and nonalcoholic fluids between meals to hydrate the oral tissues. Sucking on hard sugarless candies or chewing sugarless gum can stimulate saliva secretion. In addition, squirting a fine mist of water into the mouth with a spray bottle is soothing to the oral tissues.

Commercially prepared saliva substitutes can be used to lubricate the oral tissues. These products are convenient and usually contain carboxymethyl cellulose that forms a slippery film on the tissues. Oralbalance (Laclede Inc., Rancho Dominguez, CA) has been reported by radiation oncology nurses to be well tolerated by patients with xerostomia and provides longer-lasting relief of dryness as compared with other similar products.[19–21] Other lubricating agents such as a teaspoon of olive oil or a small pat of butter can be smeared in the mouth to provide comfort. Patients may use the oil or butter in the mouth at bedtime to enhance comfort during sleep and to minimize the potential of waking up with their tongue adhered to the roof of their mouth. Emollients on the lips are recommended to prevent drying and chapping. Lemon-glycerine products should be avoided, however, as they can cause further drying and irritation.

Papain is the proteolytic enzyme found in papayas. The patient may be instructed to consume papayas or papaya juice, or to create a solution of crushed papain tablets in water to liquefy the thick saliva. Papain is also the active ingredient found in meat tenderizers. Patients may make a solution of meat tenderizer combined with a small amount of water. Instruct the patient to rinse and expectorate this mixture before meals to help dissolve thick saliva.

With xerostomia, dentures are less stable on the gingival surface and can cause tissue breakdown. Denture liners can help cushion the prosthesis against the gingiva. The patient's dentist may need to evaluate denture fit and stability and modify the prosthesis to improve denture retention.

Late

Xerostomia can be a chronic condition. The patient may need to utilize combinations of the measures described to minimize oral discomfort and complications associated with xerostomia. Pilocarpine, a cholinergic parasympathomimetic agent, is effective in minimizing the chronic effects of xerostomia following a course of head and neck irradiation by stimulation of residual functional salivary gland tissue.[22-24] Pilocarpine has also been found to be helpful in treating xerostomia due to graft-versus-host disease (GVHD) and total body irradiation used in the bone marrow transplant setting.[25] Pilocarpine administered three times a day is reported to produce significant improvement of xerostomia. Common side effects associated with pilocarpine include sweating, rhinitis, headache, nausea, and urinary frequency. Pilocarpine is contraindicated for patients with uncontrolled asthma, acute iritis, or narrow-angle glaucoma. Zimmerman et al.[26] report that concomitant use of pilocarpine at a dose of 5 mg four times a day with head and neck irradiation can help to decrease the incidence of postradiation xerostomia.

Increased esophageal acidity, esophageal reflux, and esophagitis has been associated with chronic xerostomia. Use of histamine receptor antagonists such as nizatidine or famotidine can be effective in inhibiting acid secretion.

Evaluation of Therapeutic Approaches

Assessments of therapeutic approaches for xerostomia are performed through treatment and in follow-up visits. Xerostomia can be a chronic condition with significant effects on quality of life, nutrition, and dental health. Mouth assessments are perfomed by the clinician to evaluate the condition of the mouth as well as the benefit of measures taken to relieve the xerostomia. A nutritional assessment is completed to determine weight loss and dietary modifications used to accommodate the xerostomia. A dental evaluation by the dentist is also important to assess for cavities and periodontal disease.

Resources

Support for People with Oral and Head and
   Neck Cancer (SPOHNC)
P.O. Box 53
Locust Valley, NY 11560-0053
(516) 759-5333
http://www.sphonc.org

Oral Cancer Website
http://www.oralcancer.org

Oncolink
http://www.oncolink.upenn.edu

Conclusion

Patients and families benefit from understanding that xerostomia occurs as a result of the illness and its treat-ment. It is important to instruct the patient and family about the time that xerostomia may be expected to occur as well as about methods used to alleviate dryness and minimize complications. Xerostomia may become a chronic problem, and the patient and family need to understand the necessity for its long-term management. The patient may otherwise expect the xerostomia to resolve soon after the treatment is over and become extremely disappointed if the symptom persists.

During follow-up visits, xerostomia and its potential complications need to be assessed and managed. Patients and families can be assisted by creatively using different interventions to find solutions to address their unique needs. By utilizing good oral care measures, the patient will be able to achieve oral comfort, improve nutritional status, and prevent or minimize the occurrence of chronic problems such as periodontal disease or tooth decay.

References

1. Atkinson JC, Wu AJ: Salivary gland dysfunction: Causes, symptoms, treatment. *J Am Dent Assoc* 125:409–415, 1994
2. Beck SL: Prevention and management of oral complications in the cancer patient. *Curr Issues Cancer Nurs Pract Updates* 1:1–12, 1992
3. Dose AM: The symptom experience of mucositis, stomatitis, and xerostomia. *Semin Oncol Nurs* 11:248–255, 1995
4. Greenspan D: Xerostomia: Diagnosis and management. *Oncology* 10(suppl 3):7–11, 1996
5. National Institutes of Health: Oral complications of cancer therapies: Diagnosis, prevention, and treatment. *Consensus Development Conference Statement* 7:1–11, 1989
6. Poland J: Prevention and treatment of oral complications in the cancer patient. *Oncology* 5:45–50, 1991
7. Iwamoto RR: A nursing perspective on radiation-induced xerostomia. *Oncology* 10(suppl 3):12–15, 1996
8. Saunders RH, Handelman SL: Effects of hyposalivatory medications on saliva flow rates and dental caries in adults aged 65 and older. *Special Care in Dentistry* 12:116–121, 1992
9. Nagler R, Marmary Y, Krausz Y, et al: Major salivary gland dysfunction in human acute and chronic graft-versus-host disease (GVHD). *Bone Marrow Transplant* 17:219–224, 1996
10. Ramirez-Amador V, Silverman S Jr, Mayor P, et al: Candidal colonization and oral candidiasis in patients undergoing oral and pharyngeal radiation therapy. *Oral Surg Oral Med Oral Pathol* 84:149–153, 1997
11. Korsten MA, Rosman AS, Fishbein S, et al: Chronic xerostomia increases esophageal acid exposure and is associated with esophageal injury. *Am J Med* 90:701–706, 1991
12. Mossman K, Shatzman A, Chencharick J: Long-term effects of radiotherapy on taste and salivary function in man. *Int J Radiat Oncol Biol Phys* 8:991–997, 1982
13. Valdez IH, Atkinson JC, Ship JA, et al: Major salivary gland function in patients with radiation-induced xerostomia: Flow rates and sialochemistry. *Int J Radiat Oncol Biol Phys* 25:41–47, 1993
14. Garg AK, Malo M: Manifestations and treatment of xero-

stomia and associated oral effects secondary to head and neck radiation therapy. *J Am Dent Assoc* 128:1128–1133, 1997

15. Radiation Therapy Oncology Group (RTOG), American College of Radiology, Philadelphia, PA

16. Cacchillo D, Barker GJ, Barker BF: Late effects of head and neck radiation therapy and patient/dentist compliance with recommended dental care. *Spec Care Dentist* 13:159–162, 1993

17. Dreizen S, Brown LR, Daly TE, et al: Prevention of xerostomia-related dental caries in irradiated cancer patients. *J Dent Res* 56:99–104, 1977

18. Epstein JB, McBride BC, Stevenson-Moore P, et al: The efficacy of chlorhexidine gel in reduction of *Streptococcus mutans* and *Lactobacillus* species in patients treated with radiation therapy. *Oral Surg Oral Med Oral Pathol* 71:172–178, 1991

19. Blevins L: Practice poser. *The Boost: Radiation Special Interest Group Newsletter* 3:2, 1992

20. Takah J: Practice poser. *The Boost: Radiation Special Interest Group Newsletter* 3:2, 1992

21. Headley M: Practice poser. *The Boost: Radiation Special Interest Group Newsletter* 3:4, 1992

22. Johnson JT, Ferretti GA, Nethery WJ, et al: Oral pilocarpine for post-irradiation xerostomia in patients with head and neck cancer. *N Engl J Med* 329:390–395, 1993

23. LeVeque FG, Montgomery M, Potter D, et al: A multicenter, randomized, double-blind, placebo-controlled, dose-titration study of oral pilocarpine for treatment of radiation-induced xerostomia in head and neck cancer patients. *J Clin Oncol* 11:1124–1131, 1993

24. Rieke JW, Hafermann MD, Johnson JT, et al: Oral pilocarpine for radiation-induced xerostomia: Integrated efficacy and safety results from two prospective randomized clinical trials. *Int J Radiat Oncol Biol Phys* 31:661–669, 1995

25. Singhal S, Powles R, Treleaven J, et al: Pilocarpine hydrochloride for symptomatic relief of xerostomia due to chronic graft-versus-host disease or total-body irradiation after bone-marrow transplantation for hematologic malignancies. *Leuk Lymphoma* 24:539–543, 1997

26. Zimmerman RP, Mark RJ, Tran LM, et al: Concomitant pilocarpine during head and neck irradiation is associated with decreased posttreatment xerostomia. *Int J Radiat Oncol Biol Phys* 37:571–575, 1997

Dry Mouth

Patient Name: _____

Symptom and Description   Your mouth may become dry as a result of your cancer therapy. (The medical name for this is xerostomia.) For some, the dryness may be mild and can be relieved with a drink of water. For others, the dryness may be more severe and cause problems while eating, talking, and sleeping. A dry mouth can be uncomfortable.

A dry mouth increases the chances of your developing dental cavities. A dry mouth could also be a sign of an infection in your mouth.

If you smoke or chew tobacco, or drink alcoholic beverages, the dryness will be worse.

Learning Needs   You will need to learn how to inspect your mouth and what to report to your health caregiver. You will need to learn how to care for your mouth and ways to increase the moisture in your mouth. In some instances, you will learn about applying fluoride to your teeth. You will also learn how to adapt your diet to the changes in your mouth.

Prevention   It is not likely that you can prevent this symptom completely. You may be able to lessen the effects if you:

- Follow the mouth-care guidelines
- Avoid use of mouth irritants such as tobacco and alcohol
- Visit your dentist regularly
- Use medication (pilocarpine) if prescribed for you to help increase the saliva in your mouth

Management   Depending on your situation, good oral hygiene, care in selecting the foods that you eat, and seeing your dentist on a regular basis will help this problem.

1. *Mouth care*: Brush your teeth with a soft-bristle brush before and after each meal and at bedtime. If you usually floss your teeth and your gums are not sore, floss your teeth at bedtime. During the day, rinse your mouth with a cup of salt water (one-fourth teaspoon of salt in one cup of water) every 2 hours or more frequently.

2. *Fluoride application*: Your dentist may have you use fluoride on a daily basis. If your dentist has given you fluoride trays or carriers to use, use these items as instructed. If instructions have not been given, after brushing and flossing your teeth at bedtime, brush the fluoride on your teeth, spit out the extra fluoride, and do not eat or drink for 30 minutes afterward.

3. *Diet*: Eat soft, moist foods such as custards, foods with sauces and gravies, and stewed foods. Avoid hard, dry, and sticky foods such as crackers, chips, and peanut butter. Avoid spicy or acidic foods such as citrus fruits and juices. Drink liquids such as water and nonacidic juices with your meals. Avoid alcoholic

beverages because these can increase your mouth dryness. Avoid tobacco products.

4. *Use of saliva substitutes and other lubricants:* Many different products are available. The product you choose should be low in sugar content and comfortable to use. Talk with your dentist or other healthcare provider for suggestions. Place a small pat of butter or a teaspoon of olive oil in your mouth at bedtime to decrease the dryness in your mouth during the night. Keep a container of water at your bedside to sip on during the night.

Follow-up

- Be sure you understand what to expect, what to do about it, and when to call your doctor, dentist, or nurse.
- Have emergency phone numbers available.
- If you are unsure of any instructions, be sure to ask your doctor and nurse.
- See your dentist on a regular basis.
- Call your dentist if you develop mouth or tooth pain. If you have cavities or discomfort in your mouth, you need to see your dentist.
- By following these guidelines, you will minimize mouth problem and cavities and be better able to eat and maintain your weight.

Phone Numbers

Nurse: _____ Phone: _____

Physician: _____ Phone: _____

Other: _____ Phone: _____

Comments

Patient's Signature: _____ Date: _____

Nurse's Signature: _____ Date: _____

Source: Iwamoto RR: Xerostomia, in Yarbro CH, Frogge MH, Goodman M (eds): *Cancer Symptom Management* (ed 2). Sudbury: Jones and Bartlett, 1999. © Jones and Bartlett Publishers.

PART IV

Symptoms of Disturbances of Protective Mechanisms

CHAPTER 16

Alopecia

Dianne M. Reeves, RN, OCN®

The Problem of Alopecia in Cancer

Hair loss as a result of anticancer therapy has been described in the medical literature for 40 years. Our present body of knowledge about alopecia has been built largely by nurses who believe that, while it may not be classified as a life-threatening or dose-limiting side effect, it is one of the most tangible, difficult, emotionally painful side effect our patients experience.

Incidence in Cancer

Alopecia or epilation is a common side effect of radiation therapy and many chemotherapeutic agents. Descriptions of hair loss associated with single agents such as busulfan began to appear in the medical literature in the late 1950s.[1] By the 1960s, the number of reports of therapy-related epilation increased as chemotherapy was prescribed for more patients. The trend toward combining two or more agents with differing mechanisms of action (combination therapy) increased the likelihood of producing alopecia. With many current drug regimens, the likelihood is high that patients receiving multiple agents in a repetitive sequence (cycle or course) will experience some degree of alopecia over the ensuing weeks.

Radiation-induced hair loss is more variable and less predictable than drug-induced loss. Scalp epilation occurs only when the head is included in the radiation port; this point must be stressed to fearful radiation therapy patients who apply the experiences of chemotherapy patients to their own situation. Doses of 500 cGy can produce some hair loss as treatments progress; higher doses yield more profound alopecia and retarded patterns of regrowth.

The media, consumer education movements, and the increased availability of medical information have sensitized the public to the many side effects of cancer therapy. Ironically, this sensitivity has made it more difficult for some patients to hide evidence of their anticancer treatments. Yet others benefit from society's willingness to discuss the difficulties of these treatments and the stressors and burdens the patient must face. A supportive environment that empowers the patient to be productive and active throughout cancer therapy and beyond should be the goal of the health care and lay communities.

Impact on Quality of Life

Many oncologic references state that alopecia is an assault to physical appearance, body image, sexuality, and self-esteem. The way we look and the image we project says a great deal about the ways in which we value ourselves; when those values include portions of our physical appearance that are altered by therapy, anxiety ensues. Yet the competing factor in this inner struggle for equilibrium as physical appearance changes is the cancer patient's drive for survival. Because most people would do almost anything to live, the patient must adapt or maladapt to physical changes instead of forgoing treatment. Even though there are references in the literature suggesting that alopecia is a side effect that can affect patient compliance and ultimately survival, studies to verify these empirical statements are not available.

The concept of *therapeutic index*—the benefit of a therapy to the patient as compared with the costs in the form of side effects—is key in any discussion of treatment. Traditional study end points such as response, survival, and disease-free survival are being supplemented by qualitative and quantitative information about toxicities that have an impact on patients' perceptions of quality of life. Quality of life is multidimensional and difficult to define and measure, yet alopecia accompanied by disturbances in body image and self-esteem can have a negative impact on quality-of-life measurements.

Wagner and Bye[2] measured the impact of drug-induced alopecia on body image in 77 patients with cancer. Two groups were created from this population: one group had clinical signs of chemotherapy-induced alopecia; the other had none. The subjects completed a body image and social activity questionnaire to test the researchers' expectation that alopecia would negatively affect body image and social activities. Those expected outcomes were not confirmed. Although subjects with alopecia decreased their social activities more than those without obvious hair loss, body image and social activity scores between the groups showed no significant difference.

Patients' perceptions related to hair loss due to chemotherapeutic intervention may be linked to events beyond the physical loss of hair. Munstedt et al.[3] measured self-esteem, problem-solving ability, general health, and physical fitness in 29 patients with gynecologic cancer who were preparing for combination chemotherapy. Repeated measurements did not return to baseline, even after hair had regrown. The researchers suggest that differences in those domains are not exclusively due to hair loss but may also be related to the stressors and coping processes that remain long after the completion of a therapy regimen.

Etiology

Normal Hair Growth Patterns

A single human hair comprises a hair bulb that contains a proliferating pool of undifferentiated cells, the hair root, and the hair shaft. Active division of matrix cells occurs in the lower portion of the bulb, which pushes the hair up from the root and projects it through the surface of the scalp. A strand of scalp (or terminal) hair is composed of rows of tightly compacted, keratinized cells. Approximately 100,000 such strands cover the human scalp, with an average loss of 100 of these hairs daily.

Phases of hair growth and rest normally vary with age and body region; they can also be affected by physiologic and psychological events. Normal hair growth phases are tricyclic and are not synchronized. At any single point in time, 88% of human scalp hair is in the growing (anagen) phase, and 12% is in the transitional (catagen) and resting (telogen) phases. Anagen lasts from 2 to 5 years, producing hair growth at a rate of 0.35 mm/day. As hairs approach catagen (which lasts up to 2 weeks), the hair root separates from within the hair bulb and is pushed out of the bulb. During the resting phase or telogen, there is no hair growth for approximately 3 to 5 months. Events that initiate catagen and the resultant telogen are not clear. As telogen ends, there is a repeated increase in RNA synthesis as follicles reenter anagen.

Chemotherapeutic Agent Mechanisms of Action on Hair Follicles

Because chemotherapeutic agents make no distinction between cancer and normal cells, all sites of energetic mitotic activity are prone to their chemical insult. The bone marrow, GI tract, and rapidly proliferating cells of the hair and skin surfaces are particularly vulnerable to these effects. Not all drugs within a single pharmacologic classification produce equal degrees of epilation; the reason that some agents and not others produce alopecia is unclear.

Many drugs can produce alopecia (Table 16-1). Although some agents are more chemically identified as epilating due to their frequent appearances in the medi-

TABLE 16-1 Chemotherapy Agents That Produce Alopecia

High Potential to Produce Alopecia	
Cyclophosphamide	Ifosfamide
Daunorubicin	Paclitaxel
Doxorubicin (>50 mg)	Taxotere
Etoposide	

Moderate Potential to Produce Alopecia	
Cisplatin	Mitomycin
Dactinomycin	Mitoxantrone
5-Fluorouracil	Topotecan
Idarubicin	Vinblastine
Mechlorethamine	Vincristine
Methotrexate	Vindesine
Mithramycin	Vinorelbine

Low to No Potential to Produce Alopecia	
Bleomycin	L-Asparaginase
Busulfan	Lomustine
Carboplatin	Melphalan
Carmustine	6-Mercaptopurine
Chlorambucil	Procarbazine
Cytosine arabinoside	Suramin
Dacarbazine	6-Thioguanine
Gemcitabine	Thiotepa
Irinotecan	

cal literature (e.g., doxorubicin and cyclophosphamide), the degree of hair loss produced by any agent is influenced by the dose delivered, the schedule, and the route of administration.[4,5] Elevated blood levels of chemotherapeutic agents achieved through bolus-dosing schedules may be more injurious to the hair bulb and follicle than a cumulative dose delivered over an extended period of time.

Pathophysiology

Most hair follicle injury is caused by anagen arrest. Because mitosis is brisk in the hair bulbs of the follicles on the scalp, hair follicles are vulnerable to cytotoxic drugs. When a dose of an epilating drug is given, the cells of the hair bulbs absorb a proportion of the drug. Cellular division and protein synthesis can be suppressed or halted. If cellular activity is completely halted, the hair enters telogen (resting phase) prematurely. The hair is free to be shed at some future point, and regrowth occurs in approximately 3 to 5 months, the normal length of telogen. This sequence of events can explain the hair regrowth that some patients experience even while continuing to receive chemotherapy; it is the normal hair cycle that was precipitously interrupted by a dose of chemotherapy but which resumes if there is no further insult by additional doses of drug.

If a dose of drug is not sufficient to halt anagen, there may instead be inhibition of mitosis in the hair bulb, causing narrowing or constriction of the hair shaft; these narrow sections can be viewed as the follicle grows. Additional doses of drug can cause repeated areas of stricture, reflecting each exposure to the causative agent. These structural abnormalities are weakened sites and become points of breakage during normal activities such as shampooing or brushing the hair.

Alopecia connotes a diffuse shedding of hair. To be noticeable, at least 50% of the hair must be lost. While most discussions about this toxicity of many anticancer drugs focus on the loss of scalp hair, epilating effects can include the axillary, pubic, body, and facial hair, including the eyebrows and eyelashes. Agents that cause alopecia differ in their ability to do so through a variety of routes, doses, and schedules; high peak blood levels produced by pulse drug doses may cause great disruption in the mitotic activity of anagenic hair cells, whereas continuous infusions of lower daily doses of drug can increase the cell's length of exposure to the causative agent. The literature notes that one agent classically linked to alopecia, doxorubicin, causes significantly more epilation at doses of ≥50 mg/m².[6,7] Much of the literature reporting interventions to reduce alopecia has focused on doxorubicin, due to the high frequency with which this drug is pre-scribed and the nearly 100% reported occurrence of alopecia extending to the eyebrows and eyelashes.

Hair loss typically begins to appear 2 to 3 weeks after the first exposure to drug, with continued loss over the next 3 to 4 weeks; but there can be dramatic exceptions to this guideline. Paclitaxel alopecia appears 2 to 3 weeks after the beginning of therapy and is often sudden and cumulative, involving the entire body when given at doses of 135 mg/m². Total hair loss can occur over a 24-hour period.[8] Typically hair on the crown and the sides of the head above the ears disappears first, possibly due to mechanical friction, as these areas come into contact with bed linens, pillows, and head coverings.

Exposed scalp can be sensitive, and must be protected. Regrowth may be seen in 3 months as cells catapulted prematurely into telogen recover and reenter anagen. As hair repopulates the scalp, it may be damaged again by additional drug doses, or it may continue to grow slowly. Bierman's[1] early report on 14 patients with neoplastic disease who received a single infusion of busulfan noted that alopecia appeared in 6 of the 14, with slow regrowth. He also noted that alopecia was unrelated to clinical response. In fact, there was no alopecia seen at lower doses of the drug that were also therapeutically effective.

Hair loss is nearly always temporary when caused by anticancer drugs. Reports have cited numerous changes in new hair growth, ranging from color to texture alterations. Straight hair can regrow waved or curly, and consistency can alter from thick to fine. The literature is in agreement that hair returns without interruption once all systemic therapy has been halted.

Assessment

Instruments That Measure Alopecia

The ability to measure a phenomenon such as drug-induced alopecia is critical for three reasons:

1. To precisely describe alopecia in terms of severity, onset, duration, and recovery

2. To standardize descriptors of alopecia so that information from multiple studies/settings can be compared and contrasted

3. To evaluate responsiveness to therapeutic measures

WHO Toxicity Grading Criteria

The World Health Organization (WHO) convened meetings in 1978 and 1979 attended by representatives from 13 nations. The purpose of the meetings was to standardize reporting criteria for cancer clinical trials, especially those focused on the reporting of toxicities. WHO criteria related to alopecia that were derived from the meetings and adapted to the trials of the European Organization for Research on Treatment in Cancer (EORTC) are:

Grade 0	Grade 1	Grade 2	Grade 3	Grade 4
no change	minimal loss	moderate, patchy loss	complete alopecia but reversible	nonreversible loss

ECOG Grading Criteria

WHO grading criteria for the measurement of toxicity have not been rapidly accepted by United States clinical trials groups. A number of cooperative group tools to assess a variety of therapy side effects have been developed. One commonly used tool is a grading scale from the Eastern Cooperative Oncology Group (ECOG):[9]

Grade 0	Grade 1	Grade 2	Grade 3	Grade 4
none	alopecia (mild)	alopecia (severe)	———	———

The ECOG grading system for alopecia is simplistic, and allows for interrater scoring differences.

Cancer Therapy Evaluation Program (CTEP) Common Toxicity Criteria (CTC)

The Cancer Therapy Evaluation Program (CTEP) of the National Cancer Institute (NCI) developed Common Toxicity Criteria (CTC) in 1988 to provide a set of repetitive measures of commonly experienced side effects of clinical trials that could be used for all U.S. cooperative groups. The guidelines were revised in 1998 to expand the categories, more precisely define clinical phenomena, and remove the subjectivity of measures whenever possible.[10] The resulting alopecia scale is as follows:

Grade 0	Grade 1	Grade 2	Grade 3	Grade 4
normal	mild hair loss	pronounced hair loss	———	———

CTEP criteria are nearly identical to those used by ECOG. In both the ECOG and CTEP scales, the maximum score for alopecia severity is grade 2. With the recent revision of the CTEP CTC, standardization throughout cooperative groups participating in oncologic clinical trials is a realistic goal.

Dean Protection From Hair Loss Scale

Dean's important report on the use of scalp hypothermia required that a tool be used to produce standardized scores for multiple data points. The scale below, which measures response to scalp hypothermia, was combined with routine serial photographs.[11]

Poor	Moderate	Good	Excellent
75–100% loss	50–75% loss	25–50% loss	0–25% loss

Dean's scale can be converted easily into one with numerical equivalences, yet it should not be compared with the toxicity grading criteria scales already presented.

Instruments that measure and describe patterns of alopecia reduce the hazards of descriptors such as "good amount of protection" or "acceptable loss." Using vague terms such as these makes it impossible for researchers to compare patient responses across several studies or to make assumptions about the generalizability of intervention studies.

Physical Assessment of Alopecia

Patients who have alopecia or who receive epilating drugs are examined at serial time points to document patterns of hair loss. The physical exam must include:

* Description of patterns of hair loss on the scalp and over entire body
* Density of remaining hair
* Shape of the front hairline
* Length, texture, and curl/wave of hair
* Color—dull or bright
* Condition of the scalp

Additionally, hair can be gently pulled to test for excessive loss. The patient should be questioned about finding hair on pillows or bed linens. Fine regrowth of hair may be noted between treatments or approximately 3 months after the initiation of epilating therapy. Precise documentation of the patterns of hair loss and recovery is vital and often overlooked. The global description "alopecia" on each patient visit is not sufficient, as it overlooks important patient information about hair loss patterns that could be definitive for a new anticancer drug or drug combination. Diaries or other patient recording devices may allow patients the chance to track daily observations and may provide the professional with precise data that could fuel future research studies.

Symptom Management

Prevention

The controversy over the preventability of chemotherapy-induced alopecia has raged since 1966, when reports of scalp tourniquet use appeared in the medical literature.[12] Since those first publications, interventions to prevent or minimize the loss of hair during therapy have been of three major types:

* scalp tourniquets
* scalp hypothermia or cooling
* pharmacologic agents

Scalp tourniquets occlude the superficial blood flow to the scalp, decreasing the amount of drug that reaches the hair follicles. Pressure is typically applied using a narrow sphygmomanometer cuff inflated 10 mmHg about systolic pressure. The tourniquet is left in place for 5 to 15 minutes after injection of all drugs; it is hypothesized that by that time most of the drug has been cleared from the circulation.

Scalp pressure to retard hair loss is accompanied by risks and is not a recommended practice. It is unclear how long the tourniquet needs to stay in place and extended use can cause damage to delicate superficial facial nerves. The possibility of creating a drug-free area that could be a site of later relapse is an important risk to consider, perhaps more so in cancers that recur in the skin. Peak plasma drug levels are not always cleared within 15 minutes; additionally, the extended need for protection makes the scalp tourniquet impractical during continuous drug infusions. Pressure around the hairline for an extended period of time can also be very uncomfortable.

Scalp hypothermia or cooling applies the concept of creating a drug-free area through the use of ice or temperature-controlled devices to decrease drug uptake to the scalp. Scalp cooling may also alter the metabolism of agents in the cell. Numerous reports have shown varying degrees of success using hypothermia to retard hair loss.[11,13–18] Published reports are often difficult to analyze and compare, however, because they:

- are frequently nonrandomized studies, with no control group
- use vague or unreported scales by which to measure success
- do not adequately define assessment periods and criteria to judge success
- group together patients receiving a variety of different drugs and schedules
- have not reported follow-up on patients once alopecia occurs
- report small patient numbers

Giaccone et al.[17] reported in a controlled study of 35 patients that 37% who received scalp hypothermia had some prevention of hair loss, but 100% alopecia appeared in the control group. Tollenaar et al.[18] similarly reported on 35 patients receiving breast cancer adjuvant combination chemotherapy, who were treated with scalp hypothermia. Only 11% of patients had no to minor loss of hair, and all patients required a wig. The authors concluded that because the chemotherapeutic regimen included doxorubicin, cyclophosphamide, and 5-fluorouracil, scalp cooling has no place in treatment plans that include more than an anthracycline agent (e.g., doxorubicin).

The success of scalp cooling may be linked to:

- *Ability to cool the scalp sufficiently.*[16] "Therefore the fit, temperature, and length of application are important.

- *The drugs administered.*[11,18] Doses of doxorubicin >50 mg are more difficult to protect through scalp cooling.

- *Liver function.*[13] Scalp hypothermia may not be effective in cases of observed liver dysfunction with biochemical signs of disease. Many patients with impaired liver function may have prolonged plasma drug levels after the drug administration.

- *Concerns of patient safety.* Although reports of latent scalp metastases following scalp hypothermia or cooling are reported to be less than 1%,[13,19] the risk of placing a patient at risk for later, perhaps resistant, sites of disease recurrence may make this intervention untenable for some healthcare professionals.

Scalp hypothermia is described as uncomfortable by some patients; in addition, benefits usually become less obvious over time for patients who use it for repeated chemotherapy treatments. The intervention also requires time expenditure by the staff, who must apply and maintain these devices.

Pharmacologic agents represent an area of intervention that is new and exciting for professionals who are frustrated by the risks and failure rates associated with scalp tourniquets and scalp hypothermia. In 1985, Wood[20] reported that tocopherol may protect against doxorubicin-induced alopecia. These results have not been replicated in other studies, but tocopherol remains under investigation. Imuvert, a biological response modifier made from the bacteria *Serratia marcescens,* offered some protection against epilation from cytosine arabinoside and doxorubicin but not against cyclophosphamide epilation, when tested in rat models.[21] Interleukin-1 (IL-1) also offered excellent protection against cytosine arabinoside–induced alopecia but not cyclophosphamide-induced epilation when tested in these same rat models.[21]

Minoxidil is an orally active peripheral vasodilator used to treat severe hypertension that produces a side effect of enhanced hair growth. It has been tested for its ability to retard the loss of hair during chemotherapy treatment and to accelerate the regrowth of lost hair. Hussein[22] reported in 1995 that when injected locally the drug offered good protection against cytosine arabinoside but not against cyclophosphamide-induced alopecia in rat models. Duvic et al.[23] found a place for minoxidil in the regrowth of hair of women receiving adjuvant chemotherapy after breast cancer surgery. Compared to a control group, women using a 2% topical minoxidil solution showed a significant reduction in the period of time required from maximum hair loss to the point of hair regrowth (mean 50.2 days).

In summary, a variety of interventions aimed at chemotherapy-related alopecia reported since 1966 have shown a range of results. Scalp hypothermia or cooling using gel packs, ice caps, or a variety of commercially available devices remains the most commonly used scalp preservation intervention reported in the literature. There are no clear prescriptive guidelines as to which patient groups would clearly benefit from scalp preservation interventions throughout treatment. Instead, a number of considerations are proposed for the clinical practitioner's evaluation.

1. Scalp hypothermia cannot be predicted to be successful. Patients who may benefit the most are those who receive doxorubicin in doses of <50 mg, or drugs with low to moderate potential for producing alopecia.

2. Clinically apparent liver dysfunction may prolong plasma drug levels, making the success of hypothermia unlikely.

3. Scalp hypothermia appliances must fit snugly and be maintained at a uniformly low temperature. Some institutions report that wetting the hair before applying a scalp device gives a tight seal and a uniform cooling pattern. Patients must be assessed frequently throughout the cooling process for their comfort.

4. Scalp tourniquet is a historic and not-recommended practice that has been largely replaced by hypothermia units.

5. Pharmacologic approaches are relatively new, and results are now appearing in the medical literature with increasing frequency. Their ability to retard or prevent hair loss remains unproven.

Therapeutic Approaches

Because alopecia is unavoidable in many patients who receive chemotherapy treatment, patients must be prepared for the rapid onset and transient nature of this side effect. The appearance of hair on bed linens typically begins 2 weeks after the initiation of chemotherapy, but the onset can occur sooner. Loss can be rapid and complete, resulting in a totally defoliated scalp within 3 to 4 weeks after the beginning of treatment. Patients should be advised to purchase a wig or head coverings early in their treatment schedule, while enough hair is present to allow a good match of color and style.

Unprotected scalp and body areas are extremely sensitive to the effects of sun and temperature. Patients must be advised to use sun protection factor (SPF) products of at least SPF 15 when exposed to sunshine for more than brief periods of time. Patients may complain that their scalp hurts or has heightened sensitivity during alopecia; these are common complaints that should be heard and documented, but interventions are seldom necessary.

Patients who experience an uneven pattern of hair loss may express the desire to shave or cut the remaining hair. This can enhance a person's physical and emotional well-being, as a more symmetrical and acceptable body image is produced. Caregivers should alert the patient to avoid cuts or nicks to the scalp when sections of hair are cut. Symptomatic relief may also be obtained by using scalp heat, lotions, massage, and other locally soothing approaches. Although the medical literature offers no guide to these practices, patients may gain relief from them, provided their safety is not jeopardized. By reassuring patients that their hair will return when systemic therapy is halted, some of their anxiety may be redirected toward adaptation and recovery.

Patients who experience alopecia as a side effect of their chemotherapy regimens do not necessarily have problems with treatment compliance. But those who have difficulty with the altered self-image that alopecia imposes may suffer.[48] Healthcare professionals should be alert to patient and family reports of interference with activities because of alopecia, loss of appetite, withdrawal from family and significant others with verbalized feelings of loss of libido and attractiveness, depression, fatigue, and sadness. Classes such as "Look Good, Feel Better," a series sponsored by the American Cancer Society, can help patients accept a different, perhaps transient, view of themselves until they recover from this obvious effect of their therapy program. Appendix 16A provides a self-care guide for individuals experiencing alopecia.

References

1. Bierman HR, Kelly KH, Knudson AG Jr, et al: The influence of 1,4-dimethyl sulfonoxy-1,4-dimethylbutane (CB 2348, Dimethyl Myleran) in neoplastic disease. *Ann NY Acad Sci* 68: 1211–1222, 1958

2. Wagner L, Bye M: Body image and patients experiencing alopecia as a result of cancer chemotherapy. *Cancer Nurs* 5: 365–369, 1979

3. Munstedt D, Manthey N, Sachsse S, et al: Change in self-concept and body image during alopecia induced cancer chemotherapy. *Support Care Cancer* 5:139–143, 1997

4. Chabner BA, Collins JM: *Cancer Chemotherapy: Principles and Practice.* Philadelphia: Lippincott, 1990, pp. 2394–2395

5. Chambers JT, Chambers SK, Kohorn EI, et al: Uterine papillary serous carcinoma treated with intraperitoneal cisplatin and intravenous doxorubicin and cyclophosphamide. *Gynecol Oncol* 60:438–442, 1996

6. Wilkes GM, Ingwersen K, Barton-Burke M: *Oncology Nursing Drug Reference.* Sudbury: Jones and Bartlett, 1994, pp. 101–103

7. Kennedy M, Packard R, Grant M, et al: The effects of using ChemoCap® on occurrence of chemotherapy-induced alopecia. *Oncol Nurs Forum* 10:19–24, 1983

8. Lubejko BG, Sartorius SE: Nursing considerations in paclitaxel (Taxol®) administration. *Semin Oncol* 20(suppl 3): 26–30, 1993

9. Oken MM, Creech RH, Tormey DC, et al: Toxicity and response criteria of the Eastern Cooperative Oncology Group. *Am J Clin Oncol* 5:649–655, 1982

10. Cancer Therapy Evaluation Programs: *Common Toxicity Criteria Version 2.0.* Bethesda, MD: National Institutes of Health, National Cancer Institute, March 1998

11. Dean JC, Salmon SE, Griffith KS: Prevention of doxorubicin-induced hair loss with scalp hypothermia. *N Engl J Med* 301: 1427–1429, 1979

12. Simister JM: Alopecia and cytotoxic drugs. *BMJ* 2:1138, 1966

13. Dean JC, Griffith KS, Cetas TC, et al: Scalp hypothermia: A comparison of ice packs and the Kold Kap® in the prevention of doxorubicin-induced alopecia. *J Clin Oncol* 1:33–37, 1983

14. Hunt JM, Anderson JE, Smith IE: Scalp hypothermia to prevent Adriamycin-induced hair loss. *Cancer Nurs* 1:25–31, 1982

15. Satterwhite B, Zimm S: The use of scalp hypothermia in the prevention of doxorubicin-induced hair loss. *Cancer* 54: 34–37, 1984

16. Tierney A: Preventing chemotherapy-induced alopecia in cancer patients: Is scalp cooling worthwhile? *J Adv Nurs* 12: 303–310, 1987

17. Giaccone G, DiGiulio F, Morandini MP, et al: Scalp hypothermia in the prevention of doxorubicin-induced hair loss. *Cancer Nurs* 11:170–173, 1988

18. Tollenaar RAEM, Liefars GJ, Repelaer Van Driel OJ, et al: Scalp cooling has no place in the prevention of alopecia in adjuvant chemotherapy for breast cancer. *Eur J Cancer* 30: 1448–1453, 1994

19. Seipp C: Scalp hypothermia: Indications for precaution. *Oncol Nurs Forum* 10:12, 1983

20. Wood LA: Possible prevention of Adriamycin-induced alopecia by tocopherol. *N Engl J Med* 312:1060, 1985

21. Hussein AM: Chemotherapy-induced alopecia: New developments. *South Med J* 86:489–496, 1993

22. Hussein AM: Protection against cytosine arabinoside-induced alopecia by minoxidil in a rat animal model. *Int. J Dermatol* 34:470–473, 1995

23. Duvic M, Lemak NA, Valero V, et al: A randomized trial of minoxidil in chemotherapy-induced alopecia. *J Am Acad Dermatol* 35:74–78, 1996

24. Richardson J, Marks G, Levine A: The influence of symptoms of disease and side effects of treatment on compliance with cancer treatment. *J Clin Oncol* 6:1746–1752, 1988

Alopecia

Patient Name: _____

Symptom and Description   Alopecia, or hair loss, occurs with certain chemo-therapy drugs that have a good chance of causing hair loss. Hair loss can begin 10 to 21 days after drugs are begun, with total loss in 1 to 2 months. Hair on your head is often lost first, but hair over the entire body can be lost. If a wig is to be used, it is important to be fitted for a wig right away. Regrowth may begin while you are still on chemotherapy, although it will be slow. Full regrowth happens when chemotherapy is finished.

Learning Needs   You may need to learn to protect your scalp and skin with head covers and skin protection factor (SPF) products. You will need to learn when to expect hair loss, how it may happen, and where to go to find a wig or other acceptable head covering.

Prevention   Stopping hair loss may be impossible. Your doctor or nurse may be able to describe some measures that can slow or lessen the loss of hair. These are not always successful, however, and may be used less with some drugs. Prevention of hair loss may be difficult because chemotherapy drugs are meant to reach throughout your body via the blood. When this occurs, we cannot stop them from reaching hair cells.

Management

- Think about getting a wig, hat, or scarf early in your treatment schedule, *before* you lose your hair.
- Remember that skin suddenly exposed can be sensitive and must be protected.
- Always remember that hair loss is a *temporary* side effect of chemotherapy.
- Hair loss may change the way you feel about yourself. If your feelings are stopping you from doing important things, share them with your doctor or nurse.

Follow-up   The American Cancer Society offers "Look Good, Feel Better" classes for people who have hair loss during cancer treatment. There is a lot of information to help you to cope during this difficult time in your life. Discuss with your doctor or nurse at least each cycle of therapy how you are coping with hair loss while on treatment.

Phone Numbers

Nurse: _____ Phone: _____

Physician: _____ Phone: _____

Wig Vendors: _____ Phone: _____

Other: _____ Phone: _____

(continued) 283

Comments:

Patient's Signature: _____ Date: _____

Nurse's Signature: _____ Date: _____

Source: Reeves DM: Alopecia, in Yarbro CH, Frogge MH, Goodman M (eds.). *Cancer Symptom Management* (ed 2). Sudbury: Jones and Bartlett, 1999. © Jones and Bartlett Publishers.

CHAPTER 17

Bleeding

Julie Pruett, RN, MS

The Problem of Bleeding in Cancer

Bleeding is a common complication for many people with cancer. The problem is complex due to the diversity of causes and exacerbating factors involved in the disease and its treatment, which often makes it difficult to diagnose and manage a bleeding problem. There can be multiple bleeding abnormalities, all occurring concurrently. The type of neoplasm, location of the tumor, treatment courses and modalities, and toxic effects of treatment all have an impact on the risk of bleeding. Any organ may be affected. The extent of bleeding may vary from being virtually undetectable to life-threatening. Due to the diversity of hemostatic abnormalities and the potential sites for hemorrhage, there are many differences in presentation, management, and clinical implications when caring for the patient with cancer who has bleeding problems.

Incidence in Cancer

Neoplasms increase the risk for bleeding. Malignancies carrying a higher probability for hemorrhage include leukemias, especially acute promyelocytic leukemia, and mucin-producing adenocarcinomas. Individuals with hematologic malignancies, such as acute leukemias, are more prone to bleeding complications than those with solid tumors. This is due to the tumor involvement of the bone marrow, usually resulting in thrombocytopenia or platelets with altered function. In an attempt to eradi-

cate the tumor cells, the bone marrow itself becomes the target of the antineoplastic treatment. Increased bleeding may be due to factors other than thrombocytopenia, such as leukostasis, leukemic infiltration, and qualitative platelet defects. The incidence and severity of the bleeding in the patient with acute leukemia is also much greater. Fifty-two percent of those dying from acute leukemia will have a fatal hemorrhage, whereas only 1.5% of those individuals dying from solid tumor cancers have a fatal hemorrhage.[1]

Gaydos et al.[2] demonstrated that there is an increased incidence and severity of bleeding with a decreased platelet count. It was shown that, for the patient with leukemia, gross hemorrhage rarely occurred when the platelet count was kept greater than 20,000/mm^3. It was then postulated that keeping the platelet count greater than 20,000/mm^3 with platelet transfusions would significantly decrease the frequency of significant bleeding. More frequent, serious, life-threatening hemorrhage occurs when platelet counts drop below 10,000/mm^3.[2-4]

The relationship between platelet count and incidence of bleeding has been studied less in cases of solid tumors. The duration of thrombocytopenia due to therapy is relatively short in treatment for solid tumors. Platelet nadirs of less than 20,000/mm^3 are less frequent in this population (11%).[5] When the platelet count is greater than 10,000/mm^3, the incidence of bleeding in the solid tumor population is less than 12%; however, fatal or severe hemorrhage can occur with platelet counts greater than 10,000/mm^3. Fifty percent of bleeding that occurs is considered superficial, confined to skin, nose, and gingiva. Serious and life-threatening hemorrhage is most frequently associated with tumor extension or metastases, abnormal coagulation, or septicemia in this population.[5,6] Solid tumors more prone to having hemostatic abnormalities include the mucin-producing adenocarcinomas: gastric, lung, pancreas, and prostate. Abnormalities in coagulation laboratory tests have been reported in up to 92% of patients with cancer.[7] Most of these are consistent with overcompensated intravascular coagulation with fibrinolysis, elevated fibrin degradation products, thrombocytosis, and hyperfibrinogenemia.[8]

Impact on Quality of Life

The impact that bleeding has on the patient's quality of life depends on the acuity and the site of the hemorrhage. Bleeding might be chronic and unnoticeable to the individual who is experiencing it, such as the person who has guaiac-positive stools but is not experiencing any symptoms of bleeding. Bleeding is frequently one of the signs that brings an individual in to seek medical attention. Hemorrhage or rectal bleeding has been associated with an improved prognosis in colorectal cancer due to the early manifestation of surface erosion, which can lead to early intervention and prolonged survival.[9,10] Bleeding can also cause increased discomfort with a relatively small amount of blood loss, as in hematuria. Low-level bleeding results in anemia, causing fatigue and weakness. Hemorrhage may be dramatic and life-threatening, as in rupture of the carotid artery due to cancers of the head and neck. The location of the bleeding may be more significant in determining its severity than the volume of blood loss, such as in intracranial hemorrhages.

Etiology

Normal Hemostasis

Hemostasis is the solidification of the fluid component of blood into a clot, thus minimizing the amount of blood escaping from the injured blood vessel. Normal hemostasis is an interaction between blood vessel, platelets, and coagulation factors. Bleeding disorders occur when there is an alteration in one or more of these three components, qualitatively or quantitatively. The intact blood vessel endothelium produces substances to inhibit platelet aggregation during normal blood flow (e.g., prostacyclin, antithrombin III, and protein C activator), thus preventing hemostasis.[11–13] An injured blood vessel exposes the subendothelial connective tissues matrix, which is extremely thrombogenic, causing platelet adherence to the exposed subendothelial tissue. The blood vessel injury allows binding sites for factor XII, activating it and initiating the intrinsic pathway. The injured cells of the vessel release tissue injury factor (thromboplastin), which interacts with factor VII, activating the extrinsic pathway of the coagulation cascade (Figure 17-1).[12] As the blood vessel heals, the clot is modified and eventually dissolves to restore normal structure and function. The clot is dissolved by an enzymatic process called *fibrinolysis*. Endothelial cells near the thrombus produce plasminogen activators that convert circulating plasminogen to plasmin, thus initiating thrombolysis and dissolving the thrombus.[12]

Hemorrhage

Bleeding occurs when a blood vessel is injured and blood escapes. Hemostasis may be altered if the platelet function or the coagulation pathways are abnormal. There are multiple mechanisms altering vascular integrity, platelet function, and coagulation in the individual with cancer. Vascular integrity may be altered by an invasion of the tumor into the vessel wall or an increasing fragility of the wall due to therapy, such as radiation therapy or steroid treatment. Platelet dysfunction might be due to abnormal platelet counts from disease, medications, or therapy. Infection, liver disease, and high-viscosity proteins expressed by the tumor can alter the coagulation pathway, leading to an increased risk of bleeding.[12–14] Individuals may have one or multiple causes for altered hemostasis.

Hemorrhage caused by tumor

The tumor itself can affect bleeding tendencies in three different ways. First, as in solid tumors, the tumor may invade surrounding structures or blood vessels, causing extravasation of blood. Second, the tumor may invade and occupy the bone marrow (*myelophthisis*). These individuals may present with mild bleeding, such as gingival oozing, or be asymptomatic with diminished blood counts. Thirdly, the cancer may cause disseminated intravascular coagulation (DIC) by producing high-viscosity proteins. These individuals are frequently very ill when this diagnosis is made, as in acute DIC. Bleeding is difficult to control due to the lack of platelets and coagulation factors.

Tumors may invade the local tissues or blood vessels. Tumors that erode into mucous membranes, such as oropharyngeal, genitourinary, gastrointestinal, or gynecological tumors, are prone to cause bleeding by local tissue disruption. Tumors lying in close proximity to large blood vessels put the individual at high risk for bleeding, as the tumor may erode into the vessel and cause sudden massive hemorrhage. One of the most dramatic hemorrhages may occur if a head and neck cancer invades the carotid artery.

Leukemias and lymphomas are the most common cancers invading the bone marrow, although it has been seen in other cancers. The malignant cells are overproduced, crowding out normal hematopoietic cells, resulting in thrombocytopenia, anemia, and frequently neutropenia. The marrow's space and resources are spent making an abundance of malignant cells, causing normal cells to be underproduced.

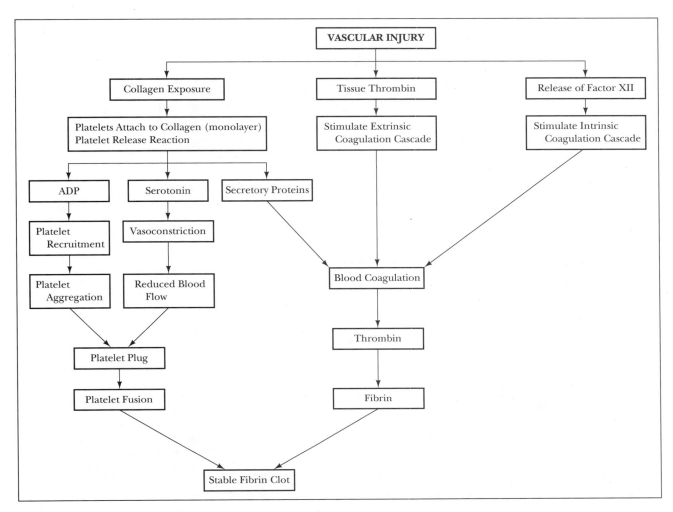

FIGURE 17-1 Mechanism of normal hemostasis. (ADP = adenosine diphosphate.)

Neoplasms may cause DIC by producing abnormal high-viscosity proteins that obstruct capillary blood flow, prompting clotting, then fibrinolysis in the microvasculature. When this is widespread and systemic, the overstimulation of the hemostatic and fibrinolytic systems uses up the coagulation factors and platelets faster than the body is able to replace them, thus increasing bleeding tendencies. Acute promyelocytic leukemic cells contain granules that induce DIC when released into the bloodstream. Excessively high white blood cell counts can cause leukostasis in patients with acute leukemia and obstructed capillary blood flow and can initiate DIC.[14,15]

Hemorrhage caused by antineoplastic therapy

Antineoplastic therapy frequently increases the risk for bleeding. Chemotherapy and radiation therapy can cause myelosuppression, including thrombocytopenia. Damaged marrow that is slow to recover or unable to fully recover after antineoplastic therapy limits the aggressiveness of further treatment for the person with cancer. Doses are diminished or eliminated because of marrow suppression. Less intensive chemotherapy may be administered in future treatments. Therapy can damage normal tissue, as well as bone marrow, making the individual more prone to bleeding. Chemotherapy and radiation therapy may cause ulcerations of the mucous membranes. Tumor necrosis, after treatment, may cause bleeding if the tumor involves any blood vessel. Corticosteroids irritate the gastric mucosa, impair wound healing, and make skin thin and fragile.

Hemorrhage due to infection

Infection may be the cause of local ulceration and bleeding or systemic bleeding. If infection occurs near a vessel, bleeding may occur. Risk of bleeding is twice as high in the thrombocytopenic patient who has fevers compared to the noninfected thrombocytopenic patient. This is due to the activation of the coagulation cascade by complement. Sepsis can stimulate the coagulation cascade, prompting DIC. This is most frequently seen in gram-negative sepsis due to the endotoxins released from the bacteria (Figure 17-2). DIC has also been seen in

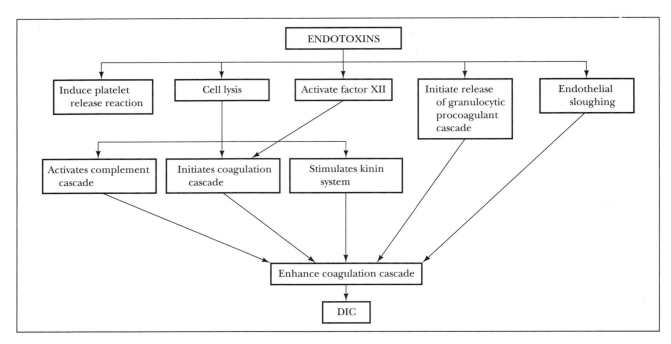

FIGURE 17-2 Sepsis triggering disseminated intravascular coagulation (DIC).

gram-positive and fungal sepsis.[16,17] Systemic diseases, such as sepsis and DIC also put the individual at higher risk for gastritis and potential bleeding. Some viruses can cause myelosuppression or thrombocytopenia. Viral and bacterial infections may irritate or ulcerate linings of the GI or genitourinary tracts, causing bleeding.

Hemorrhage due to vitamin K deficiency and liver disease

Malnourished individuals or those who have significant disease in the liver may have a vitamin K deficiency or coagulation defects. The liver is the major site of synthesis of many coagulation factors. Vitamin K is necessary for the formation of factors II, VII, IX, and X in the coagulation cascade.[13,15] If deficient, the cascade is disrupted, and coagulation is impaired. Dietary deficiency, biliary obstruction, malabsorptive syndromes, liver disease, warfarin therapy, and intestinal sterilization by antibiotic therapy all contribute to the depleted stores of vitamin K.[13,15,18,19] Liver impairment may result in decreased synthesis of these factors, leading to coagulation defects. Chronic liver disease may cause increased portal hypertension, thus leading to esophageal varices.[12] Liver failure frequently is associated with altered platelet function and abnormal production of fibrinogen.[13]

Medications interfering with hemostasis

There are numerous drugs that have an impact on platelet numbers and platelet function. Platelet dysfunction combined with another mild hemostatic abnormality can have a cumulative effect, resulting in serious hemorrhage.[13,18,19] Aspirin is the most common medication taken that is associated with platelet dysfunction. Aspirin and other nonsteroidal antiinflammatory drugs (NSAIDs) inhibit the platelet secretory process, diminish collagen-induced aggregation, and diminish the second phase of adenosine diphosphate (ADP)- and epinephrine-induced aggregation.[14,19] Alteration in platelet aggregation from aspirin may last 4 days after ingestion, until there is sufficient platelet turnover, replenishing the system with new platelets having normal function. Other NSAIDs have a more transient inhibition of platelet function, lasting only as long as the drug is circulating through the bloodstream.[19]

After aspirin, antibiotics are the drugs most associated with causing bleeding. High-dose β-lactam antibiotics, such as carbenicillin (20–40 g/day), ticarcillin (16 g/day), and penicillins (10–40 million U/day), impair the aggregation of platelets and prolong bleeding time within 1 day by blocking platelet receptors for ADP.[18–20] Maximal platelet dysfunction is reached 3 to 5 days after the initiation of therapy and resolves 3 to 4 days after the antibiotics are ceased.[13,18,21] Cephalosporins and moxalactam inhibit platelet function like penicillin, and also affect the abdominal flora, diminishing the vitamin K absorption and thus affecting coagulation.[18,21] Vitamin K may be given parenterally to counter this effect. Uremic patients have the largest incidence of antibiotics causing bleeding problems.

Other medications such as phenothiazines, tricyclic antidepressants, heparin, cimetidine, thiazide diuretics, and estrogen may suppress platelet activity.[19,20,22] If bleeding or prolonged thrombocytopenia becomes a problem, these medications should be altered. The chemotherapeutic drugs mithramycin, carmustine, and daunorubicin are associated with abnormal platelet aggregation.[23] Mithramycin (25–50 μg/kg/day for 5 or more days) is associated with developing bleeding disorders. Thrombocytopenia, platelet function abnormalities, prolonged prothrombin time and prolonged partial thromboplastin time, reduced platelet ADP stores, and reduced factors II, V, VII, and X have all been reported with mithramycin administration.[21]

The mucin-producing adenocarcinomas are associated with hypercoagulability. Anticoagulants are used in treating clotting complications. Heparin binds to antithrombin III, enhancing its inhibiting effect, inactivating thrombin, and neutralizing activated factors IX, X, XI, and XII.[12] Monitoring the partial thromboplastin time (PTT) assesses the efficacy of the anticoagulation heparin provides. Heparin does not dissolve existing clots but prevents new clots from forming. It has short half-life of 1½ hours in plasma. Low-molecular-weight heparins are being used with increasing frequency over the unfractionated heparin in the initial treatment of deep vein thrombosis (DVT). Studies suggest that enoxaparin, a low-molecular-weight heparin, is safe and an effective alternative to the traditional heparin therapy for treating DVTs.[24] Enoxaparin has a longer plasma half-life, less variability in the anticoagulation response, and less toxicity (less bleeding).[24,25] It has little effect on the activated partial thromboplastin time (a PTT). Enoxaparin is given in 1 mg/kg doses *subcutaneously* every 12 hours. Warfarin therapy is started concomitantly. The enoxaparin is administered until the International Normalized Ratio (INR) is over 2.0. It should be noted that all low-molecular-weight heparins may not be equally effective. Warfarin is an oral anticoagulant that suppresses hepatic synthesis of vitamin K–dependent clotting factors II, VII, IX, and X. It has no effect on platelets, and its action is cumulative and prolonged. The half-life of warfarin is 1.5 to 2.5 days, with steady state reached around day 4. It mostly affects the extrinsic pathway, therefore the prothrombin time (PT) may be monitored. A more reliable and standardized measurement for monitoring the effectiveness of orally administered anticoagulant is the INR. As the thromboplastin is different from institution to institution, the individual's measured PT needs to be compared to the institution's PT for that batch of thromboplastin. The INR provides a consistent ratio that can be used universally. An INR of 2.0 to 3.0 is generally accepted for prophylaxis and treatment of DVT and for pulmonary embolism prophylaxis.[15] Warfarin has many drug interactions affecting its efficacy. Individuals with polypharmacy need to be monitored closely when medications are added or deleted.

Hemorrhage associated with uremia

Abnormal bleeding is a common complication of uremia. Uremic plasma inhibits normal platelets' response to ADP, collagen, and epinephrine, causing a prolonged bleeding time and impaired platelet function.[13,14] The most frequent sites of bleeding for the person in renal failure occur in the mucocutaneous areas: ecchymosis, purpura, epistaxis, and gastrointestinal bleeding. The best way to control or diminish the risk of bleeding in the individual in renal failure is by dialysis, which corrects or at least improves the bleeding time. In emergencies, administration of cryoprecipitate normalizes bleeding times temporarily.[21]

Pathophysiology

Normal coagulation is dependent on normal levels of clotting factors and the function of cellular blood components, platelets, and the integrity of the blood vessel wall. If any of these components are deficient, bleeding will occur. Platelet and small blood vessel disorders frequently present as purpura, with pronounced cutaneous and mucosal bleeding. Thrombocytopenia and altered platelet function feature prolonged bleeding from superficial cuts and abrasions. Severe deficiencies in coagulation factors are characterized by deep hematomas and bleeding into the joints.[11]

Alterations in Vessels

Common etiologies of vessel wall weakening in the individual with cancer include hyperviscosity or dysproteinemias, infection, and atrophy due to treatment. Small blood vessels may become damaged from obstruction due to hyperviscosity, causing small vessel hemorrhage. Weakening or damaging of the endothelium may occur due to the chronic use of corticosteroids, which causes atrophy of the dermal collagen, weakening the supporting tissue of the small blood vessels of the skin.[12] Vessels in the field of radiation therapy become more fragile and friable. Infection may cause vessel damage by toxic damage or immune complex–type hypersensitivity.[11,16] Tumors may disrupt the wall integrity by eroding into the blood vessel.

Alteration in Platelet Function

Thrombocytopenia

Platelet disorders seen in the individual with cancer are due to decreased platelet numbers (thrombocytopenia) or defective platelet function. Thrombocytopenia may be due to a decrease in platelet production, sequestering of platelets in the spleen, or increased platelet consumption. Tumor infiltration of marrow, myelosuppressive antineoplastic therapy, drug toxicity, or viral infections all can diminish platelet production. The degree and duration of the thrombocytopenia secondary to chemotherapy depends on the type of chemotherapy, dose, and interval between cycles. The extent of myelosuppression after radiation therapy is dependent on amount of bone marrow in the radiation field. Recombinant human interleukin-11 (rhIL-11) has been studied for prevention of chemotherapy-induced thrombocytopenia. Studies suggest that it reduces treatment-induced thrombocytopenia and platelet transfusions significantly for those individuals undergoing dose-intensive chemotherapy.[26] It does have side effects of which the patient and the practitioner need to be aware. More than 60% of patients experience significant fluid retention. Dyspnea was also a common side effect. Pleural effusions, conjunctival infections, tachycardia, and atrial arrhythmias have also been reported.[26] Most side effects have been rated as mild to moderate, but close assessment should be done on individuals with underlying cardiopulmonary disease.

After leaving the bone marrow, platelets are taken up by the spleen. Eventually, they equilibrate with the circulating platelets, approximately one-third of circulating platelets held in the spleen at any given moment. If the spleen is enlarged or congested, the platelet are retained within the spleen for a longer period of time. The spleen may become so congested and enlarged that the sequestration causes thrombocytopenia. The marrow tries to respond to the thrombocytopenia by increasing platelet production. Platelets continue to be sequestered in the spleen, increasing the splenomegaly.

Thrombocytopenia may also be caused by destruction of platelets by immune or nonimmune mechanisms. Immune thrombocytopenia is due to antibody-mediated destruction of the platelets. The immunoglobulin G (IgG)–sensitized platelets are phagocytized by macrophages and monocytes of the reticuloendothelial (RE) system, removing them prematurely from circulation. The rate of destruction is dependent on the quantity, subclass of IgG on the platelet, the amount of complement, and the efficiency of the RE system to clear the platelets.[27] An individual developing autoantibodies to platelets, as in idiopathic thrombocytopenic purpura (ITP), is initially treated with corticosteroids, which improve platelet survival by inhibiting the RE phagocytic activity and synthesis of the pathogenic antibody. If the platelet count does not respond to corticosteroids and immunoglobulin therapy, a splenectomy is frequently performed, as the spleen is the major organ of the RE system. High-dose immunoglobulin therapy has increased the platelet count in about 75% of patients with chronic ITP.[11] The mechanism of action is thought to be the blockage of Fc receptors on macrophages in the reticuloendothelial system.[28]

The person who has received multiple transfusions in the past or the multiparous female may form antibodies to human leukocyte antigens (HLA) due to prior exposure through blood transfusions. Approximately 38 to 100% of platelet transfusion recipients who have received multiple platelet transfusions make antibodies against many foreign antigens (become alloimmunized), eventually impairing their response, or becoming refractory to platelet transfusions.[29] HLA-matched platelets may be required to achieve an increase in platelet count. Steroids and high-dose immunoglobulin therapy have shown a limited response, prolonging the life span of the transfused platelet.

Nonimmune destruction of platelets, or consumption, includes DIC, thrombotic microangiopathy (thrombus forming in the arterioles and capillaries), and platelet loss during hemorrhage. Massive transfusions of fresh frozen plasma postoperatively can also cause thrombocytopenia due to dilution.

Altered platelet function

Individuals with cancer may experience occasional bleeding, despite normal platelet count and coagulation factors. Many people with myeloproliferative diseases, acute leukemias, chronic lymphocytic leukemia, multiple myeloma, uremia, liver disease, and microglobulinemia have been found to have malfunctioning platelets.[13] Most commonly, the abnormality is a diminished procoagulant activity of the platelets.[23] In leukemia, platelets show less adhesiveness and aggregation in response to ADP secretion.

Platelet response to trauma occurs in four distinct stages; alteration in function of platelets may interfere in any of those stages. First, the adhesion of a monolayer of platelets to the injured vessel wall occurs. The second stage is the release reaction and can be stimulated by epinephrine, ADP, arachidonic acid, and thrombin. The substances released from the platelets cause them to swell and recruit more platelets. Platelet adhesion and cohesion are mediated by membrane glycoprotein receptors; this is the third stage of platelet response. Alteration or blocking of these glycoproteins inhibits platelet function. It is at this point that the β-lactam antibiotics interfere with the ADP activity on the platelet membrane and on aggregation.[19,20,30] Finally, the platelet membrane functions as a procoagulant, enhancing many steps in coagulation.

Hemolytic uremia syndrome (HUS) is a clinical syndrome in which thrombocytopenia and hemolytic anemia occurring in the renal microvasculature cause thrombi, resulting in acute renal failure. In adults, HUS is rare and is usually associated with irreversible renal failure. It is not a single disease and is caused by a variety of conditions, both infectious and noninfectious. In addition, an association with immunosuppressive drugs has been described with HUS. These drugs include cyclosporine and several cytotoxic drugs, including mitomycin-C and 5-fluorouracil.[21] The end result is extensive endothelial injury of the renal microvasculature. Treatment for HUS is mainly treating the renal failure with dialysis and removal of the offending agent. Blood and platelet transfusions should be avoided, as lysis and thrombus formation will continue and further complicate renal function.

Closely related to HUS is thrombotic thrombocytopenic purpura (TTP) and microangiopathic hemolytic anemia (MAHA). Similar vascular injury occurs simultaneously in many organs, and the associated hematologic findings are correspondingly more severe. Renal failure is found to be milder in TTP. Initial injury in TTP is so severe that injury to endothelium is conspicuous, and platelet involvement in not just morphologically visible but can be measured in the circulation.[21] Thrombocytopenia is believed to be due to both platelet activation and consumption at sites of endothelial injury. HUS, TTP, and MAHA are characterized by localized microvascular thrombosis, or localized intravascular coagulation. It is unusual for coagulation factors to be consumed sufficiently for clotting times to be prolonged. Blood vessels have a limited number of ways to respond to injury. This group of hemolytic anemias is part of a group of conditions in which thrombosis and necrosis of intrarenal vessels occur in the absence of cellular inflammation.[14,21] Transfusions should be avoided if possible.

Alterations in Coagulation

Acquired coagulation disorders usually involve multiple coagulation factor deficiencies. Vitamin K deficiency, liver disease, overdose with anticoagulants, and DIC are the most frequent causes of bleeding associated with coagulation disorders. Bleeding associated with hypocoagulative disorders is not as frequent a problem as hypercoagulopathies. Diminished coagulation factors secondary to vitamin K deficiency or liver dysfunction were discussed previously. People with hypercoagulative states may, however, experience anticoagulant overdose, which can cause severe bleeding.

DIC is the most common life-threatening hypercoagulopathy in the individual with cancer.[20] DIC is not a disorder itself but is a process caused by a variety of underlying diseases. It may be triggered by a number of mechanisms, such as malignancy, sepsis, hemolytic transfusion reactions, or shock. The most common cause is infection.[20] In acute DIC, there is exaggerated overstimulation of the normal coagulation, in which both thrombosis and hemorrhage may simultaneously occur. Two major mechanisms can initiate DIC: the invasion of foreign particles into the bloodstream and vascular endothelium injury.[16] Systemic coagulation is triggered, and thrombin is deposited intravascularly. The excessive thrombin activates both clot formation and fibrinolysis.[13,14,16] Coagulation factors are consumed rapidly with the widespread thrombin formation. Thrombin converts fibrinogen to fibrin. Fibrin thrombi may lodge in the microvasculature of various organs, consuming platelets and stopping blood flow. Organ damage frequently occurs due to the hypoxemia and necrosis caused by these fibrin thrombi. Due to the rapid clot formation, both platelets and clotting factors are consumed.

The excess thrombin formation then also increases fibrinolysis. Thrombin stimulates fibrinolysis by converting plasminogen to plasmin, which is responsible for the breakdown of fibrin and fibrinogen into fibrin degradation products. The increased circulating fibrin degradation products interfere with platelet function and formation of fibrin clots, as well as being potent anticoagulants.[14,16,20] Bleeding occurs secondary to the consumption of platelets and coagulation factors in clot formation, and to the anticoagulation activities of fibrin degradation products produced in fibrinolysis.

Simultaneous activation of the complement and kallikrein systems enhances the clotting activity. These systems increase vascular permeability, arteriolar constriction, and capillary dilatation, trapping blood in the capillary beds.[14,16] This induces an environment of stagnation, acidosis, and concentration of procoagulants, prone to clot formation. The cycle is self-perpetuating, simultaneously forming clots and bleeding.

Assessment

Assessment of the individual with cancer for bleeding should be a thorough procedure. First, the practitioner needs to take a complete patient and family history. Because bleeding is a common disorder, close attention should be paid to anything that might suggest blood loss. The history should include any bleeding tendencies, such as petechiae, easy bruising, pain, headaches, or nosebleeds. An evaluation of nutritional status can identify any vitamin K deficiency or generalized malnutrition. Reviewing all medications, including over-the-counter drugs, may uncover an interference with coagulation. Information regarding recent transfusions, possible reactions, and response to transfusions is important. Individuals with a history of prior transfusions and multiparous women are at risk of alloimmunization. A family history of any bleeding disorders should be noted.

Recognition of risk factors of hemorrhage is the first step in treating the individual with altered hemostasis. Risk factors include: leukemia, especially acute promyelocytic leukemia; mucin-secreting adenocarcinomas (lung, pancreas, stomach, and prostate), hepatic metastases, recent chemotherapy, surgery, immunologic disorders; anticoagulation therapy; acute bacterial or viral infections, transfusion reactions, or hemolysis due to infection; and shock.

Measurement Tools

A number of tools are used in the assessment of bleeding. Such tools include the Hemoccult tests of stools and excreta, urine dipstick to quantify microscopic hematuria, actual quantification of gauze or other material used to absorb the blood, and volume measurement of melena or hematemesis. Scans are also used in measurement of internal hemorrhage. Laboratory values are frequently the most useful for assessing the risk of bleeding and determining the potential pathophysiology. Treatments and transfusion replacement are based on these values. Common screening laboratory tests, normal ranges, and the meaning of their measurements are shown in Table 17-1.

Laboratory values

Tests used to determine platelet disorders include the platelet count, bleeding time, platelet function studies, and bone marrow aspirate. Those laboratory tests used for screening coagulation disorders include the prothrombin time, partial thromboplastin time, INR, fibrin degradation products, fibrinogen, levels of specific coagulation factors, and thrombin time. The hematocrit (Hct) is used in determining blood loss. Individuals with cancer have a tendency to run on the low side of the normal ranges, frequently being somewhat anemic. A sudden drop in hematocrit, however, indicates an acute blood loss. Normally, red blood cell transfusions are given to keep the hemoglobin above 7 to 8 g/dL and the hematocrit above 21 to 24 mL/dL. Cardiopulmonary compromise can occur when levels fall below this.

Quantitative and qualitative measurement of platelets

The platelet count is the best indicator of the potential risk of bleeding in the person with cancer. The platelet count is the actual quantification of platelets in a blood volume. A count below 100,000/mm³ is indicative of thrombocytopenia. Spontaneous bleeding has been prevalent in acute leukemics when the platelet count falls below 20,000/mm³.[2] In solid tumors, spontaneous bleeding due to thrombocytopenia is less prevalent until the platelet count drops below 10,000 to 15,000/mm³.[1,6,23]

The bleeding time is a measure of time taken to stop bleeding from a small skin incision. This is dependent on platelet count, function, and the vasoconstriction capability of capillaries. Prolongation suggests there is a deficiency in the platelets or a severe factor deficiency. A prolonged bleeding time is seen with thrombocytopenia, von Willebrand's disease, tumor infiltration of the bone marrow, consumption of platelets in DIC, and with the use of medications affecting platelet function.

A bone marrow aspirate is done to determine the etiology of thrombocytopenia. If platelets are low due to underproduction, the megakaryocytes in the bone marrow will be few. If the platelets are being destroyed in the periphery by the immune system, the megakaryocytes in the marrow will be normal to elevated, in an attempt to provide more platelets to the periphery.

Measurement of coagulation

Laboratory tests may quantify specific factors or screen for efficacy of a pathway along the coagulation cascade. The PT screens for coagulation deficiency along the extrinsic and common pathways and may be prolonged due to a deficiency in factors I, II, V, VII, or X.[14] This might be due to liver disease, vitamin K deficiency, obstructive biliary disease, or warfarin therapy. PTT screens for defi-

TABLE 17-1 Common Screening Laboratory Tests for Assessment of Hemostasis

Laboratory Test	Normal Range	Evaluates
Platelet Evaluation		
Platelet count	150,000–400,000/mm³	Quantification of platelets in blood
Bleeding time	1–9 min	Platelet plug formation
Bone marrow aspiration	Megakaryocytes present	Thrombopoiesis in bone marrow
Coagulation Evaluation		
Prothrombin time (PT)	Varies; compare with normal control (approx. 70–130%)	Coagulation mechanism via extrinsic and common pathways
Partial thromboplastin time (PTT)	Varies; compare with normal control (approx. 21–40 sec)	Coagulation mechanism via intrinsic and common pathways
International normalized ratio (INR)	Less than 2.0; 2.0–3.0 considered anticoagulated	Anticoagulation via manipulation of the extrinsic and common pathways
Fibrin degradation products (FDP)	Less than 10 μg/mL	Presence of FDP in serum, assessing fibrinolysis
Fibrinogen	200–400 mg/dL	Plasma concentration of fibrinogen
Specific factor assays	50–150% activity in pooled normal plasma	Concentration of functional factors in plasma
Thrombin time	10–15 sec	Estimated plasma fibrinogen levels

ciency along the intrinsic and common pathways. A prolonged PTT occurs when there is a diminished quantity of any factors, except VII or XIII. This may occur due to heparin therapy, increased fibrin degradation products, and consumption of the clotting factors. If either PT or PTT is prolonged, then the hemostatic defect is probably along the specific coagulation pathway. If both are prolonged, the defect is most likely along the common pathway. If both PT and PTT are within normal limits, then either the platelets or the blood vessel is defective. The INR is a more standardized measurement, used for assessing the anticoagulation status. An INR greater than 2.0 is considered anticoagulated enough for prophylaxis and treatment of DVT and pulmonary embolus.

Other measurements of coagulation include fibrin degradation products (FDP), thrombin time, fibrinogen, and specific factor levels. The FDP measures the breakdown of fibrin and fibrinogen activity. An elevated FDP (>10 μg/mL) can result from surgery, obstetric complications, various medical problems, and DIC. A positive D-dimer test indicates specific evidence of intravascular fibrin formation as opposed to primary fibrinolysis (lysis in absence of fibrin formation).[13,16] Positive test results are seen in individuals with DIC, pulmonary and cerebral embolism, phlebitis, thrombosis, and postoperative prethrombotic risks. Thrombin time estimates the plasma fibrinogen. This can be prolonged due to heparin, streptokinase, or urokinase therapy, liver disease, DIC, or fibrinogen deficiency.[12] Fibrinogen may be low due to congenital or acquired hypofibrinogenemia, DIC, fibrinolysis, severe liver disease, malignant processes, or obstetrical trauma.[12] It may be elevated in some malignant or inflammatory disorders. Measuring the specific factor levels in the plasma identifies individual or group factor deficiencies, aiding in the diagnosis of the bleeding disorder.

Physical Assessment

The individual at risk for bleeding needs routine assessment of all body systems. Physical assessment can detect early signs of bleeding. Some of these signs may be subtle, others overt. Bleeding can be internal or external, mild or life-threatening, occurring anywhere in the body. Most common sites of hemorrhage include the gingiva, nose, bladder, GI tract, and brain.[18,19] Because bleeding frequently occurs internally, it is essential to investigate all complaints of weakness, pain, or discomfort in the person at risk. General performance status is evaluated and might identify the effects of the disease or presence of complications. Signs or symptoms of anemia, such as fatigue, malaise, weakness, headaches, pallor, orthostatic hypotension, or tachycardia may be indicative of undetected long-term blood loss. The physical assessment of the patient at risk for bleeding must be thorough, since bleeding can occur anywhere in the body (Table 17-2).

Diagnostic Evaluation

Diagnostic evaluation of the mechanism of hemostasis can be clarified by laboratory data. Site of bleeding and extent of damage to surrounding tissues is determined by a variety of tests, depending on what system is affected by the bleed. Physical examination can be used in overt bleeding, such as in oozing from wounds, epistaxis, oral bleeding, or menses. Hemoccult and urine dipstick—body fluids sent for cell counts—demonstrate presence or absence of bleeding, although the extent and exact location may be unknown.

Tests assessing internal hemorrhage include CT scans, MRI, X-ray, and ultrasound. A funduscopic examination is the first line of testing in diagnosing intraocular hemorrhage. The diagnosis of the site in the GI tract is usually done by visualization. Endoscopy is the procedure of choice for visualizing the location of the site of bleeding in the upper GI tract. Upper GI series are also sometimes used in diagnosis of ulcers or obstruction; points of bleeding are best seen by endoscopy or angiography, however. For lower gastrointestinal bleeding, diagnostic evaluation may include a colonoscopy, flexible sigmoidoscopy, or proctoscopy. A digital rectal exam can diagnose bleeding internal hemorrhoids. Occult blood is also detected by guaiac-positive stool and excreta; however, the exact location of the bleeding in the GI tract would need to be diagnosed by endoscopy.

Degrees of toxicity

The Eastern Cooperative Oncology Group established the following degrees of toxicity in regards to hemorrhage. The scale runs from 0 (no bleeding) to 4 (life-threatening). Detectable bleeding requiring no blood transfusions per episode is rated grade 1, or mild. Hemorrhage that requires 1 to 2 units of blood per hemorrhagic episode is rated a grade 2. Hemorrhage that requires 3 to 4 units of blood per bleeding episode is rated a grade 3, and an episode that requires more than 4 units of blood is rated a grade 4.

Symptom Management

Individuals at high risk for bleeding need to receive instructions concerning how to prevent and manage bleeding. (See Appendix 17A for a self-care guide.) This includes guarding against trauma. For the thrombocytopenic person, environmental safety, such as receiving assistance when gait is unsteady or when mildly sedated or confused, is required. Potential sources of injury are avoided. Efforts to preserve natural barriers, such as skin and mucous membranes, are essential. Use of electric razors for shaving is preferred.

Table 17-2 Physical Assessment for Patient at Risk for Bleeding

Organ	Assessment
CNS: Symptoms dependent on site and size of extravasation	Headache, nausea/vomiting, retching, mental status changes (restlessness, confusion, lethargy, obtundation, coma), vertigo, seizures, changes in pupil size and reactivity; eye deviations, sensory or motor strength alterations, speech alterations, paralysis
Eyes	Visual disturbances—blurring, diplopia, absent or altered fields of vision, nystagmus, increased injections in sclera, conjunctival hemorrhage, periorbital edema; note if sclera are icteric
Nose	Petechiae, blood-tinged drainage, epistaxis
Mouth	Petechiae of oral mucosa, pain, dysphagia, hematemesis, bleeding gums/mucosa, blood-tinged secretions, ulcerations with frank bleeding
Upper gastrointestinal: Esophagus/stomach	Dysphagia, hematemesis, blood-tinged secretions, substernal burning and pain, epigastric discomfort (burning, tenderness, or cramping), coffee ground emesis, nausea, vomiting, fever, weakness, anorexia, melena, hyperactive bowel sounds
Lower gastrointestinal: Duodenum/anus	Pain (location, occurrence, duration, quality), nausea, vomiting, tarry stools, diarrhea, bowel sounds (hyper- or hypoactive), cramping, occult blood in stools, frank blood in stools (rectum or lower), blood around anus, frequency and quantity of stools, pain with bowel movements (hemorrhoids)
Lungs	Tachypnea, dyspnea, air hunger, respiration rate, depth, and exertion Crackles, rubs, wheezing, diminished breath sounds, hemoptysis (frothy BRB sputum—major airway bleeding), stridor, tickling in throat or chest with desire to cough
Cardiovascular	Tachycardia and hypotension (characteristic of anemia and acute blood loss) Changes in VS, color and temperature of extremities, peripheral pulses (present, quality), and changes in peripheral perfusion Pericardial effusions: dyspnea, cough, pain, orthopnea, venous distension, tamponade (muted heart sounds, hypotension, pulsus paradoxus, tachycardia, angina, palpitations)
Abdomen	Hepatomegaly (liver disease—possible coagulation disorder), RUQ pain, abdominal distension Splenomegaly (increased risk for bleeding): Assess for any h/o trauma; if spleen ruptures, rapid hypovolemic shock ensues; left flank or left shoulder pain Retroperitoneal bleeding: vague abdominal complaints, ecchymoses over flank, occasional bulging flanks and tenderness; associated with hypovolemia
Genitourinary	Decreased urinary output due to massive bleeding is associated with hypovolemia and shock Hematuria: dysuria, burning, frequency, pain on urination, suprapubic pain and cramping, gross blood in urine, clots Menorrhagia: suprapubic pain and cramping, gross blood in urine, clots (may need to straight catheterize female patients to distinguish between urinary or vaginal bleeding) Frequency and size of clots, number of sanitary napkins used, and color of urine are important in measuring bleeding
Musculoskeletal	Bleeding into the joints is usually associated with alterations in coagulation; swollen, warm, sore joint with decreased mobility (active and passive ROM); usually unilateral; tapping the joint's synovial fluid is frequently required to distinguish infection from bleeding
Skin	Petechiae, ecchymosis, purpura, hematoma; oozing from venipuncture sites, central lines, catheters, injection sites, incisional sounds, nasogastric tubes Gangrene, alterations in skin color (e.g., pallor, cyanosis), alterations in skin temperature

BRB = bright red blood; VS = vital signs; RUQ = right upper quadrant; ROM = range of motion.

Once bleeding begins, the site of the bleed and its cause need to be identified as quickly as possible so treatment to stop the bleeding may be given. All the precautionary actions continue to be in effect. Blood counts and coagulation are monitored. Vital signs are closely monitored as well. Transfusions of platelets, red blood cells, and coagulation factors are administered as needed. As bleeding intensifies, precautions are still maintained and transfusion and volume replenishment are necessary. Accurate assessment and monitoring of laboratory values, vital signs, renal status, and neurologic symptoms are essential.

Therapeutic Approaches

Assessment for potential hemorrhage is essential in diagnosis and prompt treatment since bleeding can occur in any system or organ and has different signs and symptoms depending upon the site of the bleed. Refer to Table 17-2 for physical assessment of the patient at risk for bleeding.

Integumentary

Prevention Personal hygiene is essential for maintaining maximum skin integrity. Venipunctures are to be kept to a minimum, along with intramuscular and subcutaneous injections. If injections are absolutely necessary, the smallest gauge needle possible is recommended. Paper tape is recommended over plastic or cloth tape to prevent trauma to the skin.

Management Direct pressure is applied to sites of bleeding from venipuncture, wound incisions, and sites of catheters. Pressure must be applied for a longer period of time than for those who do not have platelet or coagulation abnormalities. Cold compresses may assist in causing vasoconstriction. If bleeding does not stop with direct pressure, topical thrombin may be used.

Eyes

Individuals with acute leukemia, especially acute promyelocytic leukemia, have a higher tendency to have ocular abnormalities. Thrombocytopenia and severe anemia are critical factors in the mechanism of the intraorbital hemorrhage.[31] Other factors affecting intraocular infarction and hemorrhage include hyperviscosity due to high blast cell counts and disease duration.[32] Bleeding in the optic fundus can result in permanent vision damage (Figure 17-3).

Prevention For the individual with significant thrombocytopenia or altered coagulation status, transfusion of blood products may prevent or minimize the bleeding. Avoiding increased intracranial pressures also reduces the risk of bleeding.

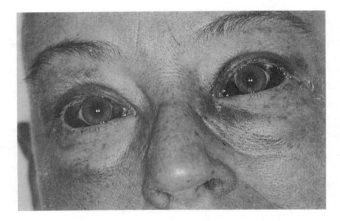

FIGURE 17-3 Scleral bleeding due to thrombocytopenia.

Management For intraocular hemorrhage, transfusion of blood products assists in controlling the bleeding. Scleral bleeding is made worse by rubbing the eyes. The eyes will feel dry and burning. Eyedrops to moisten the eye frequently helps relieve the burning and itching.

Central nervous system (CNS)

Individuals with brain cancer, leukemia, or those undergoing bone marrow transplantation have the highest risk of developing hemorrhage into the CNS. Alterations in level of consciousness, irritability, confusion, mental status changes, seizures, and coma may occur with impaired tissue perfusion of the brain or intracranial hemorrhage. Intracranial hemorrhage may occur due to tumor invasion, thrombocytopenia, or coagulopathy accompanied by hypertension or increased intracranial pressure. Hemorrhages usually occur over a matter of minutes, unless the bleeding is due to anticoagulant therapy, which may develop over 24 to 48 hours.[33] The individual may complain of a severe sudden headache. Edema around the tissue injury of the hemorrhage often leads to an increased compression and worsening clinical state. Symptoms are dependent on the location and extent of the bleed. A life-threatening intracranial hemorrhage requires little to no red cell transfusions. Toxicity is based on the patient's neurologic symptoms. "Life-threatening" implies that the individual is comatose or requires intubation.

Prevention It is imperative to avoid activities that increase intracranial pressure to help prevent intracranial hemorrhage. Maintaining platelet levels greater than 20,000/mm³, correcting coagulopathies, controlling nausea and vomiting can decrease the risk of bleeding.

Management The first line of treatment for intracranial bleeding is transfusion of platelets or coagulation factors. Corticosteroids are also administered to control edema from the tissue injury, thus preventing more elevated intracranial pressure and worse neurologic deficit. Close neurologic assessments are done, vital signs and neurologic signs are monitored, and protective measures are instituted in the event that the patient is confused or hallucinating.

Cases involving more severe hemorrhage may require emergency bur holes or drains to release the pressure on the brain tissue, in addition to the first-line treatments just described. If done early enough, before pressure builds, drains could prevent more damage to brain tissue. However, because intracranial bleeds usually occur rapidly over a matter of minutes, a severe bleed is likely to result in irreversible damage. The person may become comatose with or without requiring intubation. Provision for a calm environment, explanation of actions, and pain medication for the severe headache are important to reduce anxiety.

Nose and mouth

Assessment   Chemotherapy, radiation therapy, neoplastic disease, and oral infection all put individuals at risk for mucous membrane bleeding (Figure 17-4).

Prevention   Good oral hygiene is important. An established routine for mouth care, using a soft-bristle toothbrush while platelets remain above 50,000/mm³ and then using soft toothettes, or swabs, when the platelet count drops below 50,000/mm³ will help avoid trauma to the gums and oral membranes. An alcohol-free, nonirritating mouth rinse is recommended. Dentures or dental prostheses that do not fit well should not be used when the oral membranes are irritated or while the high risk for bleeding remains. Forcefully blowing and picking one's nose is avoided to prevent epistaxis.

Management   For epistaxis, the individual is put in high Fowler's position, with direct pressure on the nare that is bleeding. Cold compresses may help in vasoconstriction and stopping the hemorrhage. If the bleeding has not stopped with pressure in 10 to 15 minutes, topical thrombin or topical epinephrine may be applied to the nare to help hemostasis occur. Nasal passages may need to be packed to stop the hemorrhage, or the vessel is cauterized with a laser.

Bleeding oral lesions need to be kept clean; therefore, increasing the frequency of mouth care is important. Diminishing infection of oral lesions decreases damage to the mucosa, allowing for more rapid healing of the ulcerations. Gentle suction may be necessary to clear out thick bloody secretions, while rinsing with cool saline helps vasoconstriction. Topical thrombin may be applied to oral lesions to help control excessive bleeding episodes. In severe bleeding from mucositis, intubation may be necessary to keep the airway open from clot formation.

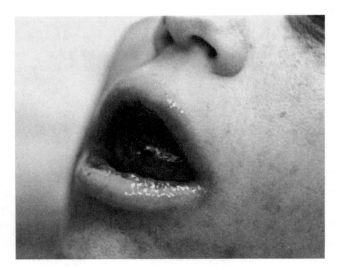

FIGURE 17-4   Drug-induced purpuric hemorrhage of lips and tongue.

Gastrointestinal

Assessment   The person with cancer is prone to have hemorrhagic complications along the GI tract. Bleeding can be negligible to a massive hemorrhage along the GI tract. Hematemesis usually indicates bleeding proximal to the duodenum, since blood entering the GI tract below that cannot enter the stomach.[34] Melena usually indicates bleeding from the esophagus, stomach, or duodenum. Approximately 60 mL of blood is required to produce a single black stool and must remain in the gut for at least 8 hours to produce melena.[34] One acute episode of blood loss may produce melena for up to 3 days. Once the stool color has returned to normal, the stool may remain guaiac positive for 1 week. Breakdown of blood proteins to urea by the intestinal bacteria elevates blood urea nitrogen levels. Blood in the GI tract is cathartic, increasing the motility with increased volume of the hemorrhage.

The four most common causes of upper gastrointestinal hemorrhage are: peptic ulceration, erosive gastritis, varices, and esophageal mucosal tear.[34] Most peptic ulcers are found in the duodenum, with hemorrhage frequently being the first indication. Irritation and erosion of the gastric mucosa may be secondary to chemotherapy, pain medications, corticosteroids, vomiting, major trauma or surgery, and severe systemic disease, such as sepsis or DIC. Bleeding from esophageal varices is usually acute and massive. Presence of varices represents long-standing portal hypertension from liver disease. Hypotension, tachycardia, anxiety, and changes in level of consciousness are symptoms of variceal bleeding. Esophagogastric mucosal tear (Mallory-Weiss) is the mucosal laceration at the esophagogastric junction caused by prolonged and violent retching. It is characterized by retching or nonbloody vomiting, followed by hematemesis. The colon and rectum are not common sites of massive hemorrhage in the cancer patient, unless there are serious bleeding abnormalities.

Prevention   Antiemetics will decrease the potential for tearing mucosa and esophagitis from vomiting. Individuals who have poor oral intake or are on corticosteroids are put on H₂ blockers to decrease the acid secretion in the stomach, thus reducing the risk for upper gastrointestinal bleeding. Indwelling catheters and tubes should be eliminated unless absolutely necessary. Rectal manipulation, such as digital examination, rectal thermometers, medications, and tubes should be avoided in the thrombocytopenic individual. Stool softeners may be used so straining and constipation are avoided. Proper diet and exercise will also help prevent constipation.

Management   Antiemetics are important to keep the gastric juices from irritating the esophagus and stress in the mucosa. Individuals with hiatal hernias and reflux esophagitis can develop significant bleeding with ulceration. This is especially prevalent with corticosteroid therapy or with prolonged vomiting. Antacid treatment, H₂ blockers, and dietary management usually provide sufficient control. Bleeding from esophageal varices is usually acute and massive. The first line of treatment is intravenous vasopressin. Blood components and fluids are administered to keep pressure stable. If bleeding continues, the varices may be repaired with endoscopic sclerosis or by balloon tamponade.[34] For a Mallory-Weiss tear, continued use of antiemetics and H_2 blockers are appropriate. If bleeding is significant, gastric decompression may be necessary, as blood in the stomach can cause nausea and vomiting. Intraarterial vasopressin may control excessive bleeding from a Mallory-Weiss tear or from a gastric ulcer. Gastric and duodenal ulcers are initially treated with antacids, or H_2 blockers, antibiotics, and coating agents like sucralfate. A peptic ulcer causing an arteriole bleed may be stopped by endoscopic coagulation using a laser, heater probe, or electrocautery.[34] In cases of severe hemorrhage, with large ulcers unresponsive to endoscopic coagulation or bleeding tumors, surgical resection may be necessary.

Pulmonary

Assessment   Respiratory assessment is an important measure of the anemic state of the individual who is bleeding, indicating the respiratory system's attempt or inability to compensate for a diminished blood supply. Bleeding can occur in the major airways, the pleural space, and the alveoli. Hemoptysis occurs when there is bleeding into the major airways. Malignant pleural effusions are frequently bloody. Many cancers may cause pleural effusions. Most notable are lymphomas and lung and breast cancer. The severity of the symptoms is frequently associated with the rate at which the effusion fills the pleural space.

Those who are severely immunosuppressed and have some kind of coagulation abnormality are most likely to bleed into the alveoli. These individuals are usually bone marrow transplant recipients or have leukemia. The alveoli fill with blood, thus prohibiting gas exchange. The person becomes hypoxic. During bronchoscopy, if more bleeding occurs when washings are taken, saline is injected into the airway and aspirated; this is indicative of alveolar hemorrhage.

Management   Intrapleural bleeding may be tapped to eliminate the fluid if it is causing symptoms of dyspnea. Frequent thoracentesis to relieve reaccumulating fluid may be needed. Sclerosis may be necessary if the effusion and bleeding return too rapidly. Malignant pleural effusions are frequently treated by treating the disease with chemotherapy.

Hemoptysis is usually very scant and will stop spontaneously within a short period of time. Codeine or hydrocodone for cough suppression might help, as coughing is an aggravating factor of increased bleeding. For treating substantial hemoptysis, the individual needs to be kept calm and on bed rest. Antianxiety medications and cough suppressants may be used. Unnecessary procedures should be eliminated. The person is placed on his or her side, with the side of hemorrhage dependent, so as not to cause asphyxiation by draining the blood into the other lung. Suctioning and intubation are imperative to control severe hemorrhage. Intubation may be done using a technique that isolates the hemorrhaging lung and protects the other lung from aspiration of blood. This is done by proper placement of a balloon catheter into the affected bronchus.[35] Laser therapy and arterial embolization are two palliative treatments for the severe hemorrhage.

Alveolar hemorrhage is much more diffuse and more difficult to treat. Bleeding occurs in the alveoli, diminishing or preventing gas exchange between the alveoli and the surrounding capillaries. Respiratory support with oxygen is required. Glucocorticoids are used to control acute bleeding, but this is not a long-term therapy of choice, as the response to keeping the bleeding suppressed or prevention is unknown.[8] Acute respiratory failure is associated with severe alveolar hemorrhage. Mortality associated with bleeding of this magnitude in the bone marrow transplant population ranges from 79 to 100%.[36] For the dying patient, oxygen and pain medications are appropriate; antianxiety medications, such as lorazepam, diazepam, or midazolam, may also be given, as anxiety increases as dyspnea becomes more acute. Positioning the individual in the high Fowler's position often decreases dyspnea. Assistance is necessary due to fatigue. The person with severe alveolar bleeding is commonly intubated. This complication is often fatal.

Cardiovascular

Assessment   The hemorrhaging individual frequently shows changes in vital signs, color and temperature of extremities, and peripheral pulses. Tachycardia and hypotension are characteristic of anemia and acute blood loss. A wide pulse pressure is suggestive of an increased intracranial pressure.

Pericardial effusions may occur with metastasis to the pericardium. Tumors that metastasize there include tumors of the lung and breast, leukemia, and lymphoma. Bloody fluid is commonly seen with tumor involvement of the pericardium, but it may also be associated with anticoagulant therapy or with uremia, especially endstage renal failure. Pericardial hemorrhage has limited space into which to bleed; rapid pericardial hemorrhage causes tamponade and is life-threatening.

Management   Severe bleeding into the pericardium can occur in patients who are thrombocytopenic or have other coagulation alterations. Due to the risk of cardiac surgery, a cardiac window is not suggested until the pericardial hemorrhage is risking tamponade. An aspiration may be attempted but is a risky procedure. A "window" procedure may be necessary to relieve pressure and allow the heart to regain its normal functioning capacity. Heart rate, blood pressure, pulsus paradoxus, and peripheral pulses are closely monitored.

Abdominal

Assessment Abdominal bleeding can result from tumor invasion, necrosis, or severe ulceration. Abdominal bleeding is frequently vague in presentation, yet bleeding can be severe.

Management Transfusions of blood, platelets, and plasma are required. Fluids to maintain the blood pressure may also be necessary. Surgery might be required as in a ruptured spleen. Thrombocytopenia is present, which makes surgery more dangerous, but the splenectomy will frequently resolve the thrombocytopenia.

Genitourinary

Bleeding of the genitourinary system can result from direct tumor involvement, side effects of treatment or ulceration.

Assessment Laboratory analysis to detach hematuria is the most reliable method to assess urinary bleeding. Fatigue, pain, and abdominal tenderness are common symptoms. Frank or gross hematuria is an indication of serious bleeding.

Prevention Cyclophosphamide and ifosfamide are frequent causative agents for hemorrhagic cystitis. On the days of treatment, proper hydration, frequent (q1–2h) voids, and use of a uroprotective agent (Mesna) will reduce the risk of chemotherapy-induced hemorrhagic cystitis. For high-dose cyclophosphamide or ifosfamide infusion, continuous bladder irrigation is sometimes used to decrease the exposure of the bladder lining to irritant.

Management The causative agent must be determined for hemorrhagic cystitis, whether it be infection, bacterial, or viral, or therapy such as cyclophosphamide, ifosfamide, and radiation therapy. If infection is the cause, antibiotics should be started. Viral infections, most frequently seen in immunosuppressed individuals, may be more difficult to treat, as viruses do not always respond well to antiviral medications. However, ganciclovir may be used in cytomegalovirus (CMV) infections; vidarabine has been shown to be somewhat effective in treatment of polyomavirus and adenovirus associated with acute hemorrhagic cystitis.[37,38]

In chemotherapy-induced hemorrhagic cystitis, the chemotherapy should be discontinued if bleeding is severe. It is not uncommon for the urine to become heme-positive during the infusion or shortly after the infusion of these antineoplastics. Increased hydration and frequent voiding, with or without diuretics, may be needed. Bleeding may become more severe later in the course for those individuals whose thrombocytopenia is severe and prolonged from the chemotherapy.

Hydration and frequent voids will help clear blood and clots from the bladder. Phenazopyridine hydrochloride may decrease pain and burning, while oxybutynine chloride can help relieve spasms of the urethra and bladder. Measurement of blood in the urine by urinalysis or 24-hour urine may be necessary. Platelets are transfused, if needed, and counts monitored until full recovery is seen.

Significant blood loss can occur due to hemorrhagic cystitis. A number of agents are used to try to stop the hemorrhage. Continuous bladder irrigation with saline or alum may be used. Bed rest is recommended at this time, as the catheter may cause more irritation due to trauma. If continuous irrigation does not stop the hemorrhage, the individual may be taken to surgery for sclerosing by formalin, silver nitrate, or prostaglandins. Pain management, hydration, and assessment for continued bleeding are important interventions postoperatively. If hemorrhage continues after multiple attempts, eventually a cystectomy is recommended.

Women may have their menses suppressed with pharmacologic agents when they are experiencing or anticipating severe and prolonged thrombocytopenia, as large volumes of blood may be lost vaginally. Suppression is generally accomplished with progestational medications. Sanitary napkins, not tampons, should be used to absorb the blood. A close count of pads will help measure the blood loss.

If hemorrhage is severe, high-dose progestational hormonal therapy is attempted when lower doses do not inhibit the bleeding. High-dose therapy, along with platelet transfusions, is usually successful. The problem with this approach is that the lining of the uterus thickens greatly with the high dose of hormones, such that when the hormones are reduced, the lining will be sloughed, entailing further blood loss. Ideally, the platelet count will have become sufficient to control the hemorrhage when hormones are reduced. If the bleeding is life-threatening and unresponsive to hormonal therapy, a hysterectomy may be necessary.

Musculoskeletal

Assessment Bleeding into joints is indicative of a coagulation deficit. Joints may be swollen, warm, and sore, with diminished mobility for both active and passive range of motion. It is difficult to distinguish between infection and bleeding into the joints without tapping the joint.

Management Coagulation factor deficits may be corrected by administering vitamin K, improving nutrition, and by administering plasma or specific coagulation factors. Physical therapy and pain medications may be necessary if the hemorrhage into the joint is substantial.

Disseminated intravascular congulation (DIC)

Assessment Individuals who have leukemia, especially acute promyelocytic leukemia (APL), sepsis, a hemolytic transfusion reaction, or have had a hypotensive episode or shock are at risk for acute DIC. In solid tumor patients (mucin-producing adenocarcinomas), DIC has a heterogeneous presentation. Some solid tumors may present with excessive bleeding and venous thromboembolism, while others maintain the chronic or low-grade type, evidenced only by altered laboratory values.[7]

Prevention Prevention of DIC may be difficult, as it has many etiologies. Infections should be treated, especially in the granulocytopenic person. Infection is the most common initiating factor of DIC; systemic infections also activate the complement and kallikrein systems, increasing the risk. Treating infections promptly diminishes the risk of DIC. Prophylactic heparin is infused for the person with APL during induction chemotherapy. This is one case in which prophylactic heparin appears to be effective in decreasing DIC incidence and diminishing the mortality rate due to fatal hemorrhage.[7]

Management The initial treatment of DIC is to always treat the causative agent, whether it is infection, hemolytic transfusion reaction, shock, malignancy, anaphylactic reactions, widespread tissue damage following surgery or trauma, or obstetric complications. DIC is frequently associated with tumor lysis syndrome. It can vary in severity, and coagulopathy correction is dependent on the elimination of the initiating event. After treating the cause of DIC, supportive measures are similar: fluid, blood, and blood component support of vascular volume, and replenishment of coagulation factors and platelets that have been consumed.[37,38] Heparin is a controversial treatment for DIC, as it involves using an anticoagulant on an individual who is already bleeding. It is used when there is definite thrombotic evidence and damage to tissues. Heparin combines with antithrombin III, inactivating thrombin and neutralizing activated factors IX, X, XI, and XII.[13,20,39] Others prefer to use transfusion therapy, replacing coagulation factors and platelets as needed.[39,40]

Transfusion therapy

Transfusing blood components replenishes deficiencies in the individual who either has bleeding or is at significant risk for bleeding. Advances in blood banking and transfusion therapy permit the individual with cancer to receive aggressive therapy while minimizing the morbidity and mortality of this therapy. To reduce the possibility of serious bleeding, prophylactic platelet transfusions are commonly administered to patients with leukemia when the platelet count is less than 20,000/mm^3, and to the individual with a solid tumor when the count is 10,000/mm^3.[1–4,23] Bleeding is controlled or prevented with the supplementation of platelets and coagulation factors received through transfusions. The advances in apheresis have made the collection of platelets from a single donor safe and simple, thus increasing the use of single-donor platelets. Blood component therapy still has significant risks, but with prudent use of transfusions, the imminent risk of hemorrhage for some people with cancer has diminished greatly. Common blood components, a description of the component, and the indications are found in Table 17-3.

Blood components

Whole blood The use of whole blood has decreased with the fractionation of the unit of whole blood into its different components, now making up less than 10% of all transfusions.[40] It is rarely used in the individual with cancer unless a massive bleed occurs, requiring both volume and red cell replenishment. Whole blood makes up less than 10% of all transfusions.

Red blood cells The decision to replace red blood cells is made according to the physiologic effects of anemia. Anemia in the patient with cancer may be due to decreased red cell production in the bone marrow or to bleeding. Anemia may present as fatigue, pallor, tachypnea, tachycardia, or shortness of breath on exertion. If an individual is bleeding substantially, red blood cells are needed for replacement. Without active bleeding, the transfusion of 1 unit of packed red blood cells, or 1 unit of whole blood, should increase the hematocrit by 3% or the hemoglobin by 1 gm/dL.

Platelets The transfusion of platelets is used in preventing and controlling hemorrhage. Transfusion is recommended for the individual with decreased platelet production, consumption of platelets due to bleeding, and platelet dysfunction. Thrombocytopenia caused by alloimmunization will destroy replacement platelets, unless HLA-matched platelets are provided. In some cases, the individual has developed antibodies to platelet antigens, and therefore will not respond to platelet transfusion. Platelets must be stored and transfused properly for the person to acquire the appropriate transfusion increment; mishandled platelets may cause transfusion failure. Platelets should be stored at room temperature with gentle agitation. The shelf life of the unit will depend on the collection method and the storage bag used. Two types of storage bags exist, 24-hour and 5-day bags.

If infection or a rapidly decreasing platelet count is present, the individual should be closely monitored for bleeding. The life span of a platelet is approximately 7 to 10 days once released from the bone marrow. Generally, if an individual is not producing any platelets and is not bleeding, the requirement of transfusions should be approximately one platelet pack every 3 days. Bleeding time is prolonged with thrombocytopenia because of the lack of platelets to form the initial temporary platelet plug. The goal of platelet therapy in active bleeding is to keep the platelet count greater than 50,000/mm^3 and thereby correct the bleeding time. A platelet count between 50,000 to 100,000/mm^3 should return the bleeding time to normal.[8]

Plasma The transfusion of plasma or specific coagulation factors found in the plasma is usually used for

TABLE 17-3 Commonly Transfused Blood Products for the Bleeding Individual

Blood Component	Description	Indication	Transfusion Considerations
Whole blood	Entire contents of blood	Massive hemorrhage for which volume is needed along with red cell replacement	Assess for fluid overload
Packed red blood cells (PRBCs)	Red blood cells with most of plasma and platelets removed; 70% more Hct than whole blood	Anemia, bleeding, replacement of red blood cells without the volume	Transfuse over 2–4 hours, assess for fluid overload
Fresh frozen plasma (FFP)	200 mL plasma, plasma proteins, and clotting factors	Bleeding, deficiency in coagulation factors, volume expander	Transfuse as rapidly as tolerated (usually less than 30 min)
Cryoprecipitate	10–20 mL fibrinogen, factors VIII, XIII, von Willebrand's factor	Severe von Willebrand's disease, hypofibrinogenemia	Transfuse rapidly, less than 30 min
Platelets			
Random donor platelets (RDPs)	Platelets taken from 4+ units of whole blood, approx. 200 mL	Bleeding and bleeding prophylaxis with thrombocytopenia (less than 20,000/mm^3)	Transfuse rapidly to prevent clot formation (usually 20–30 min)
Single-donor platelets (SDPs)	Platelets from one donor obtained by apheresis, approx. 200–300 mL	Long-term platelet transfusion, bleeding, refractory to RDP	Transfuse as for RDP
HLA-matched platelets	Platelets pheresed from one donor, HLA matched, approximately 300 mL	Refractory to RDP and SDP	Transfuse as for other platelets; more difficult to get matched platelets

coagulation disorders. The amount and frequency of the transfusions depend on the severity of the deficiency, the specific factor deficiency, the risk of bleeding, and the duration of the therapy. For the person not actively bleeding, with a coagulation factor deficiency that can be resolved with the parenteral administration of vitamin K, vitamin K should be given instead of using fresh-frozen plasma.

Complications of transfusion therapy Blood component therapy is not without risk. There are a variety of complications that may occur due to transfusions. Transfusion reactions are due to an immune response to the blood product itself. Other complications may be due to the age of the unit transfused, citrate toxicity, hypocalcemia, and hyperkalemia. Hypothermia can occur when refrigerated blood is transfused too quickly. Circulatory overload can occur due to the high osmotic density of the blood in an individual whose cardiopulmonary status cannot respond quickly to an increase in volume. Bacterial contaminants in transfused blood are rare but may occur, causing sepsis and shock. Transmission of disease organisms, particularly viruses, such as hepatitis viruses, rotavirus, Epstein-Barr virus, CMV, HIV-1 and HIV-2, and human T-cell lymphotropic virus (HTLV) is a threat, although all blood is tested for these viruses. Transfusion reactions are the more common complication of blood component therapy. There are three basic

types of transfusion reactions: hemolytic, febrile nonhemolytic, and allergic reactions (Table 17-4).

Manipulation of blood products may help prevent some of the complications associated with transfusion therapy. For those individuals receiving long-term transfusions, or for those who have had a number of nonhemolytic reactions in the past, the unit of red blood cells and platelets can have the number of leukocytes reduced. Leukocyte reduction of blood products is performed by manually washing or by filtration. This helps prevent alloimmunization to HLA antigens, diminishes exposure to CMV for the severely immunosuppressed, and diminishes the antigenic (leukocyte) load, which is likely to produce a reaction. Individuals likely to benefit from leukocyte reduction are those with long-term transfusion needs and those who have a history of numerous nonhemolytic transfusion reactions.

Washing the cells with saline helps prevent allergic reactions. Washing rids the unit of plasma, suspending the cells, either red blood cells or platelets, in saline. Washing is indicated for those individuals who have had repeated mild allergic reactions of hives or pruritus or a single episode of wheezing and respiratory compromise.

The severely immunosuppressed individual requires two extra considerations when transfusing blood components. The immunocompromised individual is at risk for graft-versus-host disease (GVHD) when transfused with immunocompetent lymphocytes, which are present in

TABLE 17-4 Blood Transfusion Reactions

Transfusion Reaction	Mechanism	Physical Findings	Management
Hemolytic Onset is usually within 15 min	• Ab-Ag reaction to major blood incompatibility, causing intravascular hemolysis • Ab-Ag complex activates classical complement pathway, lysing RBCs within the vasculature	• Fever, temp rise > 1°C • Chills/rigors • Chest pain/back pain • Hypotension • Nausea • Flushing • Dyspnea • Diffuse bleeding • Anemia • Oliguria • Hemoglobinuria	• Stop transfusion • Notify MD • Monitor VS • Maintain BP with fluids if necessary • Obtain and send blood and urine samples • Follow transfusion reaction protocol of institution • Return product to blood center • Document occurrence
Delayed hemolytic Onset occurs between 7 days to weeks after transfusion	• Ab-Ag reaction to minor RBC antigens • Extravascular hemolysis (RE system)	• Decreasing Hgb without bleeding • Low-grade fevers	• Obtain blood samples to assess for antibody against minor RBC antigens • Transfuse as needed
Febrile nonhemolytic Onset is immediate to 6h post-transfusion (prevalent in those exposed to multiple WBCs and platelet antigens)	• Ab directed against WBC or platelet antigens previously exposed to (may be HLA specific, WBC specific, or platelet specific)	• Fever, temp rise > 1°C • Rigors • Nausea • Pallor • Flushing	• Stop transfusion • Notify MD • Follow blood transfusion reaction protocol of institution • Send unit back to blood center • Document occurrence
Allergic Onset immediate to 1h posttransfusion (the more severe the reaction, the more immediate)	• Ab reaction to plasma proteins in the blood product	Mild: • Hives • Pruritus Anaphylactic: • Flushing • Dyspnea • Wheezing • Hypotension • Shock	Mild: • Slow transfusion • Administer antihistamines or corticosteroids • Complete transfusion Anaphylactic: • Stop transfusion • Notify MD • Administer fluids, respiratory support as required • Epinephrine may be required • Monitor VS • Follow transfusion reaction protocol of institution • Obtain and send blood and urine samples • Send unit back to blood center • Document occurrence

VS = vital signs; RE = reticuloendothelial; HLA = human leukocyte antigen.

any transfusion. The T-lymphocytes attack the body tissues of the immunosuppressed host after transfusion. The lymphocytes may attack the liver, skin, gut, or bone marrow. This is a potentially fatal complication. The population at risk usually includes bone marrow transplant patients and individuals with leukemia. Irradiating the blood product with 1500 to 3000 cGy makes the lymphocyte incapable of proliferating.

CMV infection is relatively harmless in the immunocompetent person but can cause serious complications in the immunocompromised patient. For the person who has been exposed to this virus before, the virus can be reactive. It is important to transfuse the individual who has never been exposed to the virus with blood products that are CMV negative. Removal of leukocytes from the unit also helps prevent CMV transmission, as CMV usually lives within the white blood cell.

Evaluation of Therapeutic Approaches

Laboratory values are an excellent measure of response to therapy. Platelet levels increasing in response to transfusion, coagulation factors replenished, correction of PT and PTT, and a hematocrit no longer dropping document the response of the patient to the therapy. Other measurements may include amount of melena and rate of decrease of overt bleeding. Evaluation depends on the organ system affected by the bleeding and the associated symptoms. Most measurements will parallel those described in the assessment section. In acute or massive hemorrhage, bleeding usually slows with medical treatment, as opposed to suddenly stopping. Documentation of this slowing should be recorded consistently. Documenting relief of symptoms also provides important information, such as decreased frequency, bladder spasms, and pain in hematuria. Increased energy and strength are indicators, too. However, these indicators may lag behind the abatement of bleeding.

Conclusion

Bleeding is a common complication for the person with cancer and may be caused and exacerbated by multiple factors. It can be caused by the cancer itself or by the treatment of the cancer. Bleeding can be internal or external, occult or frank, undetectable or life-threatening. Transfusion therapy has made it possible to treat the individual with cancer aggressively, controlling and sometimes preventing bleeding. Early detection of bleeding is important and should be diagnosed and treated before further complications arise. Control of bleeding

decreases morbidity and mortality in this patient population.

References

1. Belt R, Leite C, Haas CD, et al: Incidence of hemorrhagic complications in patients with cancer. *JAMA* 239:2571–2574, 1978
2. Gaydos LA, Freireich EJ, Mantel N: The quantitative relation between platelet count and hemorrhage in patients with acute leukemia. *N Engl J Med* 266:905–909, 1962
3. Freireich EJ, Kliman A, Mante N, et al: Response to repeated platelet transfusion from the same donor. *Ann Intern Med* 59:277–287, 1963
4. Roy AJ, Jaffe N, Djerassi I: Prophylactic platelet transfusions in children with acute leukemia: A dose response study. *Transfusion* 13:283–290, 1973
5. Heyman MR, Schiffer CA: Platelet transfusion therapy for the cancer patient. *Semin Oncol* 17:198–209, 1990
6. Dutcher JP, Schiffer CA, Aisner J, et al: Incidence of thrombocytopenia and serious hemorrhage among patients with solid tumors. *Cancer* 53:557–562, 1984
7. Rickles FR, Edwards RL: Activation of blood coagulation in cancer. Trousseau's syndrome revisited. *Blood* 63:14–31, 1983
8. Bunn PA, Ridway EC: Paraneoplastic syndromes, in Devita VT, Hellman S, Rosenberg SA (eds): *Cancer: Principles and Practice of Oncology* (ed 3). Philadelphia: Lippincott, 1989, pp. 1896–1940.
9. Cohen AM, Shank B, Friedman MA: Colorectal cancer, in DeVita VT, Hellman S, Rosenberg SA (eds): *Cancer: Principles and Practice of Oncology* (ed 3). Philadelphia: Lippincott, 1989, pp. 895–964
10. Steinberg SM, Barkin JS, Kaplan RS, et al: Prognostic indicators of colon tumors: The gastrointestinal tumor study group experience. *Cancer* 57:1866–1870, 1986
11. Hoffrand AV, Pettit JE: *Atlas of Clinical Hematology.* London: Gower, 1988
12. Benditt EP, Schwartz SM: Blood vessels, in Rubin E, Farber JL (eds): *Pathology* (ed 2). Philadelphia: Lippincott, 1994, pp. 455–501
13. Zieve PD: Disorders of hemostasis, in Barker LR, Burton JR, Zieve PD (eds): *Principles of Ambulatory Medicine* (ed 4). Baltimore: Williams & Wilkins, 1995, pp. 608–616
14. Bonner H, Erslev Ajj: The blood and lymphoid organs, in Rubin E, Farber JL (eds): *Pathology* (ed 2). Philadelphia: Lippincott, 1994, pp. 995–1096
15. Zieve PD, Waterbury L: Thromboembolic disease, in Barker LR, Burton JR, Zieve PD (eds): *Principles of Ambulatory Medicine* (ed 4). Baltimore: Williams & Wilkins, 1995, pp. 616–624
16. Secor VH: The inflammatory/immune response in critical illness. *Crit Care Nurs Clin North Am* 6:251–264, 1994
17. Bone RC: Gram-positive organisms and sepsis. *Arch Intern Med* 154:26–34, 1994
18. Hochman R, Clark J, Rolla A, et al: Bleeding in patients with infections. Are antibiotics helping or hurting? *Arch Intern Med* 142:1440, 1982
19. Clagett GP: Preoperative assessment of hemostasis, in Rossi

EC, Simon TL, Moss GS (eds): *Principles of Transfusion Medicine*. Baltimore: Williams & Wilkins, 1991, pp. 453–460

20. Manson SD, Elson S: Alterations in body defenses, in Shekleton ME, Litwackk (eds): *Critical Care Nursing of the Surgical Patient*. Philadelphia: Saunders, 1991, pp. 356–377

21. Rosove MH, Schwartz GE: Hematologic complications of cancer and its treatment, in Haskell CM (ed): *Cancer Treatment* (ed 3). Philadelphia: Saunders, 1990, pp. 850–868

22. Holguin M, Caraveo J: Thrombocytopenia and granulocytopenia. *Postgrad Med* 76:171–182, 1984

23. Gobel B: Bleeding disorders, in Groenwald SL, Frogge MH, Goodman M, Yarbro CH (eds): *Cancer Nursing: Principles and Practice* (ed 4). Sudbury: Jones and Bartlett, 1997, pp. 604–639

24. Levine M, Gent M, Hirsch J, et al. A comparison of low-molecular-weight heparin administered primarily in the home with unfractionated heparin administered in the hospital for proximal deep-vein thrombosis. *N Engl J Med* 334: 677–681, 1996

25. Grosset AB, Spiro TG, Beynon J, Rodgers GM. Enoxaparin, a low-molecular-weight heparin suppresses prothrombin activation more effectively than unfractionated heparin in patients treated for venous thromboembolism. *Thromb Res* 86:349–354, 1997

26. Isaacs C, Robert NJ, Bailey FA, Schuster MW, et al. Randomized placebo-controlled study of recombinant human interleukin-11 to prevent chemotherapy-induced thrombocytopenia in patients with breast cancer receiving dose-intensive cyclophosphamide and doxorubicin. *J Clin Oncol* 15:3368–3377, 1997

27. Warkentin TE, Kelton JG: Immune thrombocytopenia and its management, in Rossi EC, Simon TL, Moss GS (eds): *Principles of Transfusion Medicine*. Baltimore: Williams & Wilkins, 1991, pp. 233–249

28. Parsons L, Klopovich PM: Immunoglobulin therapy. *Semin Oncol Nurs* 6:136–139, 1990

29. Galel SA, Grumet FC: Platelet alloimmunization, in Rossi EC, Simon TL, Moss GS (eds): *Principles of Transfusion Medicine*. Baltimore: Williams & Wilkins, 1991, pp. 271–277

30. Ey FS, Goodnight SH: Bleeding disorders in cancer. *Semin Oncol* 17:187–197, 1990

31. Guyer DR, Schatat AP, Vitale MHS, et al: Leukemic retinopathy: The relationship between fundus lesions and hematologic parameters at diagnosis. *Ophthalmology* 96:860–864, 1989

32. Richards EM, Marcus RE, Harper P, et al: Intra-ocular haemorrhage, a frequent complication of acute promyelocytic leukaemia. *Clin Lab Haematol* 14:169–178, 1992

33. Kistler JP, Ropper AA, Martin JB: Cerebrovascular disease, in Wilson JD, Braunwald E, Isselbacher KJ, et al (eds): *Principles of Internal Medicine* (ed 12). New York: McGraw-Hill, 1991, pp. 1977–2002

34. Richter JM, Isselbacher KJ: Gastrointestinal bleeding, in Wilson JD, Braunwald E, Isselbacher KJ, et al (eds): *Principles of Internal Medicine* (ed 12). New York: McGraw-Hill, 1991, pp. 261–264

35. Braunwald E: Cough and hemoptysis, in Wilson JD, Braunwald E, Isselbacher KJ, et al (eds): *Principles of Internal Medicine* (ed 12). New York: McGraw-Hill, 1991, pp. 217–220

36. Jules-Elysee K, Stover DE, Yaholom J, et al: Pulmonary complications in lymphoma patients treated with high-dose therapy and autologous bone marrow transplantation. *Am Rev Respir Dis* 146:485–491, 1992

37. Spach DH, Bauwens JE, Meyerson D, et al: Cytomegalovirus-induced hemorrhagic cystitis following bone marrow transplantation. *Clin Infect Dis* 16:142–144, 1993

38. Chapman C, Flower AJE, Durrant STS: The use of vidarabine in treatment of human polyomavirus associated with acute haemorrhagic cystitis. *Bone Marrow Transplant* 7:481–483, 1991

39. Feinstein DI: Treatment of disseminated intravascular coagulation. *Semin Thromb Hemost* 14:351–361, 1988

40. Goodnough LT: Management of disseminated intravascular coagulation, in Rossi EC, Simon TL, Moss GS (eds): *Principles of Transfusion Medicine*. Baltimore: Williams & Wilkins, 1991, pp. 373–382

Bleeding

Patient Name: _____

Symptom and Description   Bleeding occurs when blood escapes from a blood vessel. Bleeding can happen anywhere in your body. It can happen as an open cut, nosebleed, or bleeding hemorrhoid, or it may occur inside your body, such as in your stomach, lung, brain, or bladder. Slow bleeding can have little effect or can make you tired, weak, and short of breath. Sudden bleeding can cause severe weakness, dizziness, and pain.

Bleeding most often occurs in the person who has cancer when platelets (cells and the blood that help stop bleeding) are low. This may be a problem for people with leukemias or other tumors involving the bone marrow, as well as for those receiving chemotherapy or radiation therapy.

The risk of bleeding increases with infection, especially when the platelets are low or are dropping quickly.

Learning Needs   You will need to learn the signs and symptoms of bleeding and what to report to your doctor. The signs and symptoms of bleeding may be obvious, as with a nosebleed, or more subtle. You should report any of the following signs of bleeding to your doctor.

- Skin: A fine red rash that looks like pinpoint dots, usually appearing on the feet and legs; increased bruising
- Eyes: Bleeding into the whites of the eyes, inability to see normally
- Mouth and nose: Blood blisters, blood oozing from gums, blood-tinged saliva, bleeding mouth sores, nosebleeds
- Digestive system: Blood in vomitus, blood in stools, black tarry stools
- Urination/genitals: Blood in urine, pain or burning on urination, cramping, and frequency; vaginal bleeding
- Other: Severe headaches; increased weakness; difficulty waking up; pain in joints and muscles

Prevention   Your skin and the lining of your mouth are protective barriers for your body. Keeping them clean and free of debris is important in decreasing infection and risk for bleeding.

1. Skin:
   - Bathe and clean the perineal (crotch) area daily
   - Use skin lotion to prevent dryness and breaks in skin
   - Protect skin from cuts and scrapes and sharp objects
   - Shave using an electric razor
   - Trim and cut nails
   - Avoid falling and contact sports

(continued) 305

2. Mouth care:
   - Cleanse your mouth after each meal and before bedtime
   - Use a soft-bristle toothbrush
   - If your platelets are low, you may need to use toothettes, or swabs, instead of a toothbrush
   - Use mouthwash that does not contain alcohol, which can be drying
3. Digestive system:
   - Promote normal bowel patterns, avoiding straining and constipation
   - Use stool softeners or laxatives
   - Maintain proper diet and exercise
   - Avoid rectal suppositories and enemas
   - Avoid taking rectal temperatures

Management

- If bleeding does occur, stay calm; sit or lie down
- If bleeding is external, such as a cut, wound, or nosebleed, apply pressure for at least 10 to 15 minutes
- If bleeding is on a leg or arm, raise the limb above your heart
- Use an ice pack for 5 to 10 minutes to help slow the bleeding
- If oral bleeding occurs, increase the frequency of mouth care
- If blood is in vomitus, take your prescribed antiemetics, antacids, or medications to decrease acid in the stomach; avoid spicy or acidic foods and caffeine
- If blood is in urine, increase fluids; note color and amount of urine for reporting to your doctor
- If bleeding vaginally, note if the bleeding is heavy or abnormal and the size of clots; do not use tampons; keep track of how many sanitary napkins are used for reporting to your doctor

Follow-up   Notify your nurse and/or physician if any of the following occur:

- Blood in stool, urine, or vomitus
- Unusually heavy vaginal bleeding (or *any* bleeding if you are past menopause)
- Blood in sputum, shortness of breath, or problems breathing
- Dizziness, severe headaches, or changes in mental status

Phone Numbers

Nurse: _____ Phone: _____

Physician: _____ Phone: _____

Other: _____ Phone: _____

Comments

Patient's Signature: _____ Date: _____

Nurse's Signature: _____ Date: _____

Source: Pruett J: Bleeding, in Yarbro CH, Frogge MH, Goodman M (eds): *Cancer Symptom Management* (ed 2). Sudbury: Jones and Bartlett, 1999. © Jones and Bartlett Publishers.

CHAPTER 18

Infection

Debra Wujcik, RN, MSN, AOCN

The Problem of Infection in Cancer

Patients with cancer who undergo treatment with chemotherapy, radiation, or surgery are at significant risk for infection. This risk is related to compromised host defenses and sequelae of treatment due to absence of neutrophils, infection barrier disruption, and shifts in microbial flora. The mortality attributed to infections has decreased over the years because of the development of β-lactam and fluoroquinolone antibiotics, the increased use of prophylactic antifungals and antivirals, and the use of colony-stimulating factors in selected patients.

In response to more effective drug therapy, the types of infections have changed as resistant and opportunistic organisms emerge. Strategies to minimize and prevent infection in patients with mild to moderate short-term neutropenia are generally successful. However, complete prevention or elimination of infection has not been accomplished in high-risk patients such as those undergoing bone marrow transplantation or intensive chemotherapy.

Incidence in Cancer

Fever in patients with cancer can be due to infection (80%) or tumor (20%).[1] The risk of infection is directly related to the depth and length of *neutropenia* or lowered white blood cell count. More than 60% patients with neutropenia will become infected. If the absolute neutrophil count is <100/mm³, approximately 20% of febrile patients will have a documented bacteremia.[2] Most infections are due to bacteria, and fatal infections are usually due to fungal infections.[3]

Impact on Quality of Life

The impact of infection on the patient may be minimal to quite severe. During a period of short-term neutropenia, activities may be restricted to avoid crowds or individuals with infection. Strategies to decrease colonization of bacteria, such as diet changes and extra attention to personal hygiene, cause minimal interruption in normal routines.

The hospitalized patient who develops fever or the patient who is admitted for treatment of infection is generally confined to his or her room. Visitors and diet are restricted, and intravenous antibiotic therapy must be endured. There is close monitoring and frequent reassessment of the person until the fever and neutropenia resolve.

Although studies have addressed quality-of-life issues for patients undergoing treatment for cancer, none has specifically addressed the impact of infection.[4] The use of expensive hematopoietic growth factors to decrease the risk of infection has led to studies of the cost-effectiveness of this therapy. The debate has focused on the cost of inpatient treatment of infection rather than the effect of hospitalization on quality of life.[5-8] The assumption is that most patients are willing to endure the short-term toxicity of therapy in the hope of achieving a sustained remission of cure.[9]

Etiology

The etiology of infection in cancer is multifactorial. The immunocompromised individual may have multiple defects that are variable across the treatment continuum. In general, the patient experiences defects related to the disease in combination with a variety of insults related to the treatment for the disease.[10]

Malignancy-Related Immunosuppression

Certain malignancies cause specific defects in the immune response, resulting in increased risk for infection (Table 18-1).[11,12] Bone marrow infiltration with leukemic cells results in decreased numbers and altered functioning of neutrophils. Humoral immunity is modified in patients with chronic lymphocytic leukemia or multiple myeloma, causing them to be at risk for respiratory infec-

tions with encapsulated bacteria such as *Streptococcus pneumoniae* or *Haemophilus influenzae*. When cellular immunity is impaired, as in patients with Hodgkins' disease or those undergoing bone marrow transplantation, viral and fungal infections are common.

Treatment-Related Infection

The nature, duration, and sequence of therapy for cancer influence the risk infection. Chemotherapeutic drugs cause mild to severe myelosuppression (Table 18-2).[13,14] When bone marrow production is interrupted by chemotherapy, there is a decrease in the number of white blood cells, red blood cells, and platelets. Short-term neutropenia is defined as lasting less than a week while long-term neutropenia exceeds 1 to 2 weeks.[15,16] Although patients with fever and short-term neutropenia are usually treated with intravenous antibiotics, they quickly respond to the intervention and can be discharged to the home.[15] Patients receiving higher dose chemotherapy, such as those undergoing bone marrow or peripheral stem cell transplantation, have much longer periods of neutropenia and are at risk for more serious infections.

Some chemotherapeutic agents are stomatotoxic, causing ulceration and breaks in the oral and gastroin-

TABLE 18-1 Etiology of Infection in Patients with Cancer

Factor	Defect	Types of Infection
Malignancy		
Acute leukemia	Neutropenia Qualitative defects	Bacterial, fungal, viral
Chronic lymphocytic leukemia, multiple myeloma	Humoral immunity	*Streptococcus pneumoniae* *Haemophilus influenzae*
Hodgkin's diseases, non-Hodgkin's lymphoma	Cellular immunity	Viral, fungal
Treatment		
Myelosuppressive chemotherapy	Neutropenia Altered mucosal barrier	Bacterial, fungal, viral Gram-negative colonization
Radiation	Neutropenia Altered skin integrity Altered mucosal barrier	
Corticosteroids	Immunosuppression	
Bone marrow transplantation	Neutropenia Immunosuppression	Bacterial, fungal, viral Cytomegalovirus *Pneumocystis carinii*
Protein-Calorie Malnutrition	Immunosuppression	
Nosocomial		
Tunneled central venous catheters, invasive procedures	Altered skin integrity	*Staphylococcus aureus*
Food, plants	Colonization of endogenous organisms	
Air	Airborne *Aspergillus*	

TABLE 18-2 Chemotherapeutic Agents Causing Myelosuppression and Stomatitis

Classification	Generic Name	Other Name	Myelosuppression	Stomatitis
Alkylating agent	Altretamine	Hexamethamelamine	Mild	
	Busulfan	Myleran	Moderate to severe	Moderate to severe[a]
	Carboplatin	Paraplatin	Mild	
	Chlorambucil	Leukeran	Mild to moderate[a]	
	Cisplatin	Platinol	Mild	
	Cyclophosphamide	Cytoxan	Mild to moderate	
	Dacarbazine	DTIC	Moderate	Rare
	Ifosfamide	IFEX	Severe	Mild
	Mechlorethamine	Nitrogen mustard	Moderate	
	Melphalan	Alkeran	Moderate	Rare
	Procarbazine	Matulane	Moderate	Rare
	Streptozocin	Streptozotocin	Mild	
	Thiotepa	TESPA	Moderate to severe[a]	Moderate to severe[a]
Plant alkaloid	Amasacrine	AMSA	Mild	
	Irinotecan	Camptosar	Severe	Mild
	Etoposide	VP-16	Moderate	Moderate to severe[a]
	Paclitaxel	Taxol	Moderate to severe[a]	Moderate[a]
	Docetaxel	Taxotere	Moderate to severe[a]	Mild
	Teniposide	VM-26	Severe	Rare
	Topotecan	Hycamtin	Moderate to severe[a]	Rare
	Vinblastine	Velban	Mild	Rare
	Vincristine	Oncovin	Rare	
	Vindesine[b]	Eldesine	Moderate	Rare
	Vinorelbine	Navelbine	Moderate	
Antimetabolite	Chlorodeoxyadenosine	2-CdA	Moderate	
	Cytarabine	Ara-C	Severe	Severe
	Edetrexate[b]	10-EDAM	Moderate	Severe
	Floxuridine	FUDR	Moderate	Moderate to severe[a]
	Fluorouracil	5-FU	Moderate	Moderate to severe[a]
	Gemcitabine	Gemzar	Moderate to severe	Mild
	Hydroxyurea	Hydrea	Mild	Rare
	Mercaptopurine	6-MP	Moderate	Mild
	Methotrexate	Mexate, MTX	Moderate[a]	Moderate to severe[a]
	Mitoquazone[b]	Methyl-GAG	Mild	Moderate to severe[a]
	Pentostatin	2,Deoxycoformycin	Severe	Mild
	Thioguanine	6-TG	Moderate	Mild
	Trimetrexate	TMTX	Mild	Moderate to severe
Antibiotic	Dactinomycin	Actinomycin	Moderate	Rare
	Daunorubicin	Daunomycin	Moderate	Moderate
	Doxorubicin	Adriamycin	Moderate to severe	Moderate
	Epirubicin[b]	4,Epidoxorubicin	Severe	
	Idarubicin	Idamycin	Severe	Mild
	Mitomycin	Mutamycin	Moderate	Rare
	Mitoxantrone	Novantrone	Severe	Moderate
Nitrosoureas	Carmustine	BCNU	Moderate to severe	
	Lomustine	CCNU[a]	Moderate to severe	Rare

[a] Dose-related toxicity.

[b] Investigational drug.

testinal mucosa (see Table 18-2). These breaks allow *bacterial translocation,* which is the movement of endogenous flora into the bloodstream.[17] Radiation therapy may damage skin integrity causing open, weeping skin.[18] The gastrointestinal mucosa can be damaged as well. Radiation to sites of active bone marrow, such as the sternum, pelvis, or long bones, may result in depressed hematopoiesis.

Corticosteroids used in many treatment protocols further suppress immune function and mask signs and symptoms of infection. The numbers of white blood cells are decreased, and their function is impaired. In addition, corticosteroids can diminish neutrophil adherence to epithelial cells, blocking the first step of delivery of neutrophils to the site of inflammation. Finally, lymphocytes, monocytes, and eosinophils are redistributed to extravascular spaces and away from sites of infection.[11]

Procedures such as intravenous therapy, venipunctures, biopsies, and catheters cause breaks in skin integrity and further assault the normal defenses. The infection rate associated with long-term central venous catheters is as high as 60%, depending on the disease and type of treatment.[19,20] The infections include exit-site infections, port pocket or tunnel track infection, and bacteremia. Because the combination of skin colonization with specific organisms such as *Corynebacterium* species, prolonged neutropenia, and skin breaks produces bacteremia and even death, some have assessed the benefit of a skin hygiene program to reduce the risk.[21]

The net state of immunosuppression of the person determines the actual risk of infection.[22] A patient who is severely immunosuppressed due to disease and treatment side effects can become infected with minimal exposure to nonpathogens. A delicate balance is easily tipped toward illness as exposure to pathogens can be quickly life-threatening.

One of the difficulties in treating neutropenic febrile patients is the range of organisms capable of causing infection.[23] More than half of all infections in neutropenic patients are attributed to colonization of organisms acquired from the local environment.[10] These organisms, which are usually nonpathogenic, produce disease in patients who are severely immunosuppressed.

This colonization of organisms begins with aerobic gram-negative organisms. Soon after empiric antibiotics are initiated, colonization by *Candida* spp. occurs.[15] Both endogenous and exogenous organisms contribute to the colonization. The major sources for colonizing organisms are food (uncooked fruits and vegetables), water, inhaled airborne organisms (*Aspergillus*), and organisms passed through direct contact between caregivers and the neutropenic person. Opportunistic infections are invasive infections caused by nonpathogens (e.g., *Pneumocystis carinii*) or by organisms that usually cause very minimal infection (e.g., herpesvirus). Once colonization has occurred, it is easy for microorganisms to migrate through mucosa denuded by the effects of chemotherapy or radiation or through specific breaks in the skin caused by catheters, venipunctures, or procedures.

In the 1960s and 1970s, the predominant organisms causing infection in neutropenic persons were gram-negative pathogens.[10,22] Gram-negative sepsis was frequently life-threatening since the broad-spectrum antibiotics used (e.g., carboxypenicillins, first-generation cephalosporins, and aminoglycosides) were less effective than those used today (e.g., third-generation cephalosporins, fluoroquinolones, and antifungals). In addition, less serious gram-positive infections are more prevalent now.[24] This change in the type of infecting organisms and improved antibiotic therapy allows for the consideration of monotherapy and shorter courses of combination therapy in appropriately identified low-risk persons.[23–25]

Pathophysiology

Neutropenia is well established as the greatest predictor of infection in patients with cancer.[23,26–28] The mature neutrophil is the first line of defense against bacterial infection. In general, the person with a normal total white blood count (WBC) of 4000/mm³ to 10,000/mm³ is able to fight infection. Neutropenia is defined as an absolute neutrophil count (ANC) less than 1000/mm³. The ANC is calculated by multiplying the WBC by the percentage of bands and segmented neutrophils (Figure 18-1). The ANC is used to identify persons at risk for developing infection. The risk of infection is significant when the ANC ≤ 500/mm³ and high when the ANC < 100/mm³ (Table 18-3). The rate of development and the length of the neutropenia also influence the risk of infection. Persons with a rapid decline in the neutrophil level have an increased risk of infection.

The period of neutropenia after chemotherapy is relatively predictable (Figure 18-2).[12] The nadir, or lowest WBC after treatment, usually occurs 10 to 14 days after therapy. As the bone marrow stem cells mature and are released into the peripheral blood, the blood counts rise, and full recovery is generally seen at 3 to 4 weeks after therapy. When combinations of several myelosuppressive drugs are used or high-dose therapy is employed, the nadir becomes a phase lasting several days to weeks. When the patient with underlying immunosuppression due to

---

1. Determine the white blood count (WBC), percentage of segmented neutrophis and bands from the laboratory results.

2. Use the following formula to determine the ANC:

$$ANC = \frac{(\% \text{ segments } + \% \text{ bands}) \times WBC}{100}$$

Example

$$ANC = \frac{(24 + 1) \times 4000}{100}$$
$$= 1000/mm^3$$

FIGURE 18-1 Calculating the absolute neutrophil count (ANC).

TABLE 18-3 Common Toxicity Criteria for Infection

Grade	WBC/mm³	ANC/mm³
0	>4000	>200
1	3000–3900	150–190
2	2000–2900	100–140
3	1000–1900	50–90
4	<1000	<50

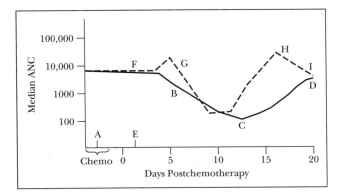

FIGURE 18-2 Infection risk and prophylaxis in patients receiving myelosuppressive chemotherapy. Chemotherapy is administered with varying combinations of drugs (A). In response to interrupted blood cell production, the absolute neutrophil count (ANC) begins to decrease (B) (*solid line*). The nadir, or lowest ANC, usually occurs 10 to 14 days after chemotherapy (C). Recovery of ANC is seen 3 to 4 weeks after chemotherapy (D). Prophylactic antibiotics may be given to protect the patient throughout the period of neutropenia (E). Hematopoietic growth factors (HGFs) may be administered daily beginning 24 hours after therapy (F). A rise in the ANC occurs due to the release of reserve cells from the marrow (G) (*broken line*). After a nadir that occurs earlier than without HGFs is of shorter duration and is less severe, the ANC recovers rapidly (H). The HGF is discontinued when the ANC > 10,000/mm³. The ANC decreases by half in the 24 hours after discontinuation, then continues normal levels (I). (Adapted from Wujcik D: Infection control in oncology patients. *Nurs Clin North Am* 28:641, 1993.[12]) (Reprinted with permission.)

disease receives myelosuppressive treatment, additional insult is added.

The pathogens responsible for infections in patients with cancer are divided into two groups: (1) those responsible for the initial infection and (2) those responsible for second or subsequent infection.[29] Bacterial infections quickly develop in the neutropenic person and account for 85% to 90% of the pathogens associated with febrile neutropenia.[30] The organisms generally arise from the endogenous flora colonizing the skin, respiratory, genitourinary, and GI tracts.[24] Breaks in the integrity of the mucosa caused by the effects of chemotherapy of intravenous catheters allow bloodstream infections. The most serious infections are attributed to gram-negative organisms, generally *Enterobacteriaceae* or *Pseudomonas aeruginosa*.

In the last decade, gram-positive infections with *Staphylococcus* spp., *Streptococcus* spp., *Corynebacteria*, and *Clostridia* spp. have increased[1,31] because of common use of implanted catheters and the increased use of prophylactic antibiotics.[2,22] A catheter-associated infection is diagnosed when there are positive blood cultures from both a catheter lumen and a peripheral venipuncture.[15]

Bacterial pneumonia is a common infection in immunocompromised persons due to a combination of variables.[1] Gram-negative bacteria colonize in the upper airway. Aspiration with chemotherapy-induced vomiting is common. Once pneumonia develops, the severity is determined by the depth and length of neutropenia and the virulence of the organism. In addition, if the neutropenia continues, secondary invasion of opportunistic organisms may occur.

Herpesvirus infections have a great impact on the immunocompromised patient as well.[22] Included are herpes simplex virus 1 and 2 (HSV-1, HSV-2), varicella-zoster virus (VZV), cytomegalovirus (CMV), and Epstein-Barr virus (EBV).[3] Each of these viruses has the characteristic of latency; that is, a primary infection with the virus results in a lifelong dormant infection capable of being reactivated during a period of immunosuppression. Herpes simplex viruses often cause an initial infection in neutropenic persons. Reactivation of viral infections are most common in patients with hematologic malignancies and those undergoing bone marrow transplantation.[32]

If fever persists 5 to 7 days after the initiation of broad-spectrum antibiotics, and no source of infection has been identified, a secondary infection is presumed. *Candida albicans* is the predominant fungal infection in patients with solid tumors, while non-albicans candida is common among patients with hematologic disorders.[33] A positive blood culture for *Candida* in a neutropenic patient is considered indicative of disseminated candidiasis.[3,10] Cytomegalovirus and filamentous fungi (*Aspergillus*) are common causes of secondary infection in severely immunosuppressed persons.[33]

Assessment

Measurement Tools

Fever has long been established as the primary symptom of infection in neutropenic patients.[1,30] Fever is defined by three oral temperatures above 38°C or 100.4°F in a 24-hour period or one temperature above 38.5°C or 101.3°F.[1,34] Endogenous pyrogens are produced by macrophages in response to microbial invasion. These, in turn, produce fever. Although only about half of all infections in patients with cancer can be attributed to a definite source, all febrile neutropenic patients should receive prompt attention. Frequently the patient becomes febrile at home. The nurse is often in a key position to conduct a telephone assessment and recommend appropriate interventions (Figure 18-3).[35]

Physical Assessment

The diagnosis of infection in the person with cancer should be made with a complete physical assessment and

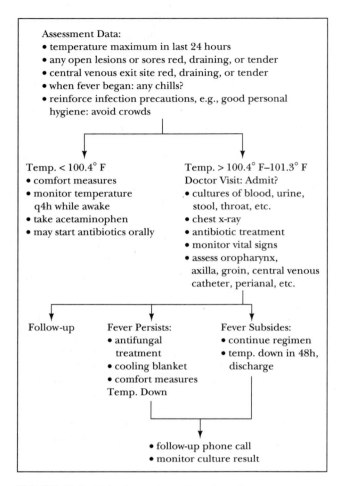

Assessment Data:
- temperature maximum in last 24 hours
- any open lesions or sores red, draining, or tender
- central venous exit site red, draining, or tender
- when fever began: any chills?
- reinforce infection precautions, e.g., good personal hygiene: avoid crowds

Temp. < 100.4° F
- comfort measures
- monitor temperature q4h while awake
- take acetaminophen
- may start antibiotics orally

Temp. > 100.4° F–101.3° F
Doctor Visit: Admit?
- cultures of blood, urine, stool, throat, etc.
- chest x-ray
- antibiotic treatment
- monitor vital signs
- assess oropharynx, axilla, groin, central venous catheter, perianal, etc.

Follow-up

Fever Persists:
- antifungal treatment
- cooling blanket
- comfort measures
Temp. Down

Fever Subsides:
- continue regimen
- temp. down in 48h, discharge

- follow-up phone call
- monitor culture result

FIGURE 18-3   Telephone triage flow sheet for assessment of fever. (From Camp-Sorrell D: Chemotherapy: Toxicity management, in Groenwald SL, Frogge MH, Goodman M, Yarbro CH (eds): *Cancer Nursing: Principles and Practice* (ed 4). © 1997 Sudbury: Jones and Bartlett Publishers, p. 395. Reprinted by permission.[33])

diagnostic studies. In the neutropenic patient, the usual objective signs of infection (redness, swelling, and pus formation) are absent. Pain and tenderness may be the only indicators of infection. High-risk areas for infection, such as the perirectal area, oral mucosa, sinuses, lung, and skin, are carefully assessed.[1,29,31]

The mucous membranes are inspected for signs of infection such as redness, tenderness, ulceration, or pseudomembranes.[36] Because drug-induced mucositis can easily progress to secondary infection, oral cultures for fungus and virus should be obtained. The manifestations of drug- and virus-induced mucositis are often clinically indistinguishable. However, without antiviral therapy, viral mucositis can be quite severe and prolonged.[15]

Any breaks in the integrity of the skin are inspected for subtle signs of infection. Tenderness and erythema along the subcutaneous tunnel of the indwelling catheter

may indicate a tunnel infection.[15,19,20] The only sign of perirectal abscess may be pain on defecation.[37]

Diagnostic Evaluation

Chest radiographs (CXRs) may be inconclusive or reveal diffuse infiltrates. Serial CXRs have proved to be useful to determine subtle changes in patients with prolonged neutropenia.[38] Other techniques such as chest tomography or indium scans are being evaluated for their usefulness in detecting infection in febrile neutropenic patients.[38,39]

Blood cultures are obtained at the first fever and may continue daily as long as the patient remains febrile, until the source of infection is identified or the neutrophil count has returned to normal. The implanted catheter is used for cultures until a positive culture is received. Then, separate cultures are drawn from the peripheral blood and each lumen of the catheter to differentiate bacteremia from an infected catheter. Two cultures obtained in close intervals are recommended to increase the yield for detecting bacteremia. In addition, blood cultures should be obtained when the fever is rising or the person is having a shaking chill, to maximize the chances of obtaining microorganisms.[40] One or two cultures from two different sites are usually adequate to document infection.

If diarrhea is present in the patient with neutropenia, a specimen is tested for *Clostridium difficile*. This bacteria causes toxin release and is treated with oral vancomycin or metronidazole.[1] Patients with prolonged neutropenia are also at risk for neutropenic enterocolitis, an inflammation of the small intestine or colon that can progress to bowel perforation and septic shock.[41]

The neutropenic patient is reevaluated daily until an infectious organism is identified, the patient is afebrile, or the neutrophil count returns to normal.

Degrees of Toxicity

Patients with neutropenia and fever are treated aggressively because it is difficult, if not impossible, to differentiate low-risk patients from high-risk patients. The common toxicity criteria for infection (see Table 18-3) simply grades the depth of neutropenia after treatment. However, the grade of toxicity does not always correlate directly with the incidence of infection, as there are other factors, such as host resistance and length of neutropenia, to be considered. Historically, any patient with fever and neutropenia was hospitalized and treated with a minimum course of 5 to 7 days of intravenous antibiotics. More recently, there has been interest in identification of neutropenic febrile patients as belonging to low-risk and high-risk categories.

Low-risk patients are those with evidence of impending bone marrow recovery indicated by increasing ANC, monocytes, or platelets >75,000/mm³.[42–44] This indication of returning marrow function can be seen 4 to 5 days before the ANC exceeds 500/mm³, potentially decreasing the length of parenteral antibiotics and hospitalization. Low risk may be determined at the onset of fever, during hospitalization, or at the time of possible discharge. For the latter, the criteria would include patients whose fever has resolved, whose blood cultures are negative, and who clinically appear well.[25,45] Although these criteria are not yet proven, there is increasing interest in strategies to decrease the length and cost of hospitalization of neutropenic febrile patients.[45] Other management options for low-risk patients may be to continue daily intravenous antibiotics in the home or outpatient setting.[25,46]

High-risk patients are those with febrile neutropenia and one or more high-risk factors such as mucositis, diarrhea, clinical instability, advanced disease, or overt organ dysfunction.[25] Underlying comorbidity (cardiac or renal disease) and inpatient status at onset of fever have also been identified as high-risk factors for serious infection.[44,47]

Symptom Management

Prevention

Multiple strategies are used to minimize infection in neutropenic patients. These include identification of patients at risk for infection; patient, family, and staff education to avoid practices that increase colonization; and fewer invasive procedures. Using knowledge of the disease and side effects of treatment, the nurse can identify patients at risk for infection.[48,49] Laboratory results are collected as appropriate and assessed to determine risk for and presence of neutropenia.

The hospitalized neutropenic patient is assessed by checking vital signs every 4 hours and a full physical assessment twice daily. The patient/family are advised to reduce room clutter and screen all visitors to minimize colonization of organisms. Thorough handwashing by staff and family alike contributes to reduced colonization. Good personal hygiene is emphasized along with an oral care protocol. Most institutions use a protective protocol that eliminates uncooked fruits and vegetables. Live plants and flowers are removed from the environment. Ambulation and aggressive pulmonary hygiene are encouraged to promote lung expansion. Colonization of bacteria in the axillae is avoided by not shaving and by using deodorants instead of antiperspirants.[10] Gastric antacids may be prescribed to lower the gastric pH; this decreases the colonization of the small and large intestine by *Candida* spp.[50]

The patient at home who is at risk for neutropenia has regular blood specimens drawn and is reminded to check his or her temperature twice daily if he or she feels warm. It is recommended to initiate procedures to decrease colonization (diet changes, avoiding those with infection) *before* the patient is neutropenic.[16] The patient must be reliable enough to call the physician if any fever or change in clinical status occurs and live close enough to a medical facility to receive prompt intervention.

Prophylactic treatment of infection with oral antibiotics in neutropenic patients is being evaluated closely. The fluoroquinolones have potent activity against gramnegative aerobes with little effect on anaerobes. Prophylactic administration has been evaluated and shown to decrease temperatures in patients with hematologic malignancy and those undergoing bone marrow transplantation.[51] However, the use of these drugs is controversial. The fluoroquinolones do not prevent gram-positive infections and outbreaks of resistant coagulase-negative staphylococcus have been reported.[52,53]

A newer method to prevent infection decreases the period of risk for infection—the period of neutropenia, which is the period of highest risk of infection. This is accomplished through the use of hematopoietic growth factors (HGFs).[54] These glycoproteins activate the production and maturation of distinctive cell lineages. Specifically, granulocyte colony-stimulating factor (G-CSF) prompts neutrophil activity and granulocyte-macrophage colony-stimulating factor (GM-CSF) stimulates neutrophils and macrophages. In addition, the activity of mature neutrophils—phagocytosis, oxidative burst, antibody-dependent cytotoxicity, and chemotaxis—is enhanced. These actions allow the neutrophils to be more aggressive and effective in destroying pathogens.

HGFs are administered daily beginning 24 hours after chemotherapy (see Figure 18-2). Although they do not eliminate the period of neutropenia, the duration and severity of neutropenia after therapy are lessened; therefore, the period of risk is shortened. HGFs have proved effective in patients with solid tumors receiving myelosuppressive chemotherapy and those undergoing bone marrow transplantation.[55,56]

Other uses for HGFs in the management of infection are being investigated. Macrophage-CSF (M-CSF) is being evaluated for treatment of fungal infections and for minimizing the period of neutropenia.[57–59] Combinations of G-CSF and interferon-γ or GM-CSF with amphotericin may be effective in treating disseminated fungal infections.[60] Preclinical and clinical studies indicate interleukin-1 has benefit for immunocompromised patients with serious infections.[61]

Therapeutic Approaches

Empiric therapy

Traditional early treatment of infection in the neutropenic patient is with empiric antibiotic therapy that continues until bone marrow recovery.[15] Empiric therapy is antibiotic therapy started before the infecting organism is identified. This clinical practice began in the 1970s after it was demonstrated that nearly 75% of febrile neutropenic patients eventually had a proven site of infection.[30] Antibiotics that cover both gram-positive and gram-negative organisms are initiated. The usual combination includes an aminoglycoside plus an extended-spectrum cephalosporin or a broad-spectrum penicillin. The goal of empiric therapy is to prevent the morbidity and mortality associated with inadequately treated infections.[24] The decision of which antibiotics are selected includes knowledge of the common pathogens in the institution.[23,31,50] It is to be expected that modifications are made according to the ongoing clinical assessment, most often due to persistent fever. Table 18-4 cites the most common antibiotics used to treat infection in neutropenic patients.

Aminoglycosides interfere with cell wall synthesis to destroy bacteria and are effective against gram-negative organisms.[23] Gentamicin, amikacin, and tobramycin are commonly prescribed. Close monitoring of drug levels is essential because the aminoglycosides have a narrow therapeutic-to-toxic ratio. Renal function is assessed daily through laboratory values and close monitoring of fluid status.

TABLE 18-4 Common Antibiotics Used to Treat Neutropenic Infection

Classification	Generic Name
β-lactams	
Penicillins	Carbenicillin
	Methicillin
	Ticarcillin
Cephalosporins	Ceftazidime
Carbapenems	Imipenem-cilastatin
Monobactams	Aztreonam
Aminoglycosides	Amikacin
	Gentamicin
	Tobramycin
Fluoroquinolones	Ciprofloxacin
	Norfloxacin
Glycopeptides	Vancomycin
Antivirals	Acyclovir
	Foscarnet
	Ganciclovir
Antifungals	Amphotericin B
	Clotrimazole
	Fluconazole
	Itraconazole
	Ketoconazole
	Miconazole
	Nystatin

The cephalosporins are a class of drugs that also interfere with cell wall synthesis and activate bacterial cell autolysis. The third-generation cephalosporins provide potent activity against gram-negative aerobic organisms such as *Pseudomonas aeruginosa,* as well as limited gram-positive coverage.[62,63] Ceftazidime has been evaluated for initial management of the neutropenic, febrile patient and is an acceptable alternative to combination therapy.[64]

The penicillins also provide coverage for gram-negative organisms. For patients who are allergic to penicillin, aztreonam, a synthetic monobactam, may be substituted.

The most frequent cause of bacteremia is now coagulase-negative staphylococci and viridans streptococci.[24] Vancomycin is effective in treating resistant gram-positive organisms and *Staphylococcus epidermidis.*[65] Vancomycin is frequently added as empiric therapy in patients with indwelling catheters who are undergoing myelosuppressive therapy.

Finally, broad-spectrum monotherapy with agents such as cefperazone or imipenem is being evaluated in many centers.[23,24] Imipenem is a carbapenem, a subclassification of β-lactam antibiotics. Imipenem has a very broad spectrum of coverage, including aerobic gram-negative rods and the Enterobacteriaceae, most gram-positive pathogens, and anaerobes.[24] One side effect of note with imipenem is a decrease in seizure threshold in elderly patients or those with central nervous system pathology.[66]

The fluoroquinolones are a class of synthetic antibiotics. The mechanism of action is unique to this classification; therefore, cross-resistance between fluoroquinolones and other commonly used antibiotics is uncommon.[24,51] The fluoroquinolones are very effective against gram-negative organisms, especially *P. aeruginosa.* Ciprofloxacin has been evaluated as part of empiric therapy for febrile neutropenic patients, but does not have a particular advantage over other drug combinations. The best use seems to be in treatment of patients with multiple resistant, gram-negative infections.[24]

The neutropenic patient continues to be carefully assessed until the bone marrow recovers. Therapy may need to be modified the longer the patient remains neutropenic due to breakthrough of organisms not covered by the initial therapy or that have become resistant to the therapy. As neutropenia continues, the patient is more susceptible to infections from other bacteria, viruses, protozoa, and fungi.

Institutions vary in their practice of modifying therapy based on persistent fever in the absence of other clinical data.[15] Modification of the initial regimen may be guided by specific clinical events. For example, a new pulmonary infiltrate may indicate a fungal infection or severe oral mucositis may require a specific antiaerobic drug.[31] Fever alone is not considered justification for adding other antimicrobials.

Empiric antifungal therapy is initiated when the patient remains febrile 5 to 7 days after empiric therapy is begun. Amphotericin B has been the drug of choice for treating fungal infections for over two decades, despite significant toxicity. Common side effects of this agent are nephrotoxicity (90%); fever, chills, and rigors (80%–90%); anorexia (50%); headache (45%); vomiting; and anemia.[67] A 1-mg test dose is administered to rule out anaphylaxis. If tolerated without cardiac or pulmonary compromise, the first dose is given. The dose is then escalated daily until the desired dosage is reached. Because fungal infections are so serious and difficult to treat, some centers are now evaluating the effectiveness of prophylactic amphotericin B. The usual dosage is 0.5 mg/kg/day.[15]

Low-dose amphotericin B, 0.1 to 0.5 mg/kg/day, has been evaluated mainly in bone marrow transplant recipients. Although there is a trend toward fewer respiratory infections, too few patients have been studied to form firm conclusions.[68] A meta-analysis of 24 trials with 2758 patients where antifungal agents were given prophylactically or empirically showed no survival benefit in patients with treatment-induced neutropenia.[69]

New formulations at amphotericin B, such as small unilamellar vesicles, lipid complex, or colloidal dispersion, are being evaluated.[70]

Imidazoles are antifungal agents that block the enzymes required to synthesize a component of the fungal cell membrane. Ketoconazole, miconazole, and clotrimazole are imadazoles given to prevent fungal infections. Fluconazole and itraconazole are triazoles with good oral absorption and penetration into cerebrospinal fluid.[65] Two large trials of fluconazole 400 mg/day for bone marrow transplant recipients reduced the number of candidal infections.[71,72] Although these drugs are useful in preventing *Candida* infections, none has proved effective in preventing or treating *Aspergillus* infections.

Herpesviruses are a group of viruses that become latent in the body after a primary infection and reactivate after varying periods of time. HSV infections are problematic in certain types of cancer such as Hodgkin's disease or acute leukemia. Oral acyclovir of doses 1 to 2 g/day are given in these patients to prevent reactivation during intensive chemotherapy.[24] When used to treat active infection, acyclovir decreases the duration of symptoms, length of viral shedding, and time of healing.

Varicella-zoster viruses (VZVs) include chickenpox and shingles and are tenfold less sensitive than HSV to the effects of acyclovir. Patients with VZV receive higher dosages of acyclovir (600–800 mg PO 5 times daily or 500 mg/m[2] IV) to prevent dissemination of the infection. If the patient is hospitalized during an outbreak of VZV, he or she is isolated to prevent spread of the virus to other immunocompromised patients.[24]

Cytomegalovirus infections are generally problematic only in patients undergoing bone marrow transplantation.[32] To add to the difficulty of dealing with CMV infec-

tions, diagnosis using traditional buffy coat specimens can take up to 6 weeks. Faster methods have been developed to diagnose CMV in urine and bronchoalveolar lavage specimens.[73] Ganciclovir, which is 30 times more potent than acyclovir, is used to treat CMV.[74]

If the source of infection is the implanted central catheter, every attempt is made to treat the infection before removing the catheter. The current recommendation is to remove the catheter only when the tunnel appears to be infected or when signs of infection are visible at the exit site.[23] It is important to rotate the antibiotics through all lumens of the catheter in order to treat the infection effectively. If the patient remains febrile on antibiotics and there appears to be no resolution of the symptoms of the tunnel infection (redness, swelling), the catheter is removed.[15]

A consensus statement from the Infectious Diseases Society of America recommends a minimum of 5 to 7 days parenteral antibiotic therapy after resolution of fever.[2] Negative effects of prolonged hospitalization and treatment with parenteral antibiotics include toxicities of antimicrobials, higher costs than for outpatient treatment, exposure to nosocomial pathogens, risk of superinfection with fungal pathogens, and altered quality of life when home, work, or school life is interrupted. Many believe selected low-risk patients can safely be switched to oral antibiotics and discharged before the ANC is greater than 500/mm[3].[23,25]

Late therapy

The neutropenic patient with fever can quickly become septic if left untreated. If the neutropenia continues and empiric antibiotic coverage is not adequate, septic shock develops. Mortality rates from septic shock are between 30% and 80%.[75] Gram-negative bacteria are the most common cause. The results are diminished cardiovascular function, microvascular perfusion, and oxygenation of tissues. If untreated, multisystem organ failure develops. About 10% of patients with bacteremia due to *Streptococcus mitis* develop adult respiratory distress syndrome, especially those who received high-dose cytarabine. The mortality rate is 60%.[76]

Gram-negative bacteria release endotoxins that react with cell membranes.[75] Complement, coagulation, and kinin systems are activated. Activated coagulation results in microthrombi formation and altered blood flow. At the same time, fibrinolysin is released, dissolving clots and consuming clotting factors and platelets. Disseminated intravascular coagulation (DIC) results.[77]

Endotoxins activate the complement system, causing vasodilation, capillary leakage, chemotaxis, and increased neutrophil activation. The kinin system, when activated, produces bradykinin, causing further vasodilation and increased vascular permeability.[75]

As blood is shunted to main organs, peripheral tissue perfusion diminishes. Fluid shifts to extravascular spaces,

FLOW SHEET—NEUTROPENIA AND FEVER

DATE:			
TIME:			
INITIALS:			

A = Axillary   103°
R = Rectal

102°

101°

100°

99°

(normal)

98°

Circle pulse if
apical (below)   97°

HEART	RATE	
	RHYTHM	
BP	SYST	
	DIAS	
RESP	RATE	

SHIFT ASSESSMENTS

1. NEUROLOGIC	
2. CARDIOVASCULAR	
3. PULMONARY	
4. MUSCULOSKELETAL	
5. GASTROINTESTINAL	
6. GENITOURINARY	
7. INTEGUMENT	
8. ORAL	
9. PSYCHOSOCIAL	
10. SAFETY	
11. COMFORT	
SIGNATURE	SIGNATURE
SIGNATURE	SIGNATURE

(continued)

FIGURE 18-4 Documentation flow sheet and assessment standards for patient with neutropenia and fever.

ASSESSMENT STANDARDS

The following parameters will be considered a negative assessment and constitute the use of a "✓":

1. Neurologic assessment—when awake is alert, oriented to person, place, and time, pupils equal and reactive.

2. Cardiovascular—regular apical pulse, capillary refill time < 2 sec, skin turgor appropriate, no edema, pedal pulses present and equal.

3. Pulmonary assessment—respirations regular, rate 10–20 at rest, bilateral breath sounds clear. No O_2 in use.

4. Musculoskeletal—normal range of motion all joints, no muscle weakness.

5. Gastrointestinal—abdomen soft, nontender, active bowel sounds, bowel movements within own pattern and consistency, no nausea or vomiting.

6. Genitourinary—empties bladder without difficulty, or Foley patent and draining. Urine clear and yellow to amber.

7. Integument—skin warm, dry, and intact with no rashes, central venous catheter exit site or IV site(s) without redness, swelling, or tenderness, and dressing dry and intact. Skin color appropriate.

8. Oral assessment—oral mucosa pink, moist, and intact without lesions or ulcerations; adequate saliva production.

9. Psychosocial—affect and emotional status appropriate for this patient and consistent with stage of disease.

10. Safety—call light within reach, ID band present and legible, bed in low position, safety equipment at bedside (ambu, mask, airway).

11. Comfort: a "✓" indicates patient is free of discomfort. Level of discomfort is measured with the analgesia scale:
    1 = sleep, 2 = comfortable, 3 = mild discomfort, 4 = pain, 5 = severe pain.

FIGURE 18-4   (continued)

especially in the lungs, resulting in pulmonary edema. As oxygen supply decreases and the metabolism switches to anaerobic metabolism, lactic acid is produced, causing metabolic acidosis. As hyperventilation continues, respiratory alkalosis develops.

There are four stages of septic shock.[78] During the *initial* stage, cellular changes are under way, and there are no obvious clinical signs and symptoms. Quickly, neural, hormonal, and chemical *compensatory mechanisms* are activated. These responses are evidenced by elevated heart rate and respirations; cool, pale, moist skin; and a patient who is restless and confused. As the compensatory mechanisms begin to fail, the patient enters the *progressive* stage. Level of consciousness is severely depressed; the skin becomes cold and mottled. Blood pressure begins to drop while the heart rate and respirations are very rapid. In the *terminal*, or *refractory* stage, the heart rate slows, becomes irregular, and eventually stops.

The nursing care focus is on astute assessment of the parameters of tissue perfusion: level of consciousness, urine output, skin, and vital signs.[49,78] Antibiotic therapy continues, and supportive management is focused on adequate ventilation and oxygenation, maintenance of intravascular fluid volume, cardiac output, and restoration of metabolic environment. Careful assessment and intervention at an early stage may inhibit progression to later stages of shock.

Evaluation of Therapeutic Approaches

Documentation tools

Because fever is the most significant indicator of infection, the individual's temperature is recorded every 4 hours.[34] A graphic display is useful to identify patterns and specific causes of temperature elevations, such as a febrile response to blood products, amphotericin B, HGFs, or tumor (Figure 18-4). The graph of temperature may indicate when the patient is beginning to defervesce in response to effective antibiotic therapy.

Other information to document are the data from a full physical assessment conducted twice daily as long as the patient remains febrile and neutropenic. Subtle physical changes may be identified that help to pinpoint the source of infection and perhaps alter therapy.

The documentation of temperature and physical assessment provides the basis for evaluation of infection resolution. It is assumed that once both fever and neutropenia have resolved, the patient is recovered from infection. It is usually not necessary to have patients record daily temperatures at home. However, it is vital that the patient and family recognize the signs of infection and period of risk and report them immediately to the healthcare team.

Educational Tools and Resources

A variety of teaching aids have been developed to meet the standard for protective mechanisms established by the Oncology Nursing Society.[79] All teaching should focus on providing the patient and family with knowledge to prevent and manage problems related to alterations in protective mechanisms. The criteria are that the client and family will:

1. List measures to prevent infection
2. Identify signs and symptoms of infection
3. Contact appropriate health team member when initial signs and symptoms of infection occur
4. State measures to manage infection

The National Cancer Institute publishes a free booklet, *Understanding Chemotherapy*, that provides useful guidance for patients on avoiding and treating infection. Many pharmaceutical companies that manufacture antibiotics and hematopoietic growth factors also provide patient education material.

However, many health professionals develop their own materials that reflect the specific practice of their institution. Any such materials should include specific instructions related to managing the environment, diet, activity, and personal hygiene.[48,49,80] Appendix 18A, Self-Care Guide: Infection, and Appendix 18B, Self-Care Guide: Herpes and Varicella, are two patient guides you may use. A small card the patient may post on the refrigerator may serve as a useful reminder of the signs of infection to report (Appendix 18C).

Most institutions, clinics, and offices that provide care for patients with cancer adopt a set of guidelines or a protocol for neutropenic patients. The components of the protocol should also specify interventions for the prevention and management of infection. Table 18-5 provides one such clinical guide for the nurse.

Conclusion

Infection persists as a problem for patients with cancer. The etiology of infection is multifactorial, with variables related to both the malignancy and the treatment. The degree of toxicity of the infection is influenced by the type of pathogen and the host susceptibility. Multiple strategies are used to prevent and treat infection, including patient/family teaching, antibiotic therapy, and the use of HGFs. Newer treatment strategies focus on providing as much care in the home or outpatient areas as possible. However, the emphasis remains on teaching patients/families to minimize the risk of infection.

TABLE 18-5 Nursing Clinical Guide

- Policy: The nurse or physician will initiate neutropenic precautions when the absolute neutrophil count drops below 1000/mm³.
- Purpose: To prevent or decrease the incidence of infection in persons with low white blood cell counts.

Precaution	Principle
Strict handwashing by all persons before and after contact with patient.	Decrease amount of bacteria transported to patient.
Provide additional instruction regarding personal hygiene.	Aids in preventing self-infection. Increases person's participation in care.
Instruct person in preventive oral care.	Decrease oral colonization.
Modify diet to avoid uncooked fruits and vegetables.	Minimize bacterial colonization.
Eliminate fresh flowers, live plants, and sources of stagnant water from environment.	Minimize bacterial colonization.
Patient wears a mask when out of room or in home environment.	Decrease amount of exposure to respiratory organisms.
Instruct patient in preventive pulmonary hygiene.	Promote ventilation and decrease respiratory colonization.
Visitors should be limited and patients should avoid anyone with signs of infection.	Protect patient from potentially life-threatening infections.
Nothing per rectum (including suppositories, thermometers, enemas). Initiate bowel regimen with daily stool softeners to avoid constipation.	Prevent fissure and infection.
Vital signs q4h and complete assessment q12h for hospitalized patient.	To detect fever and early signs of pending septic shock.

References

1. Freifeld AG, Walsh TJ, Pizzo PA: Infections in the cancer patient, in DeVita VT, Hellman S, Rosenberg SA (eds): *Cancer: Principles and Practice of Oncology* (ed 5). Philadelphia: Lippincott, 1997, pp. 2659–2704

2. Hughes WT, Bodey GP, Feld R, et al: Guidelines for the use of antimicrobial agents in neutropenic patients with unexplained fever. *J Infec Dis* 161:381–396, 1990

3. Sugar AM: Empiric treatment of fungal infections in the neutropenic host: Review of literature and guidelines for use. *Arch Intern Med* 150:2258–2264, 1990

4. Osoba D: Lessons learned from measuring health-related quality of life in oncology. *J Clin Oncol* 12:608–616, 1994

5. Gleeson S: Reimbursement of biotherapy: Present status, future directions—Perspectives of the third-party payer. *Semin Oncol Nurs* 8(suppl):13–16, 1992

6. Glaspy JA, Bleecker G, Crawford J, et al: The impact of therapy with filgrastim (recombinant granulocyte colony-stimulating factor) on the healthcare costs associated with cancer chemotherapy. *Eur J Cancer* 29A(suppl):S23–S30, 1993

7. McCabe MS: Reimbursement of biotherapy: Present status, future directions—Perspectives of the hospital-based oncology nurse. *Semin Oncol Nurs* 8(suppl):3–7, 1992

8. Xistris D: Reimbursement of biotherapy: Present status, future directions—Perspectives of the office-based oncology nurse. *Semin Oncol Nurs* 8(suppl):8–12, 1992

9. Cella DF: Quality of life as an outcome of cancer treatment, in Groenwald SL, Frogge MH, Goodman M, Yarbro CH (eds): *Cancer Nursing: Principles and Practice* (ed 4). Sudbury: Jones and Bartlett, 1997, pp. 210–213

10. Schimpff SC: Infections in patients with cancer: Overview and epidemiology, in Moosa AR, Schimpff SC, Robson MC (eds): *Comprehensive Textbook of Oncology* (ed 2). Philadelphia: Williams & Wilkins, 1992, pp. 1720–1732

11. Robinson BE, Donowitz GR: Infections in patients with cancer: Host defenses and the immune-compromised state, in Moosa AR, Schimpff SC, Robson MC (eds): *Comprehensive Textbook of Oncology* (ed 2). Philadelphia: Williams & Wilkins, 1992, pp. 1733–1739

12. Wujcik D: Infection control in oncology patients. *Nurs Clin North Am* 28:639–650, 1993

13. Finkbiner KL, Ernst TF: Drug therapy management of the febrile neutropenic cancer patient. *Cancer Pract* 1:295–304, 1993

14. Wilkes GM, Ingwersen K, Burke MB: *1997–1998 Oncology Nursing Drug Handbook*. Sudbury: Jones and Bartlett, 1997

15. Lee JW, Pizzo PA: Management of the cancer patient with fever and prolonged neutropenia. *Hematol Oncol Clin North Am* 7:937–961, 1993

16. Wade JC, Schimpff SA: Epidemiology and prevention of infection in the compromised host, in Rubin RH, Young LS (eds): *Clinical Approach to Infection in the Compromised Host* (ed 3). New York: Plenum, 1994, pp. 5–40

17. Carter LW: Bacterial translocation: Nursing implications in the care of patients with neutropenia. *Oncol Nurs Forum* 21:857–865, 1994

18. McDonald A: Altered protective mechanisms, in Hassey-Dow K, Hilderley LJ (eds.): *Nursing Care in Radiation Oncology*. Philadelphia: Saunders, 1992, pp. 96–125

19. Groeger JS, Lucas AB, Cort D: Venous access in the cancer patient. *Princ Pract Oncol Update* 5:1–14, 1991

20. Goodman J, Riley MB: Chemotherapy: Principles of administration, in Groenwald SL, Frogge JH, Goodman M, Yarbro CH (eds): *Cancer Nursing Principles and Practice* (ed 4). Sudbury: Jones and Bartlett, 1997, pp. 317–384

21. Eagan JA, Blevins A, Armstrong D: Prevention of skin colonization and subsequent bacteremia with CDC-JK organisms in patients with cancer. *Cancer Pract* 1:325–328, 1993

22. Rubin RH, Ferraro MJ: Understanding and diagnosing infectious complications in the immunocompromised host. *Hematol Oncol Clin North Am* 7:795–812, 1993

23. deLalla F: Antibiotic treatment of febrile episodes in neutropenic patients: Clinical and economic considerations. *Drugs* 53:789–804, 1997

24. Freifeld AG: The antimicrobial armamentarium. *Hematol Oncol Clin North Am* 7:813–839, 1993

25. Buchanan GR: Approach to treatment of the febrile cancer patient with low risk neutropenia. *Hematol Oncol Clin North Am* 7:919–933, 1993

26. Meunier F: Infections in patients with acute leukemia and lymphoma, in Mandell D, Bennett JE, Dolin B (eds): *Principles and Practice of Infectious Diseases* (ed 4). New York: Churchill Livingstone, 1995, pp. 2675–2686

27. Pizzo PA: Management of fever in patients with cancer and treatment induced neutropenia. *N Engl J Med* 328:1323–1332, 1993

28. Rubin M, Walsh TH, Pizzo PA: Clinical approach to infections in the compromised host, in Hoffman R, Benz EJ, Shattil SJ, et al (eds): *Hematology: Basic Principles and Practice*. New York: Churchill Livingstone, 1991, pp. 1063–1114

29. Wade JC: Management of infection in patients with acute leukemia. *Hematol Oncol Clin North Am* 7:293–315, 1993

30. Pizzo PA, Robichaud KJ, Wesley R, et al: Fever in the pediatric and young adult patient with cancer: A prospective study of 1001 episodes. *Medicine* (Baltimore) 61:153–165, 1982

31. Pizzo PA: Combating infections in neutropenic patients. *Hosp Pract* 22:93–110, 1989

32. Zaia JA: Viral infections associated with bone marrow transplantation. *Hematol Oncol Clin North Am* 4:601–623, 1990

33. Viscoli C, Castagnola E, Machetti M: Antifungal treatment in patients with cancer. *J Intern Med* 740:89–94, 1997

34. Henschel L: Fever patterns in the neutropenic patient. *Cancer Nurse* 8:301–305, 1985

35. Camp-Sorell D: Chemotherapy: Toxicity management, in Groenwald SL, Frogge JH, Goodman M, Yarbro CH (eds): *Cancer Nursing Principles and Practice* (ed 4). Sudbury: Jones and Bartlett, 1997, pp. 385–425

36. Berger AM, Kilroy TJ: Oral complications of cancer therapy, in DeVita VT, Hellman S, Rosenberg SA (eds): *Cancer: Principles and Practice of Oncology* (ed 5). Philadelphia: Lippincott, 1997, pp. 2714–2725

37. Glenn J, Cotton D, Wesley R, et al: Anorectal infections in patients with malignant diseases. *Rev Infect Dis* 10:42–52, 1988

38. Feusner J, Cohen R, O'Leary M, et al: Use of routine chest radiography in the evaluation of fever in neutropenic pediatric oncology patients. *J Clin Oncol* 11:1699–1702, 1988

39. deKleijn EM, Oyen WJ, Corstens FH, et al: Utility of indium-111 labeled polyclonal immunoglobulin G scintigraphy in fever of unknown origin. The Netherlands FUO Imaging Group. *J Nucl Med* 38:484–489, 1997

40. Elliott TSJ, Faroqui MH, Harmstron RF, et al: Guidelines for good practice in central venous catheterization. *J Hosp Infect* 28:163–176, 1994

41. Smith LH, VanGulick AJ: Management of neutropenic enterocolitis in the patient with cancer. *Oncol Nurs Forum* 19:1337–1342, 1992

42. Griffin TC, Buchanan GR: Hematologic predictors of bone marrow recovery in neutropenic patients hospitalized for fever: Implications for discontinuation of antibiotics and early discharge from the hospital. *J Pediatr* 121:28–33, 1992

43. Mullen CA, Buchanan GR: Early hospital discharge of children with cancer treated for fever and neutropenia: Identification and management of the low-risk patient. *J Clin Oncol* 8:1998–2004, 1990

44. Talcott JA, Siegel RD, Finberg R, et al: Risk assessment in cancer patients with fever and neutropenia: A prospective two-center validation of a prediction rule. *J Clin Oncol* 10:316–322, 1992

45. Wacker P, Halperin DS, Wyss M, et al: Early hospital discharge of children with fever and neutropenia: A prospective study. *J Pediatr Hematol Oncol* 19:208–211, 1997

46. Rubenstein EB, Rolston K, Benjamin RS: Outpatient treatment of febrile episodes in low-risk neutropenic patients with cancer. *Cancer* 71:3640–3646, 1993

47. Talcott JA, Finberg R, Mayer RJ, et al: The medical course of cancer patients with fever and neutropenia: Clinical identification of a low-risk subgroup at presentation. *Arch Intern Med* 148:2561–2568, 1988

48. Brandt B: Nursing protocol for the patient with neutropenia. *Oncol Nurs Forum* 17(suppl):9–15, 1990

49. Ellerhorst-Ryan JM: Infection, in Groenwald SL, Frogge JH, Goodman M, Yarbro CH (eds): *Cancer Nursing Principles and Practice* (ed 4). Sudbury: Jones and Bartlett, 1997, pp. 585–603

50. DePauw BE: Practical modalities for prevention of fungal infections in cancer patients. *Eur J Clin Microbiol Infect Dis* 16:32–41, 1997

51. Hooper DC, Wolfson JC: Fluoroquinolone antimicrobial agents. *N Engl J Med* 324:384–394, 1991

52. Kotilainen P, Nikoskelainen J, Huovinen P: Emergence of ciprofloxacin-resistant coagulase-negative staphylococcal skin flora in immunocompromised patients receiving ciprofloxacin. *J Infect Dis* 161:41–44, 1990

53. Oppenheim BA, Harley JW, Lee W, et al: Outbreak of coagulase-negative staphylococcus highly resistant to ciprofloxacin in a leukaemia unit. *BMJ* 299:294–297, 1989

54. Wujcik D: Overview of colony-stimulating factors: Focus on the neutrophil, in Carroll-Johnson R (ed): *A Case Management Approach to Patients Receiving G-CSF*. Pittsburgh: Oncology Nursing Society, 1992, pp. 8–11

55. Brugger W, Clause JF, Lindemann A, et al: Role of hematopoietic growth factor combinations in experimental and clinical oncology. *Semin Oncol* 19:8–15, 1992

56. Crawford J, Ozer H, Stoller R, et al: Reduction by granulocyte colony-stimulating factor of fever and neutropenia induced by chemotherapy in patients with small-cell lung cancer. *N Engl J Med* 325:164–170, 1991

57. Roilides E, Lyman CA, Mertins SD, et al: Ex vivo effects of macrophage colony-stimulating factor on human monocyte activity against fungal and bacterial pathogens. *Cytokine* 8:42–48, 1996

58. Ohno R, Miyawaki S, Hatake K, et al: Human urinary macrophage colony-stimulating factor reduces the incidence and duration of febrile neutropenia and shortens the period required to finish three courses of intensive consolidation therapy in acute myeloid leukemia: A double-blind controlled study. *J Clin Oncol* 15:2954–2965, 1997

59. Maruhashi T, Takahashi T, Yakushiji M, et al: Clinical usefulness of macrophage colony-stimulating factor (M-CSF) after chemotherapy for ovarian cancer: A well controlled randomized study. *Proc Am Soc Clin Oncol* 16:123, 1997 (abstract)

60. Roilides E, Uhlig K, Pizzo PA, et al: Neutrophil oxidative burst in response blastoconidia and psuedohyphae of *Candida albicans*: Augmentation by granulocyte-colony-stimulating factor and interferon-γ. *J Infect Dis* 166:668–673, 1992

61. Veltri S, Smith JW: Interleukin 1 trials in cancer patients: A review of the toxicity, antitumor and hematopoietic effects. *Stem Cells* 14:164–176, 1996

62. Allan JD: Antibiotic combinations. *Med Clin North Am* 71: 1079–1091, 1987

63. Link D: Antibiotic therapy in the cancer patient: Focus on third-generation cephalosporins. *Oncol Nurs Forum* 14: 35–41, 1987

64. Sanders JW, Powe NR, Moore RD: Ceftazidime monotherapy for empiric treatment of febrile neutropenic patients: A metaanalysis. *J Infect Dis* 164:907–916, 1991

65. Armstrong D: Empiric therapy for the immunocompromised host. *Rev Infect Dis* 13(suppl):S763–S769, 1991

66. Calandra G, Lydick E, Carrigan J, et al: Factors predisposing to seizures in seriously ill infected patients receiving antibiotics: Experiences with imipenem/cilastatin. *Am J Med* 84: 911–918, 1988

67. Bodey DP: Tropical and systemic antifungal agents. *Med Clin North Am* 72:637–659, 1988

68. Riley DK, Pavia AT, Beatty PG, et al: The prophylactic use of low-dose amphotericin B in bone marrow transplant patients. *Am J Med* 97:509–514, 1994

69. Gotzsche PC, Johansen HK: Meta-analysis of prophylactic or empirical antifungal treatment versus placebo or no treatment in patient with cancer complicated by neutropenia. *BMJ* 314:1238–1244, 1997

70. Hiemenz JE, Walsh RJ: Lipid formulations of amphotericin B: Progress and future directions. *Clin Infect Dis* 22:133–144, 1996

71. Goodman JL, Winston DJ, Greenfield RA, et al: A controlled trial of fluconazole to prevent fungal infections in patients undergoing bone marrow transplantation. *N Engl J Med* 326: 845–851, 1992

72. Slavin MA, Osborne B, Adams R, et al: Efficacy and safety of fluconazole prophylaxis for fungal infections after marrow transplantation—a prospective, randomized double-blind study. *J Infect Dis* 171:1545–1552, 1995

73. Chou S: Newer methods for diagnosis of cytomegalovirus infections. *Rev Infect Dis* 12(suppl):S727–S736, 1990

74. Cole N, Balfour H: In vitro susceptibility of cytomegalovirus isolates from immunocompromised patients to acyclovir and ganciclovir. *Diagn Microbiol Infect Dis* 6:255–261, 1987

75. Glauser MP, Heumann D, Baumgartner JD, et al: Pathogenesis and potential strategies for prevention and treatment of septic shock. *Clin Infect Dis* 18(suppl 2):S205–S216, 1994

76. DePauw BE, Raemaekers JM, Schattenberg T, et al: Empirical and subsequent use of antibacterial agents in the febrile neutropenic patient. *J Intern Med* 740:69–77, 1997

77. Thijs LF, deBoer JP, deGroot MC, et al: Coagulation disorders in septic shock. *Intensive Care Med* 19(suppl 1):S8–S15, 1993

78. Rice V: The stages of shock. *Crit Care Nurse* 11:74–82, 1989

79. *Standards of Oncology Nursing Practice.* Kansas City, MO: American Nurses' Association and Oncology Nursing Society, 1987

80. Carter LW: Influences of nutrition and stress on people at risk for neutropenia: Nursing implications. *Oncol Nurs Forum* 20:1241–1250, 1993

Infection

Patient Name: _____

Symptom and Description   Infection is a problem of cancer treatment that can be lessened and treated. You may be at risk for infection due to cancer or from the side effects of treatment. If signs of infection are ignored, you can become very ill.

The body has many ways to protect you from infections. Skin, acid in the stomach, and coughing are some ways that the body protects itself. White blood cells destroy germs after they enter the body. Neutrophils are the special white blood cells that fight infection. When the number of neutrophils is lowered, you are said to be "neutropenic" and very prone to infections. Even mild infections such as cold sores can cause life-threatening illness.

Some persons, such as those with leukemia or lymphoma, are at risk for infection because the cancer has affected the body's own defenses. Others are at risk when treatment (either chemotherapy or radiation therapy) has affected the making of white blood cells, which fight infections. If you are neutropenic for only a few days, the risk of infection is small. If the neutropenia lasts for a week or longer, the risk of infection is very high.

Learning Needs   There are some important points that you need to learn about infection. You need to learn the following:

- What to do to decrease your chance of infection
- The signs and symptoms of infection
- When infection is most likely to occur
- How to manage infection if it does occur

Your doctor will tell you when you are getting treatment that may cause your white blood count to be lowered. You may go to the office or have a nurse come to your home to have blood drawn for testing during the time when your blood count is expected to be low. Take your temperature any time you feel hot *or* chilled. If your temperature is above 38.5°C or 101.3°F, call your doctor or nurse immediately.

Prevention   Infection cannot be completely prevented. However, there are many things you can do decrease the risk of infection.

- Avoid large crowds or anyone with signs of infection.
- Keep your body very clean by bathing daily and washing hands after using the bathroom.
- Keep your mouth very clean by brushing your teeth twice daily and flossing once daily. Your doctor or nurse may suggest that you rinse your mouth with a special cleansing solution as well.
- Avoid uncooked fruits and vegetables.
- Avoid constipation and straining to have a bowel movement by using a medication that softens the stool. Drink 2 quarts of fluid a day. Do not use laxatives or enemas unless approved by your doctor.

- Remove fresh flowers and live plants from the rooms where you stay.
- Do not change cat litter or clean up excreta from animals yourself; have someone else do it.

Management   Infection is usually marked by a temperature greater than 38.5°C or 101.3°F. Symptoms of infection are as follows:

- Fever
- Cough with or without sputum production (spitting)
- Burning on urination
- Pain at the site of an intravenous catheter or tunneled catheter
- Sore mouth
- Any area with redness or swelling

Your doctor will decide the best way to treat your infection. If your temperature is less than 100.4°F, your doctor may order oral antibiotics. You should take your temperature every 4 hours while awake and inform your doctor of any increases in temperature. You may take acetaminophen (Tylenol) to control the fever, and you should drink plenty of fluids.

Your doctor may tell you to come to the office or hospital for a complete exam. This usually includes blood tests, chest x-ray films, and other tests such as urine or sputum. If you are admitted to the hospital, antibiotics will be given by vein. You should continue the same actions to decrease infection that you were doing at home.

Follow-up   If you have fever or any of the signs of infection, call your doctor or nurse immediately. Be prepared to tell them the following facts:

- Last treatment
- Highest temperature in the last 24 hours
- Any chills
- Any symptoms of infection

Phone Numbers   Listed below are people to contact if you develop infection at home or if you have questions. If you call after normal working hours, a message service will respond and contact the physician on call.

Physician: _____ Phone: _____

Primary Nurse: _____ Phone: _____

Home Health Nurse: _____ Phone: _____

Other: _____ Phone: _____

Comments

Patient to call if: _____

_____

Next appointment: _____

Patient's Signature: _____ Date: _____

Nurse's Signature: _____ Date: _____

Source: Wujcik D: Infection, in Yarbro CH, Frogge MH, Goodman M (eds): *Cancer Symptom Management* (ed 2). Sudbury: Jones and Bartlett, 1999. © Jones and Bartlett Publishers.

Herpes and Varicella

Patient Name: _____

Symptom and Description   Herpes and varicella are viruses that often cause infections in patients who are getting treatment for cancer. Herpes appears as fever blisters and varicella is seen as chickenpox or shingles.

Most of us have been exposed to these viruses at some time in our lives. When our immune systems are normal, the viruses are simply "in our system" and do not cause any problems. During treatment for leukemia or lymphoma and bone marrow transplants or other organ transplants, the normal functions of the immune system are damaged. During this time, the viruses can become active ("reactivated") and can cause fever blisters, shingles, or more serious problems such as lung infections.

Often, these viruses will become active in the patient without any symptoms that can be seen. They may cause fever, a flulike symptom, or pain and redness at the site(s) where they are starting. Herpes occurs around the mouth or the genitals. Shingles appears along a nerve track and so seems to be following a line on the skin. Tear-shaped blisters may form at the sites of redness. If blisters occur, they will dry and become crusty within 10 days after the start of treatment.

Learning Needs   Your doctor will tell you if you are likely to have an infection with a herpes or varicella virus. You should inform your doctor or nurse if any of these occur:

- Temperature greater than 38.5°C or 101.3°F
- Pain or redness of the skin or mucous membranes of the mouth or genitalia or in a line anywhere on the body
- You are around anyone who has fever blisters, chickenpox, or shingles
- You are around anyone who has been exposed to someone with the active virus

Prevention   If you have ever had fever blisters, shingles, or chickenpox, please inform your healthcare team. Also, you may have blood samples taken at the start of your treatment to see if you have been exposed to these viruses in the past.

Herpes and varicella are catching during the first stages, until the blisters become crusty. Since your immune system is not working well, the most likely way the virus spreads to you is from visitors or members of the healthcare team. You should avoid:

- Anyone with a cold sore, chickenpox, or shingles
- Children who have not had chickenpox and are in day care or grade school. They can often be exposed to the virus without knowing it.

Management   The diagnosis of herpes or varicella is made by what the blister looks like and by taking a test or "culture."

The goals of treatment are to relieve symptoms and to control the growth of the virus. Acyclovir is the medicine used most often for treatment. Acyclovir can be given as a pill or through the vein, or put on the blisters as a cream. It is important to take the medicine just the way the doctor has written the prescription.

Follow-up   As the immune function improves, the infection slowly heals. At this time, it is said to be "dormant" or at rest and should no longer cause any problems.

Phone Numbers   Listed below are people to contact if you develop infection at home or if you have questions. If you call after normal working hours, a message service will respond and contact the physician on call.

Physician: _____ Phone: _____

Primary Nurse: _____ Phone: _____

Home Health Nurse: _____ Phone: _____

Other: _____ Phone: _____

Comments

Patient to call if: _____

_____

Next appointment: _____

Patient's Signature: _____ Date: _____

Nurse's Signature: _____ Date: _____

Source: Wujcik D: Infection, in Yarbro CH, Frogge MH, Goodman M (eds): *Cancer Symptom Management* (ed 2). Sudbury: Jones and Bartlett, 1999. © Jones and Bartlett Publishers.

Patient Reminder Card

You are most at risk for infection _____ through _____.
Call immediately if you have:

- Temperature greater than 100.4°F
- Chills
- Any other signs of infection (cough, increase in sputum, burning with urination, pain or soreness around any wound, or mouth sores).

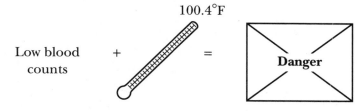

Patient Name: _____

If fever occurs, call: _____

Source: Wujcik D: Infection, in Yarbro CH, Frogge MH, Goodman M (eds): *Cancer Symptom Management* (ed 2). Sudbury: Jones and Bartlett, 1999. © Jones and Bartlett Publishers.

CHAPTER 19

Mucositis

Susan L. Beck, PhD, AOCN, APRN

The Problem of Mucositis in Cancer

The mucous membranes serve as an important protective mechanism. These soft, smooth, and moist layers of epithelial cells and connective tissue line body passages and cavities that have direct or indirect contact with the external environment. The intact mucosal membranes of the GI, genitourinary, and respiratory tracts serve for protection, support, nutrient absorption, and secretion of mucus, enzymes, and salts.

The mucosal lining is self-renewing. Stem cells, which form a basement membrane, replicate and differentiate to form the various cells of the epithelial surface. These cells live for about 3 to 5 days, resulting in a turnover of the outer epithelial lining every 7 to 14 days.[1] This pattern of cellular proliferation makes the mucosa extremely vulnerable to sources of irritation, trauma, or cellular damage, such as that caused by the cytotoxic effects of cancer treatment. The result is *mucositis,* a general term referring to an inflammation of the mucosa.

Incidence in Cancer

Oral mucositis, sometimes called stomatitis, is one of the most common and troublesome forms of mucositis in individuals with cancer. This inflammatory and ulcerative response of the oral mucosa results from the physiologic effects of multiple stressors, including cancer and its treatment. Forty percent of all people newly diagnosed with cancer will develop oral complications related to the disease or its treatment; the most common of these complications is mucositis.[2]

The oral mucosa, the moist and continuous lining of the mouth, serves an important protective function. This epithelial membrane is an integral component of the body's first-line defense against the environment. The mucosa joins the skin and the lining of the digestive tract to form a complete barrier to external organisms. Alterations in the integrity of the mucosal lining provide an entryway for microorganisms, causing localized infection that has the potential to spread via the bloodstream. Thus the oral cavity may serve as a portal of entry for life-threatening systemic infections.[2] This likelihood increases in individuals with a compromised immune status due to cancer treatment. In such individuals, the ability to fight infection is limited by a decreased neutrophil count resulting from the cytotoxic effects of cancer treatment on the stem cells of the bone marrow. Thus, normal endogenous flora of the mouth, including gram-positive and gram-negative bacteria, fungi, and viruses, can infect areas of disrupted mucosal integrity. Localized infections can easily be transmitted into the bloodstream via the rich capillary beds that perfuse the mucosa; septicemia results. In fact, studies have related septicemia to oral infections in up to 54% of neutropenic individuals.[3] In one institution, an upward trend in gram-positive bacteremia was significantly related to an increase in oral mucositis.[4]

Impact on Quality of Life

The oral mucosa also receives and transmits tactile stimuli, a function that gives the mouth an important role in sensation and nutrition. Mucositis may alter the taste receptors, causing unpleasant taste sensations, known as *dysgeusia,* or absent taste sensation, termed *ageusia.*

Oral pain almost always accompanies oral mucositis. Pain results from the denuding of the epithelium lining, ulceration, and edema. Neurotransmitters released as part of the inflammatory response stimulate the vast bed of nociceptive fibers in the mucosa. The resulting oral pain makes it difficult to eat, talk, and swallow.

Manifestations and outcomes of oral mucositis include ulceration, xerostomia or a dry mouth, ageusia, pain, infection, bleeding, and an altered nutritional status. General approaches to these symptoms are discussed in detail in other chapters. Mucositis is not a simple phenomenon—it can be viewed as one component of a fairly intricate symptom complex. As additional symptoms develop, the intensity and duration of the mucositis are enhanced. The negative impact of mucositis on the individual's comfort, ability to eat and communicate, and generalized well-being can significantly diminish quality of life.

Etiology and Pathophysiology

Risk Factors

Oral mucositis is a significant and common problem in individuals with cancer. The etiology of mucositis is related either to the cancer itself or to the direct and indirect effects of cancer treatments. These primary causes are enhanced in some individuals by the existence of a variety of factors that increase the risk for oral complications (Table 19-1).[5]

Cancer

The oral mucosa can be disrupted by a variety of disease entities. For example, oral tumors disrupt the integrity of the mucosa and often become inflamed and infected.[5] Squamous cell carcinomas are the most predominant type, accounting for 90% of oral cancers.[6] Most oral carcinomas are diagnosed in the advanced stages and often present as ulcerated and necrotic masses. In individuals with leukemia, sloughing of the mucosa can result from infarction due to capillary infiltration with malignant cells. Individuals with acquired immunodeficiency syndrome (AIDS) frequently develop oral lesions due to Kaposi's sarcoma or non-Hodgkin's lymphoma, two common neoplasms in this population.[7]

Oral cancers account for less than 5% of all tumors;

the more common causes of oral mucositis are treatments for cancer, including chemotherapy, radiation therapy, and bone marrow transplantation.

Chemotherapy

Chemotherapy is believed to have a direct and indirect stomatotoxic effect. The direct effect on the oral mucosa occurs at the cellular level. The process of constant epithelial renewal renders the mucosa very vulnerable to the effects of antineoplastic agents.[8] Many of these drugs cause destruction of cells that are actively reproducing, by interfering with DNA, RNA, or protein synthesis. Areas that have a high rate of proliferation, such as the stem cells of the oral mucosa, are particularly sensitive to the direct cytotoxic effects of antineoplastic agents. Reduced production, decreased differentiation, and accelerated detachment of epithelial cells result and lead to a denuding of the mucosa.[9] Once the continuity of the epithelial lining is disrupted, a painful and debilitating mucositis results from a sequence of tissue destruction, inflammation, and infection.[10]

The indirect effect of chemotherapeutic drugs is believed to occur as the bone marrow function is suppressed during the nadir of treatment. The nadir is the time at which the platelet and granulocyte counts are lowest due to the cytotoxic effect of the drugs on the precursor cells of the bone marrow. The individual is immunosuppressed and extremely susceptible to infection during this time. Research indicates that an increased stomatotoxicity is associated with the decrease in granulocyte counts that occurs during the nadir. Indirect stomatotoxicity is thus believed to be mediated through a suppressed immune response.[10]

Not all chemotherapeutic drugs cause mucositis, and it is thus important to identify the specific drugs included in the treatment regimen (Table 19-2). The drugs with the highest stomatotoxic potential include the antimetabolites, certain DNA-interactive agents especially the antitumor antibiotics, and tubulin interactive agents.[11]

The mucositis caused by chemotherapy can be profound (Fig. 19-1). The pattern of mucositis varies both by drug regimen and individual. Inflammation resulting from direct stomatotoxicity can first occur anywhere from 2 to 14 days from the time of drug administration. Intensity and duration vary not only by the types of drugs but also by dosage and frequency of administration. The intensity of mucositis increases with higher dosages of cytotoxic drugs; even drugs that are not usually stomatotoxic (e.g., cyclophosphamide) can cause cellular damage to the mucosa at high doses. The duration of mucositis may be prolonged with frequent administration, as there is no time for cellular recovery and healing.

Most individuals receive a combination of drugs, and there has been little research to describe systematically the patterns of response for varying protocols. As previously described, the inflammatory response causes de-

TABLE 19-1   Factors That Increase Risk for Oral Mucositis in Individuals with Cancer

Risk Factor	Mechanism of Action	Prevention Strategies
Age		
Children	• Increased prevalence not well understood but may be due to immature immune response, increased cellular proliferation, and higher prevalence of hematologic malignancies	• Careful and frequent oral hygiene
Elderly	• Degenerative changes: decreased salivary flow, diminished keratinization of mucosa, and increased prevalence of gingivitis	• Careful and frequent oral hygiene • Adequate hydration • Mouth moisturizers • Avoid trauma • Dental treatment of gingivitis
Exposure to alcohol and tobacco	• Chronic irritation of mucosa	• Avoid or limit alcoholic beverages and tobacco products, especially during treatment
Poor oral hygiene	• Increased debris breads infection • Lack of stimulation to enhance circulation	• Careful and frequent oral hygiene, including brushing tongue and gums
Oxygen therapy	• Moisture drawn from mucosa into oxygen causing a drying of mucosal lining	• Humidify oxygen • Mouth moisturizers • Adequate hydration
Oral or nasogastric suctioning	• Catheter and suctioning process cause traumatic breaks in mucosal integrity	• Minimize suctioning frequency and duration
Changes in breathing patterns	• Tachypnea and mouth breathing dry the mucosa	• Careful and frequent oral hygiene • Room humidifier
Certain drugs		
Anticholinergics and antihistamines	• Decrease salivary flow	• Careful and frequent oral hygiene
Phenytoin	• Gingival hyperplasia	• Avoid these drugs if possible
Steroids	• Fungal overgrowth	
Ill-fitting dentures	• Movement irritates mucosa and breaks integrity	• Reline dentures • Remove dentures at night and use only for eating until healing occurs
Hot, acidic, or spicy foods	• Thermal and chemical irritants inflame and traumatize mucosa	• Bland, soft foods • Avoid acidic, peppery, and spicy foods • Let hot food cool before eating
Poor nutritional status	• Refined sugars increase dental decay • Protein/calorie malnutrition delays healing • Vitamin deficiencies cause oral complications	• Minimize refined sugars • Well-balanced daily diet including fruits, vegetables, grains, and sources of protein • Daily vitamin supplement
Dehydration	• Dryness and cracking result when fluid is drawn from mucosa and lips as a protective mechanism	• Daily fluid intake of at least 2000 mL

creased taste, pain, and difficulty swallowing. The response usually becomes intensified as the individual enters the nadir of treatment. Ulceration, severe inflammation, infection, and bleeding develop due to the loss of mucosal integrity, cellular destruction, neutropenia, and thrombocytopenia. The timing and duration of the nadir vary by drug protocol, and combination therapy often results in prolonged periods of immunosuppression as the nadir of one drug overlaps with another.

Radiation therapy

Radiation therapy is a localized treatment for cancer. Mucositis results from radiation delivered to the head and neck region if the mouth or salivary glands are included in the treatment field. An inflammatory response develops as a result of destruction of the mucosal or glandular cells and is influenced by the depth of penetration, total gray delivered, and the number and frequency

TABLE 19-2 Chemotherapeutic Agents with a High Potential to Cause Stomatitis

Antimetabolites

cytarabine
5-Fluorouracil
Floxuridine
Hydroxyurea
6-Mercaptopurine
Methotrexate
6-Thioguanine

DNA-Interactive Agents

Actinomycin D
Amgacrine
Bleomycin sulfate
Daunomycin
Doxorubicin
Etoposide
Idarubicin
Mithramycin
Mitomycin C
Mitoxantrone
Procarbazine hydrochloride

Tubulin-Interactive Agents

Docetaxel
Paclitaxel
Vinblastine sulfate
Vincristine sulfate

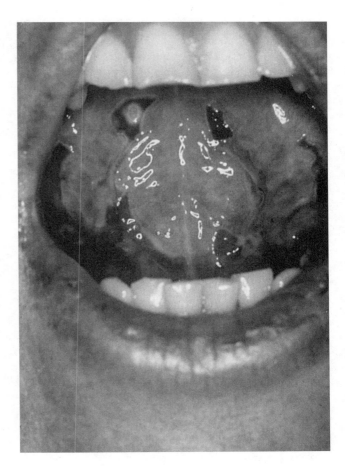

FIGURE 19-1 Chemotherapy-related mucositis.

of treatments.[12] The onset, intensity, and duration of mucositis vary with the individual but most often start in the second week of therapy or after a dose of about 2000 cGy. The mucosa in the treatment field is initially red and swollen. As treatment continues, the mucosa becomes denuded, ulcerated, and covered with an exudate.[8] Pain and burning are common and are aggravated by irritants such as acidic or spicy food. Mucositis persists for several weeks after the treatments are completed. Secondary infections, especially candidiasis, often occur and prolong the duration of mucositis.

Mucositis may be complicated by the dramatic decline in salivary production when all major salivary glands are irradiated. Decreased salivary flow, *xerostomia*, is rapid in onset and usually develops during the first week of treatment. Xerostomia can be progressive and irreversible with nearly a 95% decline in salivary production at 3 years after treatment.[13] Persistent xerostomia becomes a hazardous side effect as dental caries become rampant without adequate and aggressive oral hygiene and caries prevention.

Radiation therapy for oral cancer also causes loss of taste by damaging the microvilli and outer surface of the taste cells. The onset is rapid and progressive with ageusia or mouth blindness occurring after 3000 cGy. Taste acuity usually improves within 2 to 4 months of treatment; however, some individuals experience a permanent decrease in taste perception.

Bone marrow transplant therapy

Up to 70% of individuals receiving a bone marrow transplant develop oral complications due to the aggressive and synergistic nature of the purging pretransplant therapies.[14] Prior to transplantation, high dose antineoplastic drug regimens and total body irradiation are used in an attempt to destroy all cancer cells and induce aplasia of the bone marrow. White patchy areas, erythema, atrophy, and increased vascularity begin a few days following initiation of treatment and progressively intensify during the posttransplant period. Most ulcerations occur in nonkeratinized areas, including the tongue, buccal, and labial mucosa.[14] Immunosuppressive therapy after the transplant and the development of graft-versus-host disease (GVHD) prolong and enhance oral complications. Bacterial, fungal, and viral infections are common. Xerostomia develops as a result of the irradiation and is present throughout the posttransplant period. Pain is associated with the mucositis and peaks about 2 weeks posttransplant, when the oral cavity is usually infected and ulcerated.

In chronic GVHD, the mucosa becomes chronically irritated, mottled, and friable. There are intermittent episodes of acute inflammation often associated with bacterial, fungal, and viral infections. Xerostomia persists and the risk of caries is high.

Multimodal therapy

For most individuals with cancer, the causes of mucositis are multifactorial. Modern cancer therapy is multimodal—treatments are combined to produce the greatest cytotoxic effect. Unfortunately, this extends to normal cells, including those of the mucosa. Profound effects on the oral mucosa result. Cancer and its multiple treatments interact with risk factors present in individuals with cancer (see Table 19-1). The result is exemplified in the challenging care of an individual with an invasive oral tumor who has a history of alcohol abuse, smokes, has poor oral hygiene, and is receiving oxygen therapy. Multimodal cancer therapy, consisting of extensive surgery and a combination of radiation and chemotherapy, traumatizes the mucosa.[15] The sequelae of xerostomia, ulceration, pain, and inability to eat enhance a vicious and enduring cycle of intense inflammation and infection.

Assessment

A thorough and systematic assessment of the mouth should be a part of the comprehensive assessment of all individuals with cancer. Systematic assessment requires the proper equipment and technique (Figure 19-2).

The normal, healthy oral mucosa is pink, moist, clean, and intact. Alterations can include:

- changes in color such as pallor, erythema of varying degrees, white patches (Figure 19-3), or discolored lesions or ulcers (Figure 19-4)

- changes in moisture reflected in altered texture and shininess, an increased or decreased amount of saliva, and changes in the quality and tenacity of secretions

- changes in cleanliness represented by accumulations of debris and coating, bad odors, and changes in color of the teeth

- changes in integrity, including cracks, fissures, ulcers, blisters, or lesions that may be isolated, clustered, patchy, confluent, or generalized

- changes in perception including decreased or absent taste; hoarseness or a decrease in audible voice tone and strength; difficulty swallowing, which may be a harbinger of esophagitis; and pain, burning, or stinging

---

ORAL ASSESSMENT

1. Gather equipment
   - good source of light
   - nonsterile gloves
   - gauze
   - tongue blade
   - dental mirror (optional)
2. Wash hands.
3. Apply nonsterile gloves.
4. Remove all dental appliances. Inquire regarding the fit of dentures and any sore or painful areas.
5. Inquire regarding any changes in voice, taste, ability to eat or swallow, and comfort.
6. Systematically perform each of the following, using directed light to observe for moisture, color, integrity, and cleanliness:
   a. Observe the outer lips.
   b. Pull down lower lip and raise upper lip to observe the teeth and mucosal lining of the outer vestibule. (Note: Check teeth for color, shine, debris, and caries.)
   c. Instruct the person to open the mouth so you can observe the hard and soft palates.
   d. Use a finger to displace and examine the mucosa of the inner cheeks.
   e. Note the amount and quality of the saliva. (Note: Normal saliva is thin and watery.)
   f. Examine the top of the tongue. Then ask the person to curl the tongue up to the roof of the mouth so you can observe the underside of the tongue.
   g. Use the gauze to displace the tongue to each side to observe the lateral sides of the tongue.
   h. Ask the person to take a deep breath so you can observe the oropharynx, posterior tongue, and uvula. If this technique does not allow adequate visualization, use the tongue blade to gently depress the tongue and use the dental mirror for improved visualization.
7. Based on the results of this assessment, score each category on the assessment tool.

FIGURE 19-2 Clinical guide: performing an oral assessment.

The nurse should try to describe accurately the quality of the changes. The result of the assessment should be a specific list of nursing diagnoses or collaborative problems that are connected to a potential etiology. Table 19-3 contains a sample progress note that might result from such an assessment.

The results of this physical assessment should then be evaluated within the context of a comprehensive assessment, including a screening for the risk factors identified in Table 19-1. The plan of care should be guided by actual or potential problems.

An assessment guide such as the Guide to Physical Assessment of the Oral Cavity (Table 19-4) provides a tool to quantify the intensity of mucositis as well as to assess oral cleanliness and moisture. Nurses can repeat-

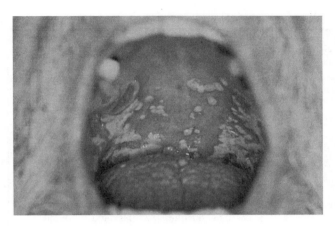

FIGURE 19-3 Oral assessment: oral candidiasis.

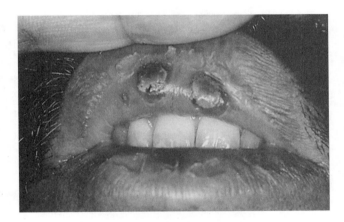

FIGURE 19-4 Oral assessment: oral lesions of herpes simplex.

TABLE 19-3 Progress Note Documenting Oral Assessment

Subjective:	Patient complains of dry lips and mouth and pain on the left side of tongue. Pain began 2 days ago and has gotten progressively worse. Pain intensity is currently 4 on a 0–10 scale. Drinking orange juice makes mouth burn. States that "nothing tastes right." Defines change in voice quality or strength.
Objective:	44-year-old white female who is 5 days postchemotherapy with 5-FU. Alert and cooperative with exam. Lips are pink, wrinkled, with a fissure on the right side. Buccal mucosa is pale, dry, and intact. Teeth shiny with minimal debris. Saliva is scanty and increased in viscosity. Tongue red and swollen with raised papillae; ulcer (0.5 cm diameter) on left lateral tongue with a purplish halo and yellow exudate. Oropharynx pink, moist, and intact. Oral exam score = 12 (moderate dysfunction).
Assessment:	Moderate mucositis and dysgeusia related to chemotherapy Pain secondary to mucositis Mild xerostomia secondary to mucositis

edly use such a tool to document patterns and evaluate changes that might occur as a result of cancer treatment or interventions. The numerical score and verbal descriptors (e.g., moderate) can be used to describe the intensity of the oral dysfunction.

Diagnostic Evaluation

The extent of diagnostic evaluation is dependent on the potential impact of the mucositis. In immunocompetent individuals, empiric therapy with a careful evaluation of improvement is the first-line approach. In the immunocompromised individual, a culture is critical for an accurate diagnosis, as neutropenia may prevent the usual presentation of inflammation in even the most common infections. Fungal and herpetic infections in particular may not present in the classical manner and can easily be missed.[16] A culture is the only precise way to diagnose the presence of infection and identify the causative organism. A culture of the oral cavity is indicated when there is a break in mucosal integrity such as a lesion, vesicle, or ulcer; in the presence of a moderate, generalized mucositis (score 11 to 15 in Table 19-4); or in the presence of an exudate.

Alterations in vital signs, such as an elevated temperature and increased heart rate, and laboratory findings (e.g., an abnormal CBC with differential) can also aid in the diagnosis of infection. In a normal individual, infection may be indicated by a shift in the differential manifested by an increased number and percentage of immature granulocytes. In an immunocompromised patient, this trend may not be evident due to the low number of white blood cells. Severe neutropenia (absolute neutrophil count <500/mm³) indicates an extremely high risk of infection. In this individual, localized oral lesions can evolve into systemic and life-threatening sepsis.

Degrees of Toxicity

Within cancer clinical trials, there are established criteria to monitor degrees of toxicity.[17] Such grading criteria are only a gross indicator of the degree of toxicity and have been criticized for the inconsistency of variables for each level. Oral assessment guides yield a numerical score that can be translated into an intensity score for mild, moderate, and severe oral dysfunction (see Table 19-4). Such scores can be graphed to evaluate patterns of mucositis over time.

TABLE 19-4 A Guide to Physical Assessment of the Oral Cavity: Numerical and Descriptive Ratings

Category	Rating	1	2	3	4
Lips	1 2 3 4	Smooth, pink, moist, and intact	Slightly wrinkled and dry; one or more isolated reddened areas	Dry and somewhat swollen; may have one or two isolated blisters; inflammatory line or demarcation	Very dry and edematous; entire lip inflamed; generalized blisters or ulceration
Gingiva and Oral Mucosa	1 2 3 4	Smooth, pink, moist, and intact	Pale and slightly dry; one or two isolated lesions, blisters, or reddened areas	Dry and somewhat swollen; generalized redness; more than two isolated lesions, blisters, or reddened areas	Very dry and edematous; entire mucosa very red and inflamed; multiple confluent ulcers
Tongue	1 2 3 4	Smooth, pink, moist, and intact	Slightly dry; one or two isolated reddened areas; papillae prominent, particularly at base	Dry and somewhat swollen; generalized redness but tip and papillae are redder; one or two isolated lesions or blisters	Very dry and edematous; thick and engorged; entire tongue very inflamed; tip very red and demarcated with coating; multiple blisters or ulcers
Teeth	1 2 3 4	Clean; no debris	Minimal debris; mostly between teeth	Moderate debris clinging to one-half of visible enamel	Teeth covered with debris
Saliva	1 2 3 4	Thin, watery, plentiful	Increase in amount	Saliva scanty and may be somewhat thicker than normal	Saliva thick and ropy, viscid or mucid
ORAL DYSFUNCTION SCORE		No Dysfunction: 5	Mild dysfunction: 6–10	Moderate dysfunction: 11–15	Severe dysfunction: 16–20
TOTAL _____					

Source: From Beck SL, Yasko, JM: *Guidelines for Oral Care* (ed 2). Crystal Lake, IL. Sage, 1993. Reprinted with permission.

Symptom Management

There are many approaches to managing mucositis, and no single agent has been shown to be more efficacious. It is not surprising that the management of mucositis varies by institution.[18] The clinician should customize care to each individual based on a dual focus—actual and potential problems—identified by the assessment and the goals of care. Specific guidelines for preventing and managing problems related to oral mucositis are thus presented in relation to five potential problems and goals (Figure 19-5). This presentation differs from guidelines based on the intensity of mucositis and is intended to facilitate designing a plan of care to meet the individual's unique response to cancer and cancer treatment.

Oral Hygiene

Effective oral hygiene can best be achieved by brushing, rinsing, flossing, and moisturizing. Brushing requires the use of a narrow, soft-bristle nylon brush and effective technique in which short, horizontal, or circular strokes are applied with gentle pressure to the junction of the gums and teeth.[19] The biting surfaces are scrubbed with longer strokes; the tongue is gently brushed to stimulate circulation and remove debris. The American Dental Association recommends a fluoridated toothpaste to prevent dental caries. Toothpastes of sodium bicarbonate are effective cleansing agents, aid in dissolving mucus, and reduce the acidity that results from inflammation.

Flossing enhances the cleansing process by removing debris between the teeth. Waxed or unwaxed floss is wrapped around the fingers, held tightly, and gently forced up and down the surfaces between the teeth from the gum line to the top of each tooth.

Recommended rinsing agents include water, saline, salt and soda, and half-strength hydrogen peroxide.[5] Commercial mouthwashes contain high percentages of alcohol that can irritate and dry the mucosa[20] and should be avoided. Water and saline are neutral, nonirritating solutions that provide a mechanical rinsing. Salt and soda, a mixture of water, salt, and sodium bicarbonate, have the added benefit of decreasing acidity and have been shown to be as effective as half-strength hydrogen peroxide.[21]

PROBLEM: MUCOSITIS, potential or actual

GOAL: TO MAINTAIN CLEANLINESS AND PREVENT INFECTION

GOAL: TO MAINTAIN INTEGRITY AND PROMOTE HEALING OF THE MUCOSA

- Brush the teeth with a soft-bristle nylon brush and a fluoridated sodium bicarbonate dentifrice within 30 minutes after eating and at bedtime. Brushing before meals can help stimulate the appetite.
- Clean and massage the tongue and oral mucosa with a soft-bristle brush and sodium bicarbonate dentifrice after brushing or removing dentures. A sponge-tipped applicator can be used to clean the teeth and the tongue if brushing causes discomfort or bleeding.
- Rinse the mouth with one ounce of saline, salt and soda, tap water or 1.5% hydrogen peroxide for 1 to 2 minutes. If saline or peroxide is used, rinse with water to enhance mechanical cleansing and minimize aftertaste.
- Remove and brush dentures within 30 minutes after eating and at bedtime, then soak dentures in 1.5% hydrogen peroxide for several minutes.
- Floss the teeth once daily after brushing. Omit flossing if it causes pain, if the platelet count is less than 40,000/mm³, or if the leukocyte count is less than 1500/mm³.
- Use special precautions to prevent aspiration in the person with a compromised gag reflex.
- Eat a high-protein diet with vitamin supplements.
- Apply agents to protect the mucosa and promote healing, such as substrates of antacids or sucralfate.
- Maintain optimal fluid and nutritional intake while avoiding foods that are irritating.
- Consult with the physician and nutritionist regarding the need for enteral or parenteral nutrition.

PROBLEM: XEROSTOMIA, potential or actual

GOAL: TO MOISTURIZE THE ORAL CAVITY

- Apply a moisturizer (e.g., petroleum jelly) frequently to lips and mucosa. Use a water soluble lubricant (e.g., K-Y Jelly or Mouth-Moisturizer) on the inside of the mouth if the person is using oxygen or if there is a danger of aspiration.
- Drink 3000 mL of fluid per day unless contraindicated.
- Apply a synthetic saliva spray, solution, or swab frequently.
- Use sugarless gum or candy to stimulate salivary flow.
- Check with physician regarding need for epilocarpinol
- Use a room humidifier.
- If xerostomia is prolonged, institute caries prophylaxis with daily fluoride/chlorhexidine.

NOTE: Do not use lemon and glycerine swabs, as they are drying and irritating.

PROBLEM: PAIN RELATED TO MUCOSITIS

GOAL: TO PROMOTE COMFORT AND MINIMIZE PAIN

- Use topical anesthetics such as benzocaine or diclonine before eating and as needed to control pain.
- Avoid irritants (e.g., alcohol and tobacco)
- Use analgesics to control pain: 1.5 hours before meals; at regular intervals around-the-clock if pain is constant.
- Avoid thermally, mechanically, or chemically irritating foods.

PROBLEM: INFECTION RELATED TO MUCOSITIS

GOAL: TO MANAGE INFECTION

- Monitor the patient's temperature every 4 hours and report any elevation over 38°C.
- Use local or systemic antibiotics, antifungals, and antiviral agents as prescribed.

NOTE: It is critical to perform an oral culture to identify the causative organism in immunosuppressed individuals.

PROBLEM: BLEEDING SECONDARY TO MUCOSITIS

GOAL: TO CONTROL BLEEDING

- Monitor vital signs every 4 hours.
- Assess platelet function from a complete blood count (CBC).
- Inspect mucosa and report any bleeding.
- Rinse mouth with ice water and/or apply pressure to an area of uncontrolled bleeding using a piece of gauze dipped in ice water or a wet tea bag that has been frozen.
- Consult with the physician regarding the need for thrombin or aminocaproic acid (use with caution in persons with thrombocytopenia, as disseminated intravascular coagulation may result).

FIGURE 19-5 Clinical guidelines to prevent and manage oral mucositis. (Data from Beck SL, Yasko JM: *Guidelines for Oral Care* [ed 2]. Crystal Lake, IL: Sage, 1993.[5])

Multiple studies have supported the use of hydrogen peroxide,[22,23] which is not only mechanically cleansing but chemically therapeutic. Salivary peroxidase liberates oxygen from the peroxide, causing a bubbling reaction that loosens mucus and debris. Hydrogen peroxide also exerts an antimicrobial effect. Yet the use of peroxide has been the focus of some controversy due to concern regarding its safety.[24] Harmful effects of 1.5% hydrogen peroxide in individuals with mucositis have not been substantiated. Further research to evaluate the safety and efficacy of peroxide is needed.

Chlorhexidine may be beneficial if the goal is to prevent infection. Chlorhexidine acts against numerous bacteria and fungi. The commercially available preparation in the U.S. contains 9.6% alcohol and causes stinging and burning. Another important side effect of chlorhexidine is a brown discoloration of the teeth; these stains are removable with oxidizing agents and abrasives. The findings of research related to chlorhexidine are inconsistent.[25,26] Although chlorhexidine may reduce potential pathogens, its effectiveness in reducing mucositis has not been clearly supported.[25–28]

Fluoride acts to decrease demineralization and increase remineralization of dental lesions. The value of daily fluoride rinses in healthy adults is controversial; however, a daily application of topical fluoride is essential in persons at high risk of developing dental caries due to irradiation of the salivary glands. Chlorhexidine rinses may augment the protective effects of fluoride in these high-risk patients.[29]

The moisture of the oral mucosa can be enhanced in several ways. Adequate hydration through frequent fluid intake is essential. Sucking or chewing on sugarless candy or gum stimulates salivary flow. Moisturizers such as cocoa butter, petroleum jelly, lipstick balms, or water-based lubricants should be applied to the lips frequently, especially at night. Research supports the effectiveness of synthetic saliva products.[30] Sprays, solutions, and swabs containing artificial saliva are neutral agents that emulate the viscosity and mineral content of saliva. Their effect is short-lived, and frequent application is needed. Pilocarpine, a sialagogue, acts by directly stimulating cells of the salivary glands. As a result of clinical trials, this cholinergic drug has now been approved for use in managing xerostomia due to radiation.[31,32]

Protective Interventions

Interventions aimed at protecting the cells of the mucosa can also be used for prevention and management of mucositis. One approach is the use of cryotherapy, sucking on ice chips for 5 minutes prior and 25 minutes following bolus administration of fluorouracil. The intent is to minimize the cytotoxic effects of the fluorouracil on the mucosa by decreasing circulation during peak blood levels. Several clinical trials supported the effectiveness

of this intervention.[33–35] Although the risk seems low, additional research is warranted.

Another intervention is the topical application of substrates of antacids or a suspension of sucralfate, a basic aluminum salt used to treat gastric ulcers. Sucralfate is believed to act by forming a protective coating over damaged surface proteins of the mucosa. It may also increase local production of prostaglandin E2, yielding increased blood flow, and production of mucus.[36] Case study reports have supported its use in individuals with mucositis. In a randomized clinical trial in children, sucralfate was associated with a nonsignificant decrease in the incidence of mucositis. Pain was significantly less in the sucralfate group.[37] Subsequent research supports the analgesic effects of sucralfate, but the findings related to its effectiveness in decreasing mucositis are conflicting.[38–41]

The use of hematologic growth factors has become a standard approach to the care of patients receiving chemotherapy that has a high potential to cause bone marrow suppression. At this time, most evidence does not support the use of growth factors to prevent mucositis.[12]

Numerous other approaches to protecting the mucosa are currently under investigation. Interventions of interest include topical vitamins, prostaglandins, oral bandages, and topical allopurinol.

Management of Complications of Mucositis

The common complications associated with mucositis include pain, infection, and bleeding. Management of each of these problems can be local or systemic in nature.

Topical anesthetics (e.g., 20% benzocaine, viscous lidocaine) and mixtures containing such anesthetics (e.g., Orabase) produce a temporary reduction in pain. The numbness that results also decreases taste and thermal perception. Oral capsaicin in the form of candy to manage oral pain is currently under investigation.[42] Oral bandages (e.g., Orahesive) and gels that congeal to form an occlusive covering (e.g., Zilactin and Oratect) provide significant pain relief lasting up to 6 hours.[43] Systemic approaches to the management of the acute and persistent pain associated with mucositis include scheduled around-the-clock analgesics. For moderate mucositis, combinations of opioid/nonopioid drugs such as acetaminophen with codeine are recommended. When pain is unrelieved or mucositis is severe, sustained-release oral doses or continuous intravenous infusions of morphine may be required until heating occurs.

Infections of the oral cavity can be bacterial, fungal, or viral in origin, and the antibiotic should be selected based on the causative organism. Antibiotics can be applied topically in ointments (e.g., bacitracin or acyclovir), swishes or pastilles (e.g., nystatin), or troches (e.g., clotrimazole). Sensitive, systemic antibiotics may also be indicated, especially in the immunocompromised individual.

The prophylactic use of the antiviral agent acyclovir is recommended in individuals who are seropositive to the herpes simplex virus and at high risk for immunosuppression, such as prior to a bone marrow transplant.[44] The use of prophylactic antifungal agents has also been reported in this population.

The risk for bleeding secondary to mucositis is especially high in the individual with a low platelet count ($<50,000/mm^3$). Local control of bleeding can be achieved by applying pressure with an icy, soaked gauze or ice water irrigations. Hemostasis results from vasoconstriction. Topical thrombin or aminocaproic acid syrup can be used to promote clotting.[45] Systemic therapy is limited to platelet transfusions.

As the intensity of mucositis increases, it is increasingly likely that more of these interventions will need to be included in the plan of care. Additionally, the frequency of intervention should increase in relation to intensity. Omission of care for even a few hours can negate previous therapeutic efforts. If mucositis is mild, oral hygiene is recommended every 2 to 4 hours. As the intensity increases, hourly care may be indicated. It is especially important to continue oral care during the night in order to sustain progress made during the day.

Dental Management

Professional dental care including examination, x-rays, cleaning, plaque removal, and application of topical fluoride is recommended at least yearly. A dental examination and prophylaxis prior to the initiation of cancer treatment can decrease the possibility of oral complications and improve the likelihood that patients will tolerate optimal doses of treatment. Treatment of caries and periodontal disease and extraction of problem-prone teeth are essential before cancer treatment such as chemotherapy or radiation to the head and neck begins. Once therapy begins, neutropenia and thrombocytopenia are contraindications to dental manipulation. Once radiation therapy is complete and acute oral side effects have diminished, a dentist should follow the patient every 4 to 8 weeks for the first 6 months.[46]

Patient Education

Patient education should acknowledge the importance of oral health and hygiene and identify the possible causes of oral dysfunction. A Self-Care Guide to help the person with cancer maintain a healthy mouth is provided in Appendix 19A. With the onset of mucositis, the approaches that are preventive in nature must be expanded to include interventions to maintain integrity and promote healing, promote comfort, manage infection, and control bleeding. Appendix 19B provides a Self-Care Guide to manage mucositis and related problems.

Evaluation

Evaluation of care results from ongoing assessment of the individual's response to treatment. The consistent use of a numerical assessment guide provides a definitive way to monitor response. Progress toward meeting the goals of care should also be monitored and documented.

Conclusion

Oral mucositis is a significant and complex symptom in the individual with cancer. A systematic approach to oral assessment will facilitate early detection and ongoing evaluation of oral complications. Cultures are indicated in immunosuppressed individuals, as typical presentations of infection may not occur. Prevention and management require a comprehensive and customized plan of care that involves the individual and caregiver in maintaining oral hygiene and managing problems such as xerostomia, infection, bleeding, and pain.

References

1. Farbman AI: The oral cavity, in Weiss L (ed): *Cell and Tissue Biology: A Textbook of Histology* (ed 6). Baltimore: Urban & Schwarzenberg, 1988
2. Fox PC: Introduction, in *Consensus Development Conference on Oral Complications of Cancer Therapies: Diagnosis, Prevention, and Treatment.* National Cancer Institute (NCI) Monographs 9:1, 1990
3. Peterson DE, Schubert MM: Oral Toxicity, in Perry MC (ed): *The Chemotherapy Source Book* (ed 2), Williams and Wilkins, 1977 pp. 571–594
4. Gonzalez-Barca E, Fernandez-Sevilla A, Carratal J, et al: Prospective study of 288 episodes of bacteremia in neutropenic cancer patients in a single institution. *Eur J Clin Microbiol Infect Dis* 15:291–296, 1996
5. Beck SL, Yasko JM: *Guidelines for Oral Care* (ed 2). Crystal Lake, IL: Sage, 1993
6. Silverman S: *Oral Cancer* (ed 3). Atlanta: American Cancer Society, 1990
7. Cheung T, Siegal FP: AIDS-related cancer, in Murphy GP, Lawrence W, Lenhard RE (eds): *American Cancer Society Textbook of Clinical Oncology* (ed 2). Atlanta: American Cancer Society, 1995, pp. 619–634
8. Dreizen S: Description and incidence of oral complications. *Consensus Development Conference on Oral Complications of Cancer Therapies: Diagnosis, Prevention, and Treatment.* NCI Monographs 9:11–16, 1990
9. Squier CA: Mucosal alterations. *Consensus Development Conference on Oral Complications of Cancer Therapies: Diagnosis, Prevention, and Treatment.* NCI Monographs 9:169–172, 1990
10. Sonis S, Clark J: Prevention and management of oral mucositis induced by antineoplastic therapy. *Oncology* 5:11–18, 1991

11. Dorr RT, VonHoff DD: *Cancer Chemotherapy Handbook* (ed 2). Norwalk, CT: Appleton & Lange, 1994

12. Berger AM, Kilroy TJ: Oral complications of cancer therapy, in Berger AM, Portenoy RK, Weissman DE (eds): *Principles and Practice of Supportive Oncology.* Philadelphia: Lippincott-Raven, 1998, pp. 223–236

13. Dreizen S, Daly TE, Drane JB, et al: Oral complications of cancer radiotherapy. *Postgrad Med* 61:85–92, 1977

14. Woo SB, Sonis ST, Monopoli MM, et al: A longitudinal study of oral ulcerative mucositis in bone marrow transplant recipients. *Cancer* 72:1612–1617, 1993

15. Beck SL: Prevention and management of oral complications in the cancer patient, in Hubbard S, Greene T, Knobf T (eds): *Current Issues in Cancer Nursing Practice.* Philadelphia: Lippincott, 1990, pp. 27–38

16. Walsh TJ: Role of surveillance cultures in prevention and treatment of fungal infections, in *Consensus Development Conference on Oral Complications of Cancer Therapies: Diagnosis, Prevention, and Treatment.* NCI Monographs 9:43–48, 1990

17. *Toxicity Criteria.* San Antonio, TX: Southwest Oncology Group, 1994

18. Mueller BA, Millhern ET, Farrington EA, et al: Mucositis management practices for hospitalized patients: National survey results. *J Pain Symptom Manage* 10:510–520, 1995

19. *Oral Health Care Guidelines for Head and Neck Cancer Patients Receiving Chemotherapy.* Chicago: American Dental Association Council on Community Health, Hospital, Institutional and Medical Affairs, 1989

20. Madeya ML: Oral complications from cancer chemotherapy. Part II. Nursing implications for assessment and treatment. *Oncol Nurs Forum* 23:808–819, 1996

21. Wujcik D: Comparison of the effects of two cleansing agents on oral condition and infection rates on patients receiving chemotherapy. *Oncol Nurs Forum* 16(suppl):221, 1989 (abstract)

22. Beck S: Impact of a systematic oral care protocol on stomatitis after chemotherapy. *Cancer Nurs* 2:185–199, 1979

23. Dudjak LA: Mouth care for mucositis due to radiation therapy. *Cancer Nurs* 10:131–140, 1987

24. Tombes M, Gallucci B: The effects of hydrogen peroxide rinses on the normal mucosa. *Nurs Res* 42:332–337, 1993

25. Ferretti GA, Ash RC, Brown, et al: Control of oral mucositis and candidiasis in marrow transplantation: A prospective, double-blind trial of chlorhexidine digluconate oral rinse. *Bone Marrow Transplant* 3:483–493, 1988

26. Samarayanake LP, Robertson AG, MacFarlane TW, et al: The effect of chlorhexidine and benzydamine mouthwashes on mucositis induced by therapeutic irradiation. *Clin Radiol* 39:291–294, 1988

27. Epstein JB, Vickars L, Spinelli J, et al: Efficacy of chlorhexidine and nystatin rinses in prevention of oral complications in leukemia and bone marrow transplantation. *Oral Surg Oral Med Oral Pathol* 73:682–689, 1992

28. Dodd ML, Larson PJ, Dibble SL, et al: Randomized clinical trial of chlorhexidine vs placebo for prevention of oral mucositis in patients receiving chemotherapy. *Oncol Nurs Forum* 23:921–927, 1996

29. Fardal O, Turnball RS: A review of the literature on the use of chlorhexidine in dentistry. *J Am Dent Assoc* 112:863–867, 1986

30. Greenspan D: Management of salivary dysfunction, in *Consensus Development Conference on Oral Complications of Cancer Therapies: Diagnosis, Prevention, and Treatment.* NCI Monographs 9:159–161, 1990

31. Greenspan D, Daniels TE: Effectiveness of pilocarpine in postradiation xerostomia. *Cancer* 59:1123–1125, 1987

32. Johnson JT, Ferrette GA, Nethery J, et al: Oral pilocarpine for post-irradiation xerostomia. *N Engl J Med* 329:390–395, 1993

33. Mahood DJ, Dose AM, Loprinzi CL, Veeder MH, et al: Inhibition of fluorouracil-induced stomatitis by oral cryotherapy. *J Clin Oncol* 9:449–452, 1991

34. Rocke LK, Loprinze CL, Lee JK, et al: A randomized clinical trial of two different durations of oral cryotherapy for prevention of 5-fluorouracil-related stomatitis. *Cancer* 72:2234–2238, 1993

35. Cascinu S, Fideli A, Fidele SL, et al: Oral cooling (cryotherapy), an effective treatment for prevention of 5-fluorouracil-induced stomatitis. *Oral Oncol Eur J Cancer* 30:234–236, 1994

36. Ferraro JM, Mattern JQA II: Sucralfate suspension for stomatitis. *Drug Intell Clin Pharm* 18:153, 1984

37. Shenep JL, Kalwinsky DK, Hutson PR, et al: Efficacy of oral sucralfate suspension in prevention and treatment of chemotherapy-induced mucositis. *J Pediatr* 113:758–763, 1988

38. Pfeiffer P, Madsen EL, Hansen O, et al: Effect of prophylactic sucralfate suspension on stomatitis induced by cancer chemotherapy. A randomized, double-blind crossover study. *Acta Oncol* 29:171–173, 1990

39. Pfeiffer Hansen O, Madsen EL, et al: A prospective pilot study on the effect of sucralfate mouth-swishing in reducing stomatitis during radiotherapy of the oral cavity. *Acta Oncol* 29:471–473, 1990

40. Epstein JB, Wong FLW: The efficacy of sucralfate suspension in the prevention of oral mucositis due to radiation therapy. *Int J Radiat Oncol Biol Phys* 28:693–698, 1994

41. Barker G, Loftus L, Cuddy P, et al: The effects of sucralfate suspension and diphenhydramine syrup plus kaolin-pectin on radiotherapy-induced mucositis. *Oral Surg Oral Med Oral Pathol* 71:288–293, 1991

42. Berger AM, Henderson M, Nadoolman W, et al: Oral capsaicin provides temporary relief for oral mucositis pain secondary to chemotherapy/radiation therapy. *J Pain Symptom Manage* 10:243–248, 1995

43. Rodu B, Russell CM, Ray KL: Treatment of oral ulcers with hydroxypropylcellulose film. *Compendium* 9:420–422, 1988

44. Woo SB, Sonis ST, Sonis AL: The role of herpes simplex virus in the development of oral mucositis in bone marrow transplant recipients. *Cancer* 66:2375–2379, 1990

45. Yasko JM, Dudjak LA: *Biological Response Modifier Therapy: Symptom Management.* Baltimore: Park Row, 1990

46. National Institute of Dental and Craniofacial Research: Oral Complications of Cancer Treatment: What the Oncology Team Can Do. Bethesda, MD: National Institutes of Health (Jan. 1999)

A Healthy Mouth

Patient Name: _____

Symptom and Description　Your mouth has an important role to play in keeping you healthy. Cancer and cancer treatment can sometimes cause a sore mouth. There are things you can do now to keep your mouth healthy.

Learning Needs　You will need to learn:

- How to keep your mouth clean and moist
- What to avoid that may be irritating
- When to see the dentist

Prevention

How to keep your mouth clean and moist:

1. Brush your teeth within 30 minutes after eating and at bedtime.
   - Use a soft-bristle, narrow nylon toothbrush and a sodium bicarbonate (baking soda) toothpaste with fluoride added.
   - Dip the bristles in very warm water to make them softer.
   - Place the brush at a 45-degree angle to the junction of the gums and teeth.
   - Brush all of the outside surfaces of the teeth using short back and forth or circular strokes. Brush the inside surfaces using only the tip of the brush. Brush the chewing surfaces with a back and forth motion.
   - Gently brush your gums, tongue, and top of mouth.
2. If you wear dentures, remove and brush them as described above.
   - Soak them for several minutes in an effervescent denture cleanser (the kind that bubbles) or flavored 1.5% hydrogen peroxide.
   - Rinse well.
   - Do not wear dentures that do not fit well. Contact your dentist to have them adjusted or relined.
   - Do not wear your dentures at night.
3. Floss your teeth at least once daily after brushing.
   - Cut a piece of dental floss 18 inches long.
   - Wrap the ends loosely around your middle fingers, leaving a few inches of floss exposed between those fingers.
   - Guide the floss with the thumbs of both hands to clean the upper teeth and with the index (first) fingers to clean the lower teeth.
   - Gently force the floss between the teeth—from your gum line to the top of each tooth.
   - Floss both sides of each tooth using a gentle up-and-down motion.

4. Rinse your mouth after brushing and flossing.
   - Use tap water, salt solution (half teaspoon of salt in 8 ounces of water), a mouthwash containing less than 6% alcohol, or flavored 1.5% hydrogen peroxide (Peroxamint) or 1 part hydrogen peroxide to 3 parts water.
   - Use your cheeks to swish the solution all around your mouth for 1 to 2 minutes.
5. Keep your lips moist.
   - Use cocoa butter, petroleum jelly, lipstick balm or lipstick, or a water-based mouth moisturizer.
   - Apply plenty of moisturizer to your lips and mouth frequently.

What to avoid that may be irritating:

- Lemon and glycerine swabs
- Mouthwashes that contain more than 6% alcohol
- Foods and drinks that are hot, spicy, or acidic
- Smoking or chewing tobacco
- Excessive alcohol

When to see the dentist:

- Visit your dentist at least every year to have a check-up and teeth cleaning.
- Make an appointment to see your dentist before you start cancer treatment or for any tooth pain.

Management   Please see the Self-Care Guide to Mucositis: A Sore Mouth.

Follow-up   Report the following to your doctor or nurse:

- Redness
- Soreness or pain
- Cracks, ulcers, blisters, white patches
- Temperature greater than 101.3°F

Phone Numbers

Nurse: _____ Phone: _____

Physician: _____ Phone: _____

Other: _____ Phone: _____

Comments

Patient's Signature: _____ Date: _____

Nurse's Signature _____ Date: _____

Source: Beck SL: Mucositis, in Yarbro CH, Frogge MH, Goodman M (eds): *Cancer Symptom Management* (ed 2). Sudbury: Jones and Bartlett, 1999. © Jones and Bartlett Publishers.

Mucositis: A Sore Mouth

Patient Name: _____

Symptom and Description   Your mouth has an important role to play in keeping you healthy. Cancer and cancer treatment can sometimes cause mucositis, a sore mouth. There are things you can do to help your mouth heal and to make it feel better.

Learning Needs   You will need to learn:

- How to know if you have mucositis
- How to keep your mouth clean and moist
- What to avoid that may be irritating
- How to control bleeding, pain, and infection
- What to eat

Prevention   Please see the Self-Care Guide: A Healthy Mouth, to learn more about how you can keep your mouth healthy.

Management

1. Examine your mouth at least once daily and report changes.
   - Use a flashlight and look in your mouth by standing in front of a mirror.
   - Look for any ulcers, pimples, sores, red areas, or patches.
   - Report these changes and any mouth pain to your doctor or nurse.
2. Keep your mouth clean and moist.
   - Clean your teeth even though your mouth is sore. If it hurts to use a soft brush, use an oral swab, a cleaning stick with a soft sponge tip.
   - Hold the swab with the grooves at a 90-degree angle to the gum line so the sponge can reach in between the teeth.
   - Gently massage your gums, tongue, and top of your mouth.
   - Do not floss when your platelet count is low or if it causes pain or bleeding.
   - Keep your dentures in only during meals.
   - Rinse your mouth with salt solution (half teaspoon of salt in 8 ounces of water) or a 1.5% hydrogen peroxide solution (1 part hydrogen peroxide to 3 parts water, or flavored 1.5% hydrogen peroxide [Peroxamint]) every 2 hours for 1 to 2 minutes. If your mouth is very sore, rinse every hour. The peroxide will foam as it cleans your mouth. This should be followed by rinsing with water.
   - Keep your lips and the inside of your mouth coated with a water-based mouth moisturizer.
   - If your mouth is very dry, drink water and other fluids frequently throughout the day. Chew sugarless gum or suck on sugarless hard candy to moisten your

mouth. Use a cool mist humidifier at night while sleeping. Artificial saliva is also available; apply frequently.

3. Avoid irritating foods, alcohol, and tobacco.

- Do not chew tobacco or smoke cigarettes, cigars, or pipes.

- Do not drink alcoholic beverages (beer, wine, or liquor).

4. Work with your doctor and nurse to control pain, bleeding, and infection.

- Ask your doctor to prescribe a medication for your sore mouth.

- Before meals and as needed for comfort, apply an anesthetic (a numbing agent), such as benzocaine or (Xylocaine), to sore areas of your mouth, using an oral swab or cotton-tipped applicator. Benzocaine can also be swished around the entire mouth. This will numb your mouth and make eating easier. However, be careful that foods are not too hot, because your sense of feeling may be changed so that you could burn yourself without realizing it.

- Take a pain medicine 1.5 to 2 hours before meals. If your mouth is constantly hurting, take the medicine at regular times around the clock (for example, every 4 hours). Liquid acetaminophen can be swished around in the mouth and then swallowed. Avoid the use of aspirin products.

- If pain is not relieved, ask your doctor about something stronger. Acetaminophen (Tylenol) with or without codeine is usually helpful. If pain is severe, morphine may be needed until healing occurs.

- If bleeding occurs, apply pressure to the site of bleeding using a piece of clean gauze dipped in ice water or a wet tea bag that has been partially frozen (the tannin in the tea will help stop the bleeding). Rinsing your mouth with ice water may also be helpful.

- If you develop an infection in your mouth, antibiotics may be needed. Some are applied directly to the mouth; others are swallowed. Follow your doctor's instructions.

5. Eat well.

- Eat a well-balanced diet. Be sure to include foods that are high in protein (dairy products, poultry, meats, and fish).

- Take a vitamin/mineral supplement daily.

- If your mouth is sore, certain foods may burn and eating may become difficult. Eat frequently and in small amounts.

- Drink at least 3 quarts (liters) of fluid a day unless you are on a fluid restriction.

- Avoid any food that is hot, rough, or coarse; highly spiced or acidic; or any other food that bothers you.

Follow-up   Report the following to your doctor or nurse:

- Redness or extreme dryness

- Soreness or pain

- Cracks, ulcers, blisters, white patches

- Temperature greater than 100°F

- Bleeding from your mouth

- Difficulty swallowing

Phone Numbers

Nurse: _____ Phone: _____

Physician: _____ Phone: _____

Other: _____ Phone: _____

Comments

Patient's Signature: _____ Date: _____

Nurse's Signature: _____ Date: _____

Source: Beck SL: Mucositis, in Yarbro CH, Frogge MH, Goodman M (eds): *Cancer Symptom Management* (ed 2). Sudbury: Jones and Bartlett, 1999. © Jones and Bartlett Publishers.

CHAPTER 20

Neurological Disturbances

Gail M. Wilkes, RNC, MSN, ANP, AOCN

The Problem of Neurological Disturbances in Cancer

Cancer complications or treatment can result in neurological disturbances, and these may occur at any point along the disease continuum, depending on the type and anatomical location of the malignancy and treatment modality(s). Symptoms are variable, ranging from subtle anxiety to obvious expressive aphasia, with onset from acute to gradual and severity from insignificant to severely disabling. The specific symptom, however, is determined by the site of injury in the nervous system, whether central, peripheral, or in the spinal cord. Many neurological symptoms are profoundly disabling, both physically and psychologically, and may further threaten an individual made vulnerable by malignancy. Through expert knowledge and skill, the oncology nurse can help the patient and family successfully manage the many problems associated with neurological disturbances.

Incidence in Cancer

Approximately 20% of patients with cancer will develop a neurological complication during the course of their disease.[1] Most disturbances result from extension of the primary tumor or metastatic disease. Primary brain tumors affect 5 individuals per 100,000 in the United States.[2] Metastatic brain tumors affect approximately 24% of all patients with cancer. Patients with lung and breast cancers have the highest incidence of neurological complications, with 40% to 65% of patients with lung cancer affected. Others at increased risk are patients with melanoma, leukemia, lymphoma, neuroblastoma, and testicular, pancreatic, prostate, gastric, and renal cancers.[3]

Meningeal carcinomatosis affects approximately 5% of patients with cancer, most commonly patients with breast and lung cancers, and lymphoma, and spinal cord compression affects an equal number. Lung and breast cancers most commonly involve the cervical and thoracic spine, whereas prostate cancer and melanoma most commonly compress the lumbosacral spine. Patients with lymphoma, cancer of unknown primary origin, sarcoma, and renal cell carcinoma are also at risk for the development of spinal cord compression.

Treatment side effects may include peripheral neuropathy and cerebellar dysfunction, especially with chemotherapy agents such as paclitaxel, cisplatin, and high-dose cytosine arabinoside. As patients survive longer with effective multimodal treatment, the incidence of neurological disturbances may increase. Chemotherapy-induced neurological toxicity can be either direct or indirect, and efforts to prevent or reduce the toxicity will change the incidence.

Finally, complications of disease, such as hypercalcemia or paraneoplastic syndromes, or of treatment, such as sepsis and central nervous system (CNS) infection, can cause neurological disturbances.

Impact on Quality of Life

Few symptoms bring a greater threat to the individual than do those related to neurological disturbances. The abilities to think, talk, and be self-reliant are intrinsic to one's sense of achievement, dignity, and satisfaction with life. The complex human CNS represents the highest level of neurological evolution. The CNS creates the very essence of a human being, that which makes each person unique.

Young and Longman[4] define quality of life as the degree of satisfaction with present life circumstances as perceived by the individual. Human functioning, the ability to perform activities of daily living and to work, may be severely threatened by neurological disturbances. For some, the neurologic disturbance is the first evidence of malignancy. The person with a primary brain tumor may present with seizures, a change in mental status, progressive weakness, aphasia, or ataxia. In addition, some of the paraneoplastic neurological syndromes precede diagnosis and suggest to the physician that a malignancy must be considered. Thus, the individual is threatened not only by the physical disability but also by the diagnosis of a malignancy. Physical disability wrought by neurological disturbances can lead to distress by thwarting the very qualifies that are quintessentially human. Loss of motor function and coordination interferes with the ability to perform self-care tasks and leads to dependency, loss of role function, and often loss of self-esteem. Communication is critical to personal relationships, to work relationships, and in caring for one's self and others. Cognitive deficits such as aphasia and dysarthria can severely impair communication. Muscle weakness, ataxia, and changes in vision or hearing alter mobility and self-protection, placing the individual at risk for injury. Loss or diminished sense of proprioception, temperature, and vibration further increase risk for injury. These threats to the intactness of the individual bring suffering, and often patients will become irritable and depressed. This may lead to estranged patient-family relationships and difficult provider-patient relationships.

What greater challenge to the patient, family, and oncology nurse can be imagined than to manage the symptoms of neurologic disturbances related to cancer and to help the individual identify and achieve meaning and quality of life?

Etiology

It is estimated that approximately 70% of lesions causing neurological disturbances result from local or metastatic tumor with subsequent direct injury to the nervous system.[1] Symptoms of memory or perceptual deficits, or aphasia may result from primary or metastatic brain tumors.

Approximately 10% to 20% of neurological symptoms arise from treatment-related toxicity, whether from chemotherapy, radiation therapy, or biological response modifier therapy. Symptoms include painful and disabling paresthesias and cognitive deficits.

Spinal cord compression is a common metastatic complication and represents an oncologic emergency. Although not usually a life-threatening problem, spinal cord compression can severely compromise quality of life.

Symptoms arising from neurological disturbances are many and are influenced by the etiology as well as the anatomical location of the underlying neurologic disturbance. This chapter presents four common clinical neurologic syndromes rather than specific symptoms:

Section A: Spinal cord compression

Section B: Increased intracranial pressure

Section C: Peripheral neuropathy (including cranial nerve and autonomic neuropathies)

Section D: Cerebellar syndromes

The following section addresses principles of neurologic assessment, which provide a foundation for assessment of each of the subsequent syndromes presented.

Principles of Neurological Assessment

History

The history starts at the highest level of functioning and moves to the lowest, and moves from the general to the specific. An enumeration of general observations is shown in Table 20-1.

Types of impairments

Primary brain tumors and brain metastases can cause impairments in cerebral functioning according to the brain area injured.[2] Injury to the *frontal lobes* can result in personality changes, memory loss, impaired judgment, and emotional lability (prefrontal). Muscle weakness results from damage to the motor area and expressive aphasia from damage to Broca's area. Damage to the *parietal lobes* may lead to tactile agnosia (inability to recognize common objects through touch) and impaired cognition. Damage to the *occipital lobes* may lead to visual agnosia (inability to recognize common objects through sight) and visual hallucinations or disturbances. Damage to the *temporal lobes* may lead to auditory agnosia (Wernicke's area, dominant hemisphere: inability to recognize common sounds, e.g., ringing telephone), visual field

TABLE 20-1 Neurological Assessment: General Observations

Quality/Function	Questions to Ask
Appearance and behavior	Is the person well groomed or disheveled? Does the person appear anxious or depressed? What is the person's posture like? Has there been a change from baseline?
Mood, facial expression, attitude	Does the person appear angry, depressed? Is the behavior appropriate? Has the patient or family noted a change from baseline?
Flow of speech, thought processes and perceptions, thought content	What is the pace and spontaneity of speech? Has the patient experienced any delusions, hallucinations, new phobias?
Orientation	Is the person oriented to person, place, and time?
Level of consciousness	Is the person alert or somnolent? Is this a change?
Attention and concentration	Can the patient count backward from 100 subtracting serial 7s with few errors?
Memory (remote)	Can the patient recall birthplace, age, history of illness, current events in last 5 years?
Memory (recent)	Can the patient recall arrival at the hospital/office?
Memory: retention and immediate recall	Can the patient recall list of objects or dates when asked to repeat the list in 3 to 5 minutes?
Calculations	Can the person do simple multiplication or addition?
Vocabulary	Can the patient define words such as *orange, metaphor, flourish*?
Abstract reasoning	Can the patient explain a simple proverb?
Similarities	Can the patient describe how a cat and a mouse are alike?
Judgment	Can the patient provide a reasonable answer to a question such as "What would you do if there was a fire on your stove?"

changes, impaired memory, receptive or sensory aphasia when the dominant hemisphere is involved, and auditory perceptual disturbances, such as inability to hear music, when the nondominant hemisphere is involved.

Apraxia may be caused by lesions in the prefrontal lobes or at the convergence of all the lobes. Cortical motor integration is required in order to perform a skill, such that the person understands how to do the task and knows where the body parts are (e.g., pick up a brush, raise the brush to the head, and brush the hair). When the person cannot coordinate skilled movements yet is not paralyzed, apraxia is diagnosed.[2]

Aphasia refers to the inability to communicate, and *dysphasia* refers to difficulty communicating. *Expressive* aphasia means that the person is unable to express thoughts or wishes orally or in writing, and *receptive* aphasia means that the person cannot understand spoken or written words.

If increased intracranial pressure (ICP) is present, a change in the level of consciousness may be the first subtle sign of neurologic disturbance. Often it is a family member who first brings this to the nurse's attention, so it is important to ask the family about changes.

Physical Exam

The nurse may or may not be involved in performing the physical exam. However, the steps of the neurological exam are presented so that the nurse is aware of the procedures involved.

Cranial nerve assessment

The cranial nerves (CNs) arise from the brain: the olfactory nerve (CN-I) from the cerebrum, and the others

from the brain stem. A protocol for examination of the cranial nerves is shown in Table 20-2. Figure 20-1 illustrates a technique for evaluating extraocular movements (cranial nerves III, IV, and VI).

Increased ICP will cause abnormalities in CN-II (decreased vision, visual field defects), CN-III through CN-V (diplopia, abnormal extraocular movements, nystagmus, unequal pupil size or light response, ptosis, difficulty chewing), and CN-VII (changes in facial sensation, weakness, or paralysis).

Some chemotherapeutic agents can damage cranial nerves (e.g., cisplatin may cause ototoxicity) and others may damage sense organs (e.g., busulfan may cause

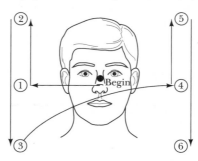

1. Ask the patient to visually follow your finger as you move it through the six cardinal gazes.
2. Draw an "H" shape in the air with your finger, moving slowly as you change direction.
3. Pause during upward and lateral gazes to identify nystagmus.

4. Normally, eyes should be conjugate (move together in the same direction). An individual may have slight nystagmus (fine, rhythmic oscillation) normally with extreme lateral gaze.

FIGURE 20-1 Testing extraocular movements (EOM).

TABLE 20-2 Physical Examination of the Cranial Nerves

Cranial Nerve	Test
CN-I: Olfactory	• This is tested by recognition of a common odor, such as coffee or cinnamon, with the eyes closed. Each nostril is tested separately.
CN-II: Optic	• To test for visual acuity, ask the patient to hold a newspaper 15–18 inches away, close one eye, and read a few sentences. Repeat with the other eye, then with both eyes open. For more accuracy, use a Snellen eye chart from 20 feet away or a hand-held chart that is comparable. • To test for peripheral vision, face the person so that your eyes are at the same level. Have the person cover the right eye while you cover your left eye, and have the person stare into your eye; then, extend your right arm out to the side and down ("5 o'clock"), point your finger, and slowly raise it into the field of vision. Ask the person to let you know when your finger is seen. Repeat with your arm extended straight out to the side ("3 o'clock") and up toward the ceiling ("1 o'clock"). Now, ask the person to cover the other eye while you do the same, and repeat your arm movements with the left arm. • The last part of the exam is done using the ophthalmoscope, which will not be discussed here.
CN-III: Oculomotor CN-IV: Trochlear CN-VI: Abducens	• These three cranial nerves are evaluated together by testing the muscle movements that rotate the eyeball. Ask the person to keep the head in one position facing you. Hold your forefinger about 12–18 inches from the person's eyes, and ask the person to follow with eyes only as you move your finger through the six cardinal gazes (see Figure 20-1). When the person's eyes have followed as far as possible, stop, hold your finger, and observe for nystagmus. Throughout, you must observe both eyes to see if they move together; disconjugate gaze suggests dysfunction in the extraocular muscles. • Observe the pupils for ptosis (CN-III controls the muscles elevating the eyelid) and for equal size and shape. • Finally, observe for pupillary light responses. Darken the room if possible. For direct response, cover one of the person's eyes and shine a penlight into the pupil in the other eye. The pupil should constrict. Repeat with the other eye. For consensual light reflex, ask the person to keep both eyes open. Shine the penlight into the right pupil from the side, and observe the left pupil constricting (both pupils should constrict); repeat in the other pupil.
CN-V: Trigeminal	• To test the motor strength of the temporal and masseter muscles, which are innervated by this nerve, place your fingers on the person's temples and ask the person to clench the teeth; then repeat with your fingers on the person's jaws. • To test the sensory tract, ask the person to close the eyes, and gently touch the skin on the forehead, cheek, and jaw bilaterally with a wisp of cotton.
CN-VII: Facial	• This nerve innervates taste buds (not usually tested) and facial muscles, which are tested for motor strength. Ask the person to frown, puff out the cheeks, smile showing the teeth, and tightly close the eyes and resist as you try to gently open the person's eyes.
CN-VIII: Vestibulocochlear (Acoustic)	• The nerve has two branches, one for hearing (cochlear) and the other for balance (vestibular). Hearing is tested by standing about 2 feet behind the person and lightly whispering a two-digit number, then asking the person to repeat it. A ticking watch can also be used and brought from a distance to just outside the ear. Ask the person to let you know when the ticking is heard. • Weber's and Rinne's tests, which help to assess lateralization and bone versus air conduction, and the use of the otoscope will not be discussed.
CN-IX: Glossopharyngeal CN-X: Vagus	• Both these nerves help regulate gag and palatal reflexes. To test motor strength, place your hand on the person's throat and ask the person to swallow. • To test the gag reflex, gently touch the back of the person's throat with a tongue depressor.
CN-XI: Spinal Accessory	• This nerve innervates the sternocleidomastoid and trapezius muscles. Test for motor strength by placing your hands on the person's right cheek and asking the person to turn the cheek against your hand as you resist. Repeat on the other cheek. Then, place your hands on the person's shoulders, and ask the person to shrug the shoulders up against the resistance of your hands.
CN-XII: Hypoglossal	• This nerve innervates the tongue. To test, ask the person to stick out the tongue, and note whether it moves in the midline and whether there is any involuntary movement or atrophy. Also note whether the uvula is midline or deviated.

cataracts). Damage to CN-VII may result in loss of hearing, tinnitus, nystagmus, and vertigo; damage to CN-IX may result in altered taste or dysphagia. Injury to CN-X may appear as hoarseness or dysphagia; to CN-XI, neck and shoulder weakness; and to CN-XII, asymmetry or fasciculations of the tongue. Vincristine may damage CN-V, causing acute jaw pain, which usually resolves within a few days and which may not recur with additional drug administration. Finally, chemotherapy-induced brain-stem injury can lead to cranial nerve palsies that can be either temporary or permanent.

Motor function assessment

Motor function is evaluated by assessing skeletal muscles for size, tone, strength, and any involuntary movements. It is important to remember that both sides of the body should be compared for symmetry and equality of motor strength. A few simple tests should be sufficient. Key techniques for assessing motor function are shown in Table 20-3. Tests of motor function are important in evaluating neurological toxicity from chemotherapy. For example, cisplatin may cause peripheral neuropathy with motor weakness, and high doses of cytosine arabinoside may cause cerebellar dysfunction.

Sensory function assessment

Sensory function is evaluated to identify alterations in the sensory cortex or pathways. Peripheral sensory receptors are located in the skin, mucous membranes, viscera, and muscles and tendons.[5] Sensory impulses are carried by peripheral nerves to the spinal cord via the posterior (dorsal) roots, and then the impulses enter either the spinothalamic tract or the posterior column and are transmitted up to the brain. Sensations of *pain and temperature* are carried via the lateral spinothalamic tract to the thalamus; *crude touch* via the anterior spinothalamic tract to the thalamus; and *position, vibration, and fine touch* via the posterior column to the medulla and then to the thalamus. At the level of the thalamus, gross sensations are registered (pain, position, temperature). Impulses are then relayed from the thalamus to the sensory cortex for precise discrimination.[5] Because the ascending tracts cross over to the opposite side of the spinal cord at the pyramids before reaching the brain, a sensory impulse on the right side of the body is interpreted by the left side of the brain and vice versa.[6] The location of the sensory loss helps to pinpoint the site of sensory damage. If the sensory cortex is damaged, the deficit will be loss of fine sensory discrimination, while the gross

TABLE 20-3 Assessment of Motor Function

Function and Assessment Technique	
Gait:	• Ask the person to walk back and forth in a room, and note the posture, body movements, and step. For example, is the step a steppage gait in which the foot is lifted high with knees flexed then dropped to the floor with a slapping sound; or is the gait staggering, unsteady, and wide-based as with cerebellar ataxia?
	• Ask the person to walk heel-to-toe along an imaginary line to test cerebellar function
Muscles:	• Starting with the upper limbs, provide fixed resistance by pushing against the extremity and ask the person to oppose it by pushing back as forcefully as possible. Grade the strength as follows: 5/5 can raise and hold limb against active resistance (push) 4/5 can raise and hold limb, but not against active resistance (push) 3/5 can raise limb, but can not hold it against active resistance (touch) 2/5 moves limb, but cannot raise or lift limb to overcome gravity 1/5 slight contraction visible (patient tries to move limb but no movement) 0/5 no movement
	• Test plantar flexion and dorsiflexion at the ankle by asking the person to push down against your hand and then to pull the foot away as you cup your hand around the foot.
	• Test for drift of the arms and legs. Have the person close the eyes and extend arms with palms facing upward for 10 seconds; ask the person to sit on the edge of a chair or bed, close the eyes, and hold both legs out in front, holding this position for 30 seconds. You should observe for any upward or downward drift of the arms or legs, wrist pronation, or curled fingers.
Involuntary Movements:	• Are tremors, spasms, or other involuntary movements observed?
Coordination:	• Test the integrity of the cerebellum, which is responsible for balance and coordination. Ask the person to sit down and then to touch the nose with a finger, first with eyes open then closed. Next, ask the person to touch your finger as you move it in different directions. This point-to-point action helps to identify intention tremors.
	• Then ask the person to alternately tap the right and left hands against the knee as quickly as possible and to alternately pronate and supinate hands and forearms.
	• Ask the person to move one foot down the shin of the other leg, and repeat this with the other leg.
	• Finally, ask the person to stand up with feet together and arms at the sides, first with eyes open then closed. If the person loses balance with eyes closed, this is a positive Romberg sign.

perceptions of pain, touch, and position will be intact. Deficits are described in terms of the *dermatomal* distribution. A dermatome is the area of skin innervated by the sensory nerve root of a spinal segment, as shown in Figure 20-2. Table 20-4 describes techniques to assess sensory function.

Patients who develop peripheral neuropathy as a side effect of chemotherapy may develop sensory abnormalities such as diminished temperature and touch sense in addition to the numbness and tingling commonly experienced. In addition, proprioceptive losses in the lower extremities can lead to ataxia if the person also has loss of reflexes. All of these can place the individual at risk for injury.

Reflex assessment

Reflexes help to assess the status of the CNS, as they indicate whether the pathway (arc) from the receptor organ to the spinal cord and back to the effector organ is intact. Observe the briskness of response. If the reflex is not elicited, have the person perform isometric exercises—for instance, cup two hands together and try to pull them apart.

The deep tendon reflexes may also be called *muscle stretch reflexes*. A procedure for examination of these reflexes is shown in Table 20-5. Patients who have developed severe peripheral neuropathies from drugs such as high-dose cisplatin or vincristine may develop footdrop and

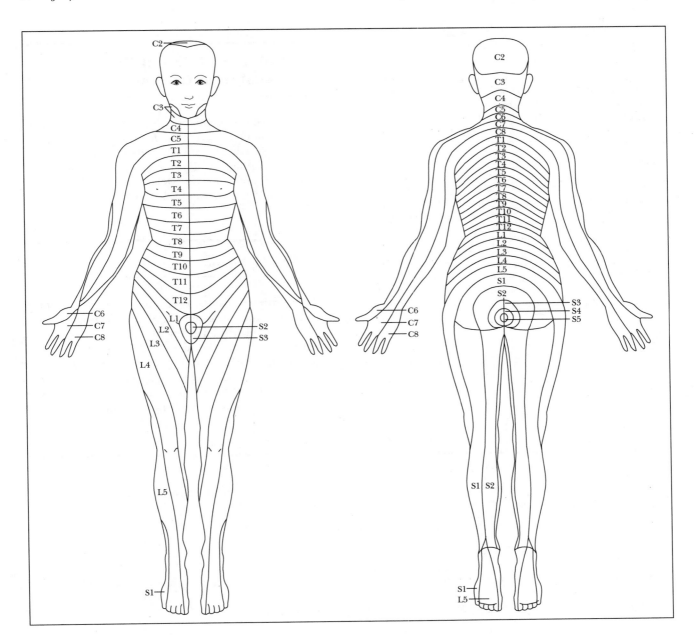

FIGURE 20-2   Dermatome chart.

TABLE 20-4 Assessment of Sensory Function

Dimension and Examination
General To begin, ask the person to keep *his/her eyes closed* during the exam. It is important to compare one side with the other throughout. Identify areas where there is decreased sensation using a washable marker.
Pain If the sensation of pain is intact, touch and temperature should be intact. Use a sterile 22-gauge needle or a safety pin cleansed with alcohol and, starting at the shoulders, gently touch the metal to the skin, asking the person to tell you when it is felt. Touch one side, then the other, and move down to the distal aspects of the arms and legs.
Light touch Using a wisp of cotton, touch the areas assessed under pain, and ask the person to tell you when the cotton is felt.
Position Grasping the person's index finger (at the last joint) from the side, move the joint up or down and ask the person whether the finger is pointing up or down. Repeat this on the opposite side as well as with each of the big toes. If position sense is impaired, move on to the next proximal joint (e.g., wrist or ankle).
Vibratory Test both sides of the body for vibratory sense using a tuning fork. Tap the tuning fork on the heel of the hand to begin vibration, then place the rounded end on the interphalangeal joint of the middle finger. Ask the patient to tell you what is felt. If pressure, then ask the patient to tell you when the sensation stops and touch the fork to stop the vibration. Repeat on the other hand. Then test the feet, placing the tuning fork on the bony joint of each great toe. If the patient has no sense of vibration, move proximally, placing the vibrating fork on the bony prominence of the wrists and the medial malleoli of the ankle joints. If still no vibration is felt, move to the elbow and knee.
Fine discrimination Place a common object, e.g., coin, in the patient's hand, and ask patient to identify it; test other hand with a different object (e.g., key). This ability is called *stereognosis*.

loss of the Achilles reflex. This results in a slapping gait and potential for injury.

Section A: Spinal Cord Compression

Associated Symptoms: back pain, leg weakness with sensory loss, loss of bowel and/or bladder function

The Problem of Spinal Cord Compression in Cancer

Spinal cord compression represents a medical emergency because prompt intervention may prevent permanent neurological disability. Spinal cord compression can result in direct injury to the spinal cord with consequent sensory and motor deficits. Delayed diagnosis and treatment can lead to permanent disability, such as paralysis.[7]

Etiology

Although primary spinal cord tumors may cause spinal cord compression, it is most commonly caused by metastatic solid tumors such as breast, lung, prostate, kidney, melanoma, or sarcoma, as well as by the hematologic malignancies multiple myeloma and lymphoma. The course of compression by primary spinal cord tumors is slow compared with the much more rapid progression of symptoms seen as a result of metastatic lesions. While

TABLE 20-5 Examination of the Deep Tendon Reflexes (Muscle Stretch Reflexes)

Reflex	Examination
General	Help the person become comfortable sitting on the edge of the bed or examining table. Use the end of the reflex hammer to gently strike the tendon. Response is graded on a 0 to 4+ scale: 4+ Very brisk, hyperactive, and abnormal 3+ Brisk, but may not be related to disease 2+ Normal 1+ Slightly diminished, but may be normal 0 No response, often abnormal
Achilles reflex	Foot should plantar flex. If there is abnormality, it may reflect a problem at nerves S-1 and S-2 of the spinal cord.
Quadriceps reflex	Elicits knee jerk, which should extend the leg. Tests nerves L-3, L-4.
Biceps reflex	Elbow should flex. Tests nerves C-5, C-6.
Triceps reflex	Elbow should extend. Tests nerves C-7, C-8.

the majority of lesions are thoracic (50%–70%), the cervical (10%–30%) and lumbosacral (20%–30%) spines can be affected as well.[8] The anatomical location of the primary tumor helps to explain the location of lesions: cervical lesions tend to be caused by primary breast tumors; thoracic by primary lung, breast, and prostate tumors; and lumbosacral by gastrointestinal malignancies and prostate cancer. Spinal cord compression can occur at any time during the disease course, from initial presentation before a diagnosis of cancer to the terminal phase of advanced disease.

Pathophysiology

Malignant lesions may directly invade the spinal cord or, more commonly, cause collapse of the vertebrae through lytic destruction of underlying vertebral bodies or pedicles,[8] as shown in Figure 20-3. Eighty-five percent of lesions compressing the spinal cord are due to tumor metastasis to the vertebral body, causing direct pressure on the epidural space or fracturing the vertebral body, which then extends directly into the epidural space.[9] The physiologic response to injury is edema and inflammation, which, together with mechanical compression causing direct neural injury to the cord, results in damaged vasculature and impaired oxygenation, ischemia, or hemorrhage. Nerve entrapment by the collapsed vertebrae may occur as well.

The extent and severity of neurological signs and symptoms depend on the rate and degree of compression. Thus, early identification and intervention are critical so that decompressive interventions can be initiated and permanent injury prevented.

Assessment

Measurement Tools

A clinical neurological assessment of the patient with suspected spinal cord compression includes evaluation of pain, sensory and motor function, and bowel and bladder function. An assessment tool is shown in Table 20-6.

Physical Assessment

Back pain, motor weakness, and decreased sensation are early symptoms of spinal cord compression. These may occur over months or within days or hours, depending on the speed or tumor growth.[8] Late signs/symptoms are

motor loss, further sensory loss, loss of proprioception and vibration sensation, and autonomic dysfunction.

Back pain

Back pain is the most common presenting symptom of spinal cord compression, occurring in approximately 95% of patients, and although back pain may occur at the time of more progressive symptoms, it also may occur weeks to months earlier.[10] Pain is gradual at first, progressively becoming more severe. Pain can be either localized or radicular. *Localized pain* occurs over the area of tumor. Usually it is found within one to two vertebrae of the compression and is caused by destruction of the vertebrae or by stretching of the bone by the enlarging tumor mass.[11] The pain is constant, may increase with the supine position, and may cause the patient to awaken at night.[12] *Radicular* pain is caused by compression of the nerve roots, and is found in the dermatome(s) of the affected nerve root(s). Thoracic involvement usually results in bilateral pain that may be described as a squeezing tight band across the chest or abdomen. Cervical and lumbosacral pain, by contrast, tend to be unilateral.[11] The pain is made worse by the supine position, sneezing, or the Valsalva maneuver, and may be relieved by sitting upright. This is the opposite of pain caused by a slipped disk.

Pain can also be *referred* (medullary pain). This pain is poorly localized due to the involvement of multiple dermatomes (refer again to Figure 20-2) and is often characterized as burning or shooting pain.[13]

Gilbert et al.[14] studied back pain and the corresponding extent of cord compression. They found that 33% of patients with back pain alone had a normal neurological exam despite greater than 75% blockage of the spinal cord. Fifty-seven percent of patients with radicular pain had greater than 75% blockage.

Motor weakness

Motor weakness involving the arms or legs is often characterized as heaviness or stiffness, and may lead to loss of coordination, ataxia, and paralysis.[12] Gilbert et al.[14] found that 95% of patients with motor weakness had greater than 75% blockage of the spinal cord; so clearly, the earlier the symptoms can be identified and evaluated, the better the prognosis.[14] Without intervention, motor weakness will progress to motor loss. Ability to walk at the time a diagnosis of spinal cord compression is made has great predictive importance, as less than 25% of patients who have paralysis at the time of diagnosis regain function.[15] Integrated motor movement is further described in Table 20-7. Assessment of motor function includes evaluation of gait, muscles, involuntary movements, and coordination.

Decreased sensation

Sensory changes are manifested initially by paresthesias (numbness and tingling of toes and fingers), pro-

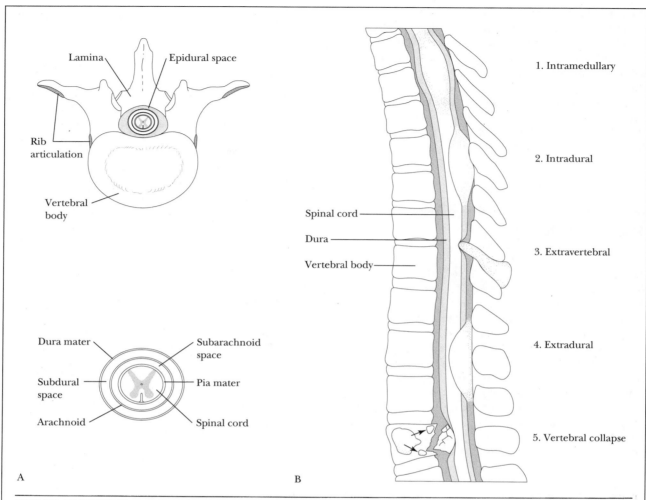

NORMAL ANATOMY: The spinal cord is encased within the vertebral column and surrounded by leptomeninges or membranes: PIA MATER surrounds the cord; the ARACHNOID MATER is the middle layer, and the DURA MATER is the outermost layer. The subarachnoid space lies between the pia mater and arachnoid mater, and provides a channel for cerebral spinal fluid (CSF). The subdural space lies between the arachnoid and dura mater, and the epidural space lies between the dura mater and the vertebral bone membrane. The spinal cord ends at nerves L1-2, and lumbar and sacral nerve roots exit the cord there (cauda equina).

MALIGNANT INVASION CAN BE DESCRIBED AS:

1. INTRAMEDULLARY: tumors originate in the spinal cord, e.g., ependymoma
2. INTRADURAL: tumor is located within the dura, arises from the meninges or from nerve roots
3. EXTRAVERTEBRAL: tumor arises outside the vertebrae, extends between the vertebrae, pushes through the intervertebral foramina into the epidural space (e.g., lymph nodes in the mediastinum from lymphoma)
4. EXTRADURAL: arise outside the spinal cord (bony metastasis to the vertebrae) and may cause
5. VERTEBRAL COLLAPSE through destruction of underlying vertebral body, pedicle, or laminae; tumor growth or bony particles are pushed into the epidural space and compress the spinal cord. This is the most common type.

FIGURE 20-3   Malignant invasion of the spinal cord.

gressing to decreased sensation to light touch and pain, then to temperature. Over time, the numbness and sensory changes ascend to the level of the compressed spinal cord. Without intervention, decreased sensation progresses to sensory loss, including losses of proprioception, position sense, vibration, and deep pressure.[16] The symptoms seen depend on the area of the spinal cord injured.

Autonomic dysfunction

Autonomic dysfunction is related to lower motor neuron functions of bowel and bladder. Difficulty initiating urination can progress to urinary retention, overflow, or incontinence. Bowel dysfunction can be manifested by loss of rectal sensation, constipation, or—very late—fecal

TABLE 20-6 Assessment of the Patient with Suspected Spinal Cord Compression

History

I. Risk factors (type of primary tumor, presence of bony metastasis)

II. Medication profile, with review of potential side effects

III. Symptom analysis: Back pain
   A. Distinguish other pain, if any, from pain due to bony metastasis: has location, intensity, character changed?
   B. Perform systematic assessment
      1. Location (is pain localized, radicular, referred? Compare with dermatome chart, Figure 20-2)
      2. Radiation? To where?
      3. Onset of pain
      4. Character (is it constant or intermittent?)
      5. Quality (have patient describe—is it squeezing, bandlike?)
      6. Intensity (have patient rate on scale from 0 to 5, with 5 being worst)
      7. Aggravating factors (lying down, coughing, sneezing, straining?)
      8. Alleviating factors (sitting up, medications?)

IV. Focused history
   A. Musculoskeletal: Has the patient noticed any weakness? Any heaviness or stiffness of the limbs? Any difficulty walking, gait disturbances? Falls? Lack of coordination? Paralysis? Onset/course?
   B. Sensory: any numbness or paresthesias? Where? Have patient describe it. Any changes in sensation to touch, temperature? Areas of no sensation? Any loss of position sense?
   C. Autonomic Function:
      1. Assess usual patterns of elimination
      2. Any bladder difficulties (urgency, initiating voiding, retention, overflow, incontinence)? Onset?
      3. Any bowel difficulties (expelling fecal contents, constipation, absence of sensation or numbness in the rectum, incontinence with loss of sphincter control)? Onset?

Physical Exam

I. General observations: orientation to person, place, time; accuracy as a historian, presence of family members.

II. Focused exam (depending on skill of the nurse)
   A. Percuss vertebrae along spinal cord—is pain elicited? Note level of pain.
   B. Ask patient to do straight leg raising (SLR) if pain in back, or on neck flexion—does this elicit pain?
   C. Evaluate urinary system. If retention, discuss with MD need for straight catheterization to evaluate postvoiding residual (residual of >150 mL considered retention).
   D. Evaluate rectal sphincter tone.
   E. Evaluate motor strengths (see text).
   F. Evaluate sensory function (see text).
   G. Evaluate reflexes: look for hyperactive deep tendon reflexes, or absence of superficial reflexes (see text).

incontinence with poor sphincter control. Key neurological assessment points are presented in Tables 20-1 through 20-5.

Diagnostic Evaluation

The clinical diagnostic evaluation begins with x-ray films of the spine. This initial screen identifies up to 85% of vertebral lesions, may show extradural masses, and is easy and inexpensive to perform. Next, magnetic resonance imaging (MRI) is performed, because the entire spine can be imaged and the precise location of spinal cord compression and paraspinal masses identified. For instance, MRI can show whether lesions are epidural, intradural, or intramedullary. This test has emerged as superior to myelogram and computerized axial tomography (CAT) scanning with myelogram because it is not invasive and does not require the injection of a contrast material. However, MRI may be problematic, as it requires the patient to lie still for 1 to 2 hours, which is difficult if back pain is severe. In addition, MRI may not show leptomeningeal spread clearly.[8]

Other tests include bone scan and, where MRI is unavailable, CAT scan with myelogram. The bone scan can be used to identify 85% of patients with spinal cord compression, even when the spinal x-ray films were normal. Limitations include injection of nuclear material and false-positive (arthritis) and false-negative (myeloma) results.[12] CAT scanning with IV contrast is useful in identifying early lesions as well as exact location of spinal cord compression and in planning the radiation treatment field, but it does not permit visualization of the entire spine. When CAT scan is combined with myelogram using intrathecal contrast, findings are greatly enhanced. Before the availability of MRI, a myelogram was the diagnostic tool of choice. However, this may involve multiple lumbar punctures, increases risk of neurological damage as it causes changes in cerebral spinal fluid (CSF) pressure, is painful, and often causes side effects such as spinal headache, dizziness, seizures, and nausea. Today, myelogram is reserved for patients for whom MRI does not explain symptoms.

Degrees of Neurologic Damage

The extent of the compression of the spinal cord determines the degree of neurological damage. Ambulatory status at the time of diagnosis of spinal cord compression is a major predictor of ability to walk after treatment, and this underscores the need for early detection and intervention. Approximately 70% of ambulatory patients diagnosed with spinal cord compression are still able to walk after treatment.[11] Unfortunately, paralysis lasting more than 24 hours before treatment is not usually reversible.[8]

Other factors influencing prognosis are primary cancer site, rapidity of onset of spinal cord compression, presence of lytic bone lesions, and location.[8] Patients with primary tumors that are responsive to cancer therapy appear to have better outcomes (for example, patients with breast and prostate cancers, multiple myeloma,

TABLE 20-7 Effects of Injury on Major Neural Pathway Function

Area of Injury	Normal Function	Dysfunction Arising from Injury
Corticospinal (pyramidal) tract	Information necessary for voluntary movement, integrated skilled movement, and muscle tone are transmitted from the brain's motor cortex to the brain stem; at the pyramids, the impulse crosses to the opposite side of the spinal cord and continues to the anterior horn, where synapses with effector neurons occur	• Loss of motor function below the level of weakness, ranging from weakness to paralysis • Loss of ability to carry out skilled movements • Increase in muscle tone • Exaggerated muscle stretch reflexes • Injury above pyramids (brain-stem crossover) results in motor loss on opposite side of body • Injury below pyramids (brain-stem crossover) results in motor loss on same side of body • Injury to cells of anterior horn results in motor loss on same side of body; muscle stretch reflexes are reduced or absent
Extrapyramidal tract	Tract carries motor movement impulses to/from cerebral cortex, basal ganglia, brain stem, and spinal cord; the information carried along this tract is essential for muscle tone and body movements, such as walking	• Increased muscle tone • Changes in posture and gait • Bradykinesia (slowing of autonomic movements)
Cerebellum	Sensory and motor input are necessary for coordinated muscle activity, posture, and balance	• Ataxia (loss of coordination) • Loss of balance • Decreased muscle tone

lymphoma). Patients with rapid onset and deterioration of neurological function do poorly compared with those whose onset is more gradual. Urinary dysfunction (e.g., retention) existing more than 24 hours before treatment is not usually reversible.[8] Patients with destroyed vertebrae plus an extradural mass have a poorer prognosis, as do patients with compressing masses anterior to the cord.

Symptom Management

Prevention

Prevention is unfortunately not an option. However, early identification of patients at risk and systematic patient and family teaching about signs and symptoms to report can help to bring about early treatment and may reduce neurological disability. Although spinal cord compression is rarely life-threatening, it can significantly reduce quality of life and thus demands rapid treatment.

Therapeutic Approaches

Treatment is aimed at palliation of symptoms and prevention of permanent disability (if instituted early). Figure 20-4 depicts a clinical pathway for the management of spinal cord compression developed by Dietz and Flaherty.[11]

Corticosteroids are introduced immediately to reduce edema within the spinal cord, leading to decreased pain and relief of neurological symptoms. High doses of dexamethasone are used initially, then gradually tapered to daily maintenance doses of 1 mg/day to 24 mg/day.[12] Dose and treatment duration are based on the patient's response to the steroids. Complications of steroids may occur and include emotional lability, hyperglycemia, fluid retention, and increased risk of infection.[17]

Radiation therapy is the treatment of choice for decompression, as radiation alone produces symptom reduction equal to combined surgical laminectomy plus radiotherapy.[18] Treatment is initiated immediately after diagnosis—and as an emergency procedure if onset of symptoms was rapid or rapidly progressive.[12] Radiation therapy doses of 3000 to 4000 cGy usually are delivered over 2 to 4 weeks to a radiation port extending two vertebrae above and below the area of compression and including any other suspicious sites.[15]

Surgical decompression is the treatment of choice for patients with tumors that are *not* radiosensitive, patients without a prior cancer diagnosis (so that biopsy can be done), recurrence within the radiated field, spinal instability, neurological deterioration during radiation therapy, and perhaps nonambulatory patients unlikely to regain motor function with radiation therapy.[19] Posterior

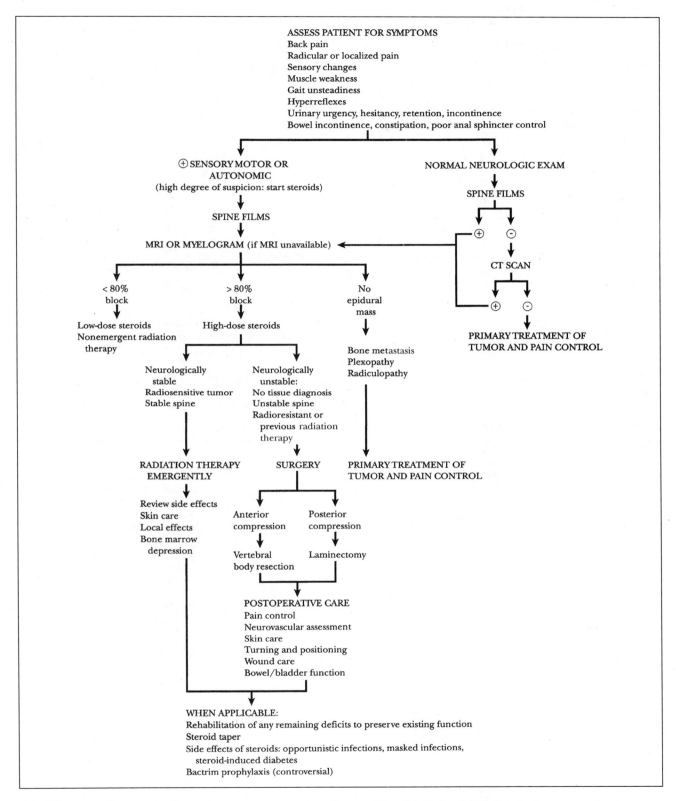

FIGURE 20-4   Clinical pathway for spinal cord compression. (Source: Dietz KA, Flaherty AM: Oncologic emergencies, in Groenwald SL, Frogge MH, Goodman M, Yarbro CH (eds): *Cancer Nursing: Principles and Practice* (ed 3). Sudbury: Jones and Bartlett 1993. p. 833. © Jones and Bartlett Publishers. Reprinted with permission.[11])

laminectomy may be performed with excision of the vertebral laminae and spinous processes, and debulking of the tumor in the exposed dural space.[12] However, residual epidural tumor often remains in the anterior spaces and is unresectable with a posterior approach. Improvements in technique and instrumentation have made the anterior approach feasible. Instrumentation with Luque rods is used for internal spine fixation, thus stabilizing the spine, correcting deformity, and replacing destroyed vertebrae.[8] Complications of surgical decompression are approximately 9% mortality, 12% further neurological deterioration, and 11% postoperative complications.[8]

Pain management must be a priority in the comprehensive plan of care. Usually decompression and steroids relieve the pain, but response to radiotherapy may take up to 5 days after treatment is initiated. Narcotic analgesics are often required. In the event of nerve root compression, phenytoin or a tricyclic antidepressant such as amitriptyline may need to be added to the analgesic regimen.[8]

Evaluation of Therapeutic Approaches

Evaluation of patient responses to treatment is a critical part of the multidisciplinary care plan. Outcomes are evaluated based on (1) prevention of neurological dysfunction by early identification and intervention, (2) relief of pain, (3) prevention of injury related to deficits, (4) recovery or preservation of neurological function if possible, and if not possible, (5) adaptation to advancing disease and management of symptoms.

Educational Tools

Nursing care is focused on symptom relief, support through therapy, and rehabilitation. Nurses must

1. be familiar with patient risk factors for development of spinal cord compression
2. be familiar with assessment techniques to evaluate back pain in patients at risk
3. institute patient/family teaching to patients at risk so that early signs and symptoms are reported in time for prompt intervention
4. advocate for and ensure that patients receive adequate pain management, and
5. use principles of rehabilitation in their practice of nursing to optimize function, minimize dysfunction, and prevent complications.

A comprehensive nursing care plan is shown in Table 20-8. A self-care guide for the patient at risk for developing spinal cord compression is provided in Appendix 20A.

TABLE 20-8 Standardized Nursing Care Plan for the Patient with Spinal Cord Compression (SCC) (actual/potential)

Nursing Diagnosis	Expected Outcomes	Nursing Interventions
I. Knowledge deficit regarding the potential risk of developing SCC in patients with myeloma, sarcoma, lymphoma, or cancers of the prostate, lung, or breast	I. Patient will describe SCC and signs/symptoms to report	I. Teach patient signs/symptoms to recognize and report immediately, or to come to the emergency room: A. Back pain (early sign) B. Back pain radiating to chest, abdomen, groin, legs, buttocks C. Leg weakness, difficulty walking D. Decreased sensation in legs E. Constipation F. Difficulty urinating or emptying the bladder G. Incontinence of bowel or bladder (late sign)
II. Impaired mobility from SCC, potential or actual	II. Patient will be without complications of immobility	II. A. Assess limitations of mobility 1. neurological status 2. leg strength, muscle tone, sensation 3. ability to bear weight 4. ability to move self in bed B. Teach patient to change position q2h as appropriate C. Discuss with team early referral to physical/occupational therapy to initiate rehabilitation as soon as possible D. Teach patient to use spine-stabilizing brace when out of bed E. Teach patient about, and place on the patient, devices to prevent foot drop

TABLE 20-8 Standardized Nursing Care Plan for the Patient with Spinal Cord Compression (SCC) (actual/potential) (continued)

Nursing Diagnosis	Expected Outcomes	Nursing Interventions
III. Altered skin integrity, potential related to bowel and/or bladder incontinence, immobility, altered sensation	III. Skin will remain intact	III. A. Assess skin integrity and risk for developing alterations (incontinence, loss of sensation, immobility) B. Consider devices to assist mobility (overbed trapeze), changes in pressure on the skin (alternating pressure mattress), and measures to protect the skin from incontinence (bowel training, catheter or intermittent straight catheterization, frequent skin care)
IV. Potential for injury related to sensory and motor deficits	IV. Patient will be free from injury	IV. A. Assess degree of risk 1. Presence of areas of decreased/absent sensation for pain and temperature 2. Presence of paresthesias 3. Changes in coordination, ability to walk, perform ADLs B. Assess environment for safety, and remove any physical hazards C. Protect patient from injury (thermal, mechanical, chemical); use log rolling while patient in bed to prevent torsion on spine D. Assist patient with ADLs as appropriate
V. Pain	V. Patient will be comfortable	V. A. Discuss analgesic regimen with team to provide control 1. Nonsteroidal antiinflammatory agents 2. Opioids 3. Dexamethasone B. Provide systematic and regular assessment of discomfort and effectiveness of analgesic regimen C. Maintain proper body alignment D. Teach patient progressive muscle relaxation, guided imagery, other relaxation techniques as appropriate E. Provide premedication prior to painful activities (e.g., moving onto stretcher for XRT)
VI. Ineffective coping, potential	VI. A. Patient will verbalize concerns related to coping B. Patient will identify strategies to assist coping C. Patient will identify resources	VI. A. Assess patient's feelings regarding potential for developing SCC; and if SCC has occurred, feelings regarding disease progression, potential for loss of function or sensation B. Assess present and past coping mechanisms and effectiveness C. Assess interaction with family members and degree of support offered D. Plan realistic short-term goals with patient and family, as appropriate E. Refer to oncologic social worker or psychiatric nurse specialist, as appropriate and needed

(continued)

TABLE 20-8   Standardized Nursing Care Plan for the Patient with Spinal Cord Compression (SCC) (actual/potential) (continued)

Nursing Diagnosis	Expected Outcomes	Nursing Interventions
		F. Discuss with the team benefit of antidepressants to improve mood, sleep, and comfort G. Teach patient how to access resources to assist in long-term coping
VII. Potential for sexual dysfunction related to altered motor functioning, muscle weakness, psychological distress	VII. A. Patient and significant other will identify alterations in sexual expression B. Patient and significant other will identify alternative methods of sexual expression	VII. A. Discuss the impact of sexual dysfunction on sexuality, social role, and self-esteem B. Discuss appropriate alternative means of sexual expression C. Refer for specific sexual counseling if diminished ability to have an erection D. Observe for changes in needs related to affection and emotional support

ADLs = activities of daily living.

Section B: Increased Intracranial Pressure

Associated Symptoms: changes in level of consciousness; drowsiness; lethargy; mental status changes; memory loss; mood changes; restlessness; headache, with or without vomiting that may be projectile; weakness; and incoordination

The Problem of Increased Intracranial Pressure in Cancer

Increased ICP is a life-threatening complication of malignancy. Untreated, it can cause herniation of the brain stem, causing cessation of life functions and death.

Etiology

There are numerous causes of increased ICP, but the principal cause is a space-occupying lesion. Primary malignancies of the brain, such as astrocytomas and glioblastomas, as well as metastasis to the brain tissue or skull from solid tumors (e.g., breast and lung cancers) can cause increased ICP. Complications of malignancy, such

as CNS infections in the neutropenic patient or the paraneoplastic syndrome of inappropriate antidiuretic hormone secretion (SIADH) in patients with small-cell lung cancer, can also increase ICP.

Pathophysiology

The brain and spinal cord exist in a closed system, and the rigid skull provides protection for the brain tissue. The pressure within this closed space is maintained within a narrow margin, and it is influenced by the volume of the brain, cerebral blood volume, and volume of CSF. Change in volume in any of these components requires a compensatory change in one of the other volumes to maintain the same pressure, because the rigid skull cannot expand to accommodate an increased volume. Increased volume can occur as a result of primary or metastatic tumor, infection, hemorrhage, or inflammation (e.g., from brain radiation therapy). Fluid movement may expand the brain mass.

Vasogenic or *extracellular cerebral edema* occurs due to increased permeability of the cerebral capillary endothelial cells, leading to a flow of fluid into the extracellular spaces, thus increasing ICP. This is amplified by damage to the blood-brain barrier, allowing the movement of water, sodium, and plasma proteins into the extracellular spaces, causing further swelling of the brain tissue.[20] Radiation may also cause this type of injury.

Cytotoxic or *intracellular edema* is swelling of the brain cells (white and gray matter) and is related to cellular hypoxia caused by disruptions in cellular metabolism in the brain. A constant supply of glucose and oxygen is required for the production of energy, and the brain cannot store substrate. Without this energy, sodium cannot be pumped out of the brain cells. As a result, sodium and water are retained, leading to swollen cells. Blood circulation to the brain may be compromised, resulting in hypoxia and cell death.[10] Hemorrhage related to severe thrombocytopenia and CNS infections are causes of intracellular edema. Infections or abscesses of the brain also cause an inflammatory response with exudate formation, which contributes to cerebral edema and increased ICP. Additionally, SIADH can cause an increase in the intracellular water and sodium content in the brain cells, resulting in swelling of the cells.[16]

Interstitial or *hydrocephalic edema* results from obstruction to flow of CSF within the ventricles of the brain by tumor (intraventricular), abscess, or obstructive hydrocephalus. As the CSF outflow is blocked, increased hydrostatic pressure forces CSF into the surrounding white matter of the brain, thus increasing the volume in the interstitial spaces.[20]

Increased cerebral blood volume increases ICP. Cerebral blood flow, although closely autoregulated during health, is increased by cerebral vasodilation due to hypoxemia, severe systemic hypertension, and decreased removal of venous blood from the brain (e.g., obstruction in bilateral internal jugular veins or the Valsalva maneuver). Blood volume in the brain is also increased with hemorrhage.

Assessment

Measurement Tools

Two available tools are the Quick Neurological Assessment for the Oncology Nurse, as shown in Table 20-9, and the Glasgow Coma Scale.

Physical Assessment

The patient experiencing increased ICP initially will show vague symptoms and signs of a *change in level of consciousness* (gradually becoming more somnolent), *change in mental status* (irritability, confusion, decreased cognition), or *restlessness*.[21] These changes may be quite subtle and require close assessment to identify. *Headache* is another early symptom, often occurring with early morning awakening. It may be associated with vomiting that may be projectile and is aggravated by the Valsalva maneuver. The headache may be dull or sharp and, as ICP rises, tends to be frontal or occipital.[22] Other signs and symptoms are dizziness, focal or generalized seizures, weakness, aphasia, ataxia, and changes in vital signs (late, and including widening pulse pressure and bradycardia).

Developing skill in neurological assessment is very important for the oncology nurse. Assessment includes history and identification of patient risk for increased ICP; evaluation of level of consciousness; and evaluation of pupillary responses, extraocular eye movements (cranial nerves III, IV, VI), and motor and sensory function. These procedures are highlighted in Tables 20-1 through 20-5.

The nurse first must identify patients at risk for increased ICP: patients with solid tumors that metastasize to the skull or brain (breast, lung, melanoma, hypernephroma) and hematologic malignancies (leukemia and lymphoma). The nursing history should evaluate the patient's level of consciousness. In the event a quick, easy assessment must be made, the Glasgow Coma Scale is helpful in assessing level of consciousness. This tool assesses and grades the person's best eye-opening response (spontaneously, to speech, to pain, or no response), best motor response (obeys verbal command, localizes pain, flexion-withdrawal, flexion-abnormal/decorticate, extension-abnormal/decerebrate, or flaccid), and best verbal response (oriented to person/place/time, conversation

TABLE 20-9 Quick Neurological Assessment for the Oncology Nurse

Area to Assess	Questions
• Flow of speech • Orientation • Memory • Thought processes • Attention span	Ask what brings the patient to the hospital at this time Ask what problems the patient has experienced, and when they began Note any restlessness, confusion, irritability, or if the patient loses interest
• Short-term memory • Visual acuity	Tell the patient you are doing a memory test Ask the patient to read his/her hospital number, and to remember it Ask the patient to repeat the number 5 minutes later
• Gait • Lower extremity motor function, coordination • Ability to follow commands	Ask the patient, if able, to walk across the room—observe gait and posture Ask the patient to sit in a chair, or on the side of the bed, and slide the right heel down the left leg—note coordination and smoothness of movement
• Upper extremity motor function, coordination • Fine motor movement	Ask the patient to unbutton his/her shirt or unzip trousers or skirt Ask the patient to pick up a dime from a flat surface
• Cranial nerves III, IV, V, VI, VII (partial exam)	Ask the patient to smile, then clench his/her teeth Observe the patient's pupils for size, equality, and reactivity to light when tested with your flashlight

confused, speech inappropriate, sounds incomprehensible, or no response).[23] The best score is a 15, the worst, 3; a score lower than 8 is considered comatose. Limitations are that the exam does not account for paraplegia or absent lower extremity function.

Consciousness is a function of arousal and awareness of self (ability to interact with the environment). Arousal is regulated by the reticular activating system in the brain stem and does not require thought to activate. Awareness, in contrast, requires a functioning cerebral cortex. If increased ICP reduces cerebral blood flow and hence oxygenation to these areas, then gradually the individual will become less responsive, more somnolent, and less able to interact with the environment. These are often the earliest signs of increased ICP. Assess awareness by observing from a distance and noting whether the patient is aware of your presence. Arousal is then assessed by calling the patient's name and noting whether the eyes open spontaneously. If not, ask the patient to open the eyes. If there is no response to verbal stimuli, assess response to touch; then if no response, to painful stimuli (sternal rub or trapezius muscle squeeze). Awareness is assessed by evaluating orientation, attention span, language, and memory.[24] Ask the patient to tell you his/her name, present location, and the current date. Observe the patient's attention span during the conversation and whether the patient loses interest. Listen to the patient's speech; is it clear, articulate, and accurate? Evaluate long-term memory by asking date of birth or some fact you can verify.[24] Short-term memory can be tested by telling the patient you need to do a memory test; tell the patient something to remember (e.g., your name or a sequence of numbers) and that you will ask for a repeat of this information in 5 minutes.

Is the patient restless—or quiet now, but restless just a while ago? These may be warning signs. Vital signs are important, although often only at a very late stage. Assess temperature, heart rate, blood pressure; note pulse pressure (difference between diastolic and systolic readings) and compare with previous readings. Widening pulse pressure is a grave sign of increased ICP. Increased ICP causes compression of the arteries supplying oxygen to the brain, resulting in ischemia. The brain-stem vasomotor center regulates life functions, and ischemia to this area causes compensatory changes. In an effort to increase oxygenation, there is increased sympathetic tone, which increases systolic blood pressure, thereby widening the pulse pressure. At the same time, parasympathetic stimulation of the heart results in a decreased heart rate (bradycardia) of 40 to 50 beats per minute. With continued hypoxia, systolic blood pressure falls as the vasomotor center ceases to activate sympathetic tone and the heart rate becomes weak and irregular.[22] The respiratory center in the medulla is equally affected by ischemia due to increased ICP, with resulting shallow, irregular respirations. Periods of apnea occur. This triad of hypertension, bradycardia, and irregular respirations is called *Cushing's triad.*[24]

Finally, increased ICP may compress the area of the hypothalamus. Temperature regulation is lost and the patient may become febrile or hypothermic. Temperature swings may occur rapidly, such as 97°F (36.1°C) to 104°F (40°C).

Selected neurological exam

Increased ICP can cause ischemia or injury in the midbrain, which will become apparent by testing the pupillary responses and eye movement (CN-III, oculomotor; IV, trochlear; VI, abducens). First, inspect the pupils with normal lighting and note size, shape, and symmetry (controlled by CN-III). Pupils should be round and equal in size, ranging from 3 to 7 mm. It has been estimated that almost 20% of the U.S. population has slightly unequal pupils.[23] If pupils are constricted, check to see whether the patient is receiving narcotic analgesics; if not, this may suggest damage to the pons in the brain stem.[20] If the pupils are dilated, determine whether the patient is receiving any atropine-containing drugs, such as diphenoxylate hydrochloride and atropine (Lomotil). Bilaterally dilated pupils suggest hypoxia. Of greatest concern, however, is a change in the patient's condition to unequal-size pupils (anisocoria) as this suggests possible herniation. As ICP increases, it can force the brain stem down through the foramen magnum of the spinal cord, and the mechanical pressure destroys the vital brain-stem functions controlling cardiac and respiratory functions. Swift intervention is required to prevent herniation, and the physician should be called immediately.

Next, test pupillary reaction to light, which helps to evaluate the optic nerve (CN-II, which carries impulses from eye to brain) and the oculomotor (CN-III, which carries impulses from the brain to eye).[25] Observe for direct and consensual pupillary light responses. Darken the room if possible. For *direct* response, cover one of the patient's eyes and shine a penlight into the pupil of the uncovered eye from the side. The pupil should constrict. Repeat with the other eye. For *consensual* light reflex, ask the patient to keep both eyes open. Shine the penlight into the right pupil from the side, and observe the left pupil constrict (both pupils should constrict); and repeat in reverse. Do the pupils constrict briskly? This is the expected response. Or is the constriction sluggish, taking a longer time to occur? Is the pupil fixed, or does it not constrict at all? Compare findings with past assessments. Note whether the patient is taking any medications that cause the pupil to dilate or whether the patient has cataracts, which can alter the response.[24] If the pupils constricted briskly before, but now one is sluggish, this reflects increased ICP and should be reported immediately to the physician.

Accommodation, or the ability of the pupils to focus at varying distances, is controlled by CN-III. Ask the patient to stare at an object in the distance, then to focus on your finger, which is held about 12 inches in front of the patient's eyes. As the patient focuses on your finger, the pupils should constrict, and the eyes should converge (come toward the center, like crossed eyes).

Extraocular eye movement is controlled by cranial nerves III, IV, and VI, and is illustrated in Figure 20-1. Table 20-2 describes cranial nerve assessment. Observe the person's gaze for *nystagmus,* a series of rapid, involuntary movements of the eyeball.[26] Prolonged lateral gaze normally may result in slight nystagmus, but greater than that should be discussed with the physician. Throughout, observe both eyes to see if they move together; *disconjugate gaze* suggests dysfunction in the extraocular muscles. Observe the pupils for *ptosis,* or drooping eyelid. If increased ICP damages CN-III (which controls the muscles elevating the eyelid), the pupil will be dilated and nonreactive, and the lid will droop. The patient will not be able to move the eyeball up, down, or inward, as is possible with normal gaze. Damage to CN-IV will result in abnormal downward and inward movement of the eyeballs; damage to CN-VI prevents upward and outward eyeball rotation.[27] Ask a family member if the patient has had previously unequal pupils, or strabismus, which might explain a disconjugate gaze.

Ophthalmoscopic assessment involves use of the ophthalmoscope, and because it requires continued practice to use skillfully, it is rarely performed by the staff nurse. However, the physician will further evaluate the neurological status of the patient using this instrument. Increased ICP causes dilation of the retinal vessels with resulting edema (papilledema) and may result in permanent damage to the optic nerve without prompt intervention to reduce cerebral edema.

Motor strength tests are used to evaluate voluntary and integrated movements. First, ask the patient to follow a command, such as raising two fingers in the air.[23] This tests normal response. If the patient cannot respond to commands, then a lower brain function response called *localizing* is tested (purposeful movement, such as removing a body part from a painful stimulus).

Motor strengths of the arms and legs are tested against active resistance and graded on a scale of 0 (no movement) to 5 (normal movement), as shown in Table 20-3. Gait and coordination should be assessed along with sensory and reflex functions.

Diagnostic Evaluation

Following a comprehensive neurological examination by the physician, the patient will have an MRI to evaluate and diagnose cerebral edema. MRI has surpassed CAT scanning because of its ability to provide high definition of areas of edema and the responsible lesions. If an MRI is unavailable, CAT scanning is performed. Lumbar punctures should not be performed, as the induced pressure changes can cause brain-stem herniation.

Degrees of Toxicity

Signs and symptoms arising from increased ICP range from early signs of restlessness and subtle changes in level of consciousness to changes in pupillary responses. Final late signs and symptoms, such as fixed and dilated pupils, coma, and Cushing's triad, may be preventable. Accurate and systematic nursing assessment can identify subtle changes early so that prompt and effective intervention can occur.

Symptom Management

Prevention

Primary prevention of increased ICP is not usually possible. Secondary prevention involves early identification of signs and symptoms of increased ICP so that prompt and early intervention can occur. The nurse, through close and ongoing assessment, can identify subtle changes or, through close professional relationships with the family, work with the family to report early, subtle changes.

Therapeutic Approaches

Treatment goals are to reduce cerebral edema and to manage symptoms. This is accomplished primarily through *drug therapy* to reduce cerebral edema and prevent seizures, and *fluid management,* as most causes are vasogenic (increased capillary permeability) and cytotoxic (neural cell swelling). Drugs most commonly used are shown in Table 20-10.

Surgical decompression may be indicated. This may be limited to the creation of bur holes in the frontal or occipital regions to drain the ventricles, or it may involve tumor resection, shunt insertion (ventricular to peritoneum), or excision of an area of the skull. Although uncommon, interstitial edema (obstructive hydrocephalus) may occur, but shunting procedures are usually not an acceptable option.

Therapeutic efforts to treat the underlying cause of increased ICP depend on the etiology. Modalities include insertion of an Ommaya reservoir for frequent intraventricular chemotherapy, radiation therapy to the brain, or specialized chemotherapy.

Evaluation of Therapeutic Approaches

Patient responses are evaluated in terms of (1) reduction of ICP and resolution of symptoms and deficits, (2) ability to treat underlying cause to prevent recurrence, (3) abil-

TABLE 20-10   Drugs Used in the Management of Increased Intracranial Pressure

Drug	Mechanism of Action	Dose	Side Effects
Dexamethasone	• Antiinflammatory • Limits capillary permeability • Some diuretic activity	• Initial: 8–10 mg IV • Then 4 mg q6h	• Emotional lability • Fluid retention • Peptic ulceration • Immunosuppression • Worsening diabetes or hypertension • Insomnia, headache
Mannitol	• Osmotic diuretic • Temporary measure	• 50–100 g/day IV given as bolus or drip; effect in 15–30 min lasting 3–10h	• Chronic use can cause rebound of increased ICP • Dehydration • Electrolyte imbalance (Na, Cl) • Hypertension with increased circulating blood volume and risk of congestive heart failure, pulmonary edema • Often combined with furosemide
Furosemide	• Systemic diuretic • Decreases CSF production	• May be used in place of mannitol • Dose varies	• CN-VIII (auditory) nerve damage with hearing loss • Dehydration • Hypotension • Be alert for overtreatment
Phenytoin	• Anticonvulsant • Inhibits seizure activity in motor cortex	• Loading dose of 1 g IV (50 mg/min) • 300 mg/day	• Rash, rarely exfoliative dermatitis • Nausea/vomiting • Nystagmus, confusion (dose-related) • Hypersensitivity syndrome
Phenobarbital	• Inhibits seizure activity in motor cortex	• 10–20 mg/kg IV infusion • Max 50 mg/min	• Drowsiness, lethargy • Rash, Stevens-Johnson syndrome • Rare angioedema

ity to perform self-care activities and need for assistance across care boundaries, (4) effectiveness of coping with changes in disease status and functional abilities, and (5) impact on quality of life.

Educational Tools

Nursing care approaches focus on early identification of neurological changes, prevention of increased ICP, prevention of seizures and consequent injury, prevention of hazards of immobility, drug administration and treatment-related interventions, and emotional support for patient and family. A standardized nursing care plan is shown in Table 20-11. A patient self-care guide for early assessment of increased ICP is found in Appendix 20B.

Section C: Peripheral Neuropathy

Associated Symptoms: dysesthetic pain, loss of temperature sensation, loss of position sense, loss of vibratory sense, paresthesias, weakness, ataxia

The Problem of Peripheral Neuropathy in Cancer

Peripheral neuropathy is inflammation, injury, or degeneration of the peripheral nerve fiber(s), and it occurs commonly in patients with cancer. Teravainen and Larsen[28] found that 48% of patients with lung cancer had peripheral neuropathy before beginning chemotherapy. A number of chemotherapeutic agents can cause peripheral neuropathy: 50% of individuals receiving vincristine will develop paresthesias of the hands and feet; depending on dose received, 20% to 90% of patients receiving cisplatin and approximately 62% of patients receiving paclitaxel will develop peripheral neuropathy.

Peripheral neuropathy can greatly diminish quality of life. Ostchega et al.[29] studied patients receiving high-dose cisplatin who developed neurotoxicity. They found that if an individual had symptomatic peripheral neuropathy, the individual had an increased likelihood for greater fatigue, malaise, and psychological distress. In addition, at 1 year posttreatment, those individuals had significantly decreased satisfaction with life, sense of well-being, and ability to work or perform ADLs.

Personal independence is greatly threatened by the various manifestations of peripheral neuropathy, such as severe, painful paresthesias and footdrop or wristdrop. Individuals who work with their hands and who lose fine

TABLE 20-11 Standardized Nursing Care Plan for the Patient with Increased ICP

Nursing Diagnosis	Expected Outcome	Nursing Interventions

Knowledge deficit regarding signs/symptoms of increased ICP	• Patient/family will verbalize signs/symptoms of increased ICP
	• Patient/family will call provider if signs/symptoms arise, or will come to ER
		• Assess patient/family understanding of disease process, risk for developing ICP
		• Teach patient/family to report:
		  Changes in affect, thought processes
		  Onset of restlessness, or quiet after long periods of restlessness
		  Headaches, with or without vomiting
		  Seizures
		  Any change from baseline

Altered intracranial fluid volume	• Early changes in ICP will be identified and treatment instituted promptly	• Assess neurologic status baseline periodically as needed, e.g., q1–4h, and compare to prior data:
		  Level of consciousness (LOC)
		  Pupillary size, symmetry, reaction to light
		  Extraocular movement
		  Motor function
		  Sensory function
		  Temperature, heart rate, BP, respirations
		• Maintain fluid restriction as ordered
		  Strictly monitor intake & output (I&O), total body balance
		• Notify MD immediately if status changes

Potential for injury related to activities that increase ICP	• ICP will remain the same or be decreased	• Maintain oxygenation to prevent hypoxia or hypercapnia; maintain patent airway
		  Monitor arterial blood gases, O₂ saturation
		  Suction only as needed, preoxygenate with 100% O₂, and limit suctioning to 10 sec
		• Elevate head of bed to 15–30 degrees or as ordered to promote venous drainage
		• Place patient on side to prevent aspiration if decrease in LOC
		• Bed rest as ordered
		• Prevent the Valsalva maneuver and isometric exercises
		  Teach patient alternative breathing, such as exhaling when turning or moving
		  Change position using pull sheet without patient pushing or pulling self
		  Monitor elimination status; institute bowel regimen to prevent constipation and strain at stool
		• Implement medical plan to prevent seizures, which increase ICP; institute seizure precautions
		• Monitor body temperature: assist in lowering temperature as ordered; prevent shivering
		• Minimize excessive environmental stimuli

Potential for alteration in skin integrity related to immobility	• Skin will remain intact	• Assess skin and bony prominences q1–2h • Use alternating pressure device • Provide gentle skin care with position changes q1–2h • Use high-top tennis shoes to protect toes and prevent footdrop: 2h on, 2h off
Potential for fatigue	• Patient will be rested	• Stagger nursing activities so patient has periods of rest between activity • Assess hematocrit, nutritional status, and discuss plan to minimize deficits
Potential for ineffective breathing patterns	• Patient will maintain normal breathing patterns if possible • Patient will remain well oxygenated	• Assess baseline respiratory pattern and breath sounds for presence of crackles, rhonchi, wheezes • Maintain oxygenation (see potential for injury related to increased ICP)
Potential for ineffective communication, related to deficits, decreased LOC	• Patient will communicate concerns if possible	• Assess patient's ability to communicate • If current communication system ineffective, develop creative alternative methods • Assess patient frequently, depending on needs

(continued)

TABLE 20-11 Standardized Nursing Care Plan for the Patient with Increased ICP (continued)

Nursing Diagnosis	Expected Outcome	Nursing Interventions
Potential for physical injury related to motor/sensory deficits	• Patient will be free from physical injury	• Assess safety risk based on motor/sensory deficits • Remove environmental hazards • Keep side rails up as appropriate, and bell cord within reach • Assist with activity as needed • Protect from thermal injury
Alteration in fluid and electrolyte balance related to diuretics	• Electrolytes will be within normal limits • Desired fluid balance will be maintained	• Assess electrolytes baseline periodically • Strictly monitor I&O, total body balance • Discuss alterations with MD
Potential for ineffective coping	• Patient will verbalize coping strategies, if possible	• Assess affect • Discuss losses, fears, strengths • Discuss previous coping strategies • Discuss alternative coping strategies • Involve social worker, chaplain, family, as appropriate
Potential for alteration in nutrition, related to decreased LOC	• Nutritional needs will be maintained	• Assess nutritional needs and ability to meet them based on physical and psychological status • Discuss nutritional alternatives with healthcare team

Data compiled from references [20,22].

motor control may have to find new employment. Rehabilitation and measures to reduce disability are critical, as is emotional support to prevent loss of self-esteem.

Etiology

Tumor, chemotherapy, or radiation therapy can each cause injury to the peripheral nerves, resulting in peripheral neuropathy. Chemotherapy (e.g., vincristine, cisplatin) can cause axonal degeneration and demyelination.

Pathophysiology

The peripheral nervous system is composed of 43 pairs of nerves: 12 pairs of cranial nerves, and 31 pairs that enter the spinal cord and become the spinal nerves.[30] All nerve fibers are enclosed within a Schwann cell, but some are more tightly wrapped in Schwann cell layers forming a myelin sheath. This enhances the speed of conduction of the nerve impulse.

The spinal nerves have both afferent and efferent fibers. The afferent fibers carry impulses from the periphery to the CNS: these fibers have their long axon and cell body outside the CNS. The sensory neuron has its cell body in the dorsal root ganglion. The efferent neurons carry impulses from the CNS to the muscles (somatic) and glands/organs (autonomic). The cell body of the somatic (motor) neuron lies within the spinal cord with the axon

in the periphery, while the autonomic neuron has its cell body in a ganglion outside the cord. This is important to know because, when the peripheral nerve is injured, it can be regenerated as long as the damage does not involve the cell body and occurs outside the spinal cord.[30] The surviving axon grows new branches to innervate muscle areas that have lost innervation due to injury.

Compression by tumor or radiation-induced injury to the brachial or lumbar plexus can cause peripheral nerve injury. Direct damage to the nerve as well as to the microvasculature results in pain.

In small-cell lung cancer, a paraneoplastic process causes the production of autoantibodies against the sensory dorsal root ganglia, causing sensory neuropathy. The symptom constellation consists of progressive loss of sensory function, loss of deep tendon reflexes, and dysesthetic pain (burning, lancinating pain).[31]

Finally, and most commonly, peripheral neuropathy is caused by the chemotherapeutic agents vinca alkaloids (vincristine), cisplatin, paclitaxel, and the podophyllotoxins (etoposide and teniposide). The sensory and motor axons are injured, as are the Schwann cells and, if involved, the myelin sheath. Demyelination reduces nerve conduction velocity, leading to loss of deep tendon reflexes. Deep tendon reflex loss is greater in the ankles than in the knees and arms.[32] Individuals at greatest risk are those with preexisting peripheral neuropathy, such as individuals with diabetes, alcoholism, or severe malnutrition.

Chemotherapeutic Agents

Vincristine is the most neurotoxic of the drugs, causing axonal sensorimotor neuropathy. The mechanism of action of this drug, as with vindesine and vinblastine, is mitotic inhibition. Apparently, the microtubules in the axon transport system are inhibited as well, resulting in axonal degeneration.[33] Initial symptoms are sequential: myalgias, painful paresthesias of the hands and feet, sensitivity to light touch and temperature, and decreased ankle reflexes.[33] Continued drug administration often leads to motor weakness in the wrist (extensors) and foot (dorsiflexors), resulting in wristdrop or footdrop, and this may occur in 22 to 34% of patients.[34] Neuropathy is usually bilateral and worse in the lower extremities, so that further motor weakness creates a broad-based stance with a slapping gait.[35] Drug discontinuance when paresthesias first appear will result in brisk resolution, whereas motor weakness may take months, and sensory loss years, to resolve.[35]

Damage to the autonomic fibers can occur, rarely resulting in dizziness (orthostatic hypotension), constipation (slowed peristalsis), abdominal colicky pain, ileus, impotence, urinary retention, and SIADH.

Cranial nerve injury can result in bilateral palsies (bilateral ptosis, diplopia), recurrent laryngeal nerve damage (vocal cord paresis and hoarseness), trigeminal nerve inflammation (jaw pain), photophobia, and transient cortical blindness.[35,36]

Although the other vinca alkaloids may also cause neurotoxicity, they are in order of decreasing risk: vincristine > vindesine > vinblastine.[36] Factors that increase risk of neurotoxicity with vincristine are (1) frequent drug administration, such as weekly; (2) dose greater than 2 mg; (3) age greater than 60 years; (4) concomitant isoniazid, teniposide, or etoposide therapy; and (5) severe liver dysfunction as the drug undergoes hepatic metabolism and clearance.[37]

Cisplatin is a heavy metal and appears to cause segmental demyelination of the large sensory nerves.[38] Extent of injury is dose related, and as cumulative doses approach 500 mg/m^2, almost 100% of patients will experience some degree of sensorimotor neuropathy.[32] Risk appears increased in the presence of hypomagnesemia.[39] As cisplatin induces renal abnormalities that cause magnesium wasting, magnesium must be repleted via the hydration solution. It is not clear whether this prevents worsened peripheral neuropathy.

Sensory deficits predominate, and the earliest sign is decreased vibratory sense.[33] Other sensory losses may include position and light touch. There may be hypersensitivity to pain. Sensory losses are usually bilateral, and follow a "glove and stocking" distribution.[34] Distal paresthesias occur next and can lead to difficulty with fine motor movement such as writing or buttoning a shirt. Decreased ankle reflexes may progress to absent reflexes with footdrop, causing a slapping gait. Motor symptoms include weakness of distal muscles and leg cramping. The patient may develop Lhermitte's sign, a sudden electric shock–like sensation as the neck is flexed. As the neuropathy progresses, neuropathic pain may develop. With se-

vere neuropathy, the individual has a broad-based stance, and as position sense becomes impaired, sensory ataxia and loss of balance result. Potential for injury and severe disability is great.

Cranial nerve injury related to cisplatin involves auditory and visual changes. The drug appears to cause loss of the hairs in the organ of Corti in the inner ear, causing *hearing loss*. Hearing loss begins with asymptomatic loss of high-frequency pure tone sounds that is manifested on audiogram. Tinnitus is the first symptom to appear and affects 60 to 70% of patients. If the drug is stopped at this point, tinnitus will resolve. With continued drug use, symptomatic loss of medium-frequency sounds occurs and may be permanent. Damage to the retina also may occur after high-dose cisplatin and can cause *blurred vision* and *impaired color vision* (color saturation and discrimination along the blue-yellow axis).[40] In a patient survey, Holden and Felde[41] demonstrated that this loss of precise color vision was extremely distressing. Other uncommon problems relating to heavy metal toxicity are *papilledema, retrobulbar neuritis* (inflammation of the optic nerve causing decreased visual acuity and eye pain), and *transient blindness.*

Although less neurotoxic, the analog carboplatin causes paresthesias in approximately 5% of patients at usual doses, and the incidence increases with high doses.[34]

Paclitaxel causes axonal degeneration and demyelination, probably related to its action of increasing microtubular accumulation in the nerve.[42] Risk of neurotoxicity is increased with the concomitant administration of neurotoxic drugs such as cisplatin, when paclitaxel is given in high doses (>200 mg/m^2), when high cumulative doses are given, and in patients with preexisting diabetes or alcoholism.

The neuropathy is primarily sensory, beginning with paresthesias of hands and feet (burning, tingling, numbness) in a glove and stocking distribution. Alterations in proprioception and vibration sense often result in difficulty climbing stairs.[43] Loss of deep tendon reflexes, leg muscle weakness, and loss of fine motor movement (e.g., difficulty buttoning clothing) may occur as well. While mild symptoms may appear 1 to 3 days after high-dose paclitaxel, resolving in 3 to 6 months after drug discontinuance, more severe symptoms may resolve only partially.[43]

Assessment

Physical Assessment

Clinical nursing parameters to be assessed for the patient with actual or potential peripheral neuropathy include sensory, motor, autonomic, and cranial nerve functions.[34]

Assessment should include the following items in the history and physical exam:

History

- Assess risk for development of peripheral neuropathy: Does the patient have a history of diabetes mellitus or alcoholism?
- Assess medication profile: Does the patient take isoniazid? If receiving cisplatin, is the patient taking other neurotoxic agents such as gentamicin? Is the patient receiving concomitant neurotoxic chemotherapy drugs (vincristine, etoposide, cisplatin, paclitaxel)?
- How well can the patient perform self-care activities? What are the limitations?

Review of systems

- HEENT (Head, Eyes, Ears, Nose, Throat): Usual vision? Any blurring of vision? Any changes in visual acuity, color perception? Any difficulty seeing traffic lights? Usual hearing? Any tinnitus? Decreased hearing?
- Gastrointestinal: Usual bowel elimination pattern? Any changes? Constipation? Colicky abdominal pain?
- Genitourinary: Usual bladder pattern? Any changes?
- Musculoskeletal: Any muscle weakness, cramping, abnormal gait, falls?
- Neurologic: Numbness, tingling of hands or feet or around mouth? Any change in ability to write name? Any loss of sensation (e.g., to temperature, vibration, touch, pain)? Any weakness or paralysis? Any pain? Ask location, intensity, character—burning, lancinating?

Physical exam

- Vital signs: Assess for orthostatic changes.
- Cranial Nerves: See Table 20-2.
- Vibration is often the first sensation lost in peripheral neuropathy. See Table 20-4.
- Motor Function: Assess gait, muscle strength and tone, reflexes, and Romberg test. See Table 20-3. Patients with early motor neuropathy may be asymptomatic and show only decreased (hypoactive) Achilles tendon reflex(es). Reflex response diminishes with continued drug administration and may disappear eventually, resulting in weakened muscles of the hands and feet (wristdrop and footdrop).

Diagnostic Evaluation

Nerve conduction studies can help identify the severity and location of peripheral neuropathy. A nerve is stimulated and response recorded either at the muscle (motor nerve) or further down the nerve (sensory nerve).[44] The results of the tests are latency period (time between stimulus and response), conduction velocity in meters per second, and amplitude of response. Testing is combined with *electromyography* (EMG) to identify early axonal degeneration (normal conduction velocity but abnormal EMG), and demyelination (reduced conduction velocity and normal EMG). Nerve conduction studies are usually performed serially. Limitations include the fact that only specific areas of the nerve are tested, and the results may not reflect all injured nerves. The procedure requires the patient to lie down for the test, which lasts 20 to 60 minutes. Paste and electrodes are taped to the skin over muscles and nerves. Mildly uncomfortable electric shocks are felt as both sides of the body are tested.[44]

Electromyography is useful in detecting early axonal neuropathy (denervation changes) and muscle atrophy related to neuropathy. Needles are inserted into muscle and electrical activity is measured (muscle action potentials, interference patterns with maximal contraction). Abnormal interference patterns (less than normal) may be due to poor effort, denervation with reduced nerve conduction to the muscle, or reduced muscle contraction ability (myopathy). Although the needles used are quite thin with only slight risk of bleeding or infection, this test may be contraindicated in patients with increased risk of bleeding. The procedure requires the patient to lie down while thin needles are inserted into the muscles. The patient feels discomfort during insertion and when the muscles contract. The test lasts 30 to 60 minutes.[44]

Audiometry assesses pure tone hearing and high- and low-frequency hearing; it includes speech audiometry, tone decay testing, and acoustic reflex testing. Baseline testing is useful for comparison with serial audiograms for patients undergoing cisplatin chemotherapy. This is especially recommended for patients with preexisting hearing loss. The patient sits in a small, soundproof testing room. The patient wears headphones to listen to varying frequencies, and the test lasts 40 to 60 minutes.

Degrees of Toxicity

Camp-Sorrell[45] suggests the following toxicity scoring method:

Neurosensory

0 = none
1 = mild paresthesias, loss of deep tendon reflexes
2 = mild or moderate objective sensory loss, moderate paresthesias
3 = severe objective loss, or paresthesias that interfere with function

Neuromotor

0 = none
1 = subjective weakness
2 = mild objective weakness
3 = objective weakness, with impairment of function
4 = paralysis

Symptom Management

Prevention

Generally, primary prevention is not possible, although pretreatment with amifostine has been shown to be effective in reducing the incidence and intensity of neurotoxicity following cisplatin chemotherapy.[46] Although the onset often cannot be prevented, progression to severe or permanent neuropathy can be averted by cessation of chemotherapy. Assessment by the nurse is crucial to early identification of toxicity and to ongoing monitoring of progress so that timely decisions can be made. The nurse must be a patient advocate, ensuring that the patient is empowered to discuss risks and benefits of drug continuance or discontinuance or of changing to another chemotherapeutic regimen.

Therapeutic Approaches

Treatment of neuropathy is symptomatic and requires input from the multidisciplinary team. Care is directed toward relief of pain, disability, and emotional distress through the use of drugs, rehabilitation, and psychosocial support.

Sensory deficits place the patient at risk for injury; thus, safety is a primary concern. For example, the patient with loss of temperature sensation should be instructed in how to assess temperature. Referral to an occupational therapist should be made to evaluate appropriate assistive devices if the patient has difficulty with hand grips. Herbison et al.[47] describe exercise therapies that may increase sensory perception (skin stimulation). Pain is often a major concern. Neuropathic (dysesthetic) pain is often unrelieved by narcotics and requires treatment with a tricyclic antidepressant agent such as amitriptyline, an anticonvulsant such as phenytoin, or carbamazepine if there is a lancinating component.

Physical therapy may help patients with motor deficits strengthen muscles that are weak. Usual exercises are range of motion, stretching, and massage.[35] In addition, the physical therapist can make recommendations for assistive devices such as orthotic braces, canes, and appropriate splints. High-top tennis shoes may help the patient with footdrop and gait disturbances.[35] Loss of fine motor movement especially may have a significant impact on quality of life, so attention to self-esteem and life satisfaction is very important.

Patient self-assessment for autonomic dysfunction (bowel and bladder) is very important, along with specific self-care measures. For example, during chemotherapy with vincristine or other vinca alkaloids, constipation can be prevented through the use of bowel regimens that promote regular bowel evacuation. Patient/family teaching should include high-fiber diet, fluid intake of 2 to 3 liters per day, and exercise, as well as the use of suppositories or cathartics as ordered.

Cranial nerve deficits include loss of hearing and visual changes. Patients at high risk for hearing loss should have audiograms performed prior to and during therapy to identify losses. If significant abnormalities appear, discussion of risk versus benefit of continued therapy should occur between the healthcare team and the patient. Patients should be instructed to report early changes in hearing such as tinnitus, and again, this will prompt risk-versus-benefit discussions between patient and provider.

Educational Tools

A standardized nursing care plan appears in Table 20-12. A patient teaching tool for early identification of peripheral neuropathy is provided in Appendix 20C.

Section D: Cerebellar Syndromes

Associated Symptoms: unsteady gait, slurred speech, dizziness, difficulty writing, loss of balance, double vision

The Problem of Cerebellar Syndromes in Cancer

The incidence of cerebellar complications in cancer is low; for example, as a side effect of 5-fluorouracil (5-FU) chemotherapy, the incidence is 3% to 7%. The consequences, however, can be severe. Cerebellar dysfunction affects the ability to perform integrated, coordinated movements; balance; and the ability to communicate verbally. Alterations in these critical human functions seriously compromise quality of life. Loss of consecutive, swift, and coordinated motor movement results in awkward, jerky movements and intention tremor and may prevent the performance of self-care activities, causing dependency on others. Ataxia may be limited to a wide, awkward gait, with risk of falling and injury, or may extend to complete truncal ataxia and immobility. Loss of coordinated speech-muscle movement results in dysarthria, which often leads to inability to communicate verbally with resulting frustration, irritability, and social isolation.

TABLE 20-12 Standardized Nursing Care Plan for the Patient with Peripheral Neuropathy

Nursing Diagnosis	Expected Outcome	Nursing Interventions
I. Potential for injury related to ↓ sensitivity to temperature, gait disturbance, ↓ proprioception	I. A. Patient will be without injury B. Patient will report changes in tactile and proprioceptive function C. Patient will develop safe measures to compensate for losses	I. A. Assess integrity of *tactile* and *proprioceptive* functions 1. Sensory perception to light touch, pinprick, vibration, temperature; vision, color vision 2. Patient's ability to tolerate light touch, cool water, presence of numbness and tingling, presence of painful sensations 3. Proprioception testing of station, gait, deep tendon reflexes, muscle weakness or atrophy, and balance 4. Patient's ability to sense placement of body parts, ability to write, evidence of muscle weakness B. Discuss alterations in sensation, proprioception, and impact on ability to do activities of daily living (ADLs) C. Discuss alternative strategies to prevent injury 1. Instruct patient in safety measures and use of visual cues 2. Encourage patient to take time to complete activities, focus attention to task 3. Use potholder when cooking 4. Use gloves when washing dishes, gardening 5. Inspect skin for cuts, abrasions, burns daily, especially arms, legs, toes, fingers D. Refer as appropriate for occupational or physical therapy, diagnostic testing using EMG E. If patient presents with S/S of peripheral neuropathy, hold chemotherapy and discuss with physician.
II. Potential for impaired self-care related to tactile and proprioception dysfunction	II. A. Patient will identify activities of self-care that are difficult B. Patient will identify strategies to meet needs	II. A. Assess patient's ability to perform ADLs such as eating, hygiene, dressing, walking, and handwriting B. Discuss and develop strategies to meet self-care needs 1. Referral to occupational therapy for splint, etc. 2. Involve family members in care planning 3. Community resource referral as appropriate (home-maker, home health aide, visiting nurse)
III. Potential for alteration in comfort related to painful paresthesias	III. A. Patient will have decreased pain	III. A. Assess comfort level and presence of severe tingling or prickling sensation, cramping or burning B. Assess intensity, quality, and frequency of discomfort C. Identify precipitating factors, such as warm or cold stimulation, and develop realistic plan to avoid precipitating factors D. Consider adjunctive analgesics with neurologic action for dysesthetic pain: amitriptyline HCl, phenytoin sodium E. Consider nonpharmacologic intervention: teach patient guided imagery, progressive muscle relaxation, massage, etc.
IV. Impaired mobility related to decreased proprioception, muscle dysfunction	IV. A. Patient will ambulate safely	IV. A. Assess level of activity, muscle strength, and mobility level prior to chemotherapy, then prior to each treatment, and at each visit once therapy is completed B. Encourage use of visual cues to determine position of body parts C. Teach measures to prevent injury D. Refer for physical, occupational therapy, and assistive devices as needed
V. Potential for sexual dysfunction related to altered tactile sensation, muscle weakness, changes in role	V. A. Patient and significant other (SO) will identify alterations in sexual expression B. Patient and SO will identify alternative methods of sexual expression	V. A. Discuss the impact of treatment-related dysfunction on sexuality, social role, and self-esteem B. Discuss appropriate alternative means of sexual expression C. Refer for specific sexual counseling if diminished ability to have erection D. Observe for changes in needs related to affection and emotional support

TABLE 20-12 Standardized Nursing Care Plan for the Patient with Peripheral Neuropathy (continued)

Nursing Diagnosis	Expected Outcome	Nursing Interventions
VI. Potential for role change with changes and alterations in self-esteem and self-concept related to sensory/perceptual dysfunction, changes in social function, changes in ability to perform occupational role	VI. A. Patient and family will demonstrate positive coping strategies	VI. A. Assess impact of sensory/perceptual dysfunction on social and work roles: ability to meet role expectations of self and family B. Discuss modifications in job and role, as appropriate and available C. Refer patient to occupational therapist/physical therapist to see if appliances available to foster rehabilitation (braces, etc.) D. Encourage independence and provide positive reinforcement for accomplishments E. Support patient as s/he grieves loss(es); assess need for support groups or counseling F. Support patient and family by providing information to help explain these behavioral responses to treatment-related dysfunction
VII. Potential for alteration in nutrition; less than body requirements related to taste distortions, anorexia, hypersensitivity to foods	VII. A. Patient will eat balanced diet from four food groups B. Patient attains ideal body weight following completion of treatment	VII. A. Assess dietary preferences, changes in food tolerances B. Teach patient to select high-calorie, high-protein foods C. Suggest dietary modifications based on taste changes: e.g., Crazy Jane Salt and spices if foods are tasteless D. Perform periodic weights prior to each treatment cycle E. Evaluate ability to do fine motor movements to feed self, cook F. Referral to nutritionist or dietitian as needed G. Monitor laboratory values, especially magnesium and calcium if on cisplatin therapy

VIII. Knowledge deficit related to self-care measures related to neuropathic changes	VIII. A. Patient identifies risk of development of neuropathy
	B. Patient identifies signs and symptoms to report to healthcare provider
		VIII. A. Teach patient regarding potential side effect(s) of neuropathy
		1. Constipation
		2. Numbness/tingling in hands/feet
		3. Motor weakness
		  a. Gait changes (e.g., footdrop)
		  b. Loss of fine-motor movement (buttoning shirt, picking up dime)
		4. Inability of males to have erection
		5. Difficulty urinating
		B. Teach patient to report the occurrence of signs and symptoms of neuropathies

Source: Barton-Burke M, Wilkes GM, Berg D, Bean K, Ingwerson K: *Cancer Chemotherapy: A Nursing Process Approach.* © 1996, Sudbury: Jones and Bartlett Publishers, pp. 177–179. Reprinted with permission.[47]

Etiology

Cerebellar syndromes can result from primary or metastatic malignancy or as a complication of chemotherapy. Antineoplastic agents that may cause cerebellar neuropathy are high-dose cytosine arabinoside (HD-ara-C) and 5-FU.

Pathophysiology

The cerebellum lies between the pons, medulla, and midbrain. It is responsible for the following human functions:[49]

- Coordination of muscle activity
- Ongoing evaluation of sensory input to correct movement
- Control of fine motor movement
- Swift, consecutive, and coordinated movements
- Balance control

Signs and symptoms of cerebellar dysfunction include *nystagmus* (rapid oscillations of the eyeball), *dysdiadochocinesia* (inability to carry out alternating movements), *dysarthria* (difficulty speaking, with slurred words, slow or irregular speech, or abnormal pauses between vowels as with scanning speech), *dysmetria* (difficulty judging distances in coordinated motor activity), *intention tremors*, and *ataxia* (staggering gait and postural imbalance).

Cerebellar degeneration rarely may be associated with breast and ovarian adenocarcinomas and appears to occur as a result of anti-Purkinje cell antibodies with resultant diffuse loss of Purkinje (neuron) cells. This paraneoplastic syndrome does not improve with treatment of the underlying disease and progresses to moderate to severe cerebellar dysfunction. Signs and symptoms include ataxia, dementia, dysarthria, and weakness related to decreased skeletal muscle tone (hypotonia).[50] Chemotherapy-induced cerebellar dysfunction is most often associated with two antineoplastic agents: high-dose cytosine arabinoside and fluorouracil.

High-Dose Cytosine Arabinoside

Also called ara-C and cytarabine, this agent causes cerebellar neuropathy at cumulative doses exceeding 36 g/m^2 (3 g/m^2, given every 12 hours for 12 doses), and this is a dose-limiting toxicity. The incidence is 11% to 28%, depending on cumulative dose. Age greater than 50 is a known risk factor, and hepatic and/or renal dysfunction, preexisting neurological dysfunction (e.g., stroke), previous cranial radiation, and intrathecal chemotherapy are suspected risks.[35] The drug readily crosses the blood-brain barrier and causes degenerative changes in the cerebellum.[51] Barnett et al.[52] describe pathological changes in severe cases: loss of Purkinje cells, loss of neurons in the dentate nucleus (motor cortex trigger, responsible for intentional and ongoing movements), and gliosis.

Toxicity usually occurs 3 to 10 days after the initiation of therapy and is reversible within 2 to 14 days after drug cessation.[53] The earliest sign is horizontal nystagmus. Other early signs are dysarthria (slurred speech), dysmetria (e.g., as shown in irregular handwriting), intention tremors, and dysdiadochocinesia.[35] If the drug is *not* stopped when nystagmus or other early signs first appear, more serious and possibly irreversible dysfunction may develop, such as gait ataxia and truncal ataxia.[51] Lethargy, confusion, memory loss, disorientation, and seizures may also appear.[54]

Fluorouracil

This agent, also called 5-FU, can cause an acute cerebellar syndrome when given in high doses as a bolus infusion. It is believed that the high peak serum drug levels are responsible, and drug regimens containing loading doses, monthly 5-day courses, or doses of 15–20 mg/kg/week are implicated.[55] The drug crosses the blood-brain barrier easily, and pathological changes in the cerebellum include chromatolysis of neurons in the olivary nucleus (densely packed nerve cells that coordinate movement) and dentate nucleus, and loss of neurons in the granular layer of the cerebellum.[56]

Signs and symptoms arise 2 to 6 months after treatment has begun.[57] Symptoms include dysmetria, ataxia (truncal and/or extremities), unsteady gait, intention tremor, slurred speech, and dizziness. Signs include

coarse nystagmus, oculomotor disturbances, and swaying or loss of balance while standing with feet together. The syndrome is reversible, with symptoms resolving 1 to 6 weeks after dose reduction or drug cessation.[55]

Assessment

Measurement Tools

A clinical neurological assessment tool that evaluates the following is appropriate:[34,35]

- Speech patterns
- Cranial nerve III (oculomotor)
- Smoothness of truncal movement
- Gait
- Posture (lying, sitting, standing)
- Rapid alternating movements
- Finger-to-nose coordination
- Balance (Romberg test)

Physical Assessment

Directed examination focuses on ocular movement, coordinated movement, and equilibrium/balance. Assess the patient's *speech pattern* and compare with baseline. Is the speech slurred? Is it slow or irregular? Is there scanning, with abnormal pauses between words or syllables?[35] Dysarthria most likely indicates cerebellar dysfunction.

Assess oculomotor function (cranial nerve III). Refer to Table 20-2 (cranial nerve assessment) and Figure 20-1 (assessment of extraocular movement). Observe for *nystagmus* (rhythmic oscillation like an ocular tremor[26]). Slight nystagmus (a few beats of fine oscillation) may be normal during extreme lateral gaze. However, coarse nystagmus may occur with cerebellar dysfunction, which can be vertical (when the patient looks up and down), horizontal (when the patient looks from side to side), or rotary.[26] Assess also for *double vision* (diplopia).

Note *posture* and *position* of the patient's body when lying, sitting, and standing. Assess successive coordinated motor function by asking the patient to do rapid alternating movements with the hands and feet. Tell the patient to lightly slap first one side and then the other side of the same hand on the thigh as rapidly as possible. Observe for speed and smooth, coordinated movement. Repeat with the other hand. If the patient has slow, irregular, or clumsy movements, this is *dysdiadochocinesia,* a symptom of cerebellar dysfunction.[26] To test the lower extremities, ask the patient to alternately tap the ball of each foot against your open hand as fast as possible.

Test point-to-point movement by asking the patient

to use the index finger to repeatedly touch first your index finger and then his/her own nose. Move your index finger so that the patient must reach to touch it. Repeat with the other hand. Then, holding your finger in place, ask the patient to touch your finger and then his/her own nose repeatedly with eyes closed. Repeat with the other hand. To test the lower extremities, have the patient put the right heel on the left knee, then slide the heel down the leg to the toes, first with the eyes open, then with them closed. Repeat with the left heel on the right leg.[26] Observe for smooth, controlled, coordinated movement. *Dysmetria* is the loss of this ability (inability to control direction, speed, and power of movement),[35] resulting in jerky, clumsy, and unsteady movements. If the movement becomes uncoordinated when the eyes are closed, this is consistent with cerebellar dysfunction: inaccuracy due to loss of position sense and overreaching (to the side or past the target called *past pointing*). Observe also for *intention tremors*, especially at the end of movement (tremor is absent at rest but appears and worsens as the finger approaches the target).

Assess the patient's *gait:* observe the patient walking across the room and back again. Is the posture erect? Is the movement balanced? Do the arms swing easily at the sides? Is the movement during the turn coordinated? Ataxia, a staggering gait and loss of postural balance, may be an early sign of cerebellar dysfunction or loss of position sense.[26] Next, ask the patient to walk heel-to-toe (tandem walking); and to walk on the balls of the feet for a few steps, then on the heels of the feet for a few steps. Other tests that may elicit ataxia include asking the patient to hop in place on first one foot, then the other; and asking the patient to do a knee bend, first with one leg, then the other.[26] If the patient is not well enough to do these tests safely, then observe the patient rising from a supine position, without using the arms for support; and stepping up onto a stool.

Last, the *Romberg* test is used to evaluate position, and if positive (present), signifies cerebellar dysfunction. Ask the patient to (1) stand with feet together, eyes open, then (2) close eyes for 20 to 30 seconds or longer without support. A slight sway is normal. The nurse must stand with arms extended around the patient lest the patient fall or lose balance. If the person can stand steadily with eyes open but loses balance when the eyes are closed, this suggests loss of position sense. In cerebellar ataxia, the patient has equal difficulty standing with feet together when eyes are open and closed.[26] The need for a broader stance may be an early sign of cerebellar ataxia; severe dysfunction is manifested by a broad-based stance with unsteady, staggering gait, and loss of balance.[35]

The test for *pronator drift* can be combined with the Romberg test or done separately with the patient sitting. Ask the patient to extend the arms with palms up, then close the eyes for 20 to 30 seconds. Observe whether the arms remain extended or if there is a downward drift of one of the arms (hemiparesis). Tap the arms downward using a brisk movement. Normally the arms should return to the original, horizontal position. If the arms overshoot the original position with jerky movements, this is consistent with cerebellar incoordination.[26]

Diagnostic Evaluation

If symptoms arise from malignancy, an MRI or CAT scan of the head, with emphasis on the cerebellum, is performed. If symptoms arise in a patient receiving chemotherapy capable of causing cerebellar dysfunction, a comprehensive neurological evaluation is performed, usually by a neurologist.

Degrees of Toxicity

Neurocerebellar toxicity can be graded as follows:[45]

    0 = none
    1 = slight
    2 = intention tremor, dysmetria, slurred speech
    3 = locomotor ataxia
    4 = cerebellar necrosis

Symptom Management

Prevention

Prevention is often possible for patients receiving HD-ara-C; for patients receiving fluorouracil, early detection of cerebellar dysfunction is the key as symptoms are reversible with dose reduction or drug cessation.

Efforts to prevent cerebellar toxicity from HD-ara-C are very important to prevent irreversible toxicity: cumulative doses should not exceed 24 to 36 g/m^2, and doses should be lowered for patients over 50 years of age (2 g/m^2, with cumulative doses of 24 g/m^2). In addition, patient's renal and hepatic status should be monitored, with dose reductions as appropriate. The drug should be withheld for 24 hours if nystagmus alone develops and discontinued entirely if nystagmus and other symptoms occur.[52]

Therapeutic Approaches

Patients receiving HD-ara-C should be assessed for cerebellar function prior to each dose (e.g., presence of nystagmus, handwriting ability, gait, rapid alternating movements, and point-to-point coordination).[58] Ongoing neurological assessment of patients will lead to early identification of symptoms, prompt intervention (drug dose reduction, delay, or drug discontinuance), and prevention of severe, irreversible toxicity.[35,36]

TABLE 20-13 Standardized Nursing Care Plan for the Patient with Potential or Actual Cerebellar Dysfunction

Nursing Diagnosis	Expected Outcome	Nursing Interventions
Potential for cerebellar injury, related to chemotherapy	Early signs/symptoms of cerebellar toxicity will be identified	1. Assess baseline cerebellar function and prior to each treatment: • Speech pattern • Gait • Coordinated movements (e.g., handwriting) • Ocular movements (presence of nystagmus) • Rapid alternating hand, foot movements • Point-to-point movement (finger to nose to finger) • Intention tremor 2. Assess patient risk for developing cerebellar toxicity (age > 50, cumulative dose of ara-C, preexisting neurologic dysfunction, renal or hepatic dysfunction, previous cranial radiotherapy or intrathecal chemotherapy) 3. Notify physician if nystagmus or any signs/symptoms appear 4. Discuss with physician withholding HD-ara-C for 24 hours if nystagmus occurs, or discontinuing drug if other signs/symptoms occur; if patient receiving 5-FU, discuss dose reduction or drug cessation
Potential for injury related to gait disturbance, loss of balance, motor incoordination, diplopia	Patient will be without injury	1. Assess patient's baseline level of activity, mobility, and ability to do tandem walking prior to chemotherapy and before each treatment 2. Assess safety features of room or home; assess need for assistive devices; keep needed objects close by 3. Refer patient to occupational or physical therapist 4. Teach patient to use wide-based stance and to walk slowly 5. Treat diplopia with patch over eye, alternating eye q4h; teach patient that depth perception will be reduced and not to drive while wearing the patch
Ineffective communication patterns	Patient will communicate effectively	1. Listen carefully to patient's conversation 2. Encourage patient to speak slowly using short and simple words 3. Use creative communication tools such as magic slates as needed 4. Refer patient to speech therapist early in care if needed
Impaired mobility related to ataxia, dysdiadochocinesia	Patient will move safely	1. Assess ability to transport self (ambulation, posture) 2. Assess need for assistive devices, e.g., wheelchair, walker 3. Refer to physical therapist as needed

Potential for self-care deficit related to dysmetria	Patient will identify activities of self-care that are difficult
	
	Patient will identify strategies to meet needs
		1. Assess patient's ability to perform ADLs such as eating, hygiene, dressing, walking, and writing
		2. Discuss and develop strategies to meet self-care needs
		  a. Referral to occupational therapist for assistive devices
		  b. Involve family members in care planning
		  c. Community resource referral as appropriate (homemaker, home health aide, visiting nurse)

Potential for role changes/ alterations in self-esteem and self-concept related to disease and deficits	Patient and family will demonstrate positive coping strategies	1. Assess impact of neurological deficits on social and work roles; abilities to meet expectations of self and family 2. Discuss modifications in job and role, as appropriate and available 3. Refer to occupational therapist/physical therapist for evaluation of rehabilitation and assistive devices 4. Encourage independence and provide positive reinforcement for accomplishments 5. Reassure patient if resolution of symptoms is realistic; otherwise, support patient during grief reaction and assess need for support group or other intervention

Patients with cerebellar toxicity from primary or metastatic malignancy will be treated with corticosteroids (e.g., dexamethasone) and radiation therapy to reduce increased intracranial pressure and symptomatology. For patients whose symptoms arise from a paraneoplastic process, symptom management is the goal, as successful treatment of the underlying malignancy alone does not improve function.[1]

Nursing care is directed toward (1) early identification of neurotoxicity, (2) enhancement of patient communication techniques if dysarthria is present, (3) prevention of patient injury, and (4) minimization of immobility. Goals are to minimize or eliminate signs and symptoms of cerebellar toxicity and to ensure patient comfort, safety, and quality of life.

TABLE 20-14 Resources

American Brain Tumor Association 2720 River Road Des Plaines, IL 60018 (800) 886-2282; (847) 827-9910
American Cancer Society 1599 Clifton Road, NE Atlanta, GA 30029-4257 (404) 320-3333; (800) ACS-2345
CAnCare Cancer Partners: A Supportive Network 2929 Selwyn Avenue Charlotte, NC 28209 (704) 489-2521
Choice in Dying 250 West 57th Street New York, NY 10107 (202) 338-9790
Corporate Angels Network, Inc. Westchester County Airport, Building One White Plains, NY 10604 (914) 328-1313
Leukemia Society of America National Headquarters 733 Third Avenue New York, NY 10017 (212) 573-8484; (800) 955-4LSA
National Brain Tumor Foundation 323 Geary St., Suite 510 San Francisco, CA 94102 (415) 284-0208
National Coalition for Cancer Survivorship 1010 Wayne Avenue, 5th Floor Silver Spring, MD 20910 (301) 650-8868
Office of Cancer Communications National Cancer Institute Building 31, Room 10A 24 Bethesda, MD 20892 (800) 4-CANCER

Educational Tools and Resources

Table 20-13 describes a standardized nursing care plan for the patient at risk for or experiencing cerebellar toxicity.

See Appendix 20D for a patient self-care guide. Table 20-14 provides a list of resources for patients with neurological disturbances.

Conclusion

There are many manifestations of neurotoxicity related to malignancy or treatment. This chapter has explored only four clinical syndromes. Nurses caring for oncology patients are in an ideal position, regardless of setting, to assess early changes in patient neurological status so that prompt and often effective intervention can occur to prevent severe disability. Nurses use the nursing process to promote rehabilitation and self-care in an effort to optimize the patient's quality of life.

References

1. Hildebrand J: *Lesions of the Nervous System in Cancer Patients.* New York: Raven Press, 1988
2. Hickey JV: *The Clinical Practice of Neurological and Neurosurgical Nursing* (ed 3). Philadelphia: Lippincott, 1992
3. Adams RD, Victor M: *Principles of Neurology.* New York: McGraw-Hill, 1993
4. Young KJ, Longman AJ: Quality of life in persons with melanoma: A pilot study. *Cancer Nurs* 6:219–225, 1983
5. Stevens SA, Becker KL: Neurologic assessment, Part 1. *Nursing 88* 18:54–61, 1988
6. Stevens SA, Becker KL: Neurologic assessment, Part 2. *Nursing 88* 18:104, 1988
7. Boogerd W, van der Sande JJ: Treatment of complications: Diagnosis and treatment of malignant disease. *Cancer Treat Res* 19:129–133, 1993
8. Dyk S: Surgical instrumentation as a palliative treatment for spinal cord compression. *Oncol Nurs Forum* 18:515–523, 1991
9. Grossman S, Lossignol D: Diagnosis and treatment of epidural metastasis. *Oncology* 4:47–54, 1990
10. Siegal TA, Siegal TE: Current considerations in the management of neoplastic spinal cord compression. *Spine* 14: 223–228, 1989
11. Dietz KA, Flaherty AM: Oncologic emergencies, in Groenwald SL, Frogge MH, Goodman M, Yarbro CH (eds): *Cancer Nursing Principles and Practice* (ed 3). Sudbury: Jones and Bartlett, 1993, pp. 801–835
12. Held JL, Peahota A: Nursing care of the patient with spinal cord compression. *Oncol Nurs Forum* 20:1507–1516, 1993
13. Raney D: Malignant spinal cord tumors: A review and case presentation. *J Neurosci Nurs* 23:44–49, 1991
14. Gilbert RW, Kim JH, Posner JB: Epidural spinal cord com-

pression from metastatic tumor: Diagnosis and treatment. *Ann Neurol* 3:40–51, 1978

15. Kim RY, Spencer SA, Meredith RF, et al: Extradural spinal cord compression: Analysis of factors determining functional prognosis. *Radiology* 176:279–289, 1990

16. Burgess KE: Neurological disturbances in the patient with intracranial neoplasm: Sources and implications for nursing care. *J Neurosurg Nurs* 54:237–242, 1983

17. Wilkes GM, Ingwerson K, Barton-Burke M: *Oncology Nursing Drug Reference.* Sudbury: Jones and Bartlett, 1997

18. Fuller B, Heiss J, Oldfield EH: Spinal cord compression, in DeVita VT, Hellman S, Rosenberg SA (eds): *Cancer: Principles and Practice of Oncology* (ed 4). Philadelphia: Lippincott-Raven, 1997, pp. 2476–2486

19. Bates D, Reuler J: Back pain and epidural spinal cord compression. *J Gen Intern Med* 3:191–197, 1988

20. Saba MT, Magolan JM: Understanding cerebral edema: Implications for oncology nurses. *Oncol Nurs Forum* 18:499–500, 1991

21. Klatzo I: Neuropathologic aspects of brain edema. *J Neuropathol Exp Neurol* 26:1–14, 1967

22. McDonnell KK: Increased intracranial pressure, in Gross J, Johnson BL (eds): *Handbook of Oncology Nursing* (ed 2). Boston: Jones and Bartlett, 1994, pp. 595–608

23. Cho DY, Wang YC: Comparison of the APACHE III, APACHE II, and Glasgow Coma Scale in acute head injury for prediction of mortality and functional outcome. *Intensive Care Med* 23:77–84, 1997

24. Lower J: Rapid neuro assessment. *Am J Nurs* 92:38–45, 1992

25. Barker E, Moore K: Perfecting the art of cranial nerve assessment. *RN* 44:62–69, 1992

26. Price MB, DeVroom BL: A quick and easy guide to neurological assessment. *J Neurosurg Nurs* 17:318, 1985

27. Bates B: *A Guide to Physical Examination and History Taking.* Philadelphia: Lippincott, 1991

28. Teravainen H, Larsen A: Some features of the neuromuscular complications of pulmonary cancer. *Ann Neurol* 2:495–502, 1977

29. Ostchega Y, Monohoe M, Fox N: High dose cisplatin-related peripheral neuropathy. *Cancer Nurs* 11:23–32, 1988

30. Vander AJ, Sherman JH, Luciano DS: *Human Physiology* (ed 5). New York: McGraw-Hill, 1990

31. Posner JB: Paraneoplastic syndromes, in Posner JB (ed): *Neurologic Complications of Cancer.* Philadelphia: FA Davis, 1995, pp. 353–355

32. Weiss RB: Miscellaneous toxicities, in DeVita VT, Hellman S, Rosenberg SA (eds): *Cancer: Principles and Practice of Oncology* (ed 4). Philadelphia: Lippincott-Raven, 1997, pp. 2796–2806

33. Forman A: Peripheral neuropathy in cancer patients: Incidence, features, and patho-physiology. *Oncology* 4:57–62, 1990

34. Furlong TG: Neurologic complications of immunosuppressive cancer therapy. *Oncol Nurs Forum* 20:1337–1352, 1993

35. Meehan JL, Johnson BL: The neurotoxicity of antineoplastic agents. *Current Issues in Cancer Nursing Practice Updates* 1:1–10, 1992

36. Kaplan RS, Wiernik PH: Neurotoxicity of antineoplastic drugs. *Semin Oncol* 9:103–129, 1982

37. Legha SS: Vincristine neurotoxicity: Pathophysiology and management. *Med Toxicol* 1:421–427, 1986

38. Berry JM, Jacobs C, Sikic B, et al: Modification of cisplatin chemotherapy with diethyliathiocarbamate. *J Clin Oncol* 8:1585–1590, 1990

39. Ashraf M, Scotel RN, Krall JM, et al: Cis-platinum-induced hypomagnesemia and peripheral neuropathy. *Gynecol Oncol* 16:309–318, 1983

40. Wilding G, Caruso R, Lawrence T, et al: Retinal toxicity after high-dose cisplatin therapy. *J Clin Oncol* 3:1683–1689, 1985

41. Holden S, Felde G: Nursing care of patients experiencing cisplatin-related peripheral neuropathies. *Oncol Nurs Forum* 14:13–19, 1987

42. Lipton RB, Apfel SC, Dutcher JP, et al: Taxol produces a predominant sensory neuropathy. *Neurology* 39:368–372, 1989

43. Noone MH, Fioravanti SG: Taxol: Past, present, and future. *Oncol Nurs* 1:4, 1994

44. Josifek LF, Bleecker MI: Peripheral neuropathy, in Barker LR, Burton JR, Zieve PD (eds): *Principles of Ambulatory Medicine* (ed 3). Baltimore: Williams & Wilkins, 1991, pp. 1155–1170

45. Camp-Sorrell D: Chemotherapy: Toxicity management, in Groenwald SL, Frogge MH, Goodman M, Yarbro CH (eds): *Cancer Nursing: Principles and Practice* (ed 4). Sudbury: Jones and Bartlett, 1997, pp. 385–426

46. Kemp G, Rose P, Lurain J, et al: Amifostine pretreatment for protection against cyclophosphamide-induced and cis-platin-induced toxicities: Results of a randomized control trial in patients with advanced ovarian cancer. *J Clin Oncol* 14:2101–2112, 1996

47. Herbison GJ, Jaweed M, Ditunno JF: Exercise therapies in peripheral neuropathies. *Arch Phys Med Rehabil* 64:201–205, 1983

48. Barton-Burke M, Wilkes GM, Berg D, Bean K, Ingwersen K: *Cancer Chemotherapy: A Nursing Process Approach* (ed 2). Sudbury: Jones and Bartlett, 1996

49. Belford K: Central nervous system cancers, in Groenwald SL, Frogge MH, Goodman M, Yarbro CH (eds): *Cancer Nursing: Principles and Practice* (ed 4). Sudbury: Jones and Bartlett, 1997, pp. 980–1036

50. Hildebrand J: Signs, symptoms, and significance of paraneoplastic neurological syndromes. *Oncology* 3:57–66, 1989

51. Rubin EH, Anderson JW, Berg DT, et al: Risk factors for high-dose cytarabine neurotoxicity: An analysis of a cancer and leukemia trial of patients with acute myeloid leukemia. *J Clin Oncol* 10:948–953, 1992

52. Barnett MJ, Richards MA, Ganesan TS, et al: Central nervous system toxicity of high-dose cytosine arabinoside. *Semin Oncol* 12:571–575, 1985

53. Chabner BA: Cytidine analogues, in Chabner BA, Longo DL (eds): *Cancer Chemotherapy and Biotherapy* (ed 2). Philadelphia: Lippincott-Raven, 1996, pp. 213–233

54. Nand S, Messmore HL, Patel R, et al: Neurotoxicity associated with systemic high-dose cytosine arabinoside. *J Clin Oncol* 4:571–575, 1986

55. Weiss HD, Walker MD, Wiernik PH: Neurotoxicity of commonly used antineoplastic agents. *N Engl J Med* 291:75–81, 1974

56. Moertel CG, Reitemeier RJ, Bolton CF, et al: Cerebellar ataxia associated with fluorinated pyrimidine therapy. *Cancer Chemo Rep* 41:15–18, 1964

57. Moore DH, Fowler WC, Crumpler LS: 5-Fluorouracil neurotoxicity. *Gynecol Oncol* 36:152–154, 1990

58. Conrad KJ: Cerebellar toxicities associated with cytosine arabinoside: A nursing perspective. *Oncol Nurs Forum* 13:57–59, 1986

Spinal Cord Compression

Patient Name: _____

Symptom and Description   Spinal cord compression is a rare but serious problem of cancer. It is caused by pressure of a tumor on the spinal cord (the bundle of nerves running inside the backbone to the brain). If treatment is not begun early, then serious injury to the spinal cord can occur. When it occurs, it can affect people with cancers of the lung, breast, prostate, and other cancers that may spread to the bone, as well as multiple myeloma and lymphoma.

Learning Needs   You should notify your doctor or nurse immediately if you have any changes in your condition or if any of the following occur:

- Pain in your back, which may move to the side. The pain may be worse when you lie down, cough, sneeze, or move.
- Numbness, tingling, "loss of feeling" in toes or fingers.
- Weakness in your legs or a change in the way you walk.
- Change in your bowel or urinary habits, such as constipation or being unable to empty your bladder.
- Loss of control of bowel or bladder (incontinence).

Prevention   While it is not possible to prevent spinal cord compression, it is possible to prevent it from getting worse. The most important thing you can do is to tell your doctor or nurse immediately if any of the above symptoms occur. If you cannot reach your doctor or nurse, go to the emergency room of your hospital, tell them that you have cancer, and tell them that you have been taught that this may be an emergency.

Management   If you develop these symptoms, your doctor will examine you carefully. Your doctor *may* then order X-ray films to help evaluate the pain and may also order a bone scan. Your doctor *will* order a test (MRI scan or CAT scan) if it appears that you have this problem; these tests will show whether there is something pressing against your spinal cord. If the tests show that you have spinal cord compression, your doctor will talk to you about treatment. Early treatment has been shown to prevent serious problems.

Follow-up   Your doctor may order rehabilitation and physical therapy to minimize loss of function.

(continued) 375

Phone Numbers

Nurse: _____ Phone: _____

Physician: _____ Phone: _____

Emergency Room: _____ Phone: _____

Comments

Patient's Signature: _____ Date: _____

Nurse's Signature: _____ Date: _____

Source: Wilkes GM: Neurological disturbances, in Yarbro CH, Frogge MH, Goodman M (eds): *Cancer Symptom Management* (ed 2). Sudbury: Jones and Bartlett, 1999. © Jones and Bartlett Publishers.

Increased Intracranial Pressure

Patient Name: _____

Symptom and Description   Increased swelling in your head can cause headache, vomiting, restlessness, and drowsiness. It can also cause changes in the way you think and remember things.

Learning Needs   There are important things that you can do to prevent the swelling from increasing:

- Do not hold your breath.
- Remember to breathe in and out when you move or change position.
- Do not strain when moving your bowels. (If you are not moving your bowels easily and regularly, talk with your nurse or doctor.)
- Report any signs or symptoms of increased pressure such as severe headache or vomiting.

Prevention   The most important thing that you can do is to prevent the swelling from getting worse. Learn to use the above tips. Tell your doctor or nurse immediately if any changes develop.

Management   If you develop increased swelling in your brain (increased intracranial pressure), you will receive medicines to reduce the pressure. In addition, you will receive treatment to shrink the tumor that is causing it and prevent the pressure from increasing again. This treatment may be radiation therapy or chemotherapy.

Follow-up   Let your doctor or nurse know if you have:

- headache
- vomiting
- restlessness
- drowsiness

Phone Numbers

Nurse: _____   Phone: _____

Physician: _____   Phone: _____

Other: _____   Phone: _____

Emergency Room: _____   Phone: _____

Comments

Patient's Signature: _____   Date: _____

Nurse's Signature: _____   Date: _____

Source: Wilkes GM: Neurological disturbances, in Yarbro CH, Frogge MH, Goodman M (eds): *Cancer Symptom Management* (ed 2). Sudbury: Jones and Bartlett, 1999. © Jones and Bartlett Publishers.

Peripheral Neuropathy

Patient Name: _____

Symptom and Description   You are receiving chemotherapy for your cancer. One of the *possible* side effects is damage to the nerves in your body. This may result in a feeling of "pins and needles" or the feeling that your hands and/or feet are asleep. You may have difficulty picking up a coin or buttoning your shirt or blouse. Another problem may be constipation. It is important to tell your doctor or nurse if these or any other changes occur. Your treatment plan can be evaluated to prevent further nerve damage.

Learning Needs   You need to learn the signs and symptoms of peripheral neuropathy. Tell your doctor or nurse if/when you develop:

- A feeling of "pins or needles" or numbness in your hands and/or your feet
- Difficulty picking up an object or buttoning your shirt or blouse
- Ringing in your ears
- Difficulty hearing
- Changes in your vision
- Pain in your hands or feet
- Constipation or other changes in your bowel or bladder function
- Any other changes

Prevention   It is important for you to prevent constipation if you receive the drug vincristine, vinblastine, or vindesine:

- Drink 2 to 3 quarts of fluid a day.
- Eat a high-fiber diet (fruit, vegetables, beans, bran, prunes).
- Do moderate exercise as tolerated.
- Take a laxative as directed by your nurse or doctor if you do not move your bowels in 1 to 2 days.

Management   Although it is not possible to prevent early nerve damage, it is possible to prevent it from worsening. The most important thing that you can do is to tell your doctor or nurse immediately if any of the above symptoms occur. Then it will be important to discuss with your doctor and nurse whether your treatment should be changed.

Follow-up   Your doctor may order rehabilitation and physical therapy to minimize loss of function.

Phone Numbers

Nurse: _____ Phone: _____

Physician: _____ Phone: _____

Other: _____ Phone: _____

Comments

Patient's Signature _____ Date: _____

Nurse's Signature _____ Date: _____

Cerebellar Toxicity from High-Dose Ara-C Chemotherapy

Patient Name: _____

Symptom and Description   A rare but important side effect that may occur from your treatment is damage to the part of brain that coordinates your muscle movement (cerebellum). This will return to normal if found early.

Learning Needs   It is important for you to tell your doctor or nurse if you develop any changes in how you walk, move, or speak. For example, these changes might be:

- Slurred speech, pauses between words or parts of words, slowed speech
- Unsteady gait, stumbling when you walk, or loss of balance
- Jerky movements, such as when you reach for an object
- Tremors in your finger as you point or reach for an object
- Difficulty writing with a pen or pencil such as jerky movements as you try to write
- Double vision

Prevention   The most important thing that you can do is to tell your doctor or nurse immediately if any changes develop. Your nurse or doctor will also examine you periodically to see if there are any changes. You will be asked to do some exercises such as walking, hand and foot movements, and eye movements. You may be asked to write your name before each of your chemotherapy treatments.

Management   If you develop changes that are due to the chemotherapy, your doctor and nurse will talk to you about stopping the medicine for 24 hours or stopping it completely.

Follow-up   Call your doctor or nurse if you develope any changes in how you walk, move, or speak.

Phone Numbers

Nurse: _____ Phone: _____

Physician: _____ Phone: _____

Other: _____ Phone: _____

Comments

Patient's Signature: _____ Date: _____

Nurse's Signature: _____ Date: _____

Source: Wilkes GM: Neurological disturbances, in Yarbro CH, Frogge MH, Goodman M (eds): *Cancer Symptom Management* (ed 2). Sudbury: Jones and Bartlett, 1999. © Jones and Bartlett Publishers.

CHAPTER 21

Skin Ulcerations

Ann E. McDonald, RN, MN

The Problem of Skin Ulceration in Cancer

Individuals with cancer often suffer from acute or chronic skin ulcers. Caused by disease, treatment, and generalized morbidity, these ulcerations can occur over the entire disease trajectory. Chronic wounds can occur as a manifestation of malignancy, from a chemotherapy extravasation, from acute and late effects of radiation therapy, or, more rarely, as a consequence of surgery. There is broad consensus that individuals with ulcerating or fungating malignant lesions have a poorer prognosis.

Chronic ulcers can become the dominant focus in a person's daily life. Their symptomatology and the regular need for dressing changes can initiate a progressive series of personal, social, and financial losses, as well as changes in roles, activities, self-image, and the home environment. The persistent wound serves as a constant reminder of the presence of cancer. Family caregivers need support and education to provide physical and emotional care to the individual.

This chapter begins with a description of the healing process in normal tissue and the cellular functions that may be altered in wounds commonly seen in patients with cancer. Next, the incidence, pathophysiology, time course, and any unique characteristics of these wounds are described. The chapter continues with a discussion of patient and wound assessment, followed by suggestions for wound care and problem solving. The aim of wound care is to promote an optimal wound environment to enhance cellular functioning.

Normal Healing and Tumor Growth

Normal healing is dependent on both microcellular and macrocellular functions. Critical individual cells are attracted to the wound, where they replicate; other cell and protein substances, including plasma, insulin, epidermal growth factor (EGF), platelet-derived growth factor (PDGF), insulin-like growth factor-1, and essential amino acids, must be present in adequate supply for the three phases of healing to progress efficiently and sequentially.[2]

On a macro level, normal healing is divided into three phases: the inflammatory phase, the proliferative phase, and the maturational phase. In normal skin these phases take up to 4 days, 3 weeks, and 1 year, respectively, and involve a complex interaction of chemical mediators and cellular function. With impaired skin or metabolism, each phase takes much longer and becomes critically dependent on available substrates and cellular function.

Injury and the blood-clotting cascade initiate the inflammatory phase by activating thrombin and platelets. In the *inflammatory phase*, blood flow to the wound is increased, and monocytes, macrophages, and fibroblasts are attracted to remove debris.[3] Polymorphonuclear neutrophils combat bacterial contamination and are found in the wound within 24 hours. They release substances to continue the inflammatory response and stimulate the transformation of monocytes into macrophages. Macrophages are the predominant cell in chronic inflammation and repair. They initiate the *proliferative phase* by secreting an angiogenic factor, which stimulates the migration of angioblasts and endothelial cells to create the neovasculature that serves as the foundation for healing tissue.

During the *proliferative phase*, granulation tissue, consisting of a dense population of macrophages, fibroblasts, and neovasculature in a loose matrix of collagen, fills the wound. Attracted by hypoxia, there is continued migration of both macrophages and mesenchymal cells that are converted into fibroblasts. The wound develops an early degree of tensile strength when the fibroblasts differentiate to orient linearly and stimulate the smooth muscles to draw in the margins of the wound. Contraction can reduce the size of the wound by up to 50%. The absence of contraction is a major problem in most oncologic wounds.

Reepithelialization follows connective tissue proliferation. Full-thickness wounds that heal by secondary intention do not have dermal appendages to supply epithelial cells as in more superficial wounds. Over a period of time, the epithelial cells migrate from the wound edges. Contact inhibition stops the lateral proliferation, and radial regeneration continues to produce a multicellular layer that resurfaces the wound.

In the *maturational phase,* there is continuous matrix formation and remodeling. Fibroblasts continue to produce collagen, while proteolytic enzymes create an active balance between synthesis and lysis of collagen. Vascularity and cellularity are reduced as scar tissue forms.

Tumor microvasculature is hyperpermeable to fibrinogen and plasma colloids. Many tumors also secrete vascular permeability factor (VPF), which is ten thousand times more potent than histamine in increasing permeability. These factors account for the large amounts of fibrous exudate secreted by malignant wounds.

Platelets are absent from tumor stroma. Their function is replaced by tumor cells, which express clotting factors and secrete growth factors that are specific to the tumor cells and damaging to normal cells. The absence of platelets in malignant wounds leads them to bleed easily.[4]

Etiology and Pathophysiology

Malignant Ulcers

Malignant ulcers evolve as infiltration of the skin by cancer cells progresses. Metastatic or recurrent disease presents more often than primary disease in the form of skin ulcerations that progress to chronic wounds.

Primary malignant skin ulcers

In a review of 135 primary malignant skin ulcers, the common histologic types included lymphoma (35%), squamous cell carcinomas (27%), basal cell carcinomas (4%–15%), and malignant melanoma (9%).[5] Figure 21-1 depicts a woman with bilateral ulcerating breast cancer. Accidental mechanical implantation of malignant cells

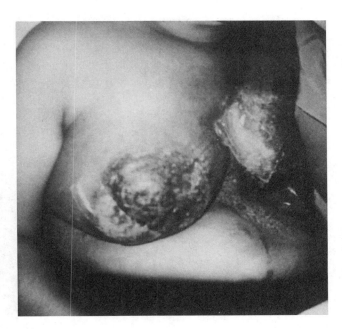

FIGURE 21-1 Bilateral ulcerating breast cancer.

during diagnostic or operative procedures can also result in cutaneous lesions.

Hematologic malignancies

Hematologic malignancies can also cause chronic wounds. One author reported 33 patients presenting with malignant ulcers.[6] Twenty of the patients had cutaneous T-cell lymphoma, ten had other types of non-Hodgkin's lymphoma, and three had leukemia. All of the patients had a poor prognosis. Most died within 9 months of the onset of the ulcers, but the average life span was 21 months.

Kaposi's sarcoma (KS)

KS, a multicentric primary, is becoming a common malignancy as a consequence of the spread of acquired immunodeficiency syndrome (AIDS). KS presents as a patch, plaque, or nodule, but can manifest as a progressive ulcer occurring anywhere on the body. KS ulcers have a necrotic base and mimic an infectious process (Figure 21-2). Following irradiation, lesions on the lower extremities are most likely to ulcerate, becoming heavily exudative. Friction, hydrostatic pressure, and the pressure of weight-bearing add to the often flawed repair process. Local radiation therapy is the most common treatment for persistent lesions.

Marjolin's ulcer

Marjolin's ulcer is the malignant transformation of a scar, usually to squamous cell carcinoma. The grade (1 to 3) predicts metastatic potential and whether a lymph

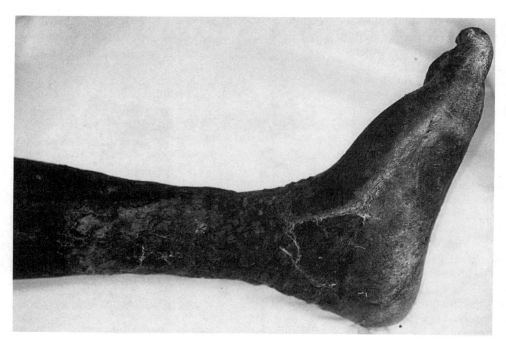

FIGURE 21-2 KS ulcer with a necrotic base.

node dissection or amputation is indicated. The overall incidence of metastasis is 35%, with a mortality rate of 33%.[7]

Pressure sore ulcer

Areas of venous stasis and chronic pressure sores are potential high-risk sites for malignant transformation. Malignancies from chronic pressure sores are usually more aggressive, well-differentiated squamous cell carcinoma with a 66% 2-year mortality rate.[8] The incidence of basal cell carcinomas in leg ulcers is reported to be as high as 9%.[9] Figure 21-3 depicts a venous stasis ulcer in a chronically lymphedematous arm.

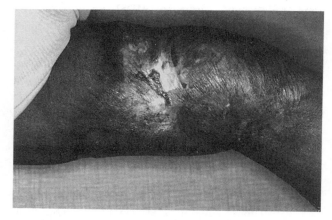

FIGURE 21-3 A venous stasis ulcer in a chronically lymphedematous arm.

Pyoderma gangrenosum (PG)

PG is a painful necrotizing ulcerative skin condition associated with systemic inflammatory diseases such as arthritis, vasculitis, infection, and inflammatory bowel disease. PG may signal malignant transformation of stable hematologic disease. Myelomas (especially IgA), polycythemia rubra vera (PRV), and acute and chronic myeloid leukemia are the most common associated diseases. Twenty-five percent of the cases of PRV transformation are fatal within the first year. With myeloma the PG usually precedes the detection of myeloma by several years.

Cutaneous metastases

Cutaneous metastases from solid tumors occur in 5% to 10% of all cancer patients with metastatic disease and may present as the initial sign of cancer.[4] Incidence of cutaneous metastasis is positively correlated with incidence rates for the primary cancer. For example, cutaneous metastases occur most frequently among women with breast cancer (18.5%–50%) (Figure 21-4) and men with bronchogenic carcinoma (3%–7.5%). These, along with melanoma, ovarian, renal, colon, gastric, and oral cavity cancers, account for 90% of cutaneous metastases. Most cutaneous metastases develop on the anterior trunk, but can be found on the pelvis, flanks, head and neck, or the posterior trunk. Cutaneous metastases often progress to necrosis and infection with ruptured capillaries, resulting in a purulent, friable, and malodorous lesion (Figure 21-5). The diagnosis and extent of disease will have an impact on the goals and expectations of healing the wound, particularly in the absence of effective cyto-

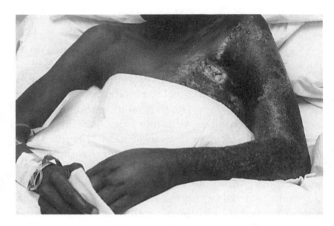

FIGURE 21-4 Cutaneous metastases from breast cancer.

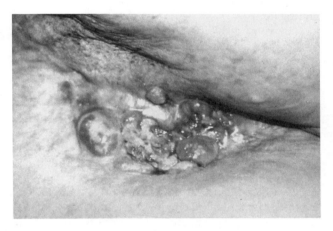

FIGURE 21-5 Cutaneous metastases from renal cell cancer.

toxic therapy. In most cases the presence of tumor in the skin occurs concurrently with other metastatic disease or generalized morbidity.

Chemotherapy Extravasation Wounds

All oncology nurses fear a chemotherapy extravasation, with the potential for pain, disfigurement, loss of function, and an ulcerative wound. *Extravasation* is defined as the accidental injection or leakage of drugs into the perivascular or subcutaneous spaces during an intravenous administration. Symptoms include pain, swelling, and erythema.

The exact incidence of extravasation has been reported in the ranges of 0.05 to 6% of all adverse effects associated with chemotherapy.[10] Only one-third of extravasations cause ulcers. A study of 329 patients reported a 6.4% incidence of local extravasation from subcutaneous ports.[11] The degree of injury is drug, dose, and concentration dependent, as well as influenced by resistance of local tissues and host factors. Extravasation injuries are most commonly induced by drugs with extreme pH, high osmolalities, high concentrations of potassium chloride and calcium salts, or the ability to induce necrosis.

A drug is categorized according to whether it is a vesicant, irritant, or nonirritant. A *vesicant* is defined as a drug that can cause tissue damage if extravasated. Most vesicants damage tissue by binding to nucleic acids, fixing to tissues, and having a prolonged noxious effect. Delayed extravasation refers to an infiltration of a drug with symptoms occurring 48 hours or more after the drug is administered. Common drugs such as potassium, nafcillin, vancomycin, norepinephrine, and dopamine can cause tissue damage, though cytotoxic agents such as doxorubicin, mitomycin C, nitrogen mustard, and vinca alkaloids are most well known. Table 20-1 lists chemotherapeutic agents by their vesicant/irritant classification.[10,12,13]

An *irritant* drug causes redness at the injection site, an inflammatory reaction in normal tissues, but no necrosis or ulceration. The effect of an irritant is briefer than that of a vesicant. It is rapidly metabolized, removed from the immediate area, and excreted.

Drug combinations may increase dermal toxicity. The interaction of methotrexate and trimethoprim is an example of a noncytotoxic agent precipitating chemotherapy toxicity and causing necrotic skin ulcers.[14] Other causes of extravasation wounds include injection sites in irradiated tissue and interferon, a drug associated with rare but serious dermatologic complications, especially in compromised tissue.

The World Health Organization developed a classifi-

TABLE 21-1 Chemotherapeutic Agents:
Vesicant and Irritant Drugs

Vesicants	Irritants
Common	**Common**
Amsacrine	Carmustine
Dactinomycin	Cisplatin
Daunorubicin	Dacarbazine
Doxorubicin	Daunorubicin, liposomal
Epirubicin	Docetaxel
Esorubicin	Etoposide
Idarubicin	Fluorouracil
Mechlorethamine	Mitoxantrone
Menogaril	Plicamycin
Mitomycin C	
Vinblastine	
Vincristine	
Vindesine	
Vinorelbine	
Rare	**Rare**
Cisplatin	Paclitaxel
Mitoxantrone	Streptozotocin
	Teniposide

cation of the toxic effects related to antineoplastic treatment. Cutaneous toxicity caused by chemotherapy is subdivided into four groups according to severity:[15]

Erythema (degree 1)

Desquamation–vesicles (degree 2)

Ulceration (degree 3)

Erythrodermas–necrosis (degree 4)

Ulceration usually does not present until 1 to 2 weeks after the injury. Gradually a dry, black eschar forms that eventually sloughs to reveal the ulcer cavity[16] (Figures 21-6 and 21-7). Local firm induration persisting for more than 24 hours indicates eventual ulceration. In some cases, the erythema does not appear for up to 2 weeks, and the entire time frame is believed to be extended. The extent of the damage is related to total dose, concentration of drug, and resistance of local tissues.

Doxorubicin acts as a radiomimetic and vesicant drug. It has a prolonged binding effect, then is released from dying cells and taken up by the adjacent cells to continue the progressive necrosis. This drug also interacts with the cell membranes and has a cell surface effect that is cytotoxic.[17]

Vasilev et al.[18] characterized the time course of a doxorubicin extravasation. Histologic evaluations revealed vasodilation and stasis at 24 hours, endothelial vacuolization at 72 hours, and ulceration of the epidermis with absence of vascularity at 5 days. The dermal ulceration is a result of collagen necrobiosis, resulting from ischemia.

The doxorubicin extravasation ulcer is typified by a necrotic, yellowish, fibrotic base, with a surrounding ring of persistent erythema. There is no significant inflammatory response with granulation tissue formation and peripheral epithelial ingrowth, which characterize normal wound healing. On histologic exam, there are multiple changes in fibroblasts. Myofibroblasts have been noted to have a normal appearance, but their action is delayed and function is altered, resulting in an absence of wound contraction.

The vinca alkaloids cause tissue damage by binding to the mitochondria of the cells, disrupting the metabolism of the cells. The tissue damage caused by these drugs has clinical characteristics similar to those of a burn.

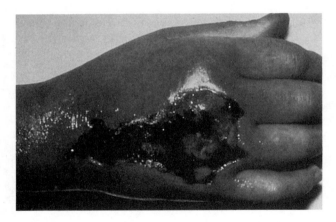

FIGURE 21-6 Doxorubicin extravasation wound depicting a characteristic eschar formation.

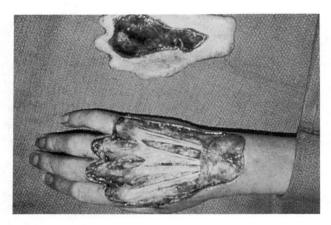

FIGURE 21-7 Surgical resection with grafting is often necessary to permit healing.

Irradiation-Induced Chronic Wounds

The chronic skin changes caused by irradiation occur more than 70 days after completing therapy. Endothelial cells and fibroblasts are the target cells for these late effects, which include atrophy, alopecia, scaling, fibrosis, necrosis, pigmentation, telangiectasis, and loss of glandular function. The incidence varies from 0% to 40% depending on treatment variables such as site, total dose, fraction size, or the use of brachytherapy. People treated with a high dose to the skin and large fractions are at greater risk of developing skin late effects. In hyperfractionated treatment of individuals with advanced head and neck cancers, grade 4 necrosis at 2-year follow-up is reported to be 5% for patients who received 6720 cGy, 10% at 7200 cGy, and 14% at 7680 cGy.[19]

Dermal and subcutaneous atrophy reflects the loss of fibrocytes and collagen reabsorption. Fibrosis becomes a progressive induration, with edema and thickening of the dermis and subcutaneous tissues. Fibrosis is usually more severe in areas that had repaired following a moist desquamation during active therapy. The onset and progression of fibrosis are also fraction-size and total-dose dependent. Once late-effect ulcers occur, they are slowly progressive. Ulcers can develop up to 20 years after irradiation.

Vascular late effects are due to a gradual loss of endothelial cells resulting in a decreased number, density, and dilation of blood vessels and the formation of telangiectasia. Medications or tobacco products that produce vasoconstriction predispose an individual to these vascular effects. The combined effect of these chronic skin changes after irradiation is a layer of skin that is intolerant of external stresses and is separated from the internal homeostasis mechanisms necessary to facilitate healing.

Soft tissue necrosis is an uncommon but serious complication of irradiation resulting from progressive ischemia. Its incidence is estimated to be 3% to 10% across tissue sites. These ulcers vary in depth and chronicity. The bed of the ulcer usually has necrotic debris and some granulation tissue but very little cellular exudate, due to fibrous necrosis of capillaries and small arteries feeding the ulcer. Radiation-related ulcers are often unable to contract spontaneously, indicating that the quality and quantity of myofibroblasts may be reduced. Damaged fibroblast stem cells may be the initial cause of the reduction in myofibroblasts, with little vascular mechanism to aid migration. Any inflammatory events that occur in the beds of these ulcers contribute eventually to further fibrosis, deformities, and stenosis. The risk of recurrent disease or a radiation-induced neoplasm needs to be ruled out prior to aggressive therapy.

Ulcers due to radionecrosis generally follow an indolent progressive course once the skin integrity is lost. The ulcers can be painful, have raised red edges and a necrotic nonvascularized base, and show no spontaneous tendency to contract or heal. In one study of 1080 individuals with radionecrosis ulcerations, 40% needed surgical treatment and most required special flaps and tissue transfer.[20] The loss of microvasculature tends to impede healing of the surgical wound.

Assessment

General Patient Assessment

A comprehensive assessment of the patient includes attention to the following important factors:

Age

Age has a strong influence on rate of healing. The dermis of the elderly has a diminished vascular supply and is covered by a thin epidermis. Older individuals may have a diminished inflammatory response, delayed neovascularity and reepithelialization, and lower tensile strength following healing due to impaired collagen deposition.

Current medications

Common drugs that adversely affect healing include corticosteroids, cytotoxic drugs (e.g., methotrexate, doxorubicin, 5-fluorouracil), and prostaglandin inhibitors. Glucocorticoids, in doses greater than 10 mg per day of prednisone, significantly inhibit wound healing by impairing inflammation, contraction, angiogenesis, fibroblast activity, and collagen formation.[21]

Nutritional status

The comorbid condition most common in cancer patients is malnutrition. Surveys show that 30% to 55% of hospitalized patients have some degree of protein-calorie malnutrition (PCM). Profound PCM is correlated with prolonged hospitalization and poor wound healing, and develops rapidly in association with catabolic stress such as neoplasms. Patients at risk for PCM include those being treated with chemotherapy or radiation therapy.

Factors to be assessed in determining risk of malnutrition include:

1. *Weight* becomes a risk factor when the individual is less than 80% of ideal body weight or has had a 10% involuntary weight loss within the last 6 months.

2. *Laboratory values* to assess include albumin, prealbumin, transferrin, total lymphocyte blood count, full chemistry panel, and a 24-hour creatinine clearance. Transferrin and prealbumin are better predictors of nutritional depletion and repletion than albumin because they have a shorter half-life and show a more rapid response to changes in protein status. Protein deficiency contributes to poor wound healing. Hypoalbuminemia prolongs the inflammatory phase and impairs fibroblast activity, resulting in decreased tensile strength. During repletion, a prealbumin level should be drawn every 2 to 3 days. Total lymphocyte count is used as a simple, inexpensive indicator of immune function and can identify malnutrition. Less than 2000/mm³ indicates progressive depletion, with less than 800/mm³ indicating severe depletion.

3. *Diet:* Protein, calorie, and fluid requirements should be calculated for each individual patient. Hypovolemia is associated with impaired healing. Inadequate volume limits distribution of oxygen, accentuating the impact of anemia. A balanced diet of fat, protein, vitamins, minerals, and carbohydrates is critical for wound healing. Dietary fats are important for the synthesis of cell membranes.

4. *Concomitant disease:* Draining wounds and infection add significant risk of malnutrition.

5. *Comorbid conditions:* Any condition that limits substrate availability will affect healing. This includes anemia, diabetes, liver disease, coagulation disorders, and malignant disease. Factors that create systemic hypoxia will also create hypoxia in the wound, as the body preferentially shunts blood to vital organs and muscles. Systemic conditions that impair the cardiovascular system and, therefore, the healing process include atherosclerosis, vasculitis, hypertension, diabetes, hypovolemia, venous stasis, and pulmonary insufficiency. Nicotine also decreases peripheral circulation. Other medications such as the nonsteroidal antiinflammatory agents, phenyl-butazone, and vitamin E disrupt healing.

Many oncologic surgical procedures involving lymph node dissection result in impaired lymph flow and function in the extremity, causing patients greater risk for developing ulcers, infections, and impaired healing. Early detection is critical for any patient developing a wound after lymph node dissection. Early detection should be followed with careful observation of wound healing and treatment with antibiotics if any symptoms of cellulitis are present.

Wound Assessment and Care Planning

The goal of wound care is to optimize the environment for healing; therefore, the nursing assessment of any wound is identical, regardless of the etiology of the wound. Figure 21-8 provides a flow chart of assessments for planning wound care including verifying or excluding the presence of malignancy; resolving any necrosis or infection while the vascular supply to the wound is being evaluated; and assessing the environment for healing. The result of the assessment should be a program of wound care that does not overburden the patient and family.

Skin lesions will not heal in the presence of tumor cells; therefore, any chronic wound should undergo biopsy to rule out malignancy. Fine-needle aspirations or conventional scraping for cytology are usually adequate to diagnose the presence of cancer cells. In a large ulcer, taking a biopsy of several areas may avoid sampling error.

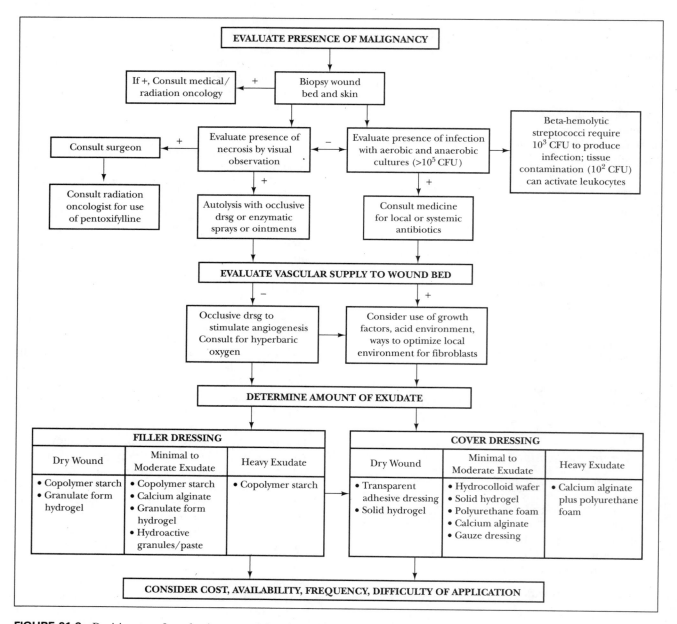

FIGURE 21-8   Decision tree for selecting wound dressings. (drsg = dressing.)

In cases of suspected lymphoma, pathologists are reluctant to make the diagnosis on skin biopsy alone because of the potential to confuse malignancy with cutaneous lymphoid hyperplasias. This is not a problem in cutaneous T-cell lymphoma or secondary cutaneous involvement of a formerly documented systemic lymphoma.[22] The medical staff will recommend any appropriate oncologic treatment following a positive biopsy. Both chemotherapy and radiation therapy will slow wound healing but not stop it.

Evaluating the vascular supply to the wound bed is important because oxygen is required for proliferation, protein synthesis, and epithelial cell migration. This can be done by observation, laser Doppler flow studies, or reflectance spectrophotometry. Wounds secondary to the late effects of irradiation are least likely to have good perfusion due to the local fibrosis.

A Late Effects of Normal Tissue Score (LENTS) has been developed to improve interrater reporting of late effects of irradiation.[23] Each type of normal tissue is assessed from subjective, objective, management, and analytic perspectives. For skin and subcutaneous tissue, the subjective scale assesses scaliness/roughness and sensation. Each is graded on a 1-to-4 scale. The objective section of the scale assesses edema, alopecia, pigmentation change, ulcer necrosis, telangiectasia, fibrosis/scar, and atrophy/contraction. Ulcers are considered grade 1 if the epidermis is ulcerated, grade 2 if the dermis is involved, and grade 3 if subcutaneous tissue is involved. Exposed bone is a grade 4 toxicity. For management, the ulcer is graded 3 if medical intervention is necessary and graded 4 if surgical intervention/amputation is necessary. The analytic aspect of the scoring system is dependent on color photographs to assess change over time.

The final considerations when planning wound care for a patient are the cost, availability of the commercial products, and the frequency and difficulty of wound care. An individual's manual dexterity becomes important if they are being asked to open small wrappers and handle syringes, scissors, or tape. Providing samples of commercial products will demonstrate their efficacy before asking the patient to incur the cost of the dressing materials. Close follow-up will provide support and problem solving for the family.

Symptom Management

Therapeutic Approaches

General wound care

Removal of necrotic tissue Like malignancy, a wound cannot heal in the presence of necrosis or infection. Necrosis is common in all types of ulcerating wounds. Malignant wounds become necrotic both by out-growing the tumor's blood supply and by destroying surrounding normal tissue, and are usually identified by a large amount of fibrous tissue and a foul odor.

There are several options available to remove necrotic tissue: autolysis, surgical excision, and chemical debridement. Surgical excision may be considered if the surrounding tissue can support the surgical wound or if the wound is the only site of disease or ulcer formation. Often a surgical debridement (debulking) followed by either of the other two methods (final dissolving) is chosen. This two-step method minimizes the potential for normal tissue damage. Autolysis is the use of occlusive dressings to facilitate the separation of the necrotic tissue from the wound bed. Moisture-retentive dressings such as hydrocolloid films work by facilitating the gathering of cells under the dressing and away from the wound itself. Lysosomal enzymes released with cell death degrade proteins and mucopolysaccharides. Hydrocolloid dressings are the dressing of choice. Chemical debridement utilizes proteolytic enzymes to dissolve the necrotic tissue. The enzyme ointments (Elase, Travase, Varidase, Streptokinase) can be introduced into an eschar either by injecting it directly or spreading it on top by scoring the eschar with a scalpel before application. An enzymatic spray has the advantage of seeping into irregular wound beds (Granulex Spray, Dow B. Hickam Pharmaceutical, TX). Chemical debriding agents such as Burow's solution (aluminum acetate), Dakin's solution (sodium hypochlorite), and potassium permanganate must be used with caution, as they will damage normal fibroblasts. Wet-to-dry dressings cause pain, bleeding, and tissue damage and are strongly discouraged. Bleeding is evidence of normal tissue damage. Nurses performing debridement at the bedside should do so under the supervision of the surgeon and should exercise exceptional caution.

Treatment of infection Infection is defined as greater than 10^5 colony-forming units (CFU) of a bacteria that may or may not be normal flora. Infection occurs when the bacteria invades normal tissue, proliferates, overwhelms body defenses, and causes toxic effects. Aerobic, anaerobic, and fungal cultures are needed as a baseline for wound care. In addition to culturing the wound bed, any sinus tracts or undermined edges should be cultured. Adequate tissue perfusion is important when considering systemic antibiotics. Treating infection is very important and can produce a rapid positive change in the appearance of the wound. Bacteria compete with macrophages and fibroblasts for limited oxygen and nutrition, delaying the healing process. Some bacteria produce ammonia, creating an alkaline environment. Measured with litmus paper, the wound pH can be used as a screening tool for infection. When a wound is kept moist, neutrophils remain viable and remove invading organisms. Povidone-iodine has shown no therapeutic benefit, is damaging to normal tissue (fibroblasts and leukocytes), and should be avoided.[24-26] Hydrogen peroxide is also toxic to fibroblasts and granulation tissue and should be avoided.

Control of odor A common problem associated with necrosis and infection is odor. A foul smell is very distressing to the patient. Resolution of the necrosis and infection will alleviate much of the odor. Occlusive dressings will contain the odor, and a dressing with imbedded charcoal will absorb it. Both types of dressings should be secured well to the skin, and if the charcoal dressing is cut to fit, it must be sealed with tape or a film dressing. Dressings have been developed to control odor and maintain a moist environment through an alginate/hydrofiber layer (CarboFlex Convatec, Bristol-Myers-Squibb Co., Princeton, NJ). Metronidazole has been used systemically as well as topically to control the odor caused by anaerobic infection, including the *Bacteroides* species. Several authors have recommended 250 mg of metronidazole administered orally three times daily.[27] Nausea is a dose-related side effect. Caution should be exercised when metronidazole is used for patients on anticoagulation therapy.[28] Metronidazole is applied topically in a 0.75% to 1.0% gel or solution form, which provides the advantages of less systemic absorption and the ability to deliver the drug to the crevices and sinus tracts of the wound.

Yogurt and buttermilk are low-cost options for odor control. Dressings are changed four times daily following thorough cleansing of the wound. The yogurt or buttermilk is left in place for 15 minutes and rinsed off.

Promotion of angiogenesis A wound with a good vascular supply allows the nurse to choose wound care products to augment healing. Occlusive dressings stimulate angiogenesis by creating hypoxia, which stimulates the macrophages to produce mediators that in turn stimulate angiogenesis. Occlusive dressings such as hydrocolloids also maintain normal temperature in the wound bed. Some commercial products, such as Granulex Spray (Hickam Pharmaceutical, TX), stimulate angiogenesis chemically. Warm whirlpool/hydrotherapy increases perfusion through heat and massage and helps keep the wound clean. Daily treatments are recommended.

Maintaining pH balance The ideal pH necessary to maintain a wound is controversial. An acid environment influences the ability of red blood cells/oxyhemoglobin to release oxygen more readily to cells in active inflammatory and fibroblastic phases. In contrast, a highly acid environment may be cytotoxic to fibroblasts. Semiocclusive dressings are able to maintain a mildly acidic wound pH.

Wound-care gels Commercially available wound-care gels contain healing stimulants such as vitamins and allantoin, an epithelialization stimulant. There has also been an increased use of aloe vera–based hydrogels. Aloe vera in concentrations of 60% to 90% has been shown to be effective against a large number of fungi as well as both gram-positive and gram-negative organisms.[29] It has also been reported that aloe significantly inactivates bradykinin in vitro, thereby potentially decreasing pain. Aloe vera also contains salicylic acid, which inhibits the produc-

tion of prostaglandins by oxidizing arachidonic acid in vitro. This inhibition may provide both an analgesic and antiinflammatory action.[30] The magnesium lactate in aloe vera inhibits histidine decarboxylase and therefore inhibits the conversion of histidine to histamine, one of the major producers of itching. A very low incidence of erythematous sensitivity is vastly outweighed by high patient satisfaction. Wound-care gels provide moisture and can act as a filler dressing.

Moisture at the wound bed is a critical factor in maintaining an optimal environment for healing-impaired tissue. Epithelial cells migrate in a moist environment. However, moist wound healing requires a balance between the absorption of excess exudate and maintaining moisture. Wounds that are dry should be dressed with products that add moisture (hydrogels). Many commercial dressings are designed to absorb exudate and remove the potentially toxic fluid while maintaining a layer of moisture at the wound bed. Some moisture-retentive dressings may actually promote fibrinolysis and production of growth factors. Refer again to Figure 21-8, which lists the categories of commercial products available to produce a balance between moisture and the presence of exudate.

Wound dressings Cover dressings alone are used on wounds that are superficial or that are almost completely filled in by granulation tissue. Examples of cover dressings commonly used are transparent adhesive film dressings and hydrocolloid wafers. Hydrocolloid dressings vary greatly in performance, in areas of absorbancy, conformability, and ability to handle fluids.[31] Semipermeable films are low-reflectance polyurethane films coated on one side with a synthetic adhesive mass. They are sterile, particle free, and very flexible. The films are permeable to water vapor and oxygen but impermeable to water and bacteria. Vapor permeability decreases the amount of exudate trapped under the dressing. Examples of nonadhesive cover dressings are solid hydrogel dressings, calcium alginate dressings, and polyurethane foam dressings, as well as the traditional gauze dressings.

Because angiogenesis is inhibited in the presence of dead space, filler dressings are used to obliterate dead space in a wound cavity and to open sinus tracts. Commonly used filler dressings include gauze, copolymer starch dressings, calcium alginate dressings, hydroactive paste, granules, and hydrogels. Calcium alginate dressings have the advantages of absorbing large amounts of exudate and being easily removable without pain. The calcium alginate fillers turn into a protective film gel in the presence of wound fluid.[32] They should not be used with dry wounds or over a thick eschar. Calcium alginate dressings are available in rope or flat gauze-like dressings. Either one can be used as a filler dressing.

The moisture in the wound and the amount of exudate will determine the appropriate filler or cover dressing. Wounds that require filler dressings also require cover dressings and a method of adhering the dressings to the skin. Elastic netting, tube dressings, or Ace wraps should be considered with impaired tissue as opposed to tape.

Hyperbaric oxygen Intermittent hyperbaric oxygen treatments have been shown experimentally to improve tissue oxygenation and promote healing. It has been used clinically in radionecrosis refractory to standard therapy alone. A review of research on hyperbaric oxygen administered to multiple sites on different individuals showed that 79% had complete resolution.[33] Hyperbaric oxygen is expensive, is administered only at select centers, and includes side effects such as a reversible myopia, significant barotrauma, claustrophobia, and cataract progression.

Wound warming Wound dressings attempt to create an optimal local environment. Hypothermia causes vasoconstriction and increases hemoglobin's affinity for oxygen, making it less available to tissue. Warm-Up Active Wound Therapy optimizes the environment by providing physiological levels of heat. It generates moist heat, raising the temperature inside the dressing to 38°C. A study of 200 surgery patients demonstrated that 19% experiencing hypothermia developed infection, while only 6% of those who received warming (three 1-hour sessions over a 5-day period) experienced infection. The hypothermia group had a 2.6 days longer length of stay.[34]

Biologic resources Blood-derived macrophages have been significantly more effective than conventional treatment of ulcerating wounds.[35] Although, currently costly to derive, the macrophages are injected at 1-cm intervals and then poured into the wound. Some wounds require a second treatment. Bovine-derived collagen has become a primary wound-care modality. It is available as dry particles, collagen gel, or collagen wafers. The triple-helical configuration of intact collagen allows it to interact with platelets and attract macrophages. Collagen requires dressing changes every other day. Collagen therapy may cause transient redness and increased drainage.

Platelet-derived growth factor and bioengineered skin equivalents have also become commercially available. Recombinant human platelet–derived growth factor (rhPDG7) is topically applied. In a trial of chronic diabetic ulcers, twice as many ulcers healed when treated with rhPDG7 compared to placebo.[36] The U.S. Food and Drug Administration has given marketing approval for bioengineered skin equivalents. Dermagraft involves cultured human dermal fibroblasts that are fashioned into a bioabsorbable scaffold (Advanced Tissue Sciences, La Jolla, CA). Diabetic foot ulcers healed within 12 weeks, and safety and efficacy was demonstrated.

Chemotherapy extravasation wounds

Preapproved physician orders should be in place for the management of extravasation. The extravasation protocol must then be put in place as soon as an extravasation is suspected. The Oncology Nursing Society has outlined recommendations for treatment of vesicant extravasation.[37] The local antidotes used currently are topical DMSO, and intradermal hyaluronidase and sodium thiosulfate. Steroids have no role, as there is little normal inflammatory response.

A drug such as DMSO is of interest because of its ability to scavenge free radicals and prevent the formation of damaging cellular products.[38,39] Fibroblast growth factor was shown to alter the vascularity of the extravasation ulcer, retarding the clinical appearance and magnitude of ulcer development.[18] Serially applied, it minimized and delayed, but did not prevent, ulcer formation.

Cold applications should be used for immediate clinical intervention in all cases except those involving vinca alkaloid extravasation. Cold topical applications for managing cytotoxic extravasation may be effective because of their vasoconstricting effect when skin temperatures approach near-freezing.[40] Heat improves the swelling and pain seen with vinca alkaloid extravasation.

A plastic surgeon should be consulted early after the injury to assess the tissues and location in addition to planning prevention of additional morbidity such as contracture. Continued pain despite conservative therapy and little evidence of healing after 2 to 3 weeks are also indications for a surgical consultation. If surgical treatment is not obtained for a doxorubicin extravasation, the wound may progress for months as the doxorubicin is taken up by the DNA of succeeding layers of cells extending peripherally, recycling the necrosing process. Excision must include all damaged tissue, including that which is reddened and painful but not necrotic. Fluorescence microscopic analysis of frozen sections is a reliable and easy method to detect and delineate doxorubicin extravasation.[41] Skin grafting is often necessary.

Radiation-induced chronic wounds

Pentoxifylline is currently being studied for the treatment of radiation-related soft tissue necrosis.[42] Pentoxifylline is a methyl xanthine derivative introduced in 1984 for the treatment of intermittent claudication, venous stasis ulcers, and cerebral insufficiency. Clinical studies have demonstrated this drug's ability to produce dose-related hematologic effects, lower blood viscosity, improve erythrocyte flexibility, and increase tissue oxygen levels. Pentoxifylline enhances red blood cell deformability, allowing cells to pass through narrowed arterioles and capillaries. It inhibits the activation of neutrophils by interleukin-1 and tumor necrosis factor-alpha, preventing the microvascular injuries of increased permeability, hemorrhage, and thrombosis. Pentoxifylline stimulates the release of prostacyclin from normal endothelial cells, which inhibits platelet aggregation, stimulates thrombolysis, and causes vasodilation. Prostacyclin decreases fibrinogen levels and increases fibrinolytic activity. Pentoxifylline indirectly inhibits the production of thromboxane, a potent vasoconstrictor and a strong stimulator of platelet aggregation. Oral pentoxifylline has been used with 30 patients who developed 37 sites of late radiation injury.[43] Nine of 12 head and neck cancer patients who developed soft tissue necrosis following radiation therapy were treated with pentoxifylline and healed completely. Mucosal pain and fibrosis was also relieved in most patients.[44] The time course of healing with pentoxifylline was significantly less than the duration of nonhealing before administration of pentoxifylline.

Psychosocial Therapeutic Approaches

Living with a chronic wound can range from a minor inconvenience to a progressive series of losses, leaving an individual depressed and isolated. In severe wounds there are social, sexual, and financial losses in addition to a dramatically changed self-image.

Individuals with chronic wounds commonly describe themselves as "feeling dirty," especially if an offensive odor emanates from the wound. The person's self-concept progressively changes, especially if the person has had any previous negative experience with someone with a chronic wound. Individuals come to define themselves in terms such as "the woman with a large leg wound."

Sexual losses occur as the individual with a chronic wound feels undesirable and unattractive to his or her sexual partner. In some circumstances, a person may choose not to allow a partner to view the area. This is similar to the situation of women who have had a mastectomy and choose not to let their partners see them naked. This lack of sharing becomes a gulf very difficult for either partner to traverse.

Social losses result when an individual withdraws from friends and social events to prevent offending others and avoid potentially embarrassing situations. He/she plans daily life around the wound: buying supplies, doing dressing changes, avoiding problems, and anticipating the home care nurse's arrival.

Family response is a critical determinant in the individual's mental health. Family members can be honest about their response to the wound in a very sensitive way, always keeping it clear that their feelings about the wound are not their feelings for the individual. Even if the individual is able to complete the dressing changes independently, family member participation provides relief and an extra pair of hands, in addition to conveying acceptance.

The financial implications of a chronic wound can be considerable. Wound care supplies are expensive; cost and reimbursement need to be considered in planning care with the patient and family, as most third-party payers do not cover the cost of wound care supplies.

Nurses caring for an oncology patient with a chronic wound need to include psychological care in addition to physiologic care to the skin. Some recommendations to keep in mind are as follows:

- Solicit from the patient what they think caused the wound. This will allow you to set education priorities. Explain the pathophysiology of the lesion formation. Provide printed information if available.

- Examine what aspect of the lesion has caused the patient the greatest emotional distress. Prioritize the wound care products to resolve that issue. By decreasing the individual's anxiety, his or her ability to learn wound care will be enhanced.

- Identify any physical limitations on the part of the individual that inhibit the ability to complete treatments or dressing changes. Arthritis or peripheral neuropathies may hinder one's ability to open jars, use spray cans, or separate dressing packaging.

- Explain the rationale of your recommendations with the goal of enhancing compliance through understanding. Provide detailed printed instructions outlining every step.

- Provide the patient with a quantity of professional samples to defray the costs while the optimal dressing materials are being selected. Individuals will be more willing to absorb the costs of the dressings once they have proved their utility.

- Return demonstrations by the individual or other caregiver(s) provide an excellent opportunity to support and reinforce good technique while providing suggestions on the fine points of how to arrange the supplies and maintain safe technique.

- Review with patients the signs and symptoms of infection, and provide them with criteria on how to make decisions if they suspect an infection.

- To enhance a personal sense of value and safety, emphasize the multidisciplinary nature of wound care. Knowing their care is being discussed among a number of trusted health professionals may add reassurance and remove doubts that other medical personnel would have done things differently. Each of the professionals can reinforce the plan of care by providing consistent information.

- At each appointment, clarify for the patient how improvement is being measured. Repeated photographs over time can be very helpful to anyone seeing the wound daily, as they will be less aware of improvement. Help the patient to establish realistic time frames based on the etiology of the wound and general health status.

- Over time, be prepared to provide alternatives if the recommended supplies are unavailable or become prohibitive due to cost.

- Reassure the patient both verbally and nonverbally that they are accepted and valued. Try to familiarize yourself with the characteristics of his or her normal daily life. Develop relationships with family members or other caregivers.

	DATE							
Wound Location:								
SIZE <u>LENGTH</u> is from top to bottom or 12 to 6 o'clock position <u>WIDTH</u> is from side to side or 3 to 9 o'clock position				TREATMENT ZONE SKIN COLOR 1. Normal for skin tone 2. Red 3. Pallor/Gray 4. Ecchymotic 5. Black/Cyanotic				
DEPTH 1. Wound closed and well approximated 2. Partial thickness, stage I or II 3. Full thickness, stage III or IV 4. Not visible due to necrosis 5. Bone involvement demonstrated as osteomyelitis				TREATMENT ZONE TISSUE EDEMA 1. None 2. Minimal demonstrated by blanching 3. Mild demonstrated by pitting edema +1 4. Moderate demonstrated by pitting edema +2 5. Severe demonstrated by pitting edema +3				
EDGES 1. Wound closed and well approximated 2. Distinct border, attached and even with wound base 3. Defined, not attached to wound base 4. Rolled under thickened, shiny, macerated 5. Thickened and hyperkeratotic, jagged, indurated, red, edematous				TREATMENT ZONE INDURATION 1. None 2. Minimal demonstrated as being easy to blanch 3. Mild demonstrated as spongy tissue 4. Moderate demonstrated as being firm and warm 5. Severe demonstrated as being hard, red, and hot or with crepitus				
UNDERMINING/TUNNELING 1. None 2. Less than 2 cm 3. Greater than 2 cm but less than 4 cm 4. Tunneling greater than 4 cm 5. Involves adjacent organs or structures				VIABLE TISSUE TYPE 1. Wound closed 2. Bright red and glossy 3. Pink and moist 4. Pale and dusky 5. None				
NECROTIC TISSUE 1. None 2. White-gray loosely adherent 3. Yellow, loosely adherent slough or fibrinous tissue 4. Loosely adherent brown or black devitalized tissue 5. Adherent black eschar				VIABLE TISSUE AMOUNT 1. 100% 2. 75% 3. 50% 4. 25% 5. None				
NECROTIC TISSUE AMOUNT 1. None 2. Up to 25% 3. 25–50% 4. 50–75% 5. 75–100%				STATUS 1. Closed 2. Significant improvement 3. Slight improvement 4. No change 5. Deteriorated				
EXUDATE TYPE 1. None 2. Serous 3. Serosanguineous 4. Bloody 5. Purulent								
EXUDATE AMOUNT 1. None 2. Scant 3. Small 4. Moderate 5. Large								
ODOR 1. None 2. Mild 3. Offensive 4. Foul 5. Extreme								
TOTAL								
DATE								
INITIALS								

FIGURE 21-9 Wound Assessment Parameter Scoring (WAPS)

Note: The #1–5 is the range entered for each date.

Source: © Kathi Whitaker, Glenda Matla

- Develop a baseline sense of what constitutes a normal activity level across social, family, and sexual dimensions. Only by having a good baseline will it be possible to identify gradual changes over time. Early intervention and support in maintaining activities will prevent the losses described above.

Evaluation of Therapeutic Approaches

A documentation tool that is comprehensive and allows both the nurse and patient to see change over time is a necessity in caring for chronic wounds. Figure 21-9 provides an example of an efficient documentation tool that summarizes the clinical history and baseline laboratory studies, while following many wound characteristics that show improvement. Photographs at regular intervals will provide evidence of change over time.

Educational Tools and Resources

Appendices 21A through 21C provide self-care guides for patients experiencing wound drainage and wound odor and those receiving hydrocolloid dressings for treatment of an ulcer.

Conclusion

The goal of treatment of a malignant ulcer will be determined by the pathology and the clinical situation. Wound care is divided into maintenance goals and healing goals. A terminally ill patient is not a candidate for an aggressive wound care regimen requiring multiple daily dressing changes. In this case it may be most appropriate to protect the wound and minimize the symptomatology. For others, a research-based program of creative wound care could lead to an ideal outcome.

Understanding and putting into practice the science of healing for the benefit of patients can truly be the domain of professional nurses. Nurses are in the best position to follow the broad multidisciplinary research that is having an impact on skin and wound care, in addition to analyzing the constant flow of new commercial products. Growth factors promise to be an exciting addition to the spectrum of commercial products.

References

1. Ivetic O, Lyne PA: Fungating and ulcerating malignant lesions: A review of the literature. *J Adv Nurs* 15:83–88, 1990
2. Gartner MH, Shearer JD, Bereiter DF, et al: Wound fluid amino acid concentrations regulate the effect of epidermal growth factor on fibroblast replication. *Surgery* 110:448–455, 1991
3. Dawes KE, Gray AJ, Laurent GJ: Thrombin stimulates fibroblast chemotaxis and replication. *Eur J Biol* 61:126–130, 1993
4. Haisfield-Wolfe ME, Rund C: Malignant cutaneous wounds: A management protocol. *Ostomy/Wound Manage* 43:56–66, 1997
5. Chang ES, Su D: Malignant ulcers: A clinicopathological review of 135 cases. *Proceedings of the American Academy of Dermatology Summer Session*, 1990
6. Helm KF, Su WPD, Muller SA, et al: Malignant lymphoma and leukemia with prominent ulceration: Clinicopathologic correlation of 33 cases. *J Am Acad Dermatol* 27:553–559, 1992
7. Novick M, Gard DA, Hardy SB, et al: Burn scar carcinoma: A review and analysis of 46 cases. *J Trauma* 17:809–817, 1977
8. Mustoe T, Upton J, Marcellino V, et al: Carcinoma in chronic pressure sores: A fulminant disease process. *Plast Reconstr Surg* 77:116–121, 1986
9. Phillip TJ, Salman SM, Rogers GS: Nonhealing leg ulcers: A manifestation of basal cell carcinoma. *J Am Acad Dermatol* 25:47–49, 1991
10. McCaffrey Boyle D, Engelking C: Vesicant extravasation: Myths and realities. *Oncol Nurs Forum* 22:57–67, 1995
11. Brothers TE, Von Moll LK, Niederhuber JE, et al: Experience with subcutaneous infusion ports in three hundred patients. *Surg Gynecol Obstet* 166:295–301, 1988
12. Herrington JD, Figueroa JA: Severe necrosis due to paclitaxel extravasation. *Pharmacotherapy* 17:163–165, 1997
13. Cabriales S, Bresnahan J, Testa D, et al: Extravasation of liposomal daunorubicin in patients with AIDS-associated Kaposi's sarcoma: A report of four cases. *Oncol Nurs Forum* 25:67–70, 1998
14. Verbov JL: Methotrexate and trimethoprim-sulphamethoxazole. *Clin Exp Dermatol* 16:231, 1991
15. WHO. *Handbook for reporting results of cancer treatment.* WHO Offset Publication. Geneva: World Health Organization, 1979, p. 48
16. Heckler FR: Current thoughts on extravasation injuries. *Clin Plast Surg* 16:557–563, 1989
17. Balsari A, Lombardo N, Ghione M: Skin and perivascular toxicity induced experimentally by doxorubicin. *J Chemother* 1:324–329, 1989
18. Vasilev SA, Morrow C, Morrow CP: Basic fibroblast growth factor in retardation of doxorubicin extravasation injury. *Gynecol Oncol* 44:178–181, 1992
19. Cox JD, Pajak TF, Marcial VA, et al: Dose-response for local control with hyperfractionated radiation therapy in advanced carcinomas of the upper aerodigestive tracts: Preliminary report of the radiation therapy oncology group protocol 88-13. *Int J Radiat Oncol Biol Phys* 18:515–521, 1990
20. Tilkorn H, Drepper H, Ehring F: Indications for the treatment by plastic surgery of the effects of radiation and radiolesions on the skin, in *Proceedings of the American Society of Plastic Surgery*, 1989
21. Stotts NA, Wipke-Tevis D: Co-factors in impaired wound healing. *Ostomy/Wound Manage* 42:44–56, 1996
22. Bueche MJ, Urba A, Lane JG: Chronic ulceration of the hand due to primary cutaneous lymphoma. *Orthopedics* 13:1385–1387, 1990
23. Archambeau JO, Pezner R, Wasserman TH: Pathophysiology of irradiated skin and breast. *Int J Radiat Oncol Biol Phys* 31:1171–1185, 1995

24. Thomas C: Wound healing halted with the use of povidone-iodine. *Ostomy/Wound Manage* 2:30–33, 1988

25. Lineaweaver W, Howard R, Soucy D, et al: Topical antimicrobial toxicity. *Arch Surg* 120:267–270, 1985

26. Rodeheaver G, Bellamy W, Kody M, et al: Bacterial activity and toxicity of iodine-containing solutions in wounds. *Arch Surg* 117:181–185, 1982

27. Rice TT: Metronidazole use in malodorous skin lesions. *Rehabil Nurs* 17:244–245, 1992

28. O'Rourke ME: Eliminating odors associated with necrotic lesions, in Powel LL (ed): *Recycling Our Ideas*. Pittsburgh: Oncology Nursing Press, 1993, p. 68

29. Robson MC, Heggers JP, Hagstrom WJ: Myth, magic, witchcraft, or fact? Aloe vera revisited. *J Burn Care Rehabil* 3: 157–162, 1982

30. Klein AD, Penneys NS: Aloe vera. *J Am Acad Dermatol* 18: 714–720, 1988

31. Thomas S, Loveless P: A comparative study of the properties of 12 hydrocolloid dressings. *WorldWide Wounds* 7, 1997 http://www.smtl.co.uk

32. Gensheimer D: A review of calcium alginates. *Ostomy/Wound Care* 39:34–43, 1993

33. Ames JW, Thom S, Goldwein J: Hyperbaric oxygen in the treatment of therapeutic radiation injuries: The University of Pennsylvania experience, in *Proceedings of the American Radium Society Mtg*, Bermuda, 1994

34. Kruz A, Sessler DI, Lenhardt R: Perioperative normothermia to reduce the incidence of surgical wound infection and shortened hospitalization. *N Engl J Med* 334:209–215, 1996

35. Danon D, Madjor J, Edinov E, et al: Treatment of human ulcers by application of macrophages prepared from a blood unit. *Exp Gerontol* 32:633–641, 1997

36. Steed DL, Donohoe D, Webster MW, et al: Effect of extensive debridement and treatment on the healing of diabetic foot ulcers. *J Am Coll Surg* 13:61–64, 1996

37. Module V: Recommendations for the management of extravasation and anaphylaxis. *Oncology Nursing Society Cancer Chemotherapy Guidelines*. Pittsburgh: Oncology Nursing Society, 1992

38. Schwartsmann G, Sander EB, Vinholes J, et al: N-acetylcysteine protects skin lesion induced by local extravasation of doxorubicin in a rat model. *Am J Pediatr Hematol Oncol* 14: 280–281, 1992

39. Alberts DS, Dorr RT: Case report: Topical DMSO for mitomycin C-induced skin ulceration. *Oncol Nurs Forum* 18: 693–695, 1991

40. Hasting-Tolsma MT, Yucha CB, Tompkins J, et al: Effect of warm and cold applications on the resolution of IV infiltrations. *Res Nurs Health* 16:171–178, 1993

41. Kjaergaard K, Chenoufi HL, Daugaard S: Fluorescence microscopic demonstration and demarcation of doxorubicin extravasation. *Cancer* 65:1722–1726, 1990

42. Perego MA, Sergio G, Artale F, et al: Hematological improvement by pentoxifylline in patients with peripheral arterial occlusive disease. *Curr Med Res Opin* 10:135–138, 1986

43. Hussey DH, Friedland JL: Second report of a pilot study of pentoxifylline in the treatment of late radiation necrosis, in *Workshop Proceedings of Pentoxifylline Leukocyte Cytokines: Potential Therapeutic Uses*. Scottsdale, AZ: 1991

44. Futran ND, Trotti A, Gwede C: Pentoxifylline in the treatment of radiation-related soft tissue injury: Preliminary observations. *Laryngoscope* 107:391–395, 1997

Wound Drainage

Patient Name: _____

Symptom and Description   You have an open sore that is draining fluid. Many open sores drain varying amounts of clear fluid. This drainage occurs for many reasons. Sores on your legs and feet drain to relieve fluid pressure. If there are cancer cells in the sore, the blood vessels around the sore may become leaky and drain large amounts of fluid. If the fluid becomes cloudy, you may have an infection. Bloody fluid is a sign of minor bleeding or tissue damage from rubbing, injury from dressing changes, or surgery.

Learning Needs   You will need to learn the signs and symptoms of infection and to report to your nurse any of the following:

- Change in smell, color, amount, or thickness of drainage
- Redness
- Warmth
- Soreness around the wound
- Puffiness or lumpiness of skin around sore

Prevention   If it is possible to keep the sore elevated above the level of your heart, this will help to decrease the amount of drainage. This is easiest to do when the sore is on an arm/hand or leg/foot. At night the sore can be kept elevated on pillows: a *gently* fastened belt may help keep an arm or leg in place on the pillow. If you need to sleep on your side, a pillow tucked against your chest and another against your back may help keep you from turning out of position.

Limiting the salt in your diet may be helpful. Discuss this with your doctor.

Keep dressings firmly on your sore to keep the fluid from leaking out.

Management   Astringent soaks, such as Domeboro solution, may help to clean, relieve pain, and decrease drainage from your sore.

- A tablet/packet is mixed with a pint of tap water. This solution should be kept covered and stored in a cool spot, and can be used for 24 hours.
- Three times a day, a clean cloth is soaked with the solution and placed in the sore for 15 minutes and then removed.
- A towel can be placed under the body part to absorb any excess. You will need to put a dressing over the sore to increase comfort and prevent sticking to the sore. The dressing needs to be changed when it becomes wet.

Follow-up   Notify your nurse if any of the following occur:

- Any change in the amount of drainage.
- If you are needing to do dressing changes more often.
- If there is any change in the color or odor of the drainage.

- If there is any bleeding with dressing changes.
- If there is any change in the feeling or appearance of the skin around the wound.

Phone Numbers

Nurse: _____ Phone: _____

Physician: _____ Phone: _____

Other: _____ Phone: _____

Comments

Patient's Signature: _____ Date: _____

Nurse's Signature: _____ Date: _____

Source: McDonald AE: Skin ulceration, in Yarbro CH, Frogge MH, Goodman M (eds): *Cancer Symptom Management* (ed 2). Sudbury: Jones and Bartlett, 1999. © Jones and Bartlett Publishers.

Wound Odor

Patient Name: _____

Symptom and Description   The most common causes of odor in chronic wounds are infection and dead tissue. Your nurse has focused on resolving these two problems. Until either of these two problems resolves, the nurse will try to use materials to absorb the odor or keep it contained. It will be a period of trial and error. The odor may go away quickly, or it may take a period of weeks to resolve. There are some things you can do at home to help with the odor problem.

Learning Needs   If you are doing your dressing changes at home, it is important to do them properly. Sticking to the schedule is also important. Your nurse will want you to be able to identify changes in the description or the strength of the odor. Your nurse will rely on you for feedback throughout this process, as you are the best person to judge what is working.

Prevention and Management   Keeping the wound as clean as possible will help prevent wound odor. Your nurse will teach you about cleansing the wound as part of the dressing change.

Either activated charcoal (¼-inch thick) or a large onion cut in half can be placed in a basin in an out-of-the-way place. The charcoal or onion should be changed every 2 or 3 days. These will help absorb odor.

Many commercial room deodorizers are available. Vanilla extract on a cloth or baking soda is commonly used. Baking soda is useful between layers of bandages as well. Maintaining some cross-ventilation in the rooms used may also be helpful.

Follow-up   Maintain contact with your nurse weekly to report any changes in the odor and condition of the wound.

Phone Numbers

Nurse: _____ Phone: _____

Physician: _____ Phone: _____

Other: _____ Phone: _____

Comments

Patient's Signature: _____ Date: _____

Nurse's Signature: _____ Date: _____

Source: McDonald AE: Skin ulceration, in Yarbro CH, Frogge MH, Goodman M (eds): *Cancer Symptom Management* (ed 2). Sudbury: Jones and Bartlett, 1999. © Jones and Bartlett Publishers.

Hydrocolloid Dressings

Patient Name: _____

Symptom and Description   Hydrocolloid dressings are used to help heal your wound and contain drainage or odor. They can do this by cutting off the oxygen from the air. It is difficult to see through them.

Learning Needs   Try to leave this dressing in place as long as you can, up to 7 to 10 days. When this type of dressing is removed, there may be a strange odor and a thick, melted paste in the wound. You may think it looks and smells like pus, but it is normal drainage.

This dressing should be applied after the wound is rinsed or cleansed. Your nurse will instruct you on how to do this. This guide will review some hints on how to keep the dressing in place for as long as you can. Before you apply the next dressing, it will be important to inspect the area for signs of infection.

Prevention and Management   After the cleansing, your nurse may want you to fill the wound with a filler dressing. If so, the nurse will provide you with specific instructions. Then dry the skin around the wound. Cut the dressing to the size and shape that best suits the body part. Cut the dressing to allow a 1-inch border of healthy skin under the dressing. Peel off the paper on the sticky side of the dressing. Flatten out any skin creases before applying the dressing. Place the dressing squarely over the wound. Make sure it is sticking down over the entire border. Any skin creases increase the chance of the dressing's leaking and defeat the goal of sealing the wound off from oxygen in the air. Edge the dressing with a 1- or 2-inch tape border.

Follow-up   If the dressing comes loose, it should be changed completely. Let the nurse know if any of the following signs of infection occur:

- Fever
- Swelling
- An increase in pain or itching around the wound
- An increase in redness
- A change in the appearance of the surrounding skin

Phone Numbers

Nurse: _____ Phone: _____

Physician: _____ Phone: _____

Other: _____ Phone: _____

Comments

Patient's Signature: _____ Date: _____

Nurse's Signature: _____ Date: _____

PART V

Symptoms of Alterations in Fluid and Electrolyte Balance

Chapter 22

Ascites

Janet Ruth Walczak, RN, MSN, CRNP
Carol S. Heckman, RN, BSN

The Problem of Ascites in Cancer

Malignant peritoneal effusions, or *ascites,* are usually associated with advanced disease and a poor prognosis; they have a devastating effect on individuals' ability to function and on their quality of life. The accumulation of fluid in the abdomen causes problems with gastrointestinal functioning, nutrition, ambulation, breathing, and sleeping, as well as psychosocial distress, all of which contribute to a decreased sense of well-being and a decreased quality of life. Individuals with ascites present a challenge to clinicians because the only way to completely eliminate the fluid accumulation is to eliminate the cancer, and for most patients this is not a realistic option. Treatment efforts therefore often focus on symptom control and supportive measures rather than on definitive therapies.

Etiology

Unlike the ascites that frequently is seen with nonmalignant liver disease, malignant ascites is always associated with a cancer. It occurs most often with ovarian cancer—in about one-third of women at the time of diagnosis and in about two-thirds at death.[1] Ascites is also associated with a variety of other primary cancer sites.

- Ovary
- Stomach
- Liver
- Uterus
- Leukemia
- Testis
- Breast
- Pancreas
- Colon
- Lymphoma
- Mesothelium
- Lung
- Unknown primary site

Malignant ascites occurs with advanced or progressive disease. Although survival is limited to months in most patients, women with primary ovarian cancer tend to have an extended survival period.[2] In this subgroup, ascites is often present at the time of diagnosis when exploratory laparotomy, tumor debulking, and initial chemotherapy offer the best opportunity for response, even if only for a limited period of time. In other cases, if ascites is associated with recurrent or progressing disease, the patient will probably already have received the optimal therapy so there is little chance for tumor response or control of the ascites.

Pathophysiology

The peritoneal cavity is enclosed by the parietal peritoneum that lines the abdominopelvic walls and the dia-

405

phragm, and the visceral peritoneum that covers the abdominal organs. A small volume of fluid lubricates the cavity and prevents the abdominal organs from adhering to the abdominal wall. Malignant ascites occurs when the amount of fluid produced exceeds the amount of fluid cleared from the peritoneal cavity. This occurs primarily from two causes: decreased (or deficient) clearance of fluid from the cavity and increased (or excessive) peritoneal fluid production.[1-5]

Tumor obstructing the main thoracic duct as well as other subdiaphragmatic lymphatic channels will impair the normal flow of fluid out of the peritoneal cavity. Widespread metastases to the liver also may cause an obstruction of the hepatic venous system, resulting in transudative ascites that is characterized by low serum albumin, low plasma oncotic pressure, and increased portal vein pressure.[1-5]

Extensive tumor seeding throughout the peritoneal cavity results in increased capillary permeability and excessive fluid exudate. Ascites is the result of tumor-induced hemodynamic changes within the peritoneal cavity. This mechanism occurs primarily in ovarian and other gynecologic cancers.[1,4,5]

Assessment

Assessment of the individual with ascites includes an evaluation of the symptoms experienced as a result of the fluid accumulation, physical signs of ascites, and diagnostic testing. Although early ascites can be subtle, the overall clinical picture of a person with advanced malignant ascites is often that of a malnourished individual with a distended abdomen, cachectic extremities, and compromised respiratory and gastrointestinal function.

Symptoms

Because the abdomen is distensible, the peritoneal cavity can accommodate large volumes of fluid. When the fluid volume becomes excessive (>500 mL), the patient becomes symptomatic. A detailed history will reveal a variety of problems. The symptoms are produced by the pressure of the increased fluid on abdominal organs, resulting in pain, discomfort, or malfunction of those organs. Individuals often describe a variety of concerns, including:

- Recent weight gain
- Clothes not fitting
- Abdominal bloating
- Lack of appetite
- Feeling full after small meals
- Indigestion
- Urinary urgency or frequency

- Constipation
- Feeling tired
- Difficulty breathing
- Inability to tolerate even limited activity
- Abdominal or low back pain
- Nausea and vomiting
- Ankle swelling

Abdominal Assessment

The presence of excessive peritoneal fluid (>500 mL) is easily discernible. The abdomen is usually distended along with bulging flanks. Skin may be shiny and tense, and the umbilicus may be everted. Percussion of the abdomen with the patient supine reveals the presence of fluid, with tympany at the upper and midabdominal region and dullness over the flanks. If the patient then turns to one side, shifting dullness occurs with tympany over the upper flank, and dullness in the lower flank can be appreciated up to the umbilicus.

The presence of a fluid wave is also characteristic of excessive fluid in the abdomen. This wave is detected by having a colleague place the ulnar surface of their hand on the midline of the patient's abdomen and applying pressure. When pressure is applied, a wave of fluid can be palpated along the patient's flank.

Gastrointestinal Assessment

Bowel sounds may be diminished, high pitched, or absent, depending on the extent of the ascites and intraabdominal tumor volume. A detailed history of frequency and consistency of bowel movements, dietary intake, and presence of nausea and vomiting demonstrates the extent to which gastrointestinal function may be impaired. Abdominal girth is measured as baseline so that response to therapy can be monitored.

Respiratory Assessment

The respiratory system can be compromised by elevation of the diaphragm and decrease of the space due to increased peritoneal fluid. Therefore, the individual will typically exhibit dyspnea, tachypnea, and orthopnea. The thoracic cavity is also assessed for effusions, as peritoneal fluid can cross through the diaphragm into the pleural space due to the increased fluid volume and pressure in the abdomen. If fluid is present within the thoracic cavity, there is a dull or flat sound in response to percussion in the lower lung field where the fluid is located. Breath sounds are diminished over the area of fluid and sounds are hyperresonant in the area above the fluid level.

Diagnostic Testing

A variety of diagnostic tests are used to determine the presence of malignant ascites. Malignant ascites can most definitively and readily be diagnosed by obtaining fluid for evaluation. A diagnostic paracentesis can both confirm the diagnosis and provide temporary symptomatic relief. The color and character of the fluid assist in the determination of the cause of the ascites:

- Bloody or serosanguineous ascites is usually associated with ovarian cancer, liver cancer, or other cancers causing intraperitoneal dissemination of the cancer[1,3]
- Chylous ascites is a milky fluid associated with lymphoma that is blocking large lymphatic channels
- Serous ascites is usually associated with nonmalignant conditions such as congestive heart failure, renal disease, or cirrhosis
- Cloudy peritoneal fluid may be due to an infection

If the origin of the fluid is unclear, fluid obtained should be cultured and analyzed for protein, glucose, lactic acid dehydrogenase (LDH), and amylase.[1,3,4] The chemistry profile of malignant ascites as compared with serum reveals elevated total protein and LDH levels. The presence of red and white blood cells, and negative Gram stains and cultures are typical of a malignant ascites.

The fluid is also evaluated with Papanicolaou staining to determine the presence of malignant cells. However, malignant cells will be found in only approximately half of all specimens examined.[1,3] Because tumor markers have been shown to be elevated with malignant ascites, levels of carcinoembryonic antigen (CEA), cancer antigens 125 (CA 125), and alpha-fetoprotein (AFP) in the fluid may also be determined.

Other studies that may be useful in making the diagnosis of ascites include an abdominal X-ray film, abdominal ultrasonogram, and abdominal CT scan. Ultrasonography and CT have the sensitivity to detect even small amounts of ascitic fluid.[1,3]

Symptom Management

Ascites is associated with advanced disease and is not a side effect of therapy; therefore, it is a sign of poor prognosis. The only way to eliminate the fluid accumulation is to eliminate the malignant disease. Due to the advanced nature of the disease when ascites is present, cure is not usually a realistic goal. As many individuals presenting with ascites have previously received cancer therapy, including surgery, radiation, or chemotherapy, standard therapeutic regimens will be of little benefit in controlling the ascites. The one exception is when the ascites is present at the time of diagnosis, such as occurs with ovarian cancer or lymphoma. In this situation, the individual usually responds to primary therapy, so the tumor and the ascites are controlled at least for a period of time. Other efforts to treat the ascites aim to palliate or control the cancer and manage the symptoms associated with the accumulated fluid.

Therapeutic Approaches

Surgical tumor debulking, chemotherapy, or radiation therapy may be used to gain control of the disease. However, once therapeutic modalities have failed to control the cancer, efforts to relieve symptoms are initiated along with supportive measures in order to improve the individual's quality of life.

Effective management of ascites is a great challenge to clinicians. Although multiple interventions have been explored, control of the fluid accumulation remains less than optimal. Interventions to enhance quality of life that can be initiated early and continued throughout the course of the disease are described in Table 22-1. The overall outcome of specific therapeutic interventions such as paracentesis, intraperitoneal therapy, and peritoneovenous shunting is less than optimal.

Paracentesis

Abdominal paracentesis is frequently used to remove accumulated fluid and relieve symptoms. It is usually reserved for individuals who have accumulated a large volume of fluid or who are very symptomatic. Because the mechanism of malignant ascites differs from that of other types of ascites, rapid removal of fluid can be accomplished without altering hemodynamic equilibrium and without increasing morbidity for the patient.[2,6] Although relief after paracentesis is immediate, the benefits are usually short in duration. Ascitic fluid tends to reaccumulate more rapidly with repeated paracenteses.[2] In addition, removal of large volumes of fluid (>2 L per paracentesis) can lead to increased protein depletion and electrolyte imbalances. It can also cause infection or injury to the peritoneal viscera resulting from perforation or fibrosis.[3,7] Although there are potential side effects and only temporary benefit, paracentesis is often employed because the patient experiences dramatic relief and is not usually a candidate for other, more aggressive efforts to control the fluid accumulation. The use of an implanted Tenckhoff catheter can facilitate the removal of the ascitic fluid and minimize the risks associated with repeated paracentesis.[8]

Intraperitoneal therapy

Intraperitoneal therapy is the instillation of a therapeutic agent directly into the peritoneal space via a temporary or permanent vascular catheter. Chemotherapy is often used with the intention of causing irritation to the exposed peritoneal surfaces to produce subsequent

TABLE 22-1 Nursing Guidelines for Management of Ascites

Management Goal	Intervention
Promote fluid mobilization	• Assess peripheral edema • Minimize sodium and fluid intake • Monitor intake and output, electrolytes, serum protein, albumin • Administer diuretics as ordered • Obtain daily weight, abdominal girth • Elevate feet/legs when sitting • Apply compression stockings, boots • Maintain high-calorie, high-protein diet, as tolerated • Assist patient in maintaining mobility
Promote respiratory function	• Elevate head of bed • Promote activity as tolerated • Provide oxygen as needed • Administer analgesics as ordered

Promote gastrointestinal function	• Maintain adequate nutrition as tolerated:
	    Small, frequent meals
	    Food supplements
	    Bland diet
	    Calorie counts
	• Obtain daily weights
	• Assess frequency of bowel movements
	• Administer antacids, H_2 blockers, antiemetics, bowel regimen, as ordered
	• Encourage oral hygiene after meals and as needed
	• Provide diversional therapy
	• Instruct in guided imagery

Promote skin integrity	• Encourage and assist in ambulation, positioning, turning • Apply lotion to relieve pruritus and dry skin • Massage bony prominences • Provide air mattress, foam cushions on bed, chairs • Encourage nutritional intake • Provide food supplements as needed
Promote safety	• Monitor blood counts, coagulation, liver function, renal function • Monitor for signs of bleeding, infection, peritonitis • Evaluate current medications based on abnormal lab results • Provide clutter-free environment • Minimize invasive procedures • Assist in ambulation
Promote comfort	• Assess severity and quality of pain, discomfort • Provide air mattress, foam cushions on bed, chairs • Instruct in relaxation techniques, guided imagery • Administer analgesics, antianxiety agents, diuretics, antiemetics as ordered • Assist in positioning for comfort • Provide uninterrupted rest periods • Provide psychosocial and spiritual support/counseling
Promote self-care	• Instruct patient/family in interventions for self-care at home and in follow-up appointments • Assess equipment/resources needed within the home • Provide appropriate referrals to home-care agency, hospice • Provide referral for psychosocial counseling as indicated

scarring and fibrosis. An additional benefit of this therapy is that a high concentration of the drug can be delivered directly to the tumor for prolonged periods and with less systemic toxicity. Agents that have been used for intraperitoneal treatment include bleomycin, doxorubicin, nitrogen mustard, and cisplatin. The use of hyperthermic intraperitoneal chemotherapy with mitomycin has been evaluated but needs further study to define its role in this patient population.[9] Radioactive colloid suspensions such as radioactive phosphorus (^{32}P) may also be administered intraperitoneally. Radioactive suspensions have become less favored because of the potential bowel damage that can occur if the radioactive fluid remains in a loculated area within the peritoneal cavity. The bowel damage can be significant enough to require surgical intervention.[3]

Another type of intraperitoneal therapy involves the use of both alfa and beta interferon.[10–13] It appears that beta interferon offers better response (up to 40%) in a variety of cancers causing ascites than does alfa interferon (no effect reported by Stuart et al.[10]). Unfortunately, the duration of response time reported was variable. This modality combined with intraperitoneal chemotherapy may offer better palliation than either intraperitoneal chemotherapy or interferons alone.

Regardless of the agent being utilized, it is important to assess for free flow of fluid throughout the abdomen prior to instillation into the peritoneal cavity. If the catheter is placed in a loculated space created by adhesions, the agent will remain concentrated in that space and can cause potential serious complications, including further adhesions, bowel obstruction, or fistula formation. Thus, care must be taken to ensure flow while the catheter is in place.

While intraperitoneal access can be obtained and therapy administered via a temporary long intravascular catheter, another option that may be considered is the placement of long-term catheter devices such as Groshong, Tenckhoff, or a Tenckhoff that is attached to an implantable port. These devices allow the administration of chemotherapy and frequent peritoneal sampling or drainage, and decrease the risks associated with repeated paracenteses, such as perforation and peritonitis. However, the catheters require care and are not without risk. They must be assessed frequently for patency and signs of infection.[2,8,14]

Peritoneovenous shunting (PVS)

Another palliative treatment modality to consider is PVS. This treatment uses a shunt to continuously rechannel ascitic fluid from the peritoneal cavity to the superior vena cava and thus into venous circulation. It is usually a treatment reserved for those in whom other attempts at management have failed. The management of the patient with a shunt is described in Table 22-2.[4]

The shunting device consists of a length of perforated tubing that is inserted into the peritoneal cavity and a length of tubing that is passed under the subcutaneous tissue and inserted into the superior vena cava. A one-way valve in the tube allows fluid to flow unidirectionally from the peritoneal cavity into the vascular system when peritoneal cavity pressure increases. When the patient inhales, the diaphragm descends, causing the intraperitoneal pressure to rise and the intrathoracic pressure to fall. This pressure gradient, which is approximately 3 to 5 cmH$_2$O higher than central venous pressure, causes the one-way valve to open, and thus the ascitic fluid flows upward into the superior vena cava circulation.[3,15]

The shunts most commonly used are the LeVeen and Denver shunts. The primary differences between these devices are valve structure and pressure sensitivity. The LeVeen shunt has a valve that opens with ≥3 cmH$_2$O pressure. The Denver shunt opens with ≥1 cmH$_2$O pressure, and its valve is enclosed inside a compressible chamber placed subcutaneously. This valve can be manually compressed if needed to irrigate the system and enhance fluid flow.[1,3,4] Physician preference, rather than the superiority of one device over another, usually determines which is used.[3,4]

Placement of the peritoneovenous shunt is a surgical procedure and not without contraindications or complications. Acute complications of PVS require adjustment in the rate of reinfusion and are seen during the first 48 to 72 hours after permanent shunt placement. Complications are due to the amount of fluid infused into venous circulation and include hemodilution, acute pulmonary edema, acute respiratory distress syndrome, and ventricular tachycardia. Coagulation abnormalities, particularly disseminated intravascular coagulopathy, may occur due to the introduction of ascitic fluid rich in proteins and clotting factors. Protein and cellular debris carried with the ascitic fluid can result in pulmonary embolus.[12] Problems with placement of the catheter itself include pneumothorax, neck trauma, laryngeal nerve trauma, leaking ascitic fluid, tubing migration, and shunt occlusion. In addition, there may be wound infection, peritonitis, and septicemia.[3,4,15] Thus, patients will need to be intensively monitored for several days after shunt placement (see Table 22-2).

Problems with PVS that occur after the postoperative period are primarily related to shunt occlusion. This results either from increased amounts of cellular debris found in the ascitic fluid or from infection, which can occur any time after shunt placement. Although treatable with antibiotics, infection usually necessitates shunt removal.[15] Finally, there is also the possibility of shunt-induced tumor dissemination as ascitic fluid containing tumor cells is infused into the venous circulation.[3,4,15]

Peritoneovenous autotransfusion

Recently, peritoneovenous autotransfusion has been used to preliminarily assess patient tolerance of shunting and to identify potential complications. The autotransfusion procedure consists of draining the peritoneal fluid

TABLE 22-2 Guide for Peritoneovenous Shunting

Management	Interventions
Before placement of shunt	• Obtain baseline vital signs, electrocardiogram, weight, abdominal girth, electrolyte panel, complete blood count, coagulation profile, pulse oximetry • Transfuse red blood cells and platelets, as ordered, prior to procedure • Administer antibiotics, anesthetics, as ordered, prior to procedure

After placement of shunt	• Monitor for first 48–72 hours after shunt placement:
	  Obtain vital signs q15 min × 4, q30 min × 4, then hourly
	  Place patient on cardiac monitor
	  Obtain central venous pressure reading qh
	  Auscultate breath sounds/pulse oximetry q4h
	  Obtain weight and abdominal girth postprocedure, then every shift
	  Obtain electrolytes, complete blood count, coagulation profiles q4h
	  Assess level of pain, discomfort q2–4h
	• Administer diuretics, blood, platelets, oxygen, electrolytes, antibiotics, and pain medications, as ordered
	• Assess surgical wound sites and catheter patency q4h

Increase fluid flow	• Lower head of bed to supine position • Encourage patient to inspire against resistance for 15 minutes 4×/day using spirometry • Apply abdominal binder • If appropriate, increase flow by manually compressing shunt as necessary if patient notes accumulation of fluid, increase in girth or weight, or difficulty breathing
Decrease fluid flow	• Have patient sit upright in bed • Administer diuretics, as ordered

Self-care	• Instruct patient/family in:
	  Interventions to increase or decrease flow
	  When to call for help
	  Follow-up appointments

Data from references.[3,15]

and transfusing it into the venous circulation via a closed external system of infusion and drainage bags, tubing primed with saline, connectors, and stopcocks (Figure 22-1). One end of the tubing is connected to a central venous catheter and the other to a peritoneal catheter. Fluid is drained by gravity from the abdomen via the peritoneal catheter into one of the collection bags. Once the bag is filled, the infusion and drainage bags are switched. The collected ascitic fluid is then allowed to infuse into the venous system. The ascitic fluid is infused rapidly unless otherwise indicated. The patient is autotransfused continuously in this manner for a period of 48 hours prior to permanent shunt placement. The procedure for this is outlined in Table 22-3. Complications of peritoneovenous autotransfusion are similar to the acute complications of PVS, described in the preceding section.

Evaluation of Therapeutic Approaches

The effectiveness of any intervention can be evaluated by collecting and evaluating data over time. Certain pa-

rameters will be useful in evaluating response. Certainly abdominal girth measurements indicate how the fluid volume is responding to the chemotherapy or shunting procedure. The interval between successive *paracenteses,* or drainages of fluid, via the peritoneal catheter indicates how well the ascites is responding to interventions: in general, the shorter the interval, the poorer the response. The volume and color of the fluid removed also are a means of evaluating response to therapy: a decrease in fluid volume and a clearing of the fluid, particularly in the presence of a decrease in a tumor marker such as CEA or CA 125, indicate a positive response. Other signs and symptoms that are useful in evaluating response are an improvement in respiratory and gastrointestinal symptoms, an increase in physical activity, and an improvement in the level of comfort experienced.

Documentation tools

Patient assessment and evaluation of interventions can easily be monitored via documentation on a nursing flow sheet (Figure 22-2). Information on this form in-

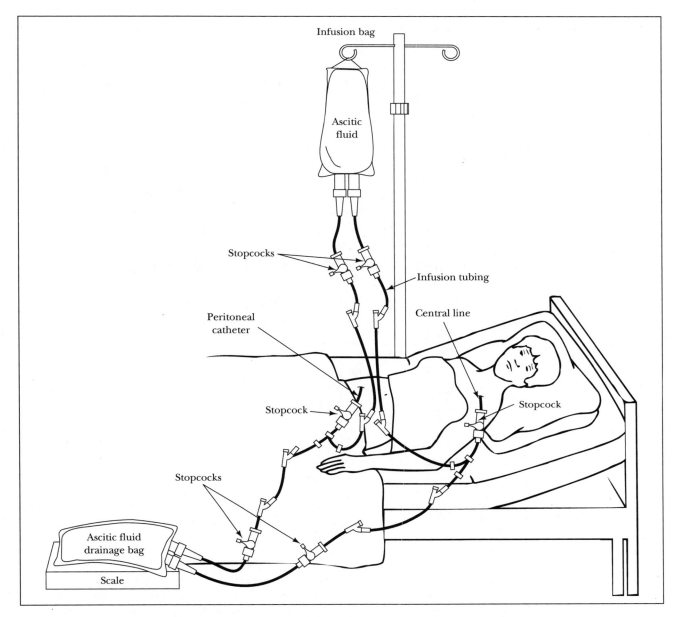

FIGURE 22-1 Peritoneovenous autotransfusion consists of draining the peritoneal fluid and then transfusing it into the venous circulation via a closed external system. Adapted from Kehoe, 1991.[4]

cludes physical assessment and measurements such as vital signs, weight, intake and output, abdominal girth, and laboratory values. Information regarding the frequency of interventions, such as paracentesis or access of peritoneal catheters for fluid sampling/drainage or chemotherapy, can also be recorded and analyzed over time. The character and amount of fluid removed from the peritoneal cavity are described in the comments section. The volume and frequency of fluid removed can be correlated with the degree and duration of symptom relief for the patient. The effectiveness of medications given to alleviate pain or discomfort can also be documented and monitored on the flow sheet.

Evaluation tools

Patients are able to evaluate their own response to therapy in a number of ways. One measure is their tolerance of routine activities of daily living. Fit of clothing can also indicate the extent of fluid loss or gain. Abdominal girth, weight, and the existence or extent of peripheral edema can be recorded and monitored over time as an indicator of response. The ability to eat and drink without discomfort or nausea as well as the frequency and amount of pain and medication can also be evaluated by the patient. However, although patients can easily monitor all of these data, it is not always in their best interests

TABLE 22-3 Guide for Peritoneovenous Autotransfusion

Management and Interventions	
Prior to autotransfusion	Prime autotransfusion tubing with sterile saline.
	Connect the central line and peritoneal catheter to the outflow/inflow tubings on the bags.
	Hang first infusion bag on IV pole to maintain central line patency; place drainage bag below the bed level.
During autotransfusion	Open clamps to peritoneal catheter and drainage bag.
	Allow drainage bag to fill.
	Close clamps on tubings from patient to drainage bag and from patient to central line.
	Record drainage time and volume on flow sheet.
	Switch positions of infusion/drainage bags.
	Open clamp to the drainage bag.
	Open clamp on infusion bag to patient.
	Infuse ascitic fluid into the central line as rapidly as patient tolerates.
	Drain ascitic fluid into new drainage bag.
	Continue to switch infusion and drainage bags.
	Be sure to clamp line to patient with each bag exchange.
	Monitor for complications/side effects:
	• Obtain vital signs qh
	• Place patient on cardiac monitor
	• Obtain central venous pressure reading qh
	• Auscultate breath sounds/pulse oximetry q4h
	• Obtain weight and abdominal girth postprocedure, then every shift
	• Obtain electrolytes, complete blood count, coagulation profiles qh
	• Assess level of pain, discomfort q2–4h
	Administer diuretics, blood, platelets, oxygen, electrolytes, antibiotics, and pain medications, as ordered.

Source: Kehoe C: Malignant ascites: Etiology, diagnosis, and treatment. *Oncol Nurs Forum* 18:523–530, 1991.[4]

to focus on symptoms or signs over which they have little control. The patient's diminishing quality of life can inadvertently be reinforced by keeping a detailed record of how he or she is doing. Thus, it is important to have patients focus on those items over which they have some measure of control, such as diet, pain, and activity.

Educational Tools and Resources

Appendixes 22A, 22B, and 22C are all tools that can be used to educate patients and families about ascites and self-care techniques. Patients without shunts should receive educational tools 22A and 22C, while patients with shunts should receive tools 22B and 22C. In addition to these tools, which can help with physical care, it is important to provide psychosocial and spiritual support for the patient and family. For this, referral to other professionals and groups may be indicated. Also, for the individ-

ual with progressive malignant ascites, it is important to consider the home-care resources available to assist in the patient's care and support. Finally, resources may be needed to present and discuss the issue of advanced directives with the patient and family if this has not already been done. Table 22-4 lists professional and community resources available to help nurses provide holistic care for patients with ascites and for their families.

Conclusion

Malignant ascites is a distressing sign of advanced and progressive disease. Although there are many approaches available to control ascites, there are unfortunately no therapies that give long-term relief except for those that control the underlying cancer. Therefore, our efforts

ASCITES FLOW SHEET

Nurse Signature _____

Nurse Signature _____

Nurse Signature _____

Nurse Signature _____

Date _____

Patient identification

Parameters	Time						
Central venous pressure							
Blood pressure							
Heart rate							
Respiratory rate							
O$_2$ saturation							
O$_2$ flow rate							
Weight							
Abdominal girth							
Ascitic fluid drained							
Diuretic							
Urinary output							
Total output							
Total intake							
Pain rating							

Comments

FIGURE 22-2 Ascites flow sheet.

TABLE 22-4   Professional and Community Resources

Professional Specialities for Resource and Referral	
Physical care:	Home nursing agencies
	Hospice
	Home equipment companies
	Physical therapy
Psychosocial and spiritual:	Psychologist
	Psychiatric clinical nurse specialist
	Social worker
	Chaplain
	Occupational therapist
	Recreational therapist
	Hospice
Community Services for Resource and Referral	
American Cancer Society:	Disease information, social services, and support groups
National Cancer Institute:	Disease and treatment information, Cancer Information service (CIS)
State Attorney General's Office:	Advanced Directives Information

must focus on interventions to control the associated symptoms and to support and enhance the patients' quality of life.

References

1. Olopade OI, Ultmann JE: Malignant effusions. *CA Cancer J Clin* 41:166–179, 1991

2. Maxwell MB: Malignant effusions and edemas, in Groenwald SL, Frogge MH, Goodman M, Yarbro CH (eds): *Cancer Nursing: Principles and Practice* (ed 4). Sudbury, Jones and Bartlett, 1997, pp. 721–741

3. Marincola FM, Schwartzentruber DJ: Malignant ascites, in DeVita Jr VT, Hellman S, Rosenberg SA (eds): *Cancer: Principles and Practice of Oncology* (ed 5). Philadelphia: Lippincott, 1997, pp. 2598–2606

4. Kehoe C: Malignant ascites: Etiology, diagnosis, and treatment. *Oncol Nurs Forum* 18:523–530, 1991

5. Parsons SL, Watson SA, Steele RJ: Malignant ascites. *Br J Surg* 83:6–14, 1996

6. Ratliff CR, Hutchinson M, Conner C: Rapid paracentesis of large volumes of ascitic fluid. *Oncol Nurs Forum* 18:1461, 1991

7. Horton J: Malignant effusions, in Moosa A, Schimpff S, Robson M (eds): *Comprehensive Textbook of Oncology* (ed 2), vol 2. Baltimore: Williams & Wilkins, 1991, pp. 1690–1696

8. Murphy M, Rossi M: Managing ascites via the Tenckhoff catheter. *MEDSURG Nurs* 4:468–471, 1995

9. Loggie BW, Perini M, Fleming RA, et al: Treatment and prevention of malignant ascites associated with disseminated intraperitoneal malignancies by aggressive combined-modality therapy. *Am Surg* 63:137–143, 1997

10. Stuart GC, Nation JG, Snider DD, et al: Intraperitoneal interferon in the management of malignant ascites. *Cancer* 71:2027–2030, 1993

11. Cappelli R, Gotti G: The locoregional treatment of neoplastic ascites with interferon-beta. *Recent Prog Med* 83:82–84, 1992

12. Bezwoda WR, Golombick T, Dansey R, et al: Treatment of malignant ascites due to recurrent/refractory ovarian cancer: The use of interferon-alpha or interferon-alpha plus chemotherapy in vivo and vitro. *Eur J Cancer* 27:1423–1429, 1992

13. Gebbia V, Russo A, Gebbia N, et al: Intracavitary beta-interferon for the management of pleural and/or abdominal effusions in patients with advanced cancer refractory to chemotherapy. *In Vivo* 5:579–581, 1991

14. Hrozencik SP, Ness EA: Intraperitoneal chemotherapy via the Groshong catheter in patients with gynecologic cancer. *Oncol Nurs Forum* 18:1245, 1991

15. Moskowitz M: The peritoneovenous shunt: Expectation and reality. *Am J Gastroenterol* 85:917–929, 1990

Ascites

Patient Name: _____

Symptom and Description   Ascites is a symptom that occurs when large amounts of fluid pool in your abdomen. The fluid can cause a sense of fullness and make your clothes fit tightly. The effects of the fluid can be managed with the care outlined in this guide.

Learning Needs   You will need to know how to live with the fluid in your abdomen. You will learn how to handle pain if it occurs. You will learn how to adjust to the symptoms and when to call for help.

Management

1. *Diet:* There are no limits to your diet. Try to eat foods high in protein and calories. Small, frequent meals (up to 6 meals a day) may be easier for you to eat.
2. *Pain control:* Rate your pain daily using a scale of 0 to 10 in which 0 equals no pain and 10 equals the worst pain that you can imagine. Select the number that best describes your level of pain.

0	1	2	3	4	5	6	7	8	9	10
no pain										worst pain

3. *Activity:* There are no limits to your activities. You should do what you feel like doing. Rest periods may be helpful. Elevate your feet/legs when sitting.
4. *Diary:* Keep a record of your daily pain rating and activity level on the Patient Data Record included. Bring this with you when you come for your next visit with your nurse or doctor.

Follow-up   Call your nurse or doctor if any of the following occurs:

- A weight gain so that your clothes do not fit
- Trouble breathing or shortness of breath
- Nausea, vomiting
- Increase in pain rating to above 4 for 2 days in a row

Phone Numbers

Nurse: _____   Phone: _____

Physician: _____   Phone: _____

Other: _____   Phone: _____

Comments

Patient's Signature: _____   Date: _____

Nurse's Signature: _____   Date: _____

Source: Walczak JR, Heckman CS: Ascites, in Yarbro CH, Frogge MH, Goodman M (eds): *Cancer Symptom Management* (ed 2). Sudbury: Jones and Bartlett, 1999. © Jones and Bartlett Publishers.

Shunt Care

Patient Name: _____

Symptom and Description   Ascites is a symptom that occurs when large amounts of fluid pool in your abdomen. The fluid can cause a sense of fullness and make your clothes fit tightly. The shunt is a tube that has been placed to reduce this fluid by draining it into your bloodstream. The excess fluid can then be eliminated via the kidneys into the urine. The fluid can be removed and the effects of the fluid managed with the care outlined in this guide.

Learning Needs   You will need to know how to live with the fluid and shunt in your abdomen. You will learn how to take care of the shunt and how to handle the effects of the shunt and fluid. You will learn how to adjust to the symptoms and when to call for help.

Management

1. *Diet:* There are no limits to your diet. Try to eat foods high in protein and calories. Small, frequent meals (up to 6 meals a day) may be easier for you to eat.

2. *Pain control:* Rate your pain daily using a scale of 0 to 10 in which 0 equals no pain and 10 equals the worst pain that you can imagine. Select the number that best describes your level of pain.

0	1	2	3	4	5	6	7	8	9	10
no pain										worst pain

3. *Activity:* There are no limits to your activities. You should do what you feel like doing. Rest periods may be helpful. Elevate your feet/legs when sitting. Wear an abdominal binder while up to increase pressure and enhance fluid flow.

4. *Fluid flow:* If you notice an increase in size around your abdomen, you may increase fluid flow into the bloodstream by any of the following:
   - Lying down flat on your back
   - Using the spirometer for 15 minutes 4 times a day
   - Wearing an abdominal binder while up to increase pressure and enhance fluid flow
   - If you have a Denver shunt in place, compress it as you were taught by your doctor or nurse

5. *Diary:* Keep a record of your daily pain rating, measurement around abdomen, and weight on the Patient Data Record included. Be careful to measure your abdomen in the same place each day. Bring this record with you to your next visit with your nurse or doctor.

Follow-up   Call your nurse or doctor if any of the following occurs:

- A weight gain or increase in abdominal size so that your clothes do not fit
- Trouble breathing or shortness of breath
- Nausea, vomiting
- Increase in pain rating to above 4 for 2 days in a row.

Phone Numbers

Nurse: _____ Phone: _____

Physician: _____ Phone: _____

Other: _____ Phone: _____

Comments

Patient's Signature: _____ Date: _____

Nurse's Signature: _____ Date: _____

Source: Walczak JR, Heckman CS: Ascites, in Yarbro CH, Frogge MH, Goodman M (eds): *Cancer Symptom Management* (ed 2). Sudbury: Jones and Bartlett, 1999. © Jones and Bartlett Publishers.

Patient Data Record

Patient Name: _____

Date							
Weight (daily)							
Abdominal girth (daily)							
Activity rating (daily)*							
Pain rating**							
Pain medication used							

*On a scale of 0 to 10, with 0 meaning you are able to do anything you wish and 10 meaning that you stay in bed all of the time and are unable to get around by yourself, write the number that best describes the amount of activity that you are able to do.

0	1	2	3	4	5	6	7	8	9	10

fully active   in bed all of the time/
                                                                            unable to get around

**On a scale of 0 to 10, with 0 meaning no pain at all and 10 meaning the worst pain imaginable, write the number that best describes the level of pain that you are having. If you are taking pain medication, indicate when you take it and the relief that you experience, using the same scale.

0	1	2	3	4	5	6	7	8	9	10

no pain   worst pain

Comments

Source: Walczak JR, Heckman CS: Ascites, in Yarbro CH, Frogge MH, Goodman M (eds): *Cancer Symptom Management* (ed 2). Sudbury: Jones and Bartlett, 1999. © Jones and Bartlett Publishers.

CHAPTER 23

Effusions

Patricia E. Lawler, RN, MS

The Problem of Effusions in Cancer

Malignant effusions, the accumulation of fluid in a serous cavity secondary to the effects of a neoplastic process, is a relatively common problem in individuals with cancer. In pleural effusions, the fluid accumulates in the pleural cavity, and in pericardial effusions, the fluid accumulates in the pericardial cavity.

Incidence in Cancer

A diagnosis of malignant effusion may be the first indication of cancer in an individual, but more often it is detected in individuals with advanced metastatic disease. Up to 50% of pleural effusions are thought to be caused by cancer.[1] It is estimated that almost 250,000 new cases of malignant pleural effusions are identified yearly in the United States due to the rising incidence of lung and breast cancer.[2] Although not as prevalent as pleural effusions, pericardial effusions are also seen in individuals with advanced disease. Autopsy studies have revealed that 0 to 21% of individuals with cancer have involvement of the heart and pericardium at the time of death.[3]

Impact on Quality of Life

Fluid accumulation in the pleural or pericardial space can inhibit normal function of the lungs and the heart. Because malignant effusions are often late complications of progressive cancer, individuals are often debilitated, with a low performance status and a short life expectancy. Malignant pleural effusions are identified in individuals with extensive tumor burdens, with a 1-month mortality of 25% to 54% and a 6-month mortality of 84%.[4] Malignant pericardial effusions likewise signify a poor prognosis.

Therapeutic approaches used in the management of malignant effusions must be able to maintain or improve the quality of life of the individual and yet take into consideration the clinical course of the disease. In some cases, aggressive therapy may eradicate the effusion and be appropriate in individuals with a high-performance status. Other individuals with end-stage disease and a low-performance status may best be managed conservatively with comfort measures.

In this chapter, symptom management of pleural and pericardial effusions will be discussed separately. Maintenance or improvement of quality of life is the most important goal in treating both types of effusions.

Section A: Pleural Effusions

Etiology

The most common tumor types associated with malignant pleural effusions are lung, breast, gastrointestinal and ovarian tumors, lymphomas, and leukemia (Figure 23-1).[5–8] With the rising incidence of breast and lung

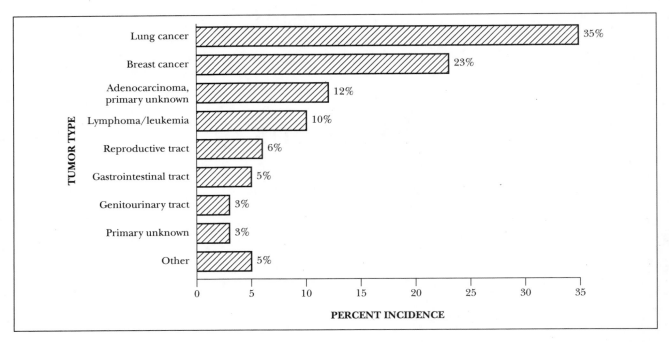

FIGURE 23-1   Tumor types associated with pleural effusions, shown as a percentage of all pleural effusions. (Source: Adapted with permission from Hausheer FH, Yarbro JW: Diagnosis and treatment of malignant pleural effusions. *Semin Oncol* 12:54–75, 1985.[6])

cancer, more than half of all malignant pleural effusions are attributed to these tumor types. In two studies, 80% to 90% of pleural effusions were ipsilateral to the primary lesion.[4,9] Bilateral effusions are most frequently detected in individuals with cancer of the ovary, breast, or lymph nodes. About one-third of individuals with malignant pleural effusions have bilateral effusions.[10]

Pathophysiology

Normal Pleural Fluid Formation

The pleura is a thin layer of mesothelium that encases the lungs on one side (*visceral pleura*) and the thoracic cavity on the other side (*parietal pleura*). The pleural space is a potential space between the visceral and parietal pleurae (Figure 23-2). Pleural fluid is a filtrate secreted by the mesothelial cells of the pleurae. Eighty to 90% of the fluid is reabsorbed. Liquid, protein, and large cells in the pleural space are primarily reabsorbed by the lymphatic system of the parietal pleura via stomata, which are 2 to 12 μm openings found on the parietal pleura.

Normally there is only 10 to 20 mL of fluid at any one time in the pleural space. It was originally thought that 5 to 10 liters of fluid move through the pleural space in a 24-hour period;[11] however, recent findings suggest that daily fluid production is closer to 200 to 500 mL in 24 hours.[5,8] Continuous pleural fluid movement is influenced by capillary permeability, hydrostatic and colloidal

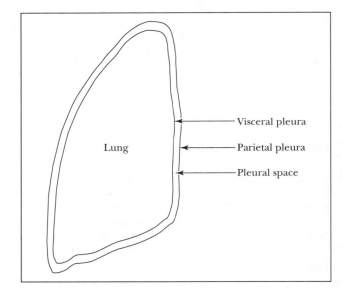

FIGURE 23-2   Structure of the pleura.

osmotic pressures, and lymphatic drainage. Changes in the balance among these parameters may result in pleural fluid accumulation.

Abnormal Pleural Fluid Formation

Cancer can alter the balance among capillary permeability, hydrostatic and colloidal osmotic pressures, and lymphatic drainage in several ways: pleural implantation, lymphatic obstruction, venous obstruction, and tumor cell suspensions.[12] Pleural implantation occurs by seeding of the primary tumor onto the serosal surface of the visceral or parietal pleura. Pleural implants lead to increased capillary permeability through inflammation of the pleural surfaces, with an increased net filtration of fluid into the pleural space.[13] This is most commonly seen in lung cancer.

Lymphatic obstruction is often seen in lymphomas and metastatic breast or lung cancer. Obstruction of the lymphatic channels interferes with fluid and protein reabsorption from the pleural space, with a resulting pleural effusion. The mediastinal lymph nodes are most commonly involved.

Pulmonary venous obstruction causes increased hydrostatic pressure at the pleurae, thereby decreasing the pressure gradient, resulting in fluid accumulation in the pleural space. This is often seen in lung cancer.

Tumor cell suspensions are malignant cells that are shed into the pleural space, changing the colloid osmotic pressure. Pleural implants result in mesothelial shedding and thickening of the pleurae. It is the number of tumor cells in the pleural space that differentiates a tumor cell suspension from a pleural implant.[10] Cytologic evaluation of the pleural fluid would indicate cell counts greater than 4000 cells/mL in a tumor cell suspension.[14] Tumor cell suspensions are seen in lung, breast, and ovarian cancer.

Assessment

Physical Assessment

A thorough history and physical examination are essential in the diagnosis of a malignant pleural effusion. Most individuals present with complaints of dyspnea, dull aching or pleuritic chest pain, and a dry, nonproductive cough. Less than 25% of individuals are asymptomatic.[4,11]

A pleural fluid accumulation greater than 300 mL may be detected on physical examination. Physical findings may include intercostal prominence, dullness or flatness on percussion, decreased breath sounds, and decreased tactile fremitus. Tachypnea, labored breathing, fever, and decreased chest wall expansion may be observed. If the effusion is large, it can cause tracheal deviation to the unaffected side.

Diagnostic Evaluation

Chest x-ray film

A chest radiograph will usually confirm fluid in the pleural cavity. Anterior-posterior films classically reveal a blunting of the costophrenic angle and a mediastinal shift if a large effusion is present (Figure 23-3). Lateral decubitus films are usually taken, as they can detect as little as 100 mL of pleural fluid accumulation, whereas anterior-posterior films can detect an effusion with a minimum of 175 to 525 mL of fluid.[1,8,11]

Thoracentesis

A thoracentesis is typically used in the diagnosis of pleural effusions, because it confirms the presence of fluid in the pleural space *and* it allows for the evaluation of the fluid. In addition, removal of the pleural fluid often relieves the physical symptoms. A thoracentesis is performed at the bedside or in the outpatient setting under local anesthetic by inserting a needle through the posterior chest wall. The posterior axillary line and the seventh intercostal space are landmarks. A chest x-ray film should be obtained after the procedure to ensure that a pneumothorax has not occurred. Large volumes of fluid can be removed, but fluid should not exceed 1500 mL in order to avoid hypotension or circulatory collapse.

Pleural fluid evaluation

At least 25 to 50 mL of fluid is needed in order to obtain an accurate diagnosis. Pleural fluids are classified as transudates or exudates (Table 23-1). Classification is diagnostic and may help distinguish between a benign and a malignant etiology. A transudative pleural effusion is low in protein and occurs when systemic factors such as cirrhosis or congestive heart failure cause fluid to leak from blood vessels into the pleural space.[16] Transudative effusions are often seen in individuals with lymphomas, although most transudates indicate a benign process.

Most malignant effusions are classified as exudates. When local factors influencing fluid formation are altered, an exudate is formed. An exudative pleural effusion is a high-protein fluid that leaks from blood vessels that have an increased permeability. The visceral and parietal pleurae are often seeded with tumor, which increases the capillary permeability. The lactate dehydrogenase (LDH) level of the fluid is elevated secondary to the tissue destruction. The chance of misclassifying an exudate is decreased when these three variables are utilized: LDH level, the ratio of pleural fluid LDH level to serum LDH level, and the ratio of pleural fluid protein to serum protein.[14]

Cytology determines the cell count and composition of the fluid. Cytology is diagnostic in 70% to 80% of individuals with malignant pleural effusions. Pleural fluid pH and glucose levels may be obtained. In 77 patients with pleural neoplasms, a low mean glucose of 66 mg/dL and pH of 7.30 correlated with greater tumor involvement and a poor prognosis.[12,17]

Thoracoscopy

Thoracoscopy is gaining favor for diagnostic purposes when cytologic evaluation is unable to confirm a malig-

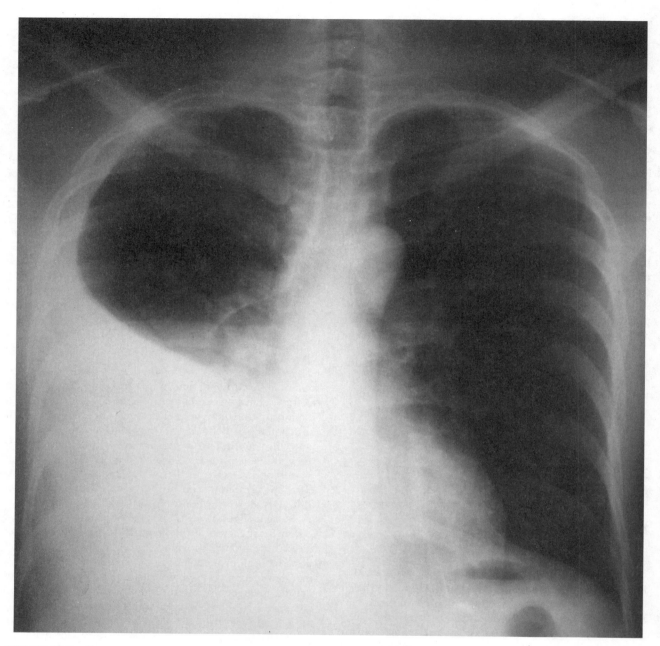

FIGURE 23-3   Chest x-ray film showing right pleural effusion. (Source: Courtesy of Rush-Presbyterian-St. Luke's Medical Center, Chicago, IL.)

TABLE 23-1   Characteristics of Transudates and Exudates in Pleural Effusions

Characteristics	Transudates	Exudates
Specific gravity	Less than 0.016	Greater than 0.016
Protein content	Less than 3.0 g/100 mL	Greater than 3.0 g/100 mL
Color	Clear or straw-colored	Cloudy, bloody, or purulent
LDH level	Less than 200 IU	Greater than 200 IU
Pleural fluid LDH/serum LDH ratio		Greater than 0.6
Pleural fluid protein/serum ratio		Greater than 0.5

Source: Gobel BH, Lawler PE: Malignant pleural effusions. *Oncol Nurs Forum* 12:49–54, 1985.[15] Reprinted with permission.

nant origin. Thoracoscopy can be done under local anesthesia with intravenous sedation. This procedure allows visualization of about 75% of the visceral and parietal pleurae, as well as the ability to obtain biopsies. Studies report that a diagnosis was obtained by this means in 80% to 96% of individuals.[18,19] It is also possible to break down loculations during this procedure, which can facilitate the success of further therapy.

Symptom Management

Therapeutic Approaches

The goal in the management of malignant pleural effusions is permanent symptom relief while maintaining or improving the quality of life of an individual. Cure is not always possible. The choice of treatment depends on several factors: an individual's age, performance status, and prognosis, as well as the site of the primary tumor. If an individual is asymptomatic with an effusion, treatment is often postponed.

Thoracentesis

Some individuals experience relief of symptoms after a diagnostic thoracentesis and no additional therapy may be indicated. In most cases, the mean time of effusion recurrence with thoracentesis alone is 4.2 days.[5,20] Repeated thoracentesis is not recommended due to the increased risk of pneumothorax, empyema, and pleural fluid loculations.

Tube thoracostomy

Chest tubes are inserted to drain pleural fluid and allow opposition of the visceral and parietal pleurae. Individuals are usually premedicated with a narcotic to decrease discomfort and help relax them before chest tube insertion. Chest tubes to a water seal drainage, with negative pressure applied, are left in place until pleural fluid drains 100 mL/day. Tube thoracostomy alone has a 30-day success rate of only 11% to 40%.[5,6]

Tube thoracostomy with sclerosing agent

After chest tube insertion, an attempt is made to eliminate the pleural space by sclerosing together the visceral and parietal pleurae in a process called *chemical pleurodesis*. Chemical pleurodesis is now accepted as the standard of care in treating malignant pleural effusions.[21] An irritant or sclerosing agent is instilled into the pleural space via the chest tubes to induce a pleuritis and obliterate the space. Chest tube drainage should be less than 100 mL per day before sclerosing is attempted. Individuals are premedicated with a narcotic agent 15 to 30 minutes before sclerotherapy. The sclerosing agent is instilled in a total volume of 30 to 50 mL of saline via the chest tube. The chest tube is then flushed with normal saline and clamped for 2 to 4 hours. The individual is repositioned every 15 to 30 minutes to distribute the agent equally throughout the pleural cavity (prone, supine, left-side, right-side). The chest tube is then unclamped and placed to suction until drainage is less than 50 to 150 mL per 24 hours. Repositioning of the individual after the instillation of the sclerosing agent is being questioned based on the findings that, with some agents, distribution of the agent throughout the pleural cavity may be rapid and complete without repositioning.[21]

Many agents have been used in chemical pleurodesis with varying degrees of effectiveness (Table 23-2). The decision as to which sclerosing agent to choose is often based on physician and institutional experience as well as patient-related factors. Nitrogen mustard, quinacrine, and thiotepa are no longer recommended or are unavailable. Injectable tetracycline and *Corynebacterium parvum* are no longer available in the United States.

Tetracycline was once the sclerosing agent of choice because of its efficiency, low cost, convenience, and low morbidity. Because of its unavailability in the injectable form, other agents, including sterilized talc, bleomycin, and tetracycline derivatives, are gaining favor.[22] Because of its similarity to tetracycline, doxycyline is being used in the treatment of pleural effusions. Doxycycline is a methacycline derivative and is thought to damage the mesothelial surfaces of the pleurae and interfere with the pleural reparative processes, thus causing a chemical pleurodesis.[23] Several studies found doxycycline (500–1000 mg) effective in 61% to 88% of cases.[23,27] In some cases, multiple instillations of doxycycline were needed. Side effects included fevers and mild to moderate pleuritic pain managed with narcotics.

One study tested the tetracycline derivative minocycline and found that six of seven individuals (86%) responded to intrapleural minocycline (300 mg).[21] The limited number of individuals in the study, as well as the possibility of vestibular side effects from minocycline intravenous doses exceeding 200 mg, necessitates further investigation of this drug.

Bleomycin is an antineoplastic agent used for pleurodesis. Its mode of action is unknown, but it is thought to cause an inflammatory chemical pleurodesis by a combination of its antineoplastic and fibrogenic effects.[21] Studies have reported that 13% to 91% of pleural effusions responded to sclerosing with bleomycin.[21,24–26,28,29] In a review of eight studies using bleomycin, Walker-Renard et al.[21] reported a complete response rate of 54% overall. The standard dose of bleomycin is 60 units. The most frequently reported side effects included pain (28%), fever (24%), and nausea (11%). Myelosuppression was unusual.[21] The cost of bleomycin is a major drawback, whereas doxycycline and minocycline are both inexpensive and easy to use with minimal morbidity. One dose of bleomycin is 15 times more expensive than tetracycline derivatives.[25]

TABLE 23-2 Success Rates in Patients Treated with Sclerosing Agents for Malignant Pleural Effusions

Sclerosing Agent	Dose	Number of Patients	% Success Rate (Complete Response)[a]
Talc	2.5–10 g	165	93
Minocycline	300 mg	7	86
Corynebacterium parvum	3.5–14 mg[b]	169	76
Doxycycline	500 mg, 1 to 4 doses	60	72
Tetracycline	500 mg–20 mg/kg[b]	359	67
Fluorouracil	2–3 g	35	66
Methylprednisolone acetate	160–820 mg, 3 doses	10	60
Bleomycin	15–240 units	199	54
Mitomycin C	8 mg	27	41
Interferon-β	5–35 million units	29	41
Cisplatin + cytarabine	100 mg/m^2 + 600 mg/m^2 or 1200 mg	44	27
Doxorubicin	10–40 mg	55	24
Etoposide	100 mg/m^2 repeated weekly × 3	9	0

[a] Complete response (CR) is defined as the absence of reaccumulation of fluid as determined by chest x-ray film or physical examination.

[b] Not available in the United States.

Adapted from Walker-Renard PB, Vaughan LM, Sahn SA: Chemical pleurodesis for malignant pleural effusions. *Ann Intern Med* 120:56–64, 1994.[21]

Thoracoscopy with talc

Talc was first used for pleurodesis in the 1950s and has recently come back into favor.[24] The talc must be sterilized and asbestos free when used for pleurodesis. Talc is administered into the pleural cavity via the chest tube and by insufflation or poudrage. A talc *slurry* consists of 5 to 10 g talc in 250 mL of normal saline and is instilled via the chest tube. The slurry is left in the pleural cavity for 2 hours. Response rates have been reported to be 100% with only one instillation.[21,30] Side effects included significant pain, fever, dyspnea, and acute respiratory distress syndrome. Talc can also be instilled directly onto the pleural surface via *poudrage*. Aerosolized talc (5–10 g) is instilled after thoracoscopy with local or general anesthesia. Recent advances in flexible video-assisted thoracoscopic surgery (VATS) with local or general anesthesia make this a viable alternative.[31,32] Pleural effusions were controlled in 85% to 100% of individuals treated by talc poudrage.[11,21,33,34] Thoracoscopy under general anesthesia is preferred for patient comfort due to severe pain experienced upon talc insufflation. The risk of fever, dyspnea, and acute respiratory distress syndrome necessitates careful monitoring of the individual.

Pleurectomy

Removal of the parietal pleura from the rib cage and mediastinum as well as abrasion of the visceral pleura is reserved for the individual who has failed other therapies and has a high performance status and long life expectancy.[25] The individual must be able to tolerate major surgery. Pleurectomy has been effective in controlling effusions greater than 90% of the time, although postoperative bleeding, pneumonia, air leak, and empyema can occur.[12] Mortality rates of 9% have been reported.[11]

Recent developments in VATS makes it possible for parietal pleurectomy to be performed without thoracotomy. VATS is performed under general anesthesia via a 2-cm incision. This minimally invasive technique warrants further study in the palliative treatment of malignant pleural effusions.[35]

Pleuroperitoneal shunt

Although less frequently used, pleuroperitoneal shunting is an alternative for those patients who fail sclerotherapy.[35] It also appears that patients with restricted lung expansion due to a thickened cortex encasing the lung (trapped lung syndrome) may benefit from pleuroperitoneal shunting.[32] A silicone rubber catheter with a one-way valve provides palliation of malignant pleural effusions. Under local or general anesthesia, the pumping chamber is placed subcutaneously; the proximal end of the catheter is placed in the pleural cavity while the distal end is placed in the peritoneum. Motivated individuals or families must then be taught to manually pump the chamber to prevent clogging. The chamber requires pumping for 10 minutes (over 100 times) four times a day. Studies report that 12 to 25% of shunts failed due to clotting, requiring replacement or removal.[31,36,37] Complications are few, so this procedure can be an alternative for some individuals.

External radiation

Individuals with lymphoma diagnosed with an effusion secondary to hilar lymphatic obstruction may benefit from external-beam irradiation. Almost 90% of individuals with lymphoma responded to this therapy.[11,38] Radiation therapy may be the primary treatment modality, or it might be combined with systemic chemotherapy.

Experimental approaches

Intrapleural immunotherapy with cytokines is being investigated. Interferon-β and recombinant interleukin-2 (IL-2) were instilled intrapleurally with response rates of 41% and 21.7%, respectively.[39,40] Response rates were similar to intravenous administration of cytokines. Additional trials are needed to assess the efficiency of intrapleural cytokines.

Robinson et al.[41] hypothesized that palliation in the treatment of pleural effusions could be achieved with minimal morbidity by attempting long-term placement of an indwelling Tenckhoff catheter (Quinton Instrument, Seattle, WA). The Tenckhoff catheter, a translucent silicone rubber tubing, was placed through the sixth or seventh intercostal space and into the pleural cavity of nine individuals under local anesthesia. The fluid was drained into a container whenever the individual became symptomatic. The volume of fluid drained was recorded daily with a mean drainage volume of 477 mL per 24 hours. No significant changes in serum albumin or total protein levels were seen. The individuals were managed at home without further hospitalization or catheter malfunction. This technique warrants further study as an alternative treatment in the palliation of malignant pleural effusions.

Supportive care

There are individuals with end-stage cancer for whom supportive care may be all that is warranted. These individuals may be in the last days or weeks of their lives and just wish to be kept comfortable. Morphine sulfate and oxygen therapy are appropriate. Nurses can help keep the patient comfortable with measures such as positioning and pulmonary hygiene.

Educational Tools and Resources

Clinical nursing guide

Nursing management of the individual with a pleural effusion is a complex process and depends on the treatment modality selected, the individual's performance status, the underlying disease process, and the extent of the effusion. The nurse plays an important role in assessing the individual, providing education, and ensuring individual comfort through select interventions.

Two potential nursing diagnoses in the nursing care of an individual with a pleural effusion are ineffective breathing patterns and impaired gas exchange secondary to pleural effusions.[42,43] Breathing patterns might be ineffective due to the inability of the lung to expand to its full extent. Compromise of the respiratory system may result in impaired gas exchange. A sample nursing care guide with appropriate interventions for these diagnoses is given in Table 23-3. Nursing interventions are geared toward maximizing the individual's ability to breathe effectively with the least amount of effort. In addition, specific nursing responsibilities related to chest tubes and chemical pleurodesis are included.

Self-care guide

The symptom management of malignant pleural effusions requires complex medical management. Individuals are often diagnosed with an effusion late in their disease process and are managed at home, in a hospice, or in the hospital. It is reassuring to the individual if they understand what a pleural effusion is and what its symptoms are. Appendix 23A includes this information for individuals at risk for malignant pleural effusion. In addition, the self-care guide Shortness of Breath (see Chapter 5, Dyspnea, Appendix 5A) will help individuals effectively manage dyspnea.

Section B: Pericardial Effusions

Etiology

Pericardial effusion is the most common cardiac complication of cancer. Lung and breast cancers were the malignancies most often associated with malignant pericardial effusion, with leukemia, lymphoma, sarcoma, melanoma, and gastrointestinal malignancies also cited[44–46] (Figure 23-4). More than 60% of malignant pericardial effusions were seen in individuals with lung or breast cancer.

Many cancer patients can develop pericardial effusions not directly attributed to their primary malignancies. Individuals treated with external radiation in doses exceeding 4000 cGy can develop pericardial effusions.[47] Pericardial effusions also can be related to anthracycline therapy, rheumatoid arthritis, renal failure, hypoalbuminemia, or hypothyroidism. Treatment of the pericardial effusion may vary depending on its etiology.

TABLE 23-3 Nursing Care Guide: Pleural Effusions

Diagnoses

Impaired gas exchange secondary to pleural effusions

Ineffective breathing patterns secondary to pleural effusions

Assessment

- Obtain baseline data: vital signs, mental status (level of consciousness and orientation), activity level.
- Observe for signs and symptoms of pleural effusion: dyspnea, tachypnea, dry nonproductive cough, fever, pleuritic pain (mild to severe).
- Assess lungs: Observe rate and depth of breathing. Findings may include intercostal prominence and signs of cyanosis, decreased tactile fremitus, tracheal deviation, decreased chest expansion, flatness over the effusion on percussion, and decreased breath sounds over the effusion.
- Monitor laboratory data: CBC, electrolytes, arterial blood gases, sputum or blood cultures, chest x-ray film, pulmonary function tests, pleural fluid analysis.
- Assess level of pain related to chest tubes, chemical pleurodesis.
- Assess chest tube drainage system: chest tubes patent, connections taped and airtight, dressing intact at entry site, gentle bubbling seen in water seal chamber (ensures proper functioning).
- Monitor character, color, and amount of pleural drainage.

Nursing Interventions

- Medicate individuals as ordered: analgesics, antianxiety, and respiratory medications. Premedicate individuals for pain 15–30 minutes prior to tests, procedures, and activity including tube thoracostomy and chemical pleurodesis.
- Position individual for optimal chest expansion (orthopneic position). Use multipositional bed and change positions frequently.
- Encourage level of activity appropriate to disease state. Allow for adequate periods of rest.
- Provide for oxygen therapy and humidification of air as needed.
- Maintain adequate nutrition and hydration (2–3 liters of fluid/24 hours unless contraindicated).
- Assist individual with pulmonary hygiene: coughing and deep breathing, mouth care, incentive spirometry, as ordered.
- Make referrals to other healthcare members as needed (respiratory therapy, home health care, hospice, social work).
- Maintain proper function of chest tube drainage system: keep tubes free of kinks and dependent loops, keep drainage system lower than individual, mark and record amount and color of pleural fluid drainage, report any abnormal changes in fluid production to the physician, keep hemostats and occlusive dressing near individual, do not clamp chest tubes, maintain fluid in suction control chamber.
- Facilitate chemical pleurodesis as ordered: premedicate individual for pain; reassure individual throughout procedure; if indicated, turn and position individual to ensure distribution of sclerosing agent (usually 15–30 minutes for 2–6 hours). Positions include prone, left-lying, supine, right-lying. Monitor chest tube drainage until less than 150 mL/24 hours.
- Decrease anxiety and stress through relaxation techniques, breathing techniques, and antianxiety medications.

Patient Teaching

- Teach signs and symptoms of pleural effusions.
- Teach pulmonary hygiene techniques.
- Discuss methods to increase effective breathing: positioning, relaxation techniques, pulmonary hygiene, hydration, scheduled rests.
- Explain procedures: thoracentesis, tube thoracostomy, chemical pleurodesis, as appropriate.

Pathophysiology

Normal Pericardial Fluid Formation

The heart and a portion of the great vessels are surrounded by the double-layered pericardium. The outer fibrous layer, or *parietal pericardium,* protects the heart and holds it in position. The inner serous layer surrounds the surface of the heart and is termed the *visceral pericardium* or *epicardium.* Between these two layers is the pericardial cavity (Figure 23-5). The pericardial cavity is lubricated by less than 50 mL fluid at any one time.[11] As with pleural effusions, Starling's hypothesis dictates that the equilibrium of pericardial fluid is maintained through four factors: capillary permeability, hydrostatic and osmotic pressures, and lymphatic drainage. Both the visceral and parietal pericardia have channels that empty into the mediastinal lymphatics.

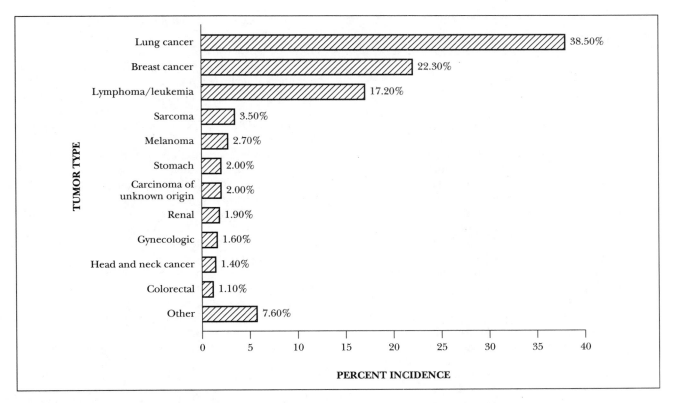

FIGURE 23-4 Tumor types associated with pericardial effusions, shown as a percentage of all pericardial effusions.

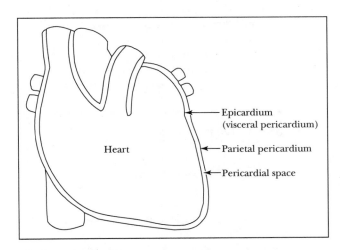

FIGURE 23-5 Structure of the pericardium.

Abnormal Pericardial Fluid Formation

An alteration in the mechanisms that control pericardial fluid formation can be caused by lymphatic obstruction, pericardial tumor implantation, or direct tumor invasion of the heart.

Lymphatic obstruction

Obstruction of the mediastinal lymph nodes with tumor, as seen in patients with lung and breast cancer, interrupts pericardial fluid flow. Capillary permeability and hydrostatic and osmotic pressures are altered, resulting in increased pericardial fluid formation. The majority of malignant pericardial effusions are the result of lymphatic obstruction.[12,46]

Pericardial tumor implantation

Tumor cells can metastasize directly to the pericardium via hematogenous spread. The pericardial surfaces are irritated, leading to a change in capillary permeability and resulting in a malignant pericardial effusion.

Direct invasion

Tumors can spread directly to the heart from mediastinal tumors. Primary tumors of the heart are uncommon but include mesotheliomas and sarcomas.

As pericardial fluid accumulates, intrapericardial pressure increases, which compresses the heart. To maintain cardiac output, the body compensates by increasing heart rate and by increasing peripheral vasoconstriction. If left untreated, these compensatory mechanisms progress, yet are unable to maintain cardiac output.

Pericardial effusions can develop slowly or have a rapid onset. If an effusion develops slowly, the pericardium can actually stretch to accommodate almost 4 liters of fluid. Rapidly developing effusions have been known to cause severe cardiac compromise with the accumulation of only 150 to 200 mL of fluid.[48]

Assessment

Physical Assessment

Many pericardial effusions go undetected as individuals remain asymptomatic throughout the course of their disease. Physical findings are present only when a pericardial effusion causes a decrease in cardiac output. Because individuals are increasingly being supported in the outpatient setting, nurses need to be familiar with the signs and symptoms of pericardial effusions.

Pericardial effusions are usually characterized by a slow onset, but in some individuals they develop rapidly as the first sign of a malignancy. In individuals first diagnosed with cancer by symptoms of cardiac tamponade, 58% of the malignancies were lung cancer.[49] Other primary tumors include stomach, pancreas, kidney, ovary, lymphoma, leukemia, breast, and mediastinal rhabdomyosarcoma.[50]

Symptoms of pericardial effusion include dyspnea, cough, chest pain, orthopnea, fatigue, weakness, and dizziness. *Cardiac tamponade* is the term used to describe the severe decrease in cardiac output caused by pericardial effusions. Symptoms include a rapid progression of dyspnea with chest tightness. Individuals are anxious and often assume a forward-leaning position to obtain relief.

Physical findings include tachycardia (over 100 beats/minute), cyanosis, tachypnea, jugular venous distention, peripheral edema, and irregular heart rate.[51] Cardiac assessment might also reveal cardiac enlargement, pericardial dullness, pericardial friction rub, and distant weak heart sounds. Hepatosplenomegaly and ascites are less common. Breath sounds usually are clear. Cardiac tamponade includes hypotension and pulsus paradoxus (a large decrease in systolic pressure, more than 10 mmHg, on inspiration). Pulsus paradoxus was identified in approximately 33% to 75% of patients.[52,53]

Diagnostic Evaluation

Many individuals with slowly developing pericardial effusions remain asymptomatic for a long time. Routine chest x-ray film and electrocardiogram may reveal subtle abnormalities, increasing one's suspicion for pericardial-effusion. Knowledge of the etiology of malignant pericardial effusions will help nurses identify those individuals at increased risk.

An anterior-posterior chest x-ray film typically reveals an enlargement of the normal contour of the heart due to the increased amount of fluid in the pericardial sac. However, a normal chest x-ray film does not rule out the possibility of a pericardial effusion. Therefore, due to its lack of specificity, chest x-ray films are combined with other diagnostic tools in the evaluation of pericardial effusions.

Some nonspecific changes noted on electrocardiogram (ECG) that are seen with pericardial effusions include sinus tachycardia, premature contractions, and diffuse ST changes and T-wave changes.[38,45] Cardiac tamponade classically produces electrical alternans, which is the change in amplitude of the P wave and QRS complex every other beat. This also is a nonspecific finding as it has been seen in only 5% of individuals with pericardial effusions.[46]

Computerized tomography (CT) can be helpful in the diagnosis of pericardial effusions. High-density areas of fluid, pericardial thickening, and pericardial masses are visualized when viewing the heart.

Echocardiography (Echo) is a quick, reliable, noninvasive diagnostic tool that can establish the presence of small amounts of pericardial fluid. An echocardiogram accurately demonstrates the effusion's effect on ventricular function. It is the most commonly used diagnostic test when a pericardial effusion is suspected. Echocardiography had a 96% diagnostic accuracy in one study.[52]

Another tool used in the diagnosis of pericardial effusion is percutaneous pericardiocentesis. This procedure is used diagnostically only for individuals with symptoms from large effusions or with cardiac tamponade.[12] It is an invasive procedure performed with the use of fluoroscopy or echocardiography in order to decrease the risk of cardiac puncture, ventricular tachycardia, and tension pneumothorax. Under local anesthetic, the pericardial sac is entered just to the left of the xiphoid process. The pericardial fluid aspirated is then classified as a transudate or an exudate and may be assessed for bacteria, fungi, and myobacteria. Cytology has confirmed malignant cells in 80% to 90% of patients with neoplastic pericarditis.[11,52]

Symptom Management

Therapeutic Approaches

The goal of therapy in the treatment of malignant pericardial effusion is to completely remove the pericardial fluid and prevent reaccumulation, with minimal morbidity. The individual's primary diagnosis, stage of disease, and performance status must be considered. Some individuals may require immediate systemic treatment of cardiac tamponade before mechanical interventions can be considered, in order to increase cardiac output. Emergency measures include intravenous plasma or colloid solutions for volume expansion and sympathomimetic agents such as isoproterenol hydrochloride.[46,47,54]

Pericardiocentesis

Therapeutic pericardiocentesis is most often utilized in the initial management of pericardial effusion. The actual procedure was discussed in the section on evaluation. Pericardiocentesis alone has been successful in removing fluid and initially alleviating symptoms in 94% to 97% of individuals.[55,56] However, more than one-half of the individuals had reaccumulation of fluid without further therapy.[52,56]

Pericardiocentesis with sclerosing agent

Pericardiocentesis with the use of sclerosing agents is often attempted in an effort to obliterate the pericardial space. Chemical agents are used for their antitumor activity or to induce an inflammatory response in the pericardium in order to achieve symphysis of the epicardium and parietal pericardium. Sclerosing agents include bleomycin, mitomycin C, cisplatin, fluorouracil, tetracycline, and doxycycline.[11,12,46,53,56–59] Many of the studies that have been conducted contained small numbers of subjects, making it difficult to compare the true efficacy of these agents. Vaitkus et al.[56] estimated the overall success rate of all sclerosing agents considered together to be 81.6%. Pain, fever, and myelosuppression are reported side effects. Randomized controlled studies need to be conducted in order to get accurate information as to the most efficacious sclerosing agents available.

Radiation therapy

Radiation therapy to treat pericardial effusions has been used most successfully in radiosensitive tumors such as lymphomas or leukemias.[11,46] Lymphomas and leukemias have had high success rates of 93.3%, whereas breast cancers and other solid tumors have had success rates of 70.6% and 45.4%, respectively, when radiation therapy was used.[56]

Chemotherapy

Systemic chemotherapy with or without external-beam radiation has been used in lymphoma, breast, and solid tumors.[52] After initial drainage of the effusion by pericardiocentesis, chemotherapy may help prevent recurrence of pericardial fluid.

Surgery

Surgery is a treatment reserved for individuals who require repeated pericardiocentesis and who can withstand the stress of surgery. It may also be necessary if the diagnosis is uncertain and a biopsy is needed. Surgical intervention includes subxiphoid pericardial window, thoracotomy with pleuropericardiotomy, and thoracotomy with pericardiectomy. Table 23-4 compares their effectiveness along with that of indwelling pericardial catheters and percutaneous balloon pericardiotomy.

The *subxiphoid pericardiectomy* (window) is performed under local anesthesia with few side effects and low morbidity.[60,61] Biopsies can be obtained with this procedure. An incision is made beneath the xiphoid process and a portion of the parietal pericardium is excised, creating a "window" to allow pericardial fluid to drain into the pleural space or subcutaneous tissue. This procedure has been effective in controlling effusions 90% to 100% of the time.[52,56]

A *thoracotomy* requires general anesthesia and a patient with a high-performance status. This approach may not be appropriate for all patients. Through a median sternotomy, the pericardium is entered, fluid is drained, and biopsies can be taken. In a *pericardiectomy* the majority of the pericardium is excised while protecting the phrenic nerves on both sides. Chest tubes are left in until drainage is minimal. Complications include arrhythmias, bleeding, infection, and hemothorax. In a *pleuropericardiotomy*, a smaller portion ("window") of the pericardium is excised.

Indwelling pericardial catheters

Catheters have been left in place to drain pericardial fluid after a successful pericardiocentesis. Indwelling pericardial catheters have been successful in 76.3% of individuals.[56] Drains remained in place for an average of 4.8 days.

Percutaneous balloon pericardiotomy

A percutaneous balloon pericardiotomy is an alternative method used to prevent the reaccumulation of

TABLE 23-4   Prevention of Recurrent Pericardial Effusions by Mechanical Approaches

Mechanical Approach	Number of Patients	% Patients with Effusion Control*
Indwelling pericardial catheter	76	76
Subxiphoid pericardiectomy (window)	165	92
Thoracotomy with pleuropericardiotomy (window)	78	86
Thoracotomy with pericardiectomy	60	83
Percutaneous balloon pericardiotomy	46	96

* Effusion was considered controlled when patient remained asymptomatic without further intervention.

Adapted from Vaitkus PT, Hermann HC, LeWinter MM: Treatment of malignant pericardial effusion. *JAMA* 272:59–64, 1994. Copyright 1994, American Medical Association. Used with permission.[56]

TABLE 23-5 Nursing Care Guide: Pericardial Effusions

Diagnoses

Decreased cardiac output secondary to pericardial effusions

Impaired gas exchange secondary to pericardial effusions

Assessment

- Obtain baseline data: vital signs, mental status (level of consciousness and orientation), activity level.
- Observe for signs and symptoms of pericardial effusion: dyspnea, chest pain or tightness, cough, fatigue, weakness, dizziness, peripheral edema. For cardiac tamponade: anxious, restless, confused, sudden severe shortness of breath and chest tightness; individual assumes a forward-leaning position, appears ashen, skin is cool and clammy.
- Assess cardiovascular system: Pericardial effusion/cardiac tamponade may present with jugular venous distention, absent point of maximal impulse (PMI), weak peripheral pulses on palpation. Narrowing pulse pressure (decreasing systolic and increasing diastolic blood pressure), weak, distant heart sounds with arrhythmias, and pulsus paradoxus (drop in systolic blood pressure greater than 100 mmHg, upon inspiration), possible friction rub.
- Assess lungs: Findings may include dyspnea, tachypnea, cough. Breath sounds usually clear.
- Assess integumentary system: Check color (ashen, pale, cyanotic), palpate for temp (cool, clammy, may be diaphoretic).
- Assess gastrointestinal system: Findings may include nausea and vomiting, vague abdominal pain, increased abdominal girth. Palpate for hepatomegaly, ascites.
- Assess genitourinary system: Monitor intake and urine output.
- Monitor laboratory data: CBC, electrolytes, arterial blood gases, chest x-ray film, electrocardiogram (arrhythmias, electrical alternans), echocardiogram.
- Assess level of pain related to chest tightness and procedures.

Nursing Interventions

- Medicate individuals as ordered: analgesics, antianxiety, cardiac and respiratory medications. Premedicate individuals for pain 15 to 30 minutes prior to tests, procedures, including pericardiocentesis and sclerosis.
- Administer blood products, plasma, saline fluids, as ordered, for cardiac tamponade.
- Maintain intake and output.
- Position individual with head of bed elevated 45 degrees or position of greatest comfort. Use multipositional bed.
- Decrease activity and schedule periods of rest as appropriate. Cardiac tamponade requires bed rest.
- Provide oxygen therapy as needed.
- Provide emotional support: Reassure and stay with individual as appropriate; reorient individual if confused.
- Keep emergency equipment near the individual.
- Provide safe environment if individual is confused (side rails, restraints, companion, as appropriate).
- Make referrals to other healthcare members as appropriate (home care, hospice, social work, chaplain).
- Maintain cardiac monitor: watch for tachycardia, arrhythmias, electrical alternans.
- Monitor and record vital signs, central venous pressure, as ordered.
- Assist with pulmonary hygiene as ordered.
- Assist with activities of daily living.
- Monitor patient postpericardiocentesis: Check pericardiocentesis dressing for drainage, monitor blood pressure, heart rate, color and temperature of extremities; medicate for comfort/relaxation as ordered; do chest x-ray film postprocedure to assess for pneumothorax.

Patient Teaching

- Teach signs and symptoms of pericardial effusions.
- Explain all tests/procedures: chest x-ray film, electrocardiogram, echocardiogram, CT, cardiac monitor.
- Teach passive range-of-motion exercise and pulmonary hygiene techniques as ordered.
- Explain appropriate treatments: pericardiocentesis, surgery, sclerosis, radiation, chemotherapy.

pericardial fluid. Using the same approach as with a pericardiocentesis, a guide is placed into the pericardial space. A balloon-dilating catheter is exchanged over the guide wire and inflated, creating a "window" in the pericardium.[62] A catheter is left in place to drain and a chest x-ray film is obtained to assess for pneumothorax. This procedure can be done under local anesthesia with a success rate of 93% to 96%.[56,63]

Pericardioperitoneal shunt

Recently, pericardioperitoneal shunts have been attempted in the palliation of malignant pericardial effusions.[64] The technique is similar to pleuroperitoneal shunting except that the proximal end of the catheter is placed in the pericardial space. The pumping chamber requires compression for 15 minutes five times a day to maintain shunt patency. This procedure is relatively new and requires further study to assess its efficacy.

Educational Tools and Resources

Clinical nursing guide

With the possibility that fluid can develop rapidly in the pericardial space, giving rise to symptoms of cardiac tamponade, nurses must have a clear understanding of pericardial effusion and its management. Nurses play an important role in the assessment of individuals in the outpatient setting, in the home, and in the hospital. Initial management may require emergency interventions. Further treatment of a pericardial effusion will depend on the stage of disease and performance status of the individual. Nurses need to educate, reassure, and comfort the individual as well as perform specific nursing interventions.

Decreased cardiac output and impaired gas exchange secondary to pericardial effusions are two potential nursing diagnoses.[43,65] Cardiac output could be impaired due to cardiac compression caused by excess pericardial fluid. Compensation by the respiratory system for the change in cardiac output could lead to impaired gas exchange. A sample nursing care guide for these complications of pericardial effusions can be found in Table 23-5. Specific nursing interventions related to pericardiocentesis are included.

Self-care guide

In some asymptomatic individuals, pericardial effusions will be detected on a routine chest x-ray film or electrocardiogram. It is very important to teach these individuals the signs and symptoms of pericardial effusions in order to prevent an emergency situation. Appendix 23B contains this information. The self-care guide may also be useful for individuals at risk for recurrence of pericardial effusions.

Conclusion

Pleural and pericardial effusions are complex problems that usually affect individuals late in the disease process but may also be the first indication of cancer. Symptom management is varied and depends on many factors related to the individual. Nurses work closely with individuals in the home, hospice, and outpatient setting. Knowledge of the etiology, pathophysiology, and therapeutic management of effusions will give nurses the ability to provide quality care to individuals in all settings and to anticipate potential problems before they arise.

References

1. Austin EH, Flye MW: The treatment of recurrent malignant pleural effusion. *Ann Thorac Surg* 28:190–203, 1978
2. Sahn S: Pleural diseases, in Bone R, Petty T (eds): *Year Book of Pulmonary Diseases*. St. Louis: Mosby, 1992, pp. 327–341
3. Markiewicz W, Borovik R, Ecker S: Cardiac tamponade in medical patients: Treatment and prognosis in the echocardiographic era. *Am Heart J* 111:1138–1142, 1986
4. Chernow B, Sahn SA: Carcinomatous involvement of the pleura: An analysis of 96 patients. *Am J Med* 63:695–702, 1977
5. Lynch TJ: Management of malignant pleural effusions. *Chest* 103:385S–389S, 1993
6. Hausheer FH, Yarbro JW: Diagnosis and treatment of malignant pleural effusions. *Semin Oncol* 12:54–75, 1985
7. Moores DWO: Malignant pleural effusions. *Semin Oncol* 18:59–61, 1991
8. Miles DW, Knight PK: Diagnosis and management of malignant pleural effusions. *Cancer Treat Rev* 19:151–168, 1993
9. Raju RN, Kardinal CG: Pleural effusion in breast carcinoma: Analysis of 122 cases. *Cancer* 48:2524–2527, 1981
10. Moores DWO: Malignant pleural effusion. *Semin Oncol* 18:59–61, 1991
11. Pass HI: Treatment of malignant pleural and pericardial effusions, in DeVita VT, Hellman S, Rosenberg SA: *Cancer: Principles and Practice of Oncology* (ed 4), vol 2. Philadelphia: Lippincott, 1993, pp. 2246–2255
12. Olopade OI, Ultmann JE: Malignant effusions. *CA Cancer J Clin* 41:166–179, 1991
13. Baker R: Pleural and pericardial effusions, in Abeloff M (ed): *Complications of Cancer*. Baltimore: John Hopkins, 1979, pp. 169–183
14. Light RW, MacGregor MI, Luchsinger PC, et al: Pleural effusions: The diagnostic separation of transudates and exudates. *Ann Intern Med* 77:507–513, 1972
15. Gobel BH, Lawler PE: Malignant pleural effusions. *Oncol Nurs Forum* 12:49–54, 1985
16. Bone R, Petty T: Pleural diseases, in Bone R, Petty T (eds): *Year Book of Pulmonary Diseases*. St. Louis: Mosby, 1993, pp. 385–397
17. Rodriguez-Panadero F, Mejics L: Low glucose and pH levels in malignant pleural effusions: Diagnostic significance and

prognostic value in respect to pleurodesis. *Am Rev Respir Dis* 139:663–667, 1989

18. Hucker J, Bhatnagar NK, al-Jilaihaur AN, et al: Thoracoscopy in the diagnosis and management of recurrent pleural effusions. *Am Thorac Surg* 52:1145–1147, 1991

19. Charbonneau MR: Thoracoscopy in the diagnosis of pleural disease. *Ann Intern Med* 114:271–276, 1991

20. Anderson CB, Philpott GW, Ferguson TB: The treatment of malignant pleural effusions. *Cancer* 33:916–922, 1974

21. Walker-Renard PB, Vaughan LM, Sahn SA: Chemical pleurodesis for malignant pleural effusions. *Ann Intern Med* 120:56–64, 1994

22. Light RW: Pleural disease, in Bone R, Petty T (eds): *Year Book of Pulmonary Diseases*. St. Louis: Mosby, 1994, pp. 395–407

23. Heffner JE, Standerfer JR, Torstveit J, et al: Clinical efficacy of doxycycline for pleurodesis. *Chest* 105:1743–1747, 1994

24. Windsor PG, Como JA, Windsor KS: Sclerotherapy for malignant pleural effusions: Alternatives to tetracycline. *South Med J* 87:709–714, 1994

25. Sahn SA: Pleural effusion in lung cancer. *Clin Chest Med* 14:189–198, 1993

26. Keller SM: Current and future therapy for malignant pleural effusion. *Chest* 103:63S–65S, 1993

27. Robinson LA, Fleming WH, Galbraith FA: Intrapleural doxycycline control of malignant pleural effusions. *Ann Thorac Surg* 55:1115–1122, 1993

28. Ostrowski MJ: An assessment of the long-term results of controlling reaccumulation of malignant effusions using intracavity bleomycin. *Cancer* 57:721–727, 1986

29. Kessinger A, Wigton RS: Intracavitary bleomycin and tetracycline in the management of malignant pleural effusions: A randomized study. *J Surg Oncol* 36:81–83, 1987

30. Webb WR, Ozman V, Moulder PV, et al: Iodized talc pleurodesis for the treatment of pleural effusions. *J Thorac Cardiovasc Surg* 103:881–885, 1992

31. LoCicero J: Thoracoscopic management of malignant pleural effusion. *Ann Thorac Surg* 56:641–643, 1993

32. Petrou M, Kaplan D, Goldstraw P: Management of recurrent malignant pleural effusions. *Cancer* 75:801–805, 1995

33. Fentiman IS, Rubens RD, Hayward JL: Control of pleural effusions in patients with breast cancer: A randomized trial. *Cancer* 52:737–739, 1983

34. Hartman DL, Gaither JM, Kesler KA, et al: Comparison of insufflated talc under thoracoscopic guidance with standard tetracycline and bleomycin pleurodesis for control of malignant pleural effusion. *J Thorac Cardiovasc Surg* 105:743–748, 1993

35. Waller DA, Morritt GN, Forty J: Video-assisted thoracoscopic pleurectomy in the management of malignant pleural effusion. *Chest* 107:1454–1456, 1995

36. Reich H, Beattie EJ, Harvey JC: Pleuroperitoneal shunt for malignant pleural effusions: A one-year experience. *Semin Surg Oncol* 9:160–162, 1993

37. Little AG, Kadowaki MH, Ferguson MK, et al: Pleuro-peritoneal shunting: Alternative therapy for pleural effusions. *Ann Surg* 208:443–450, 1988

38. McKenna RJ, Ali MK, Ewer MS, et al: Pleural and pericardial effusions in cancer patients. *Curr Probl Cancer* 9:1–44, 1985

39. Viallat JR, Boutin C, Rey F, et al: Intrapleural immunotherapy with escalating doses of interleukin-2 in metastatic pleural effusions. *Cancer* 71:4067–4071, 1993

40. Rosso R, Rionoldi R, Salvati F, et al: Intrapleural natural beta interferon in the treatment of malignant pleural effusions. *Oncology* 45:253–256, 1988

41. Robinson RD, Fullerton DA, Albert JD, et al: Use of pleural Tenckhoff catheter to palliate malignant pleural effusion. *Ann Thorac Surg* 57:286–288, 1994

42. Wood HA, Ellerhorst-Ryan JM: Ineffective breathing pattern, in McNally JC, Somerville ET, Miakowski C, et al (eds): *Guidelines for Oncology Nursing Practice* (ed 2). Philadelphia: Saunders, 1991, pp. 359–363

43. Schreiber JA: Impaired gas exchange, in McNally JC, Somerville ET, Miakowski C, et al (eds): *Guidelines for Oncology Nursing Practice* (ed 2). Philadelphia: Saunders, 1991, pp. 364–369

44. Thurber DL, Edwards JE, Achor RW: Secondary malignant tumors of the pericardium. *Ann Intern Med* 26:228–241, 1962

45. Adenle AD, Edwards JE: Clinical and pathologic features of metastatic neoplasms of the pericardium. *Chest* 81:166–169, 1982

46. Press OW, Livingston R: Management of malignant pericardial effusion and tamponade. *JAMA* 257:1088–1092, 1987

47. Miller SE, Campbell DB: Malignant pericardial effusion, in Polomano RL, Miller SE (eds): *Understanding and Managing Oncologic Emergencies*. Columbus, OH: Adria Laboratories, 1987, pp. 19–26

48. Kuhn LA: Acute and chronic cardiac tamponade, in Spodick DH (ed): *Pericardial Diseases*. Philadelphia: FA Davis, pp. 177–189, 1976

49. Chen KTK: Extracardiac malignancy presenting with cardiac tamponade. *J Surg Oncol* 23:167–168, 1983

50. Almagro UA, Caya JG, Remeniuk E: Cardiac tamponade due to malignant pericardial effusion in breast cancer: A case report. *Cancer* 49:1929–1933, 1982

51. Mangan CM: Malignant pericardial effusions: Pathophysiology and clinical correlates. *Oncol Nurs Forum* 19:1215–1223, 1992

52. Wilkes JD, Fidias P, Vaickus L, Perez RP: Malignancy-related pericardial effusion. *Cancer* 76:1377–1387, 1995

53. Liu G, Crump M, Goss PE, et al: Prospective comparison of the sclerosing agents doxycycline and bleomycin for the primary management of malignant pericardial effusion and cardiac tamponade. *J Clin Oncol* 14:3141–3147, 1996

54. Theologides A: Neoplastic cardiac tamponade, in Yarbro JW, Bornstein RS (eds): *Oncologic Emergencies*. New York: Grune & Stratton, 1981

55. Celermajer DS, Boyer MJ, Bailey BP, et al: Pericardiocentesis for symptomatic malignant pericardial effusion: A study of 36 patients. *Med J Aust* 154:19–22, 1991

56. Vaitkus PT, Herrmann HC, LeWinter MM: Treatment of malignant pericardial effusion. *JAMA* 272:59–64, 1994

57. Kohnoe S, Maehara Y, Takahashi I, et al: Intrapericardial mitomycin C for the management of malignant pericardial effusion secondary to gastric cancer: Case report and review. *Chemotherapy* 40:57–60, 1994

58. Tomkowski W, Szturmowicz M, Fijalkowska A, et al: Intrapericardial cisplatin for the management of patients with large malignant pericardial effusion. *J Cancer Res Clin Oncol* 120:434–436, 1994

59. Lee L, Yang P, Chang D, et al: Ultrasound guided pericardial drainage and intrapericardial instillation of mitomycin C for malignant pericardial effusion. *Thorax* 49:594–595, 1994

60. Prager RL, Wilson CH, Bender HW: The subxiphoid approach to pericardial disease. *Ann Thorac Surg* 34:6–9, 1982

61. Hankins JR, Satterfield JR, Aisner J, et al: Pericardial window for malignant pericardial effusion. *Ann Thorac Surg* 30:465–471, 1980

62. Jackson G, Keane D, Mishra B: Percutaneous balloon pericardiotomy in the management of recurrent malignant pericardial effusions. *Br Heart J* 68:613–615, 1992

63. Palacios I, Tuzcu E, Sizkind A, et al: Percutaneous balloon pericardial window for patients with malignant pericardial effusion and tamponade. *Cathet Cardiovasc Diagn* 22: 244–249, 1991

64. Wang N, Feikes R, Mogensen T, et al: Pericardioperitoneal shunt: An alternative treatment for malignant pericardial effusions. *Ann Thorac Surg* 57:289–292, 1994

65. Hydzik CA: Alternation in cardiac output, decreased: Related to cardiac tamponade, in McNally JC, Somerville ET, Miaskowski C, et al (eds): *Guidelines for Oncology Nursing Practice* (ed 2). Philadelphia: Saunders, 1991, pp. 422–425

Risk of Pleural Effusion

Patient Name: _____

Symptom and Description   Pleural effusions are a common problem in cancer, although pleural effusions can arise in people with other illnesses. A pleural effusion occurs when fluid collects in the space around the lungs. When this happens, the lungs cannot fully expand, and breathing may become difficult and painful. Pain, shortness of breath, and lung infections can occur if an effusion increases in amount or is left untreated.

Learning Needs   The most important thing you can do is to learn the symptoms of pleural effusions. You should report any of these symptoms to your doctor or your nurse:

- Shortness of breath
- The need to breathe fast
- A dry cough
- Chest pain, which may be slight or severe. The pain may be worse when you lie on one side or the other.
- Fever

A small number of patients never have any symptoms.

Management   If you have any of these symptoms, your doctor may want to see you. The doctor will order a chest X-ray film to see if there is fluid on the lung. If fluid is seen or suspected, a thoracentesis is done. This test removes fluid from the space around your lung. Many times, people breathe easier when the fluid is removed.

If you are short of breath or if breathing is difficult or painful, there are things you can do to help yourself breathe easier.

- Some positions allow your lungs to better expand. Sit upright, lean forward, and rest your forearms on a table.
- Sleep with the head of the bed raised or use pillows to raise your upper body. Some people are more comfortable sleeping in a recliner.
- Save your energy. Do chores early in the day (bathing, stair-climbing). Take time to rest and relax.
- The doctor may prescribe oxygen to help you breathe.
- Take your pain medication. Some medicines help to relax you and help you breathe easier.
- There is no special diet to follow. Small frequent meals (up to 6 meals per day) might be easier for you and may tire you less.
- Drink 2 to 3 liters of fluids per day, unless your doctor or nurse tells you differently.

Follow-up The fluid is sent to the lab for more tests. The doctor will talk to you about further treatment when those results are in. Let your doctor or nurse know if the symptoms are getting worse.

Phone Numbers

Nurse: _____ Phone: _____

Physician: _____ Phone: _____

Other: _____ Phone: _____

Comments

Patient's Signature: _____ Date: _____

Nurse's Signature: _____ Date: _____

Source: Lawler PE: Effusions, in Yarbro CH, Frogge MH, Goodman M (eds): *Cancer Symptom Management* (ed 2). Sudbury: Jones and Bartlett, 1999. © Jones and Bartlett Publishers.

Risk of Pericardial Effusion

Patient Name: _____

Symptom and Description   Pericardial effusions can develop in patients with cancer. A pericardial effusion occurs when fluid collects in the space around the heart. This can happen slowly or very quickly.

Learning Needs   The most important thing you can do is to learn the symptoms of pericardial effusions. You should report any of these symptoms to your doctor or your nurse:

- Shortness of breath
- Cough
- Chest pain or chest tightness
- Weakness
- Feeling dizzy
- Feeling tired all the time
- Swollen hands or feet
- Feeling restless
- A change in memory or feeling confused

Management   If you have any of these symptoms, your doctor may want to see you. The doctor will order a test to look at your heart, called an echocardiogram. A chest x-ray film and electrocardiogram may also be ordered. If fluid is seen around your heart, you will need to come to the hospital for a pericardiocentesis. This test will remove fluid from the space around your heart.

Follow-up   The doctor will talk to you about any further treatment. Further treatment will try to prevent more fluid from collecting in the space around your heart.

Phone Numbers

Nurse: _____ Phone: _____

Physician: _____ Phone: _____

Other: _____ Phone: _____

Comments

Patient's Signature: _____ Date: _____

Nurse's Signature: _____ Date: _____

Source: Lawler PE: Effusions, in Yarbro CH, Frogge MH, Goodman M (eds): *Cancer Symptom Management* (ed 2). Sudbury: Jones and Bartlett, 1999. © Jones and Bartlett Publishers.

CHAPTER 24

Electrolyte Imbalances

Lucinda A. (Cindy) Jones, RN, MS, AOCN

Introduction

Metabolic disturbances associated with malignancy, although relatively rare, may cause life-threatening conditions and have a significant impact on the quality of life of persons experiencing cancer. Some of the electrolyte imbalances, such as hypercalcemia and syndrome of inappropriate antidiuretic hormone secretion (SIADH), are associated with the tumor's ability to produce hormones that interfere with normal cellular function. Hypercalcemia occurs in 10% to 20% of patients with cancer; SIADH occurs much less frequently. Tumor lysis syndrome is a preventable complication occurring in persons with high tumor burdens who may be expected to have a rapid response to treatment. In the following chapter, each of these electrolyte imbalances will be discussed in detail in regard to the population at risk, pathophysiology, assessment, medical management, and nursing interventions.

Section A: Hypercalcemia

The Problem of Hypercalcemia in Cancer

Hypercalcemia, a potentially fatal condition, is the most commonly occurring metabolic complication of malignancy. Although the incidence varies among types of tumors, the overall incidence among individuals with cancer is estimated to be 3% to 35%.[1-4] The incidence is reported to be as high as 30% to 40% in persons with breast cancer and 20% to 40% in persons with multiple myeloma.[5] The relative incidence of hypercalcemia among the pediatric oncology population is rare.[6] In the face of slowly rising serum calcium levels, the person at risk may remain relatively asymptomatic for a period of time. However, if the serum calcium rises swiftly, a hypercalcemic crisis may ensue, putting the person at risk of death from coma, renal failure, or cardiac arrest. Prompt recognition and treatment of the disorder can result in reversal of a life-threatening condition. The overall prognosis is dependent on several factors, including response of the underlying tumor to treatment, the effectiveness of various medications used to treat the hypercalcemia, and the general condition of the patient. In advanced disease, where treatment options are limited and the aim is to alleviate suffering, a decision to withhold treatment and focus on comfort measures may be considered in conjunction with the patient, family, and physician.[7,8]

Etiology

Sources vary in their estimation of incidence,[3,9,10] but in malignancy the most common tumors associated with hypercalcemia are breast cancer and multiple myeloma, followed by lung (varies with histology, but more common in squamous cell than in adenocarcinoma or small-cell carcinoma[10]) head and neck (occurring more frequently in the tongue, oropharynx, and hypopharynx regions and less often in the larynx, floor of mouth, or tonsillar fossa areas), and renal cell carcinoma.[10,11] Hypercalcemia is relatively rare in lymphomas but does occur in individuals with adult T-cell lymphoma and may be a presenting symptom in these persons.[11] Many other factors can contribute to the development of this metabolic complication, including immobility, dehydration related to anorexia or nausea/vomiting, and renal failure.

Pathophysiology

In order to care for persons at risk for developing hypercalcemia of malignancy, it is necessary to possess a basic understanding of the normal processes that promote calcium homeostasis. Calcium is a crucial regulator of numerous cellular processes that affect multiple organ systems, including the gastrointestinal, neuromuscular, cardiac, and renal systems. Calcium balance is achieved by the hormonal influences affecting the kidney, which filters and reabsorbs ionized calcium; the gut, which absorbs dietary calcium and excretes it in the feces; and bone, which stores approximately 99% of the body's supply of calcium. The three hormones exerting an influence on the exchange of calcium between the extracellular fluid and these organs are parathyroid hormone, vitamin D, and calcitonin.[5,12–15]

Bone serves as the primary reservoir for the body's supply of calcium, containing approximately 99% of the total body content. It is a constantly changing tissue that continually undergoes a process known as bone remodeling. In this process, bone formation is controlled by cells known as osteoblasts, and bone resorption or breakdown involves cells known as osteoclasts. Bone remodeling is influenced by a number of hormonal factors.

Parathyroid hormone (PTH) is a hormone produced by the parathyroid gland in rapid response to changing levels of calcium in the extracellular fluid. It acts directly on bone by increasing the rate of bone resorption (or release of calcium). It exerts its influence on the kidney by increasing tubular reabsorption of calcium and by stimulating the kidney to produce *vitamin D,* a steroid hormone that is responsible for regulating calcium and phosphate absorption in the GI tract. *Calcitonin,* a hormone secreted in the parafollicular cells of the thyroid gland in response to high serum calcium levels, inhibits bone resorption of calcium through the inhibition of osteoclast activity. It also decreases the rate of renal reabsorption of calcium. When hypercalcemia occurs, the body tries to regain homeostasis by the suppression of PTH and vitamin D secretion and by the release of calcitonin. If the normal regulatory mechanisms are inadequate, the condition of hypercalcemia results. The hormonal regulatory functions are summarized in Figure 24-1.

Hypercalcemia of malignancy often occurs with bone metastases. The presence of tumor cells causes osteolytic activity, resulting in release of calcium into the extracellular fluid. This accounts for some hypercalcemia associated with lung, breast, or renal cell cancer and with multiple myeloma, which are tumors known for producing bone metastases. However, hypercalcemia also occurs in persons with little or no bone metastases. In these cases, known as *humoral hypercalcemia,* other substances play a role in the process of bone resorption. Identified factors include

1. Parathyroid hormone–related peptide (PTHrP), a protein produced by many solid tumors, most commonly squamous cell carcinomas, and in certain normal tissues, which acts by increasing renal reabsorption of calcium and by increasing bone resorption

2. Transforming growth factors alpha, which stimulate cell growth and replication, and beta, whose mechanism is unclear

3. Tumor necrosis factors (TNFs), cytokines that increase osteoclastic resorption by acting on osteoblasts

4. Interleukin-1 (IL-1), a cytokine that may possibly stimulate osteoblasts to proliferate and produce prostaglandin E and that also leads to bone resorption

5. Osteoclast activating factors (OAFs), found in multiple myeloma cells, which suppress bone formation and may act as mediators of osteoclast resorption.

The humoral hypercalcemia associated with certain lymphomas, primarily adult T-cell lymphoma, is believed to be mediated by ectopic production of vitamin D and tumor-producing lymphokines that have bone-resorbing activity.[16–18]

Prostaglandins were previously thought to play an important role in the development of hypercalcemia of malignancy. However, this has been found not to be the case in many tumors, as evidenced by the lack of response to prostaglandin inhibitors. The local release of these substances may act by magnifying the activation of osteoclasts at the sites.[5] It should be noted, though, that a potential for a rapid increase in serum calcium levels exists in persons with breast cancer who have recently received estrogen or antiestrogen therapy.[5,11,13]

Assessment

The regulatory processes previously discussed act to maintain serum calcium levels within a precise range, usually between 8.5 and 10.5 mg/dL. The severity of symptoms is not dependent solely on the level of serum calcium. In cases of rapidly increasing calcium levels, patients with only slight to moderate elevations (11–12 mg/dL) may present in an obtunded state. Other individuals with pro-

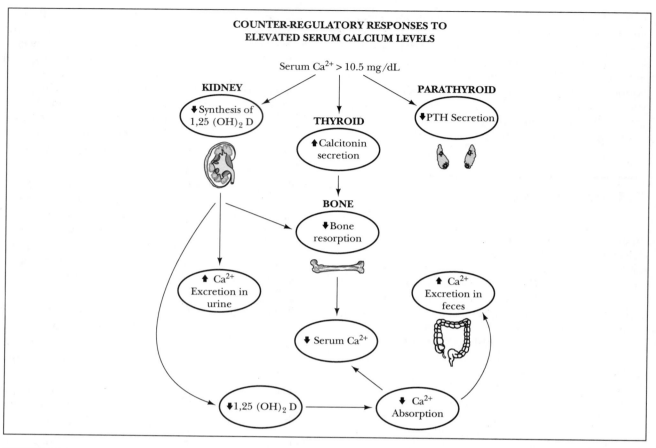

FIGURE 24-1   Elevated serum calcium levels are restored to normal by the hormonal influences of parathyroid hormone (PTH), calcitonin, and vitamin D on the renal, gastrointestinal, and skeletal systems.

longed periods of slowly rising serum calcium may tolerate levels of 13 mg/dL without becoming symptomatic. The author has observed one patient who was asymptomatic in the presence of a calcium level of 16.0 mg/dL.

Physical Assessment

Identifying the population at risk is key to determining which individuals may develop hypercalcemia. As the calcium level rises, organ systems including the neuromuscular, gastrointestinal, cardiac, and renal may be affected. Early signs may be difficult to distinguish in cancer patients who are already anorexic or experiencing fatigue, nausea, vomiting, or constipation. Other early symptoms include excessive thirst, polyuria, poor skin turgor, and dry mucous membranes. As the metabolic imbalance worsens, the clinical manifestations may include dehydration, confusion or progressive stupor, loss of deep tendon reflexes, ECG changes and orthostatic hypotension. It is therefore beneficial to have a good baseline assessment for the population at risk. A summary of symptoms can be found in Table 24-1.

TABLE 24-1   Symptomatology of Hypercalcemia by Organ System

Neuromuscular	Fatigue, lethargy, confusion, obtundation, coma, profound muscle weakness
Gastrointestinal	Anorexia, nausea, vomiting, abdominal pain, constipation
Cardiac	Arrhythmias, bradycardia, tachycardia, ECG changes
Renal	Polyuria, polydipsia, stone formation, renal failure

Diagnostic Evaluation

As previously stated, most of the body's calcium is stored in bone. The remaining 1% exists in two major forms. Approximately one-half is in the ionized or free form (Ca^{2+}) while the remainder is attached to serum proteins, primarily albumin.[4] The ionized form is the physiologically active form involved in many cellular processes. However, if the serum albumin is decreased, as occurs frequently in persons with cancer, the fraction of ionized calcium becomes greater than the fraction of the total measured calcium level. In a person who is hypoalbuminemic, the relative severity of hypercalcemia may be underestimated if a correction is not performed. The following formula is used:

- Calculate an additional 0.8 mg/dL of calcium for every 1.0 g/dL of albumin below normal (commonly 4.0 g/dL of albumin is used as normal), *or*
- Corrected total serum calcium (TSC) = Measured TSC + [(4.0 − serum albumin) × 0.8][3,19]

Example: Laboratory reports calcium of 10.5 mg/dL and albumin of 2.0 g/dL.

1. Determine albumin value

	4.0	normal albumin (low normal)
	−2.0	reported albumin value
	2.0	amount of albumin below normal

2. Correct for Ca^{2+} 2.0 × 0.8 = 1.6 mg/dL Ca^{2+}

3. Corrected Ca^{2+}

	10.5	measured TSC
	+1.6	correction
	12.1	Corrected TSC

Symptom Management

General Measures

The only effective long-term management strategy for hypercalcemia is to control the growth of the underlying tumor.[5,11,16] As hypercalcemia often occurs in persons with advanced disease for whom previous attempts at treatment have failed, many therapeutic interventions are aimed at palliation of symptoms, with the recognition that effects may be short-term at best.

Attempts at dietary restriction of calcium have been tried but are of little use. Although controversial,[20] most sources agree that the ingestion of dietary calcium has little effect on the overall problem of hypercalcemia. Calcium-restricted diets are generally unpleasant for the patient and can contribute to the chronic malnutrition often experienced by the person with cancer. An exception to this may be the person with hypercalcemia associated with lymphoma, which may be metabolized by vitamin D.[12]

Immobilization is a contributing factor to the development of the condition. Weight-bearing exercise is encouraged whenever possible, as prolonged immobilization enhances bone resorption.[1,5]

Mild hypercalcemia has been defined as a corrected calcium level of 10.5 to 12.0 mg/dL. If the patient is asymptomatic, careful observation and a trial of chronic therapy may be the treatment of choice. The presence of moderate hypercalcemia (12.0–13.5 mg/dL) in asymptomatic patients usually requires initiation of specific but nonurgent therapy. Severe hypercalcemia (>13.5 mg/dL) in addition to symptoms requires immediate treatment.[12]

When the patient presents in a hypercalcemic crisis, the immediate goal is to regain fluid and electrolyte balance. The person may be in an advanced state of dehydration, resulting from the body's attempt to eliminate excess levels of calcium in the urine as well as from prolonged nausea and vomiting. Rehydration is achieved through vigorous IV infusion of isotonic (0.9%) saline, usually at a rate of 4 to 6 liters per day. This maneuver will increase the glomerular filtration rate, thereby promoting sodium diuresis and inducing calcium excretion.[5,12,21] Caution must be observed in persons with underlying cardiac disease. Potential signs of fluid overload include a positive fluid balance as measured by intake and output values, development of shortness of breath, peripheral edema, distended neck veins, and rales on auscultation of the lungs. During rehydration, serum electrolytes (sodium, potassium, calcium, and magnesium) and indicators of renal function (blood urea nitrogen [BUN], creatinine) need to be closely monitored. Once rehydration has occurred, a loop diuretic such as furosemide may be added to further enhance renal excretion of calcium. Thiazide diuretics are contraindicated, as their use may inhibit urinary excretion of calcium. It is essential that rehydration be complete before initiation of diuretic therapy, as furosemide may worsen the hypercalcemia by promoting depletion of extracellular fluid, thus causing increased calcium resorption. Most agree that diuretics are best administered only in the presence of fluid overload or congestive heart failure. The use of IV fluids and diuretics alone may temporarily decrease serum calcium levels, but additional medications will be needed to prevent worsening or recurrence of the disorder. The degree of saline administration and forced diuresis may not need to be as vigorously employed as in the past because of the use of adjunct medications, especially the bisphosphonates. Aggressive hydration is overly toxic, as it may result in fluid overload and pulmonary edema. The resulting weight gain and lower extremity edema occurring in patients with low protein stores and advanced disease may not resolve and could negatively affect quality of life.[5]

Medications

Bisphosphonates

A number of medications are available for the treatment of hypercalcemia. Recent advances have shown the bisphosphonates (formerly called diphosphonates) to be highly effective in restoring calcium homeostasis. These drugs are derivatives of pyrophosphates that are incorporated into bone and act to inhibit bone resorption by altering osteoclast activity.[12,15,22] The two most commonly used in the United States are pamidronate and etidronate. Of these, pamidronate use far outweighs that of etidronate because of its ease of administration, generally mild side effect profile, and cost-effectiveness. Pamidronate has been shown to be effective in reducing serum calcium levels in the moderate to severe ranges by single administration doses of 60 to 90 mg, given as IV infusions of 2 to 24 hours. The most widely used regimen is a 2- to 4-hour infusion.[5,12,23–25] Its maximum therapeutic hypocalcemic effect is reached in 24 to 48 hours. It has a low side effect profile that includes transient fever within 1 to 2 days of treatment, occasional infusion site reactions, and hypocalcemia and hypophosphatemia occurring in 10% to 20% of patients.[15] The dose may be repeated in several days if response has been inadequate. One approach to maintaining normocalcemic values is the regular periodic administration of IV infusion of pamidronate. In the acute phase of treatment, when a very rapid reduction in serum calcium is urgently needed, calcitonin may be used in combination with pamidronate.[12] Effects of calcitonin are transient, usually lasting only 24 to 48 hours.

By contrast, etidronate is approved for administration in doses of 7.5 mg/kg as an IV infusion of at least 2 hours daily for 3 days.[5,19] A 24-hour single dose infusion of 25 to 30 mg/kg has been shown to be a safe and effective treatment.[26] Etidronate is less potent than pamidronate and has been shown to cause nephrotoxicity. It should be used cautiously in persons with renal dysfunction. Although available in oral form, it has not demonstrated efficacy in the control of chronic hypercalcemia. Studies comparing the relative effectiveness of these two medications have shown pamidronate to be significantly superior to etidronate in terms of normalizing serum calcium levels and prolonging time to relapse.[5,27]

Other bisphosphonates are available in Europe or are undergoing investigation in the United States. These include clodronate, alendronate, tiludronate, ibandronate, and risedronate.[3,5] Clodronate has been used in both oral and intravenous forms to reduce hypercalcemia. An IV infusion of 1.5 g in 500 mL of normal saline has been shown to be effective. Oral administration has been given adjuctantly with melphalan and prednisone in patients with multiple myeloma. This regimen reduced bone pain, progression of osteolytic bone lesions and the number of hypercalcemic episodes.[19] A recent study reports that subcutaneous infusions of clodronate may be of some benefit in reducing hypercalcemia in patients with advanced cancer.[28] Alendronate, given as an IV infusion of 10 to 15 mg over 2 hours, has been shown to be effective in lowering serum calcium levels, but this preparation in not widely available.[29] Tiludronate (currently experimental) is undergoing investigation primarily for the treatment of metabolic bone disease.[22]

The bisphosphonates have also been demonstrated to be useful in the prevention of recurrent hypercalcemia. In addition, they have been used successfully to reduce bone complications, such as pathologic fractures, and decrease the need for pain medications in persons with multiple myeloma and breast cancer.[30,31]

In general oral bisphosphonates have a very low bioavailability (<1%). Oral alendronate is in general use for the treatment of postmenopausal osteoporosis, but has not been proven effective in the control of hypercalcemia.[5] An alternative for the control of chronic hypercalcemia might be the use of oral agents such as alendronate after the initial episode has resolved. However, the use of this preparation has been associated with mucosal ulcerations in the mouth and esophagus and must be taken in accordance with the manufacturer's instructions.[12]

Gallium nitrate was originally developed as an antineoplastic agent. Preliminary studies with this agent showed an associated calcium-lowering capability. Although it has been shown to be slightly better than pamidronate in some studies,[32] its use is limited.[17] It requires administration of 100 to 200 mg/m²/day for up to 5 days given by continuous infusion associated with enough PO or IV hydration to ensure a urine output of approximately 2000 mL/day. There is also a clinical concern regarding the potential nephrotoxicity associated with this drug. Concurrent use of renal toxic medications such as amphotericin B and aminoglycosides has been discouraged. The ease of administration and cost effectiveness of other drug regimens has limited the use of this drug in the treatment of acute hypercalcemia.[12]

Plicamycin

Plicamycin (mithramycin) is one of the most potent antihypercalcemic agents and also the one with the highest toxic profile. It, too, was originally developed as an antineoplastic agent and was found to have hypocalcemic properties. It is a cytotoxic drug that exerts its effect directly on osteoclasts, thereby inhibiting bone resorption. Dosing ranges from 10 to 50 μg/kg, with the total dose usually not exceeding 1.25 to 2.0 mg. Methods of administration vary from slow IV push to an infusion of several hours' duration. No benefit in prolonged infusions has been demonstrated,[22] but caution regarding extravasation should be observed.[2,15] The onset of action is usually 24 to 48 hours after administration. Doses may be repeated, but should not be given more often than every 2 to 3 days. Potential side effects include nausea, vomiting, thrombocytopenia, and bleeding disorders with potential hemorrhage, hepatotoxicity, and renal insufficiency. Organ toxicities appear to be cumulative with repeated dosing.[2,5,22] Dose adjustments should be made in persons with concurrent liver or renal disease.[15] The use of plicamycin has been greatly reduced with the advent of the more highly effective bisphosphonates.

Calcitonin

Calcitonin, a substance secreted by the parafollicular cells of the thyroid gland, promotes a rapid decrease in serum calcium levels, usually within 2 to 4 hours of administration, by inhibiting bone resorption and enhancing urinary excretion of the mineral. A major disadvantage is its relatively short duration of action (24–72 hours) despite repeated doses.[5] It is given as a subcutaneous or intramuscular injection in doses of 4 to 12 IU/kg every 6 to 8 hours for 2 to 3 days.[2,5] Side effects include nausea, vomiting, and a potential risk for anaphylaxis. The use of calcitonin has decreased over the years as more effective treatments have been developed. However, as previously mentioned, it may be used in conjunction with pamidronate in order to achieve a rapid decline in serum calcium while waiting for the pamidronate's onset of action.[5]

Corticosteroids

Corticosteroids are often used in the treatment of hypercalcemia of malignancy despite a paucity of evidence proving their efficacy in most cases.[2,5] They have been shown to be beneficial in persons with tumors such as lymphomas that are readily responsive to the action of these drugs. The steroids act by decreasing calcium resorption from the GI tract and by inhibiting bone resorption.

Oral phosphates

Oral phosphates have been found to be a reasonable treatment for ambulatory patients who are hypophosphatemic.[2,5] They work by inhibiting calcium resorption from bone. The use of regularly scheduled dosing of bisphosphonates is the preferred form of antihypercalcemic therapy in the management of mild and chronic hypercalcemia. The recommended dose range is 0.5 to 3 g per day in divided doses. The dose-limiting toxicities include diarrhea and nausea. While IV administration of phosphates has been tried in the past, it is no longer recommended because of a high incidence of toxicities including acute renal failure, hypotension, and calcifications in such organs as muscle, lung, heart, and eye.[2] A summary of medications used in the treatment of hypercalcemia may be found in Table 24-2.

TABLE 24-2 Available Therapy for Malignant Hypercalcemia

Therapy	Dosage	Comments
Tumor ablation	Tumor-specific	Only definitive approach to long-term resolution of hypercalcemia
Saline	5–8 liter IV in first 24h, then 3 liters/day	Restores plasma volume, ↑ renal Ca^{2+} excretion; continue until Ca^{2+} is <12.0 mg/dL; may require cardiac and CVP monitoring with compromised cardiovascular or renal function.
Furosemide	Diuretic dose 20 mg q4–6h; calciuretic dose 80–100 mg q1–2h	Diuretic dose to control overhydration; calciuretic doses require ICU monitoring to replace electrolyte and fluid losses.
Bisphosphonates		
Etidronate	7.5 mg/kg/d IV over 2–3h × 3–7 days	Prevent osteoclast bone resorption; when effective, calcium level will normalize in 3–5 days; contraindicated in renal failure; given with saline hydration; adverse effects include taste perversions, nausea and vomiting, fever; osteomalacia with long-term use.
Pamidronate	60–90 mg in 1000 mL IV fluid as single dose over 3–24h	Inhibits bone resorption without impairing bone mineralization. Higher doses for more severe hypercalcemia; onset of action within 24h, longer duration of action; adverse effects same as above but dose-related, intravenous infusion site reactions in 7% of patients.
Calcitonin plus a glucocorticoid	200 MRC units q12h IM/SQ; hydrocortisone 100 mg PO q6h	Rapid onset of action; ↑ renal calcium excretion; safe in patients with cardiac or renal failure; most effective in hematologic malignancies.
Plicamycin	15–25 µg/kg (max 1500 µg) as single dose IV over 4h; can be repeated in 48h	Onset of action within 24–48h; variable duration of action; adverse effects increase with cumulative dosage and include thrombocytopenia, hepatic and renal toxicity, nausea and vomiting. Extravasation causes cellulitis at injection site.
Phosphate	1–3 g/dL in divided doses	Prevents intestinal Ca^{2+} absorption and inhibits mineral and bone matrix resorption; dose limiting toxicity usually occurs at 2 g/dL. Chronic administration accompanied by loss of effectiveness. Contraindicated in patients with renal failure and serum phosphorus levels >3.8 mg/dL.
Gallium nitrate	200 mg/m²/dL continuous IV infusion over 5–7 days	Inhibits osteoclast bone resorption. Median duration of response is 6 days. More effective than calcitonin or etidronate in achieving normocalcemia. Adverse effects include asymptomatic hypophosphatemia and nephrotoxicity. Five-day continuous treatment limits outpatient use.

Lang-Kummer JM: Hypercalcemia, in Groenwald SL, Frogge MH, Goodman M, Yarbro CH (eds): *Cancer Nursing: Principles and Practice* (ed 4). © 1997, Sudbury: Jones and Bartlett, p. 695. Reprinted with permission.[19]

Nursing Management

Patient and caregiver education is paramount in the prompt recognition and early intervention for acute hypercalcemia and recurrent episodes. The following points of nursing management each contain an opportunity for educating the patient and caregiver on measures to lessen the impact of symptoms related to hypercalcemia.

Nurses, whether in ambulatory care, home care, or acute care settings, may be the first to recognize the signs and symptoms of persons developing hypercalcemia. A state of hypercalcemic crisis may be averted when the problem is assessed in the early stages. The recognition of the population at risk, including those with actual or potential bone metastases and persons with tumors having a high rate of associated hypercalcemia, is key. Both patients and caregivers should be made aware of the symptoms of impending hypercalcemia, including changes in the neuromuscular status and the gastrointestinal, cardiac, and renal systems. (Refer again to Table 24-1 for detailed symptomatology.) The potential sequelae of untreated hypercalcemia, including severe hypertension, azotemia, renal calculi, stupor, coma, and death, should be discussed with the patient, family, and healthcare team.

The rationale for early and progressive mobility needs to be emphasized. As ambulation is often compromised by pain or generalized weakness, measures should be instituted to ensure periods of mobility. Such interventions include administration of pain medications prior to planned exercise and allowance of adequate periods of rest between activities. Canes, walkers, or other devices should be obtained to promote mobilization. The potential for pathologic fractures must be assessed when planning care for the person with impaired mobility. If complaints of bony pain are noted, especially in weight-bearing bones, the area should be evaluated for possible palliative radiation treatments or stabilization procedures.

Maintaining adequate hydration as a preventive or maintenance measure in high-risk patients is an extremely important part of nursing care. Conditions such as nausea, vomiting, or diarrhea, which may contribute to a state of dehydration, should be reported and treated as early as possible. Oral intake of 2 to 3 liters of fluid per day should be encouraged, unless advised otherwise by a physician.

The medication regimen of each person should be reviewed to identify drugs that may potentiate hypercalcemia, including thiazide diuretics, lithium carbonate, antihypertensives, and vitamin supplements, especially those containing vitamin D. Persons taking digitalis are more susceptible to the effects of increased serum calcium and should be observed for signs of digitalis toxicity.

When the person with hypercalcemia is severely symptomatic and requires rehydration with IV fluids, careful monitoring for signs of fluid overload, including development of shortness of breath, peripheral edema, distended neck veins, and rales on auscultation of the lungs, should be undertaken. Electrolytes such as sodium, potassium, and phosphorus and indicators of renal function such as BUN and serum creatinine must be closely monitored. The nutritional state should be assessed by monitoring serum albumin, as a low value may give a false normal serum calcium. The restriction of dietary calcium is usually not indicated.

Nurses must be aware of the rationale, doses, and potential side effects of the medications used for the control of chronic and acute states of hypercalcemia (refer again to Table 24-2). Hypercalcemia may become a recurring problem as the efforts at tumor control become less effective. The nurse should explore with the patient and family the effects of advanced disease and recurring hypercalcemia on the perceived quality of life. The nurse may act as a patient advocate in discussions about the decision to continue treatment.

Appendix 24-A presents a self-care guide for a patient at risk of developing hypercalcemia.

Section B: Syndrome of Inappropriate Antidiuretic Hormone Secretion (SIADH)

The Problem of SIADH in Cancer

The syndrome of inappropriate secretion of antidiuretic hormone is an endocrine disorder resulting from an abnormal production of ADH (arginine vasopressin). It is characterized by fluid retention, dilutional hyponatremia, and an inability to secrete dilute urine. The incidence is relatively low, occurring in 1% to 2% of all persons with neoplasms.[33]

Etiology

Malignancy is the most common cause of SIADH, although it is also associated with infection, pulmonary disorders such as tuberculosis, lung abscesses or pneumonia, trauma, emotional stress, hemorrhage, dehydration, pain, and central nervous system disorders, including brain tumors or abscesses and head injuries. Drugs that have been identified as possibly contributing to the development of SIADH include antineoplastics such as cyclophosphamide, vincristine, vinblastine, and cisplatin. There has been a case report of SIADH associated with levamisole and fluorouracil used in the treatment of colorectal carcinoma.[34] Other medications that have been implicated in association with SIADH are tricyclic antidepressants, narcotics, barbiturates, thiazide diuretics, oral hypoglycemics, general anesthetics, anesthetics, phenothiazines, and selected serotonin reuptake inhibitors (SSRI).[35–38] SIADH is most commonly associated with bronchogenic cancer, especially small-cell carcinoma. Individuals with small-cell carcinoma account for approximately 80% of all cases of SIADH.[39] It has also been associated with other types of malignancy including prostate, duodenal, pancreas, esophagus, adrenal cortex, thymomas, head and neck, Hodgkin's and non-Hodgkin's lymphomas, carcinoid, lymphosarcoma, and acute and chronic leukemia.[36,39–42] SIADH may occur as a presenting symptom of malignancy that resolves as the tumor responds to therapy, or it may persist as a chronic state.

Pathophysiology

The control of body fluid balance is tightly regulated and determined primarily by maintenance of plasma solute concentration (osmolality) between 285 to 295 mOsm/kg water. Overall balance is regulated by altering the intake and output of free water. When plasma volume decreases, osmolality increases. Osmoreceptors in the hypothalamus, which are sensitive to increased osmotic pressure, are stimulated and induce the thirst response and the release of arginine-vasopressin (AVP/antidiuretic hormone [ADH]) from the pituitary gland. Changes in osmolality of as little as 1% may lead to significant secretion of ADH.

ADH has two primary physiologic effects. Its primary activity is to increase permeability of the collecting ducts of the kidney to an antidiuretic state by retention of body water and the production of urine low in volume and high in solute concentration. In normal individuals, ADH is secreted only in response to high plasma osmolality, and ADH secretion is inhibited by normal or low plasma osmolality. The lack of ADH decreases the permeability of collecting ducts of the kidney, preventing reabsorption and leading to the production of dilute urine and diuresis. A secondary activity of ADH is its effect on arterial blood pressure. This action is mediated by vasoconstriction of arterioles and capillaries, but it requires large doses in excess of normal endogenous levels and therefore has a negligible effect on blood pressure in normal persons.[40]

In SIADH, ADH is secreted even though osmolality is normal or low. Clinically, this leads to inappropriate reabsorption of free water by the kidney, dilutional hyponatremia, and increased intravascular volume. A normal response of the kidney to increased intravascular volume is to increase glomerular filtration, resulting in excretion of more sodium and other solutes in the concentrated urine. The net result is a reduction of plasma osmolality,

reflected by hyponatremia and water retention. If fluid intake is continued, water intoxication may result.

Assessment

The severity of symptoms is related to the degree of hyponatremia and abnormal plasma osmolality. In mild or chronic cases, the person may be totally asymptomatic. However, in general, the severity of symptoms will increase as the serum sodium levels decrease. Presenting symptoms may include thirst, generalized weakness, lethargy, irritability, headache, and weight gain. Anorexia, nausea, and vomiting occur occasionally. Edema is rarely noted. If the hyponatremia has a rapid onset and is severe (less than 120 mg/dL), changes in mental status will ensue including confusion, psychotic behavior, seizures, coma, or occasionally death.[35,39,43,44] All of these symptoms are related to the excessive retention of free water and resulting water intoxication. The laboratory data necessary to make the diagnosis include:[2,33,40,43]

- Hyponatremia (<130 mEq/liter)
- Serum hypoosmolality (usually <280 mOsm/kg)
- Urine osmolality (>330 mOsm/kg)
- High urine sodium concentration (>20 mEq/liter)
- Absence of volume depletion
- Normal renal function
- Normal thyroid and adrenal function

Symptom Management

Prevention

SIADH is not a preventable condition. Treatment of the underlying tumor is the ideal treatment, but other measures may be undertaken to correct the metabolic imbalances.

Therapeutic Approaches

General

SIADH is a medical emergency only when the hyponatremia is severe (<120 mEq/liter) and the individual is symptomatic.[10] Mild cases are initially treated conservatively with fluid restriction (500–1000 mL/day).[2,10,33,39] This restriction of water will allow the body to normalize serum sodium concentration and osmolality, usually within 7 to 10 days.[11] Fluid restriction may present a problem when the treatment plan includes cyclophosphamide, a drug that requires additional hydration to prevent hemorrhagic cystitis and that itself may induce SIADH. Such cases may be handled by giving normal saline with furosemide diuretics and replacement of electrolytes. Careful attention must be given to the monitoring of intake and output, body weight, and frequent assessments of serum sodium levels.[39] In more severe cases of SIADH with water intoxication, an intravenous infusion of hypertonic saline (3%–5%) may be indicated. This infusion is given over several hours in order to prevent the possibility of pulmonary edema. Institutions vary as to the degree of monitoring required during the infusions of hypertonic saline. Some facilities require that the individual be transferred into a monitored setting, while others are kept on the medical-surgical unit with close observation of vital signs during the infusion. Intravenous furosemide may be administered to prevent congestive heart failure.

Medications

Demeclocycline is a derivative of tetracycline that interferes with the response of the kidneys to ADH. It has been shown to be consistently effective in the treatment of SIADH and has relatively few side effects; however, hematologic changes, photosensitivity, azotemia, nephrotoxicity, and superinfection may occur. It should be administered on an empty stomach. Its use in pregnancy is contraindicated.[36] Persons with preexisting renal or hepatic dysfunction should use this drug with caution.[11] The usual dose of demeclocycline is from 600 to 1200 mg/day.[2,11,43]

Lithium has been used in doses of 900 to 1200 mg/day for the treatment of chronic SIADH but is not generally recommended because of the significant side effects that may be seen in hyponatremic patients. It produces diabetes insipidus in 35% to 70% of persons taking this medication. Its major side effects are observed in the renal, cardiac, and central nervous systems. Because of its side effect profile, it is rarely used.

Nursing management

The symptoms of SIADH are often vague and difficult to distinguish from the effects of the underlying tumor or its treatments. As a result, the oncology nurse needs to carefully identify the population at risk for developing this metabolic complication. Nursing interventions are aimed toward controlling the symptoms associated with SIADH and correcting the underlying cause of the disorder. Presenting symptoms of SIADH include an altered sensorium such as lethargy or drowsiness, personality changes such as irritability or hostility, headache, anorexia, nausea, vomiting, muscle cramps, abdominal cramps, weakness, fatigue, unexplained weight gain, oliguria, or anuria. Patients and caregivers should be taught about signs and symptoms to report and the significance of these symptoms. The rationale for fluid restriction and explanations of dose, frequency, and potential side effects

of medications should be included in the teaching plan (see Self-Care Guide: SIADH, Appendix 24B).

Initially, nursing interventions are directed toward fluid management. Daily weights and intake and output are carefully monitored. Fluid restrictions of 500 to 700 mL may be imposed. As the person with SIADH is experiencing water retention and is at risk for congestive heart failure and fluid overload, observation for possible pulmonary edema is important. Thirst may be alleviated or controlled by the use of frequent oral hygiene, the avoidance of commercial mouthwashes containing alcohol, and the administration of artificial saliva.[44]

The only means of permanently controlling SIADH is to successfully treat the underlying disease. Systemic chemotherapy may be employed as the treatment of choice for some tumors. Antineoplastic agents such as vincristine, cyclophosphamide, and cisplatin may cause or exacerbate existing SIADH. Fluid restriction may worsen the hemorrhagic cystitis associated with cyclophosphamide administration, the nephrotoxicity associated with cisplatin, and the uric acid nephrolithiasis due to tumor lysis. Extreme care must be taken with the use of hydration in these patients. If hydration is required, normal saline is used with or without furosemide diuresis. Measurements of urine and serum sodium levels, urine and plasma osmolality, intake and output, and weight are conducted to assess the effectiveness of the treatment regimen. Resolution of SIADH is achieved when urine and serum levels of sodium and osmolality return to normal.

As the sodium level falls below 120 mEq/liter, the person's risk of seizures increases. Seizure precautions that may be employed include use of padded side rails, placement of the bed in the lowest position, and other measures to prevent injury in the event of seizure activity. Altered mental status may also occur as the sodium level decreases. Supportive care for the confused or disoriented person includes frequent orientation to place and time, raised side rails, and the use of soft restraints if applicable.

Other factors that may contribute to or worsen SIADH are pain and stress. These conditions are known to increase ADH secretion. Nurses should conduct a thorough pain assessment and administer pain medications as needed to minimize discomfort. The use of tricyclic antidepressants, narcotics, and barbiturates should be limited, as they may also cause increased ADH secretion. Alternative methods of pain relief such as distraction, heat, cold, and massage may be beneficial. Stress reduction techniques such as progressive relaxation exercises, guided imagery, self-hypnosis, or attendance at support groups can be incorporated into the plan of care if the person is able to participate.

In some situations, SIADH may become a chronic problem. Management includes the continued use of fluid restriction and the employment of prescribed medications such as demeclocycline. Patients and caregivers should be warned of the possible side effects of demeclocycline, including hematologic changes, nephrotoxicity, azotemia, and photosensitivity. They should be instructed to administer it when the patient has an empty stomach. The importance of maintaining the fluid restriction should be stressed. Discussions that assist the person to incorporate the limitations into their normal intake schedule may help them to adapt to this situation. Quality of life may be enhanced if the patient is able to accept the consequences of the treatment regimen. Untreated, SIADH will eventually lead to coma and death.

Section C: Tumor Lysis Syndrome

The Problem of Tumor Lysis Syndrome in Cancer

Tumor lysis syndrome (TLS) is a potentially fatal metabolic complication occurring in individuals with high tumor burdens who are expected to have a rapid response to treatment, especially chemotherapy. If not detected and treated early, the metabolic imbalances may lead to acute renal failure and death.

Etiology

Individuals having tumors with high growth fractions or bulky disease (greater than 8–10 cm) that are responsive to the effects of cytotoxic therapy are at high risk of developing TLS. These malignancies include lymphomas, acute leukemias with high leukocyte counts (lymphoblastic and nonlymphoblastic), chronic myelogenous leukemia in blast crisis, small-cell carcinoma, and, rarely, Ewing's sarcoma.[5,16,43] Additionally, persons with bulky tumors associated with an elevated lactate dehydrogenase (LDH) level are at risk.[43,45] Although most prevalent in patients treated with drugs having potent myelosuppressive activity, TLS has also been observed in patients receiving drugs such as alfa interferon, tamoxifen, cladribine, and intrathecal methotrexate.[5]

Pathophysiology

A collection of metabolic abnormalities results from the breakdown, or lysis, of tumor cells and the kidney's inability to clear these by-products. The intracellular components include potassium, phosphorus, and nucleic acids,

the foundation of RNA and DNA. When cellular destruction occurs, these substances are released, causing hyperkalemia and hyperphosphatemia. In normal physiology and in TLS, an inverse relationship exists between phosphorus and calcium. Therefore, hyperphosphatemia results in hypocalcemia. Rapid catabolism of nucleic acids results in increased uric acid and hyperuricemia (Figure 24-2).

The magnitude and duration of TLS are related to renal function and tumor burden. Many cellular and organ systems are involved in clearing the by-products of cell lysis, including phagocytosis, hepatic metabolism, and renal excretion.[1] As the tumor burden lessens in response to effective chemotherapy, the metabolic abnormalities gradually are corrected. If the tumor growth remains unchecked and the body is unable to clear the cellular debris, the symptoms of TLS will worsen and can result in fatal hyperkalemia, hypocalcemia, and renal failure.

Assessment

Assessment begins with identification of the population at risk for developing the syndrome. A baseline assessment should include renal function and electrolytes (potassium, phosphorus, calcium, magnesium, and uric acid). A summary of signs and symptoms associated with the metabolic abnormalities of TLS is presented in Figure 24-3. Preexisting conditions, such as dehydration, impaired renal function, acidosis secondary to sepsis, adrenal insufficiency resulting from steroid tapering, and effects of various medications, such as indomethacin, potassium supplements, and potassium-sparing diuretics, may predispose patients to hyperkalemia.[2] Metabolic imbalances can affect the normal functioning at the cellular and systemic level. The effects of hypocalcemia and hyperkalemia can be observed in cardiac irritability. Hypocalcemia is also manifested in neuromuscular irritability that may be observed as twitching, cramping, digital and perioral paresthesia, or tetany. The neuromuscular effect of hyperuricemia results in a decreased mental status or

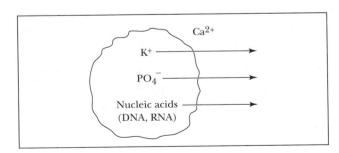

FIGURE 24-2 Tumor lysis causes release of intracellular components resulting in hyperkalemia, hyperphosphatemia, hyperuricemia, and subsequent hypocalcemia.

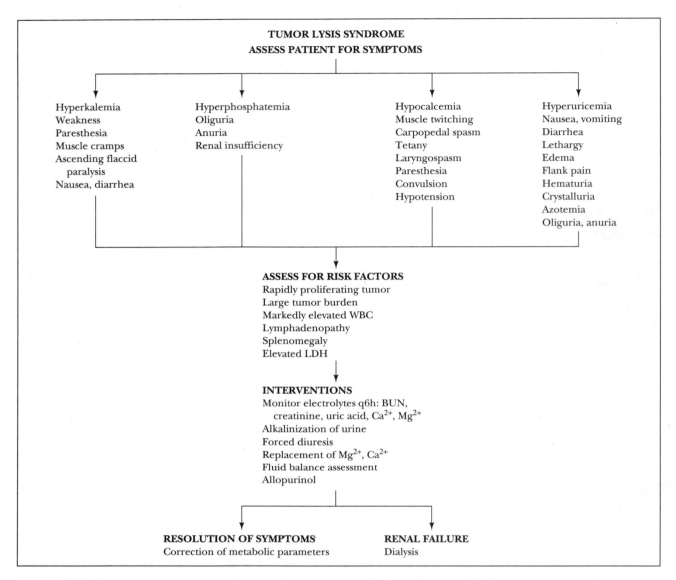

FIGURE 24-3   Clinical pathway for tumor lysis syndrome. (Source: Dietz KA, Flaherty AM: Oncologic emergencies, in Groenwald SL, Frogge MH, Goodman M, Yarbro CH (eds): *Cancer Nursing: Principles and Practice* (ed 3). © 1993, Sudbury: Jones and Bartlett, p. 825. Reprinted with permission.[2])

lethargy. Thus the physical exam focuses on neurologic function, including mental status and determination of muscle strength and changes in cardiac rate and rhythm.

Symptom Management

Prevention

TLS is most likely to occur within 24 to 48 hours after initiation of cytotoxic therapy and may last for up to 7 days after therapy. The goals of medical management

in TLS are to prevent renal failure and prevent severe electrolyte imbalance.[1] This is accomplished by increasing urine output, decreasing uric acid concentration, and increasing the solubility of uric acid in urine.[5,45]

Hydration

Aggressive IV hydration is initiated 24 to 48 hours before, and continued for at least 48 to 72 hours after, cytotoxic therapy is completed.[5,46] The purpose of diuresis is to decrease the rate of urate deposits in the kidneys and to enhance urinary clearance of urate and phosphates. A recommended IV regimen of 5% dextrose in water with one-half normal saline (D5W/0.45NS) at a rate of

3 liters/day. Diuretics such as furosemide or ethacrynic acid may be employed in elderly persons or in those with preexisting cardiac conditions that may place them at risk for fluid overload.

Allopurinol

Allopurinol is administered prophylactically to decrease uric acid concentration by inhibiting the enzyme, xanthine oxidase, that is necessary for the conversion of nucleic acids to uric acid.[5] When TLS is anticipated, a dosing regimen of 600 to 900 mg/day of allopurinol may be initiated, then decreased to 300 to 450 mg/day after several days.[2] Side effects of allopurinol result from hypersensitivity and may manifest in fevers, rash, and eosinophilia. Dose adjustments of 6-mercaptopurine or azathioprine may be needed if these drugs are administered concurrently with allopurinol.

Urinary alkalinization

The administration of sodium bicarbonate in conjunction with IV fluid hydration in order to achieve urine alkalinization is controversial.[46] Some believe that aggressive hydration and diuresis should be the primary means of controlling uric acid. Most agree that alkalinizing the urine promotes the solubility of uric acid, thus minimizing uric acid precipitation and possible stone formation in the kidneys.[5,38,43] Urine alkalinization may be accomplished by adding 50 to 100 mEq of sodium bicarbonate to each liter of IV fluid (D5W or D5W/0.45NS). The goal is to maintain a urine pH of greater than 7.

Therapeutic Approaches

Late management

Despite the initiation of preventive measures, acute TLS may occur. Monitoring of electrolytes and renal function should be conducted every 6 to 12 hours until stable for a period of 3 to 5 days.[2,43] Treatment for hyperkalemia depends on the severity of symptoms, degree of hyperkalemia, and urgency of the patient's condition. The goal of treatment is to remove potassium from the extracellular fluid. This may be done by medications such as sodium polystyrene sulfonate, orally or by retention enema, or the intravenous administration of 50% dextrose, which acts to increase plasma insulin levels and thereby force potassium back into the intracellular fluid. Calcium gluconate may be administered if neuromuscular or cardiac toxicity is evident.[5] Hyperphosphatemia is managed by the administration of phosphate-binding antacids or aluminum antacid gels. The aluminum in these substances reacts with phosphate to form an insoluble complex that is then excreted in the feces.[2] The treatment of the resulting hypocalcemia associated with hyperphosphatemia is controversial. Some sources advise giving calcium gluconate supplements only if the patient is symptomatic;[5,16]

others believe that calcium supplements are contraindicated.[47]

Despite the use of preventive and maintenance measures, some patients will remain unresponsive and will require dialysis. Failure to respond may be secondary to an obstructive problem caused by precipitation of calcium phosphate or uric acid crystals in the kidney.[1,5,48]

Nursing measures

Perhaps the most important nursing intervention for persons at risk of TLS is the recognition of this population so that preventive measures may be instituted appropriately. Nursing management requires a focus on the maintenance of fluid and electrolyte balance and observation for possible drug side effects, and includes the following:

- Administer IV hydration
- Monitor weight every day
- Measure intake and output
- Monitor for fluid overload (especially for persons with preexisting renal or cardiac disease): shortness of breath, peripheral edema, distended neck veins, and rales on auscultation of lungs
- Monitor electrolytes as indicated
- Observe for signs of hyperkalemia: weakness, nausea, diarrhea, flaccid paralysis, ECG changes, muscle cramps, paresthesias
- Observe for signs of hyperphosphatemia: oliguria, anuria, azotemia, renal insufficiency
- Observe for signs of hypocalcemia: paresthesias, muscle twitching, tetany, seizures, hypotension
- Observe for signs of hyperuricemia: nausea, vomiting, diarrhea, altered mental status, edema, hematuria, oliguria, anuria, azotemia, crystalluria
- Replace electrolytes (magnesium and calcium) as indicated
- Maintain urine pH >7 as ordered
- Observe for signs of potential side effects from allopurinol: skin rash, fever, gastrointestinal disturbances (rare), blood dyscrasias, vasculitis

Nurses play an important role in the early detection and treatment of this potentially fatal metabolic complication.

References

1. Moore JM: Metabolic emergencies, in Gross J, Johnson BL (eds): *Handbook of Oncology Nursing* (ed 2). Boston: Jones and Bartlett, 1994, pp. 675–713
2. Dietz KA, Flaherty AM: Oncologic emergencies, in Groenwald SL, Frogge MH, Goodman M, Yarbro CH (eds): *Cancer*

Nursing: Principles and Practice (ed 3). Sudbury: Jones and Bartlett, 1993, pp. 800–839

3. Pecherstorfer M, Herrmann Z, Body JJ, et al: Randomized phase II trial comparing different doses of the bisphosphonate ibandronate in the treatment of hypercalcemia of malignancy. *J Clin Oncol* 14:268–276, 1996

4. Bajorunas DR: Disorders of endocrine function, in Groeger JS (ed): *Critical Care of the Cancer Patient* (ed 2). St. Louis: Mosby-Year Book, 1990, pp. 192–225

5. Warrell RP: Metabolic emergencies, in De Vita VT, Hellman S, Rosenberg SA (eds): *Cancer Principles and Practice of Oncology* (ed 5). Philadelphia: Lippincott-Raven, 1997, pp. 2486–2498

6. McKay C, Furman WL: Hypercalcemia complicating childhood malignancies. *Cancer* 72:256–260, 1993

7. Boisaubin EV, Lynch GR, Dresser R: Hypercalcemia of advanced malignancy: Decision making and the quality of death. *Am J Med Sci* 301:314–317, 1991

8. Nussbaum SR: Pathophysiology and management of severe hypercalcemia. *Endocrinol Metab Clin North Am* 22:343–362, 1993

9. Singer FR: Pathogenesis of hypercalcemia of malignancy. *Semin Oncol* 18(suppl 5):4–10, 1991

10. Johnson BE: Paraneoplastic syndromes, in Fauci AS, Braunwald E, Isselbacher KS, et al (eds): *Harrison's Principles of Internal Medicine* (ed 14). New York: McGraw-Hill, 1998, pp. 618–622

11. Glick JH, Glover D: Oncologic emergencies, in Murphy GP, Lawrence W, Lenhard RE (eds): *American Cancer Society Textbook of Clinical Oncology* (ed 2). Atlanta: American Cancer Society, Inc, 1995, pp. 597–618

12. Mundy GR, Guise TA: Hypercalcemia of malignancy. *Am J Med* 103:134–145, 1997

13. Mundy GR: Pathophysiology of cancer-associated hypercalcemia. *Semin Oncol* 17:10–15, 1990

14. Theriault RL: Hypercalcemia of malignancy: Pathophysiology and implications for treatment. *Oncology* 7:47–50, 1993

15. Hall TG, Schaiff RA: Update on the medical treatment of hypercalcemia of malignancy. *Clin Pharmacol* 12:117–125, 1993

16. Cannellos GP: Cancer emergencies. *Sci Am Med* 3:1–8, 1993

17. Guise TA, Yoneda T, Yates AJ, et al: The combined effects of tumor-produced parathyroid hormone-related proteins and transforming growth factor-alpha enhance hypercalcemia in vivo and bone resorption in vitro. *J Clin Endocrinol Metab* 77:40–45, 1993

18. Goni MH, Tolis G: Hypercalcemia of cancer: An update. *Anticancer Res* 13:1155–1160, 1993

19. Lang-Kummer JM: Hypercalcemia, in Groenwald SL, Frogge MH, Goodman M, Yarbro CH (eds): *Cancer Nursing: Principles and Practice* (ed 4). Sudbury: Jones and Bartlett, 1997, pp. 684–699

20. Arnaud CD: The calcitropic hormones and metabolic bone disease, in Greenspan FF, Baxter JD (eds): *Basic and Clinical Endocrinology* (ed 4). Norwalk, CT: Appleton & Lange, 1994

21. Ritch PS: Treatment of cancer-related hypercalcemia. *Semin Oncol* 17:26–33, 1990

22. Warrell RP Jr: Etiology and current management of cancer-related hypercalcemia. *Oncology* 10:37–43, 1992

23. Ritch PS: The Warrell article reviewed (etiology and current management of cancer-related hypercalcemia). *Oncology* 10:47–50, 1992

24. Sawyer N, Newstead C, Drummond A, et al: Fast (4-hour)

or slow (24-hour) infusions of pamidronate disodium caminohydroxypropylidene; APD) as single shot treatment of hypercalcemia. *Bone Miner* 9:122–128, 1990

25. Gucalp R, Theriault R, Gill I, et al: Treatment of cancer-associated hypercalcemia: Double blind comparison of rapid and slow intravenous infusion regimens of pamidronate disodium and saline alone. *Arch Intern Med* 154:1935, 1994

26. Flores JF, Rude RK, Chapman RA, et al: Evaluation of 24-hour infusion of Didronel for the treatment of hypercalcemia of malignancy (HCM). *Proc Annu Meet Am Soc Clin Oncol* 12:1497, 1993 (abstract)

27. Gucalp R, Ritch P, Wiernik PH, et al: Comparative study of pamidronate disodium and etidronate disodium in the treatment of cancer-related hypercalcemia. *J Clin Oncol* 10:134, 1992

28. Walker P, Watanable S, Lawlor P, et al: Subcutaneous clodronate: A study evaluating efficacy in hypercalcemia of malignancy and local toxicity. *Ann Oncol* 9:915–916, 1997

29. Nussbaum SR, Warrell RP Jr, Rude R, et al: A dose-response study of alendronate for the treatment of malignancy-associated hypercalcemia. *J Clin Oncol* 11:1618, 1993

30. Bankhead C: Bisphosphonates spearhead new approach to treating bone metastases. *J Natl Cancer Inst* 89:115–116, 1997

31. Mayer DK, Struthers C, Fisher G: Bone metastases: part II—nursing management. *Clin J Oncol Nurs* 1:37–43, 1997

32. Bertheault-Cvitkovic F, Armand J-P, Tubiana-Hulin M, et al: Randomized double-blind comparison of pamidronate vs gallium nitrate for acute control of cancer-related hypercalcemia. *Proc 9th EORTC/NCI Symposium of New Drugs in Cancer Therapy* 140, 1996

33. Sorenson JB, Anderson MK, Hansen HH: Syndrome of inappropriate secretion of antidiuretic hormone (SIADH) in malignant disease. *J Intern Med* 238:97–110, 1995

34. Tweedy CR, Silverberg DA: Levamisole-induced syndrome of inappropriate antidiuretic hormone. *N Engl J Med* 326:1164, 1992 (letter to the editor)

35. Poe CM, Taylor LM: Syndrome of inappropriate antidiuretic hormone: Assessment and nursing implication. *Oncol Nurs Forum* 16:373–381, 1989

36. Lindaman C: SIADH—Is your patient at risk? *Nursing* 22:60–63, 1992

37. Woo MH, Smythe MA: Association of SIADH with selective serotonin reuptake inhibitors. *Ann Pharmacother* 1:108–110, 1997

38. Rohaly-Davis J, Johnston K: Hematologic emergencies in the intensive care unit. *Crit Care Nurs Q* 18:35–43, 1996

39. John WJ, Foon KA, Patchell RA: Paraneoplastic syndromes, in DeVita VT, Hellman S, Rosenberg SA (eds): *Cancer: Principles and Practice* (ed 5). Philadelphia: Lippincott-Raven, 1997 pp. 2397–2422

40. Streeten D, Moses AM, Miller M: Disorders of the neurohypophysis, in Fauci AS, Braunwald E, Isselbacher KS, et al (eds): *Harrison's Principles of Internal Medicine* (ed 14). New York: McGraw-Hill, 1998, pp. 2003–2012

41. Mesko TS, Garcia O, Yee LD, et al: The syndrome of inappropriate antidiuretic hormone (SIADH) as a consequence of neck dissection. *J Laryngol Otol* 111:449–453, 1997

42. Ferlito A, Rinaldo A, Devaney KD: Syndrome of inappropriate antidiuretic hormone secretion associated with head and neck cancer. *Ann Otol Rhinol Laryngol* 106:878–883, 1997

43. Gucalp R, Dutcher J: Oncologic emergencies, in Fauci AS, Braunwald E, Isselbacher KS, et al (eds): *Harrison's Principles*

of Internal Medicine (ed 14). New York: McGraw-Hill, 1998, pp. 624–634

44. Finley JP: Nursing care of patients with metabolic and physiological oncologic emergencies, in Clark JC, McGee RF (eds): *Core Curriculum for Oncology Nurses* (ed 2). Philadelphia: Saunders, 1992, pp. 169–192

45. Kalemkerian GP, Darwish B, Varterasian ML: Tumor lysis syndrome in small cell carcinoma and other solid tumors. *Am J Med* 103:363–367, 1997

46. Stucky LA: Acute tumor lysis syndrome: Assessment and nursing implications. *Oncol Nurs Forum* 20:49–59, 1993

47. Nace CS, Nace GS: Acute tumor lysis syndrome: Pathophysiology and nursing management. *Crit Care Nurse* 5:26–34, 1985

48. Hoffman V: Tumor lysis syndrome: implications for nursing. *Home Health Nurse* 14:595–600, 1996

Hypercalcemia (High Calcium Level in the Blood)

Patient Name: _____

Symptom and Description Hypercalcemia is an abnormal amount of calcium in the blood. Calcium is needed by the body to function properly. Calcium can affect your nerves, muscles, digestive tract, kidneys, and the way your heart functions. When the calcium level becomes too high, you may develop unusual symptoms. This may occur because your cancer has spread to the bones, causing calcium to be released, or your cancer may release certain hormones that affect the normal systems that control the calcium level in your blood. Usually, *you* do not cause the calcium level to go up too high by drinking too much milk or by eating too many dairy products; the imbalance occurs because of your cancer. The symptoms may come on gradually or may happen in a short period of time.

Learning Needs You and your family should learn which signs and symptoms to look for that mean your calcium level is getting too high. Some of these symptoms may also be caused by loss of appetite, nausea and vomiting, constipation, or confusion if you are taking strong pain medications. However, it is important for you or your family members to let your doctor or nurse know if you develop any of the following, especially if they are different from the way you usually feel:

- Fatigue (tired feeling)
- Excessive sleepiness
- Confusion
- Coma
- Extreme muscle weakness
- Loss of appetite
- Nausea, vomiting
- Stomach pain
- Constipation
- Changes in your heartbeat (too slow or too fast)
- Frequent urination
- Excessive thirst
- Dry mucous membranes (the lining of your mouth and throat)

Prevention Because changes in the calcium level in your blood are influenced by your cancer, the best way to control the calcium is to treat the cancer itself. Your doctor will discuss this with you.

Management Some people have symptoms when the calcium level is only slightly elevated, whereas others may not develop these symptoms until the level is extremely high. Many medications are available to help control the calcium level—even if the cancer is not being treated. If your calcium level is too high and you are having many problems, you may need to go in the hospital for a short period of time. If it is only mildly high, you might be able to control it at home. The decision of when to treat this condition is usually based on your symptoms, not on the exact level of your blood calcium. Your doctor or nurse will discuss this with you.

For mildly high calcium levels (10.5–12 mg/dL)

- Drink 2 to 3 quarts of fluid a day
- If you are able to walk, do it at least 2 to 3 times a day

For higher calcium levels (greater than 12 mg/dL) you may be hospitalized, and you can expect:

- Extra fluids will be given by a needle in your vein
- Medications will be given to make you urinate (this flushes extra calcium out through your kidneys)
- Frequent blood draws will be taken to check the level of calcium and other chemicals
- Calcium-controlling medications may be given by mouth, by shots, or in the vein

Follow-up

- Blood draws may be necessary
- Drink 2 to 3 quarts of fluid a day (unless directed not to by your doctor or nurse)
- Take medications as ordered
- Report any signs or symptoms of high calcium level to your doctor or nurse
- Walk as frequently as possible if you are able to

Phone Numbers

Nurse: _____ Phone: _____

Physician: _____ Phone: _____

Other: _____ Phone: _____

Comments

Patient's Signature: _____ Date: _____

Nurse's Signature: _____ Date: _____

Source: Jones LA: Electrolyte imbalances, in Yarbro CH, Frogge MH, Goodman M (eds): *Cancer Symptom Management* (ed 2). Sudbury: Jones and Bartlett, 1999. © Jones and Bartlett Publishers.

SIADH (Syndrome of Inappropriate ADH Secretion)

Patient Name: _____

Symptom and Description   Although cancer is the most frequent cause of this condition, it may also happen to people with other illnesses. ADH stands for antidiuretic hormone. This is a substance which controls the amount of water in your blood. Some cancers can produce more ADH than you need. When this problem happens, there is not enough sodium in the blood. This results in too much water being retained in the blood. If the sodium level is only slightly down, you may not notice any symptoms. However, as it continues to go down you may notice symptoms that will be described below. If your doctor or nurse suspects that this problem is occurring, you will be asked to give a urine and blood sample.

Learning Needs   You and your family should know what signs to look for. It is important to let your doctor or nurse know if any of these things happen:

- Increased thirst
- Generalized weakness
- Excessive sleepiness
- Confusion
- Feeling irritable
- Seizures
- Headache
- Weight gain (without swelling in the legs or elsewhere)

Prevention   You cannot prevent this problem from occurring. When it is caused by a cancer, only successful treatment of the cancer can make it go away. However, if you do get it, there are things that you can do to keep the symptoms from getting worse.

Management

- Limit the amount of fluids you drink. Your doctor or nurse will let you know how much you are allowed to drink. As the sodium level returns to normal, you will be able to drink more normal amounts of fluid.
- Take your medications as ordered.
- Demeclocycline, a type of antibiotic, may be given to treat this condition. It is best taken on an empty stomach. This drug may cause changes in your blood or kidneys, and you might become more sensitive to the effects of sunlight.
- Talk to your doctor or nurse about how to better cope with things that cause

stress in your life. These might include learning how to feel more relaxed or going to a support group in your area.

- If you are having pain that is not controlled with your current medicine, tell your doctor or nurse so that a better plan can be started.

Follow-up

- Keep appointments
- Notify your doctor or nurse if any of the symptoms occur or get worse
- Limit your fluid intake until told by your doctor or nurse to increase it
- Additional blood or urine samples may be needed

Phone Numbers

Nurse: _____ Phone: _____

Physician: _____ Phone: _____

Other: _____ Phone: _____

Comments

Patient's Signature: _____ Date: _____

Nurse's Signature: _____ Date: _____

Source: Jones LA: Electrolyte imbalances, in Yarbro CH, Frogge MH, Goodman M (eds): *Cancer Symptom Management* (ed 2). Sudbury: Jones and Bartlett, 1999. © Jones and Bartlett Publishers.

CHAPTER 25

Lymphedema

Barbara Hansen Kalinowski, RN, MSN, AOCN

The Problem of Lymphedema in Cancer

Lymphedema is swelling related either to an abnormality of the production of lymph fluid or to an obstruction in the circulation of lymph fluid. It is commonly classified into two categories: primary and secondary. Primary lymphedema is rare and is related to a defect at birth or a congenital lymph channel deficit. Secondary lymphedema develops from obstruction or blockage of the lymphatic system caused by tumor or trauma (e.g., infection, surgery, or radiation) to the lymphatic channels. Lymphedema can develop immediately after surgery (acute) or months to years after treatment for cancer has been completed (chronic). Acute lymphedema usually subsides after collateral circulation has developed (usually weeks after surgery) and does not result in the scarring or fibrosis that can occur with chronic lymphedema.

The common sites of lymph obstruction are the pelvic and inguinal nodes in the legs and the axillary nodes under the arms. This chapter addresses chronic secondary lymphedema of the upper and lower extremities. The physiology of lymphedema, assessment techniques used at different centers around the country, and management efforts (both standard and controversial) for mild, moderate, and severe lymphedema are presented.

Incidence in Cancer

The incidence of secondary lymphedema, particularly obstruction related to surgery, has dramatically decreased since the early 1900s. Lymphedema that occurred as a sequela of radical mastectomy was reported in the literature from 1908 to 1950 to be present 6.7% to 62.5% of the time,[1,2] with an average incidence of 40%.[3] This was the time period when the Halsted technique for mastectomy (resecting breast tissue and pectoralis major and minor, total axillary clearance, and a split-thickness skin graft[1]) was widely used. Severe lymphedema occurred in about 10% of the cases reported at that time.

More recently, the complication of lymphedema occurs at a much reduced rate of 14% to 22% with radical mastectomy and about 6% to 7% with modified radical mastectomy (removal of breast tissue and axillary node dissection, no removal of chest wall muscles). Breast-conserving surgery (lumpectomy or partial mastectomy with lymph node dissection) typically results in an even lower incidence of arm lymphedema, between 2 and 8%. Variances in incidence rate depend on surgical technique used, which may differ from center to center.[4]

Incidence of lower-extremity lymphedema following lymphadenectomy or groin dissection (e.g., gynecologic or prostate cancer surgery) is also decreasing since surgical approaches have become less drastic.[5] Lower-extremity lymphedema previously occurred in 80% of cases within 5 years after surgery; however, recent studies report the presence of only mild or moderate lower-extremity edema in about 20% of cases after groin dissection.[6]

Impact on Quality of Life

Chronic lymphedema following lymph node surgery can be particularly devastating, both physiologically and psychologically. Because the incidence of lymphedema has

457

recently decreased,[7] individuals who now experience it feel particularly "unlucky." Preconceived notions of lymphedema add to the fear people feel when it develops. They wonder if the mild swelling will turn into a huge, swollen limb.

The physical effects of the swollen extremity may range from mild discomfort to severe pain and may prevent use of the affected limb. In addition to pain, upper and lower extremity swelling can be quite visible and require changes in clothing styles or a support sleeve or stocking. Lymphedema may be precipitated or aggravated by everyday activities—picking up grandchildren, operating a computer, playing the piano, flying in a plane, lifting boxes. It may also be precipitated by factors totally out of one's control, as in environmental temperature shifts or infection in the extremity.

Research studies on the psychological impact of lymphedema are remarkably absent from the literature. Most reports are anecdotal, consisting of case reports or patient testimonials regarding a mix of physical and psychological aspects of lymphedema and its treatment. One study in England[8] involved a matched sample of 50 women diagnosed with breast cancer who had lymphedema that had been present for 12 months. The researchers found that the women with lymphedema were different from the control group in having greater functional impairment and higher scores on anxiety and depression scales. The authors conclude that the psychological differences seem to relate to the sudden, uncontrolled onset of the arm swelling, the fear and physical reminder of possible tumor recurrence, and the visibility and thus the stigma associated with the swollen arm.

Diagnosis and treatment of lymphedema can be frustrating and difficult. There is no guarantee that lymphedema will not occur following lymph node dissection or lymph node irradiation. In fact, it is a complication discussed with people before surgery or radiation. For many years, nurses have used lists of "do's and dont's after breast surgery," posted cautionary signs over inpatient beds, and emphasized hand and arm care in an effort to help the patient have some control over this occurrence. However, lymphedema is not a common complication when the surgeon makes an effort to spare nerves and preserve lymphatics, and avoids stripping the axillary vein. Still, the complication is unpredictable. Very late onset lymphedema (5 to 10 years after surgery) may be the result of the aging process on the lymphatic system.[9] If the lymphedema is not associated with an axillary or pelvic recurrence and is therefore considered to be a "benign" problem, health professionals may well relegate it to the bottom of the patient problem list.

The National Lymphedema Network, founded in California by Saskia Thiadens, was born out of the frustration of people with lymphedema. Treatment information, relevant articles, product information, and conferences are provided by this organization, as well as a hotline for emergency consultation. The services are for both patients and healthcare professionals. The National Lymph-edema Network is a useful resource for people who are at risk for the development of lymphedema.[10]

Etiology

Upper- or lower-extremity lymphedema is a potential problem for anyone who has had a lymph node dissection.[5,9] Secondary lymphedema is a result of an accumulation of lymph fluid in the subcutaneous tissue and an inability to effectively return that accumulated fluid to the circulatory system. This symptom can result from surgical trauma, obstruction of the lymphatics from recurrent tumor, radiation, infection, or scar tissue from previous surgery.

There are several risk factors that have been identified for secondary lymphedema (Table 25-1). These factors include lymph node dissection, radiation therapy, infection, obesity, and age.

Lymph Node Dissection

The extent of axillary node dissection varies from surgeon to surgeon. Studies indicate that accurate staging information can be obtained by removing level I and II axillary lymph nodes (sometimes called a limited axillary dissection).[4,10] Dissection of levels I, II, and III lymph nodes (a full axillary dissection or clearance) is not necessary for staging information and may result in increased arm edema compared with the more limited surgery.

Groin and pelvic lymph node dissections are performed for three reasons: (1) for cure (as in melanoma), (2) for staging (as in prostate or testicular cancers), and (3) for local disease control (as in advanced ovarian or vulvar cancer).[11]

Surgical extent of node dissection will continue to be controversial. A technique that is currently being investigated to potentially decrease the morbidity of axillary lymph node dissection is sentinel lymph node biopsy. This procedure allows the surgeon to identify the node at highest risk of involvement in the axilla in order to

TABLE 25-1 Risk Factors for the Development of Lymphedema

- Lymph node dissection: pelvic, groin, axillary (especially full axillary clearance of levels I, II, and III)[11,12]
- Radiation therapy: directed to site of lymph node removal (axilla, groin, pelvis)[12]
- Infections: immediately post-op or later resulting in cellulitis (usually streptococcal in origin)[13,14]
- Obesity: a disposition to fat necrosis, poor wound healing[15]
- Age: due to decreased lymphovenous connections associated with aging[9,15]

predict whether additional nodes need to be removed.[16] Nurses need to keep up to date on research results and current recommendations about the techniques and rationale for lymph node dissection. To assess a person's risk for the development of secondary lymphedema, it is important to read the pathology report as well as the surgeon's operative notes, which will outline the anatomic operation and level of dissection.

Radiation Therapy

Radiation to the draining lymph nodes following surgery is considered a significant risk factor for the development of lymphedema. Both Larson[12] and Kissin[13] reported an increase in the incidence of upper extremity lymphedema if axillary radiation was used in addition to axillary surgery. It is important for nurses to be aware that axillary radiation is not part of breast conservation therapy, although unfortunately it is still being carried out as standard practice in some centers. In one large radiation therapy center,[12] routine axillary and supraclavicular radiation therapy was done only until 1979. Axillary radiation may be done today if there are a large number of positive lymph nodes or if the tumor is at the tail of the breast near the axilla. The current treatment for early-stage breast cancer typically includes surgery removing the tumor in the breast, axillary node dissection (level I and II), and radiation to the whole breast if a lumpectomy was done.

Radiation to the pelvic or groin lymph nodes is often done instead of surgery as part of the cancer treatment plan. The status of the lymph nodes may be evaluated by CT or MRI rather than by surgical removal. Radiation alone does not seem to cause lower extremity lymphedema but when combined with surgery can be implicated as a cause.[7] To determine the extent of the radiation treatment, the nurse can review the radiation treatment plan, which will give anatomic descriptions of exactly where the radiation was delivered and the exact dosages to each area.

Infection

The protein-rich lymph fluid is a hospitable medium for bacterial growth leading to infection or cellulitis. If bacteria are introduced into the lymph environment, the bacteria are likely to disturb the delicate balance, increase blood flow, and place excessive demands on the lymphatic system. Simon[14] reviewed 26 cases of cellulitis in 15 women out of a group of 273 patients with breast cancer. In this group of 26 cases, upper extremity lymphedema was diagnosed at the same time as cellulitis or was already present when the cellulitis was noted. Researchers reported difficulty culturing the infection (either by needle aspiration or blood cultures), but also noted generally successful treatment of the cellulitis with antistreptococ-

cal antibiotics. Outside of North America, the most common cause of secondary lymphedema is filariasis, a parasitic infection transmitted by the mosquito.[14]

Obesity

Several studies have described obesity or weight gain after treatment for breast cancer as risk factors for the development of lymphedema.[15,17] This may be due to the physical demands placed on the system due to increased fluid and body fat, as well as a tendency toward poor healing and the development of fat necrosis.[9,18,19] Obesity and weight gain, in combination with other factors, increases the risk of the development of secondary lymphedema.

Age

Age has been included as a risk factor for the development of lymphedema, again in relation to and in combination with other factors. Pezner[17] found patients over 60 years of age were at risk. Gottlieb[9] speculates that this may be because "the normal compensatory mechanisms present may be age dependent, and this may explain the onset of lymphedema years later, without an obvious inciting event" (p. 822).

Pathophysiology

The Lymph System

The lymph system parallels the blood vessel system and is responsible for maintaining the delicate balance of interstitial fluid. The main function of the lymphatic system is to transport fluid and larger particles in the extravascular or interstitial spaces—plasma proteins, red cells, bacteria, lipids, etc. that have been filtered out of the vascular system or cannot be resorbed by the venules—back to the circulatory system via the thoracic duct to the subclavian vein. The lymphatic system by way of the lymph nodes also provides lymphocytes and antibodies. The superficial lymph channels drain the dermal layer and subcutaneous fat. The deep lymph channels drain the muscular compartment, joints, and synovial tissue.[20]

In a well-functioning system, fluid enters lymphatic channels, which are blind end capillaries. The capillaries are permeable and consist of single-layer endothelial cells with no basement membrane. From these superficial channels, lymph fluid is transported to larger channels with thicker walls that contract and dilate to promote flow.[7,14] The lymph fluid progresses slowly by gravity and by the contraction of skeletal muscles, which helps force the fluid through the channels. One-way valves in the lymph capillaries and along the lymph channels help keep the flow moving in one direction.

Disruption of the lymph system does not always lead to lymphedema. Acute swelling may occur after trauma (surgery, radiation, infection), but compensatory mechanisms exist,[9] and lymph fluid can be rerouted, collateral circulation can develop, and new routes of flow can be found. When these systems cannot accommodate the demand for drainage, fluid accumulates in the interstitial tissue. Increased osmotic pressure causes more fluid to be shifted from the vascular system into the interstitial spaces, resulting in swelling or edema. If the interstitial edema persists, the high concentration of protein in the fluid causes fibrosis of the subcutaneous tissue, which further inhibits lymphatic drainage. If fibrosis occurs, the damage to tissue becomes irreversible and results in brawny, stiff lymphedema that is not responsive to therapy. Dilation of the lymph channels, weakening of the one-way valves, and thickening of the lymph vessels occur, and the tissue becomes even more vulnerable to injury or infection.[7]

Assessment

The assessment of lymphedema depends on the experience and interest of the professionals involved in evaluating the problem. Typically the patient is the one who notices the swelling and brings the problem to the attention of the healthcare provider. Ideally, the extremities are measured before surgery, and these measurements are used as a baseline for the determination of lymphedema. Unfortunately, as measurements are not routinely done, assessment of the upper or lower extremity is usually initiated only after the lymphedema has been discovered.

A review of the literature indicates that there are numerous techniques to assess and quantify lymphedema. The lack of consensus about assessing lymphedema makes it difficult to generalize treatment protocols from center to center.[12,20,21] Several points to remember are:

1. Patient self-report is the most common method of presentation for secondary lymphedema (it is usually not picked up by the healthcare provider at a routine visit).

2. There is no consistent agreement about the degree of severity, but broad categories (mild, moderate, and severe) are generally used.

3. There is no consistent agreement about how to measure the swollen limbs, but some common techniques include:

   • Volumetric measurement (water displacement) seems to be the most accurate,[12] but is impractical

in an outpatient office setting. It may be available in physical therapy facilities.

   • When using tape measures, anatomic landmarks should be consistent to allow accurate replication of measurement.

Measurement Tools

The most common method of assessing the swollen extremity is to measure the circumference. For the measurement of upper extremity edema, points above and below the olecranon process are used as reference points (e.g., 6 cm above and below, at the wrist and the dorsum of the hand).[18,22] Lower extremity measurement is even less standardized, but measuring the circumference periodically, usually at the calf, can be helpful. Both left and right limbs are measured and the determination of lymphedema is based on the measured differences. A tape measure can be used but should be replaced regularly as the tape tends to stretch and will not report consistent measurements over time. One study[17] that included a control group (no lymph node surgery) found that the control group members could have a difference of up to 2 cm in arm measurements that was not considered to be lymphedema. Other studies have adjusted measurements based on hand dominance. The dominant hand and arm tend to be larger, and that factor needs to be taken into account.[17] Volumetric measure, or measuring limbs by water displacement, seems to be more accurate but is impractical in the general setting. However, for physical therapy units or for surgeons who specialize in lymphatic surgery, the water displacement technique may be practical. Whatever technique is used, progression of lymphedema should be evaluated by comparing only measurements taken by the same method at the same anatomic points—and ideally by the same person.

Physical Assessment

History

When taking a history, it is important to reiterate to the individual that the causes of secondary lymphedema are not known. Care must be taken during this interview not to blame or judge. An assessment of the following information should be included:

• Possible sources of infection (e.g., recent trauma, puncture wounds, burns, bites, cuts)

• Mobility and range of motion of nearest joint (especially a change in mobility as a result of the swelling)

• Report of recent heavy lifting, unusual activity

• Report of activity that seems to either increase (e.g., repetitive movement like typing, piano playing) or decrease (elevation, rest) lymphedema

- Time frame of swelling in relation to surgery (i.e., postoperative traumatic swelling or chronic swelling)
- General health condition (activity level, nutritional status, comorbid conditions, other illnesses)

Physical exam

The physical exam can provide valuable information about the lymphedema and contributory factors. Carefully examine high-risk areas (axillae, groin, breast, pelvis) to determine presence of suspicious masses that may indicate recurrence of tumor. Examine the skin of the extremity to determine obvious areas of inflammation or infection, warmth, erythema, redness, turgor, breakdown, necrosis. Check pulses to determine if circulation is adequate. Assess range of motion and strength of affected joints and limbs.

Take measurements by agreed-on method for flow chart comparing and evaluating treatment over time.

Diagnostic Evaluation

The goals of typical diagnostic evaluation are twofold:

1. To differentiate between lymphatic and venous swelling (such as axillary venous obstruction, thrombosis).
2. To distinguish the presence of a cancer recurrence or progression from a secondary lymphedema related to a lymph transport problem.

Diagnostic tests include, but are not limited to, CT or MRI of axilla or groin to rule out tumor recurrence. Both of these tests have a high degree of accuracy in determining presence or absence of recurrent tumor. Once tumor recurrence has been ruled out, however, the tests may not be able to assess accurately the patency of lymphatics.

Tests to determine patency of the venous system may include color flow Doppler ultrasonogram[9] or a venogram to rule out obstruction. The role of directly assessing the lymphatics via radiologic techniques is controversial at best and rarely done except in the case of impending surgery. Lymphography is an older technique that uses a contrast material to visualize the lymphatics of the affected limb. Lymphoscintigraphy is a more refined technique, although it is not useful for routine assessment. Both of these tests have been shown to be potentially harmful to the delicate lymphatics that are being illuminated and can exacerbate the problems of an already burdened system.[23]

Degrees of Severity of Lymphedema

Lymphedema is usually characterized by the degree of involvement, ranging from mild to severe. The classifications or degrees are defined as follows:

- *Mild:* Commonly characterized by a 2- to 3-cm difference in circumference from one limb to the other. The person may present with no measurable swelling but may complain of a feeling of heaviness, throbbing pain, or soreness in the limb.
- *Moderate:* Usually characterized by a 3- to 5-cm difference in circumference between the swollen and nonaffected limb. The difference in limbs is visible. The skin may be stretched and shiny, and the edema may be pitting. The tissue is usually soft. It may be difficult for the person to button sleeves or fit into shoes.
- *Severe:* There is a large difference in limb circumferences, greater than 5 cm. Skin may be stretched and discolored, purple or brownish. Skin may have a tough, brawny appearance with peau d'orange. The tissue may feel firm (fibrosis) and the edema is nonpitting. This degree of lymphedema is usually very uncomfortable and disabling.[7,24,25]

Symptom Management

The development of secondary lymphedema is related mainly to the primary treatment of the cancer (surgery and radiation) but also to the behavior of the cancer itself. Risk factors have been described that will help the oncology nurse begin to identify the potential population that has specific learning needs regarding the symptoms of lymphedema. Table 25-2 presents an overview of management options for prevention and treatment of mild, moderate, and severe lymphedema.

Attention to the psychological aspect of lymphedema

TABLE 25-2   Management Measures for Lymphedema

Measure	Prevention	Mild (<3 cm)	Moderate (3–5 cm)	Severe (5+ cm)
Exercise	+	+	+	+
Avoid heavy dependent lifting	+	+	+	+
Prevent infection	+	+	+	+
Elevation		+	+	+
Compression garment		+	+	+
Massage/ physical therapy		±	+	+
Sequential pump		±	+	+
Surgery				±
Benzopyrenes				±

+ = usually recommended.
± = optional.

at all levels (from prevention to management of the symptoms) is important for many reasons. The strategies for prevention, as well as the treatment strategies, guide the person at risk to attend to alterations in the body that are a constant reminder of cancer and the possibility of recurrence. Preventive maneuvers, and particularly techniques for management of actual lymphedema depend on the person's motivation to carry them out daily, probably for life. It is imperative that the nurse discuss the feasibility of the plan for management with the patient in terms of appropriate physical measures and also how the plan can be adapted into the person's lifestyle.

Prevention

Prevention of lymphedema is difficult because its causes are usually not under the control of the patient. The patient must rely on the expertise of the healthcare provider to make recommendations that are medically sound and that reflect current practice. In addition, the person with cancer will need assistance to anticipate what life after cancer treatment will be like to minimize the potential side effects and to deal with the consequences of lymphedema.

Nurses who care for people who are at risk for the development of lymphedema can counsel them about exercise, heavy lifting, and preventing infection (see Appendix 25A for a self-care guide on prevention).

Exercise

The benefits of exercise are well known but are worth noting for people who are recovering from lymph node surgery. Normal use of the limb on the side that has been operated on is encouraged. Gentle stretching and range-of-motion exercises are begun usually about 1 week after surgery or when the drains have been removed and the initial pain from surgery has subsided. As range of motion increases and wound healing occurs, gentle strengthening exercises can begin. People are encouraged to continue this simple exercise program through any adjuvant therapy and beyond.[26,27]

Nursing research has documented the beneficial effects of exercise for people receiving cancer treatment.[28] The physiologic benefit of exercise is particularly important for people who have had lymph node surgery. The motion of lymph fluid through the lymph channels is aided by the motion of the skeletal muscles. Deep-breathing exercises cause a drop in intrathoracic pressure, which facilitates the lymph drainage into the thoracic duct.[20] Today, many people are already participants in exercise programs before surgery, either through a health club or their own program of walking or exercise at home. The person who has had lymphatic resection can usually look forward to returning to these exercise routines after he or she has healed from surgery, or may use this time as an opportunity to begin an exercise program.[27] The nurse should review any aggressive exercise program (such as lifting heavy weights) to help the patient develop a plan for a gradual return to presurgical exercise status. See Appendixes 25B and 25C for self-care guides for upper-extremity and lower-extremity exercises, respectively.

Heavy lifting

The person who has had axillary lymph nodes removed should avoid heavy dependent lifting (heavy suitcase, briefcase, grocery bags).[10,29] People should use their presurgical condition or status as a gauge for their activity—if they were strong and in good shape before surgery, they can gradually work back to that status during the postoperative period, and eventually return to most activities.

Prevent infection

Because infection is a risk factor for the development of lymphedema, strategies to avoid infection are discussed with people who have had lymph node surgery. While nurses have traditionally used lists of "do's and don'ts" for education of women following breast surgery, there is little research that corroborates the long list of suggested behaviors. At a minimum, it is important for patient education programs to:

- Explain how the lymph system functions
- Teach the signs and symptoms of infection
- Teach the importance of reporting these signs and symptoms early
- Review possible sources of infection (puncture wounds, insect bites, venipuncture, etc.)
- Emphasize maintenance of excellent skin hygiene
- Formulate a plan for recovering and maintaining range of motion and strength in the affected extremity[7]

Therapeutic Approaches

Mild lymphedema

After infection and tumor recurrence have been ruled out, mild swelling or lymphedema usually is treated conservatively by elevation, a compression sleeve, and possibly gentle massage. Combinations of measures are often used. The strategies for prevention listed above are continued. The main goal of management of mild lymphedema is to help move the lymph fluid from the interstitial spaces into the circulation in order to prevent tissue fibrosis. Gravity, muscle movement, external support, and compression all help to promote lymphatic fluid flow. Good hygiene practices and precautions against trauma or injury are critical measures to avoid introducing bacteria into the protein-rich lymph fluid. See Appendix 25D for a self-care guide to assist the person with mild lymphedema.

Elevation   Elevating the swollen extremity uses the forces of gravity to assist in moving the lymph fluid as it progresses through the lymph channels. Elevation will usually cause a temporary decrease in the swelling of the extremity. More importantly, elevation will provide relief from the tight, heavy sensation that patients experience in the affected extremity.[20] Elevation can be accomplished by the use of pillows to bring the extremity above the level of the heart. Wedge-shaped cushions are readily available and are useful for elevation when sleeping. Simply putting the arm up on the back of a couch when sitting or propping the leg on a stool is easy to remember and can help promote lymphatic drainage.

Compression garment   Elastic stockings and sleeves have long been used for symptomatic relief of lymphedema. The effectiveness of these garments is supported by both researchers[17] and clinicians.[20,30,31] Compression garments can be custom made or ready made, and the cost ranges accordingly. Most insurance policies will reimburse for compression garments if they are medically justified and prescribed by a healthcare provider. The garment should be fitted by a professional fitter when the extremity is at its lowest point of swelling, preferably with no edema. Some fitters have a pneumatic pump and will use it to force the fluid from the limb, albeit temporarily, in order to get the correct fit. A compression garment that is too tight may cause pain or decreased circulation to the hand or foot. A loose garment will not adequately support the extremity. The sleeve or stocking should be checked periodically for size and exchanged for a new one at least every 6 months, because it will lose elasticity with repeated use.[10]

Massage/physical therapy   Manual compression of the extremity as well as massage of other areas of lymph drainage (e.g., trunk or pelvis) may be recommended for management of mild lymphedema. A physical therapist who is expert in treating lymphedema can be invaluable in assessing the person's mobility, muscle strength, posture, degree of fascial constriction, need for supervision, and in developing a plan of education, exercise, and massage techniques.

Complex decongestive physiotherapy   The literature on the treatment of lymphedema reports success with a five-stage approach to treatment called complex decongestive physiotherapy (CDT). The reports tend to be anecdotal[21,30] but the results are compelling. Parts of this "new" approach consist of therapies used previously but now used in a more intense and consistent way as part of a comprehensive program. The five stages are presented in Table 25-3. There are centers in Europe and in the United States that offer CDT. The treatments typically involve a 4-week intensive program, on either an inpatient or outpatient daily basis, followed by home maintenance. These programs are beginning to be cov-

TABLE 25-3 Components of Complex Decongestive Physiotherapy

1. Elimination of fungal infection. Skin care to prevent infection.
2. Manual lymph drainage (MLD): A special massage technique using light strokes to drain the area of congestion and to open the collateral lymphatics. It is usually done for 1 hour a day per limb.
3. Bandaging with nonelastic bandages to prevent reaccumulation of lymph fluid in the treated limb.
4. Performance of exercises while wearing the bandages to further enhance lymph drainage using muscles as a pump.
5. Use a compression garment after the course of treatment to provide support for the treated limb.

Data from Casley-Smith JR, Foldi M, Ryan TJ, et al: Lymphedema: Summary of the 10th International Congress of Lymphology working group discussions and recommendations. *Lymphology* 18:175–180, 1985.[25]

ered by insurance, including Medicare. Healthcare providers need to be proactive to help legislators understand the need to continue coverage for treatment of lymphedema. The National Lymphedema Network is a valuable resource for both healthcare professionals and laypersons. They have a listing of lymphedema treatment centers, therapists, and have a large selection of patient education materials available at a nominal cost. (call 1-800-541-3259, or visit them on the Web at http://www.lymphnet/resource/html). Many physical therapists use one of the components, manual lymphatic drainage, as one of their techniques for working with people with lymphedematous limbs. It is worth interviewing physical therapists to determine their preferred approaches.

Moderate lymphedema

As with mild lymphedema, infection or recurrence should be ruled out as a cause of limb swelling (see the assessment section). If there is no infection or recurrence, then strategies for managing moderate lymphedema will include those used for mild lymphedema (refer again to Table 25-2). In addition, a physical therapist should be consulted for massage and manual lymphatic drainage and for assessment of fascial constriction, range of motion, and strength.

A pneumatic pump is often added to the management approach at this point to enable increased frequency of massage (Figures 25-1A and 25-1B). Communication with the physical therapist and the nurses managing the person in the home is important to evaluate the success of the therapy and to determine whether changes in the therapy regimen are needed. Generally, if someone has moderate lymphedema, effort is exerted initially to mobilize the fluid to prevent and avoid the development of fibrotic tissue. Once the lymphedema has decreased for at least part of the day, then the nurse and therapist work with the person to determine the optimal schedule of exercises, pumping, and compression bandages or sleeves to keep the level of edema minimized.

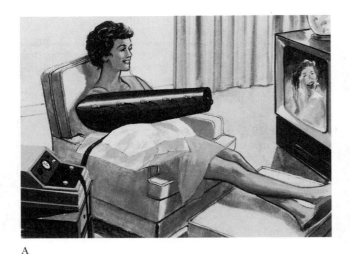

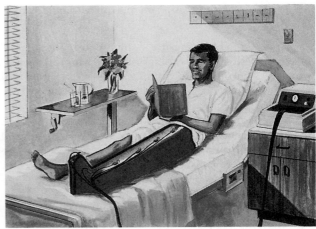

A   B

FIGURE 25-1   Gradient sequential compression pump used to actively compress lymphatic fluid from the extremities affected with moderate or severe lymphedema (A, B). The pump is easy to use, comfortable, and usually effective in decreasing edema (manufacturer: Biocompression, Model 3004). (Illustrations courtesy of Advanced Care Associates, Philadelphia, PA.)

Pneumatic pressure pumps   Recent literature contains consistent recommendations that if a pump is to be used, it should be the sequential chamber type.[7,9,31,32] These electric pumps consist of a plastic sleeve with a number of overlapping chambers that fill with air starting from the hand (or foot) and moving up the extremity in a milking action over a 45- to 90-second period of time. The pressure varies according to patient response, but usually starts at 50 to 70 mmHg. The pressure in the chambers is completely released for a 15- to 30-second period and the sequence begins again. In contrast, pumps that have a single inflatable chamber allow the fluid to travel in both the proximal (preferred) direction and the distal (against the valves) direction, thus allowing fluid to be pushed to areas that may counteract the desired lymphatic drainage.

Pneumatic pressure pumps are contraindicated for people who have infections, deep vein thrombosis, pulmonary embolism, or any cardiac syndrome that would be aggravated by an increase in venous circulation.

The decision to use a pump must be made collaboratively by the person who will be using it and the healthcare providers who will be monitoring its use (physician, nurse, physical therapist, or technician from pump company). The effectiveness of the pump depends on consistent use by the person and good communication with the healthcare providers.[9] Initially the person pumps several times a day (e.g., 2 hours in the morning, 2 hours in the evening) to produce a response in the swollen limb. Use of an elastic compression garment is important between pumpings to continue to support the edematous limb. The person slowly decreases pump time and days of pumping per week to arrive at the right amount of time needed to keep the swelling reduced.

The cost of the pump is usually a concern. Individuals need to determine whether their particular insurance

policies cover rental or purchase of lymphedema pumps. The National Lymphedema Network reports that most pumps are covered under insurance plans.[10] Unfortunately, healthcare providers may need to spend considerable time convincing insurance companies to provide equipment with the newest technology (sequential pumps vs. single-chamber pumps) so effective pumping can be accomplished.

Evaluating the effectiveness of the pump in a timely and ongoing manner is important both to make needed changes in the treatment program and to avoid unnecessary expense for equipment if pumping is not helpful or if the person is not able to tolerate the treatment. Initially the nurse should contact the individual and the pump technician (if one is involved) weekly to determine effectiveness and compliance with the prescribed regimen. Once it has been determined that the pump is helpful, the nurse can contact the patient at less frequent intervals (both by telephone and patient visits) to check progress and to measure and assess the extremity.

See Appendix 25E for a general self-care guide to assist the patient with moderate lymphedema.

Severe lymphedema

Late or severe lymphedema (greater than 5- to 6-cm difference between extremities) is not common, but it is uncomfortable and often painful as well as disabling. The strategies outlined for mild and moderate lymphedema are employed, teamed with more aggressive physical therapy consisting of massage, exercise, and pumping. For some individuals, an inpatient stay on a vascular or surgical specialty unit may be needed to provide acute intervention. Pain management is a concern and may include use of nonprescription analgesics, nonsteroidal antiinflammatory drugs (NSAIDs), use of transcutaneous electrical nerve stimulation units (TENS), and positional support such as slings. (Please refer to Chapter 9 for additional discussion of pain management.) The goal is to decrease the degree of edema of the extremity and promote lymphatic circulation. See Appendix 25F for a self-care guide to assist the person with severe lymphedema.

Severe lymphedema, however, has usually progressed to the stage of hard, fibrotic swelling and often is characterized by tough, brawny skin. The person with severe lymphedema that has not responded to conservative therapy may be referred to a surgeon for consideration of surgical techniques to help diminish the swelling and promote lymphatic circulation, with the goal of preserving functional use of the limb.

Surgery Surgery cannot cure lymphedema, but some practitioners have seen improvement of the condition with the use of surgical procedures. The number of patients treated so far with these surgical procedures is very small.[9,33] Surgery is considered if there is (1) impaired mobility of the limb, (2) pain associated with the swollen extremity, (3) recurrent infection, (4) a cosmetic reason (e.g., difficulty fitting into clothing), or (5) suspected lymphangiosarcoma (tumors of unknown etiology on the lymphedematous extremity). Characteristically, lymphangiosarcomas are purplish-blue in color and bulbous. They may be confused with melanoma and are a rare but often fatal complication of severe lymphedema.[33]

Generally, the patency of the lymphatic channels is investigated before surgery to define the surgical possibilities for each individual. This is usually accomplished with lymphoscintigraphy, a diagnostic technique done at a major medical center.

Surgical procedures for lymphedema are divided into two categories: (1) excisional or debulking procedures and (2) procedures to correct the underlying physiologic defect, as in anastomosing lymphatics. Excisional or debulking procedures, performed since the early 1900s,[34] are used to remove excess tissue and skin with the expectation that this will stop the edema. This operation results in a tightening of the skin and an increasing resistance for the lymphatic channels (similar to a compression garment) that may promote flow in the proper direction. As the number of patients who have undergone these procedures remains small, generalization to the population at large is difficult.

Several surgical procedures can be done to alter or repair the physiologic deficits causing the lymphedema. Lymphangioplasty,[34] which creates an artificial lymph channel, is one technique. Bridging procedures use autogenous tissue pedicle flaps to bring normal lymphatics to an area where lymphatic drainage is impaired. Lymphatic anastomosis is another surgical approach used. Complications of these procedures include infection, fibrosis, and scarring. Research in this area will continue, particularly as microsurgical techniques continue to improve, and a subset of patients who will benefit from the various surgical procedures will likely be identified.

Benzopyrenes Although not yet approved by the FDA, pharmacologic treatment of severe lymphedema by benzopyrenes (coumarin) is being studied in the literature.[21,35,36] Benzopyrenes stimulate macrophages, which then induce proteolysis in the interstitial fluid. The benefit has been a reduction of degree of lymphedema, but this is offset by the length of time needed to see some effect (usually only after 6 months of use) and the length of time the person needs to be on the drug (5 years to the entire life span). Researchers are encouraging more studies of pharmacologic treatments to help define which subset of patients would benefit and to describe parameters for use.[37]

Special circumstances

Because of the awareness both patients and healthcare providers have about lymphedema, circumstances can arise that may cause unnecessary anxiety for persons as they move within the heathcare system for their care.

Traditionally patients have been instructed never to allow venipuncture for blood drawing, chemotherapy administration, or any kind of injection in the affected limb. Because of the risk of introducing infection in this manner, the physiologic reasoning is sound. However, this risk is small and must be balanced by individual circumstances, such as needing chemotherapy in the presence of inaccessible veins on the unaffected side or having had bilateral lymph node dissections. Similarly, blood pressure measures on the affected limb are traditionally avoided to prevent compression of the lymphatics, but if the situation is emergent in nature, preventive considerations can be outweighed by the needs of the moment.

Nurses need to teach principles of avoiding infection and compression without presenting them as dogma such that it will cause the person to think great harm will ensue if the "rules" are broken. An effective presentation of guidelines includes avoiding trauma (such as injections) but evaluating the risk/benefit ratio for individual circumstances.

Conclusion

The incidence of lymphedema has decreased over the years due to changes in both surgical techniques and patterns of administration of radiation therapy. When lymphedema occurs, it is usually mild and is often amenable to treatment. The dramatic decrease in incidence, however, has led to a perception that this is a small problem in the spectrum of treatments and their sequelae. The oncology nurse is in an ideal position to assess the effects of this symptom on individuals and to counsel, teach, and monitor management strategies while providing support for people experiencing this lifelong symptom.

References

1. Britton RC, Nelson PA: Causes and treatment for postmastectomy lymphedema of the arm: Report of 114 cases. *JAMA* 180:95–102, 1962

2. Markowski J, Wilcox JP, Helm PA: Lymphedema incidence after specific post-mastectomy therapy. *Arch Phys Med Rehabil* 62:449–452, 1981

3. Treeves N. An evaluation of the etiological factors of lymphedema following radical mastectomy: An analysis of 1,001 cases. *Cancer* 10:444–459, 1957

4. Siegel BM, Mayzel KA, Love SM: Level I and II axillary dissection in the treatment of early-stage breast cancer. *Arch Surg* 125:1144–1147, 1990

5. Piver MS, Lele SB: Complications of pelvic and aortic lymphadenectomy, in Delgado G, Smith J (eds): *Management of Complications in Gynecologic Oncology.* New York: Wiley, 1982, pp. 199–211

6. Karakousis CP, Heiser MA, Moore RH: Lymphedema after groin dissection. *Am J Surg* 145:205–208, 1983

7. McGrath E: Lymphedema, in Dow KH, Hilderley LJ (eds): *Nursing Care in Radiation Oncology.* Philadelphia: Saunders, 1992, pp. 323–333

8. Tobin MB, Lacey HJ, Meyer L, et al: The psychological morbidity of breast cancer-related arm swelling. *Cancer* 72: 3248–3252, 1993

9. Gottlieb LJ, Patel PK: Lymphedema following axillary surgery: Elephantiasis chirurgica, in Harris J, Hellman S, Henderson IC, et al: *Breast Diseases* (ed 2). Philadelphia: Lippincott, 1991, pp. 820–827

10. Thiadens S: *Lymphedema: An Information Booklet.* San Francisco: National Lymphedema Network, 1995

11. Rogers R: Gynecology, in Schwartz SI, Shires TG, Spencer FC, et al (eds): *Principles of Surgery* (ed 6). New York: McGraw-Hill, 1994, pp. 1793–1829

12. Larson D, Weinstein M, Goldberg I, et al: Edema of the arm as a function of the extent of axillary surgery in patients with stage I–II carcinoma of the breast treated with primary radiotherapy. *Int J Radiat Oncol Biol Phys* 12:1575–1582, 1986

13. Kissin MW, Querci della Rovere G, Easton D, et al: Risk of lymphoedema following the treatment of breast cancer. *Br J Surg* 73:580–584, 1986

14. Simon MS, Cody RL: Cellulitis after axillary lymph node dissection for carcinoma of the breast. *Am J Med* 93:543–548, 1992

15. Greenfield LJ: Venous and lymphatic disease, in Schwartz SI, Shires TG, Spencer FC, et al (eds): *Principles of Surgery* (ed 6). New York: McGraw-Hill, 1994, pp. 989–1014

16. Giuliano AE, Kirgan DM, Guenther JM, Morton DL: Lymphatic mapping and sentinel lymphadenectomy for breast cancer. *Ann Surg* 220:391–398, 1994

17. Pezner RD, Patterson MP, Hill LR, et al: Arm lymphedema in patients treated conservatively for breast cancer: Relationship to patient age and axillary node dissection technique. *Int J Radiat Oncol Biol Phys* 12:2079–2083, 1986

18. Bertelli G, Venturini M, Forno G, et al: An analysis of prognostic factors in response to conservative treatment of postmastectomy lymphedema. *Surg Gynecol Obstet* 175:455–460, 1992

19. Getz DH: The primary, secondary and tertiary nursing interventions of lymphedema. *Cancer Nurs* 8:177–184, 1985

20. Brennan MJ: Lymphedema following the surgical treatment of breast cancer: A review of pathophysiology and treatment. *J Pain Symptom Manage* 7:110–116, 1992

21. Miller LT: Lymphedema: Unlocking the doors to successful treatment. *Innovations in Oncology Nursing* 10:53–62, 1994

22. Hoe AL, Iven D, Royle GT, et al: Incidence of arm swelling following axillary clearance for breast cancer. *Br J Surg* 79: 261–262, 1992

23. Svensson WE, Mortimer PS, Tohno E, et al: The use of colour Doppler to define venous abnormalities in the swollen arm following therapy for breast carcinoma. *Clin Radiol* 44: 249–252, 1991

24. Knobf MK: Primary breast cancer: Physical consequences and rehabilitation. *Semin Oncol Nurs* 1:214–224, 1985

25. Casley-Smith JR, Foldi M, Ryan TJ, et al: Lymphedema: Summary of the 10th International Congress of Lymphology working group discussions and recommendations. *Lymphology* 18:175–180, 1985

26. Lymphedema Section VIII, Practice Guidelines for Nurse Practitioners. Boston: Dana-Farber Cancer Institute, Breast Evaluation Center, 1993, pp. 141–142

27. Webb S: "Back in the Swing: Stretch and Strengthen after Breast Surgery." Exercise video, Boston: Boston Group for Medical Education, 1995

28. Winningham M: Walking program for people with cancer: Getting started. *Cancer Nurs* 14:270–276, 1991

29. Love S: *Dr. Susan Love's Breast Book.* Reading, MA: Addison-Wesley, 1990

30. Lerner R: The ideal treatment for lymphedema. *Massage Therapy Journal* Winter: 37–39, 1992

31. Richmand DM, O'Donnell TF, Zelikovski A: Sequential pneumatic compression for lymphedema. *Arch Surg* 120: 1116–1119, 1985

32. Zelikovski A, Deutsch A, Reiss R: The sequential pneumatic compression device in surgery for lymphedema of the limbs. *J Cardiovasc Surg* 24:122–126, 1983

33. Stryker S, Roth S, Hines J: Postmastectomy lymphangiosarcoma: Clinical and pathologic features. *Contemp Surg* 26: 73–76, 1985

34. Savage R: The surgical management of lymphedema. *Surg Gynecol Obstet* 160:283–290, 1985

35. Casley-Smith JR: Treatment of lymphedema of the arms and legs with 5,6-benzo-[alpha]-pyrone. *N Engl J Med* 16: 1158–1163 1993

36. Foldi E, Foldi M, Clodius L: The lymphedema chaos: A lancet. *Ann Plast Surg* 22:505–515, 1989

37. *Harvard Women's Health Watch* 2:9, May 1995

Prevention of Lymphedema

Patient Name: _____

Symptom and Description   You may develop arm or leg swelling, sometimes called lymphedema. The swelling may never occur, but it is possible after lymph node surgery. Because you have had lymph nodes removed, your body's ability to move lymph fluid has been changed. You may notice some swelling right after surgery. This is normal and will decrease as the tissues heal. Infection and stress (e.g., lifting heavy items) can cause swelling to occur.

Learning Needs   You will learn to notice and report (even if small) any signs of infection. They are as follows:

- redness or warmth
- red streaks going up or down the limb
- pain or soreness that is in one area or that came on suddenly
- swelling in your hand/arm or foot/leg (on the side where you had surgery)

Prevention   Getting back to normal use of your arm or leg is important after lymph node surgery.

- Gentle exercises that stretch your limb are important, as is strengthening your arm with small weights. Exercises should be done gently and gradually to allow the body to develop new pathways to drain the lymph fluid without creating more trauma. Once the muscles and tissues feel stretched and movable again, you should plan daily exercises. Staying in shape is the best advice, as it keeps joints and muscles in good working order. Please review your exercise sheet with your nurse to develop an exercise plan for you.
- In addition to daily stretching exercises, avoid heavy lifting on the side on which you had surgery (suitcases, heavy grocery bags).
- Skin: Keep skin moisturized and free of cuts and cracks.
- Report any signs of infection (redness, warmth, red streaks, inflamed areas) to your healthcare provider.
- Report any changes in your hand/arm or foot/leg (such as tightness of clothing or rings, numbness, pain, etc.)

(continued)

Follow-up   After surgery you should expect to regain the movement that you had before surgery. The time needed to get this differs from person to person. Please talk about your progress with your doctor, nurse, or other healthcare provider. A good time to plan for this talk is at your post-op visit. There you can discuss how you are healing, how your range of motion is moving along, and whether you need a referral to a physical therapist.

Date of next visit: _____

Phone Numbers

Nurse: _____ Phone: _____

Physician: _____ Phone: _____

Physical Therapist: _____ Phone: _____

Support/Exercise Group: _____ Phone: _____

National Lymphedema Network: (800) 541-3259

Comments

Patient's Signature: _____ Date: _____

Nurse's Signature: _____ Date: _____

Source: Kalinowski BH: Lymphedema, in Yarbro CH, Frogge MH, Goodman M (eds): *Cancer Symptom Management* (ed 2). Sudbury: Jones and Bartlett, 1999. © Jones and Bartlett Publishers.

Back in the Swing: Stretch and Strengthen after Breast Surgery

Patient Name: _____

Getting Started   Do exercises for 30 minutes every day for several weeks. You may want to divide the time into short segments at the beginning to avoid becoming tired.

- Do 10 to 15 repetitions of each exercise.
- Increase to two 30-minute sessions every day.
- Warm up before exercising—it relieves stress and makes it easier.

Loosening Up   Usually may start when drains and/or stitches are out. Check with your physician if you have questions about when to start.

1. Arm swings (warm up)
   - Stand up.
   - Put hand on chair.
   - Bend at waist.
   - Swing arm back and forth, side to side.

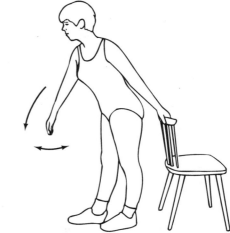

2. Front raises
   - Place good arm on opposite shoulder.
   - Massage shoulder joint with hand.
   - Raise arm up and hold 4 counts.
   - Feel stretch.

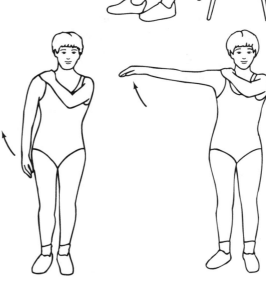

3. Side raises
  - Raise arm up from side.
  - Hold 4 counts and stretch.

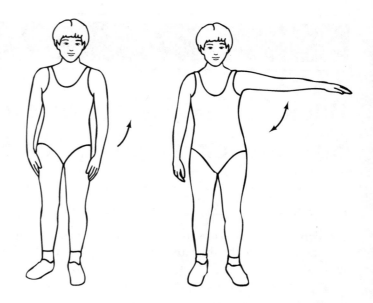

4. Turning arm out
  - Bend arm at elbow, keep at side.
  - Move arm away from body.
  - Turn hand up.

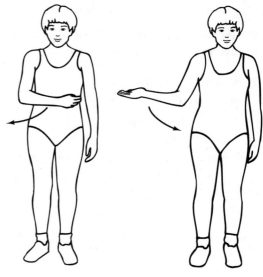

5. Back reach (stretches muscle in chest)
  - Grab wrist behind back with good hand.
  - Bend at elbow.
  - Pull arm up gently.
  - Hold 4 counts.

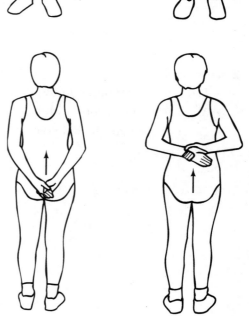

6. Shoulder shrug
- Raise shoulders to ears
- Hold 5 counts

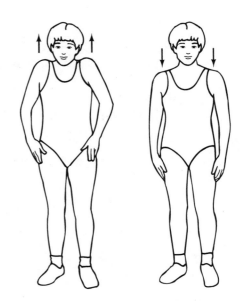

Stretching Do these exercises *slowly and gently*. Hold the positions for 5 counts, relax, and breathe.

First 5 exercises are done lying on a bed or mat

1. Stick raises
- Lie on back. Hold stick (broom handle, cane, umbrella) in both hands.
- Raise arms over your head. Let gravity do the work.
- Hold 5 counts.

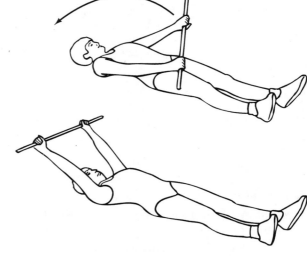

2. Forehead slide
- Lie on back.
- Place heel of hand on forehead.
- Slide hand over head (hair). Hold 5 counts. Goal is to get the bend of the elbow to the forehead. You may need to gently push the elbow with the other hand.

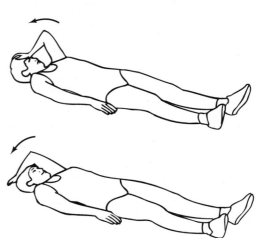

3. Snow angel

- Lie on back.
- Raise arms over head, reach as high as you can (don't let it hurt).
- Hold 5 counts.
- Lower arms slowly.

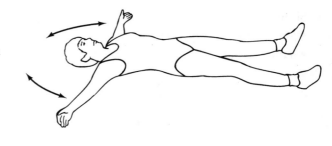

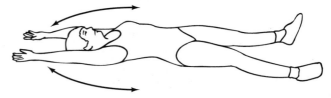

4. Sideways slide

- Still lying down, lie on unaffected side.
- Place other hand on ear, elbow up toward ceiling. Slide hand over head toward back.
- Hold 5 counts.

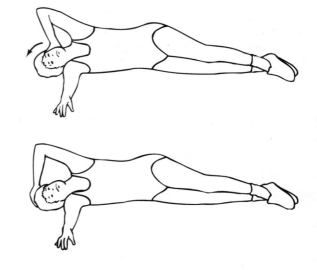

5. Bowing

- Put hands and knees on bed/mat, hands in front stretched out.
- Slide back and sit on heels. Drop head down gently.
- Come back up to hands and knees. This stretches arms and back.

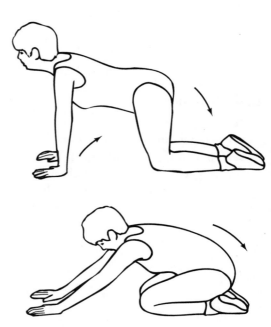

Next four exercises are done standing up.

6. Wall crawls
- Stand in front of wall. With both hands walk fingers up the wall until you feel a pull. Hold 5 counts.
- Slide hands down wall.

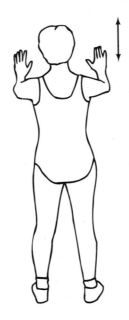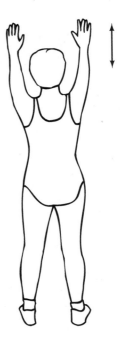

7. Side wall crawls.
- Stand sideways from wall.
- Walk fingers up the wall until you feel a pull. Hold 5 counts.
- Slide hand down the wall. Make sure you keep shoulders square with the wall.
- Step closer to the wall to increase the stretch.

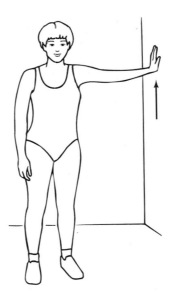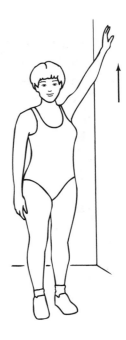

8. Corner stretch
  - Stand in a corner, hands and forearms on the wall. Lean entire body in as a unit.
  - Hold 5 counts.

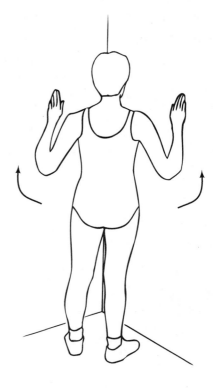

9. Door stretch
  - Put hand inside frame of a door.
  - Turn your body away from your arm.
  - Hold 5 counts.

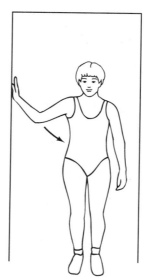 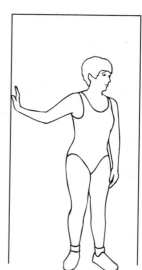

Advanced Stretches   These exercises use your own body weight to increase your range of motion.

1. Atlas
   - Stand in front of door.
   - Put hands outstretched on door.
   - Bend head.
   - Feel stretch in shoulders.
   - Take small steps back.

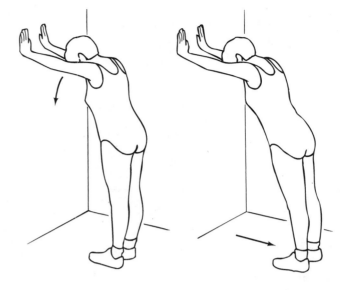

2. Champion
   - Bend at the elbow.
   - Pull arm up and over head with other hand.
   - Hold 5 counts.
   - Feel stretch down side.

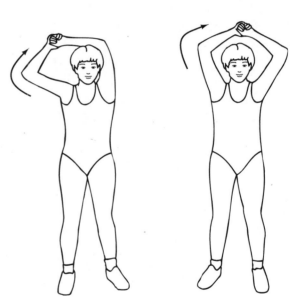

3. Elbow push
- Bend elbow.
- Raise arm.
- Push arm straight back with other hand.
- Hold 5 counts.

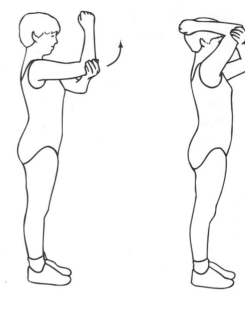

4. Stick pull
- Hold stick in both hands.
- Raise stick to side and up toward ear.
- Hold 5 counts.

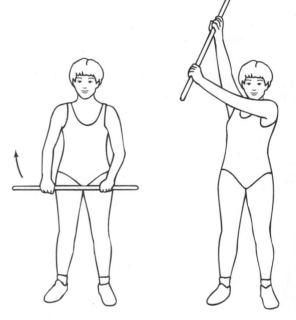

Strengthening   Use small weights, light enough to control (1 lb, such as small can of soup). Use both arms to work muscle groups evenly. Muscle groups that you will be strengthening are:

- Trapezius, deltoid (lifting muscles)
- Pectoralis (pushing out in front)
- Rhomboid, serratus (shoulder stabilizers)
- Latissimus (pulling in or down)

1. Side raises
   - Sitting, raise straight arm up and over head. Put hand on elbow to help.

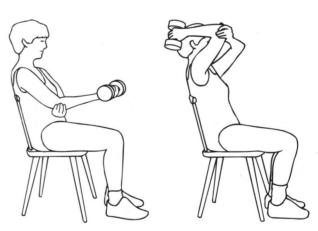

2. Overhead press
   - Sitting, bend elbow, palm out to front.
   - Put other hand on elbow.
   - Raise arm over head.
   - Work up to doing both arms together.

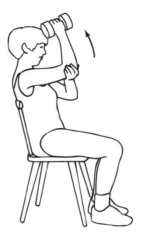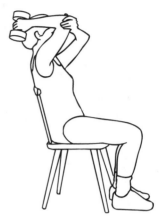

3. Floor pulls
   - Standing, put hand on chair arm.
   - Bend at waist, arm hanging toward floor.
   - Turn hand toward body.
   - Pull arm up to waist, back toward hip.

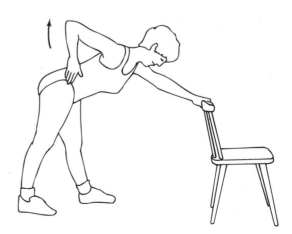

4. Side lifts
- As above, turn hand to back.
- Bend at elbow.
- Bring arm up to hip.
- Bring arm down.
- Feel squeeze in muscles between shoulder blades.

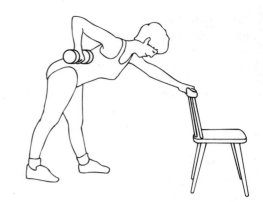

5. Bench press
- Lie on floor.
- Bend elbows, arms out to side.
- Bring arms up and over head.

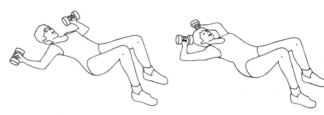

6. Crossovers
- Lying down.
- Arms out to side.
- Bring arms up and meet in middle.

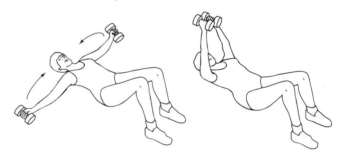

Exercises adapted from the videotape "Back in the Swing: Stretch and Strengthen after Breast Surgery." Boston Group for Medical Education, Dr. Sharon Webb, Boston, 1995. For more information call (617) 522-0008.[27]

Phone Numbers

Nurse: _____ Phone: _____

Physician: _____ Phone: _____

Physical Therapist: _____ Phone: _____

Support/Exercise Group: _____ Phone: _____

National Lymphedema Network: (800) 541-3259

Comments

Patient's Signature: _____ Date: _____

Nurse's Signature: _____ Date: _____

Source: Kalinowski BH: Lymphedema, in Yarbro CH, Frogge MH, Goodman M. (eds): *Cancer Symptom Management* (ed 2). Sudbury: Jones and Bartlett, 1999. © Jones and Bartlett Publishers.

Lower Extremity Exercises

Patient Name: _____

Getting Started   Do exercises for 30 minutes every day for several weeks. You may want to divide the time into short segments at the beginning to avoid fatigue.

- Do 10 to 15 repetitions of each exercise.
- Progress to two 30-minute sessions every day.
- Warm up before exercising—it relieves stress and makes it easier.

Standing behind the chair, holding the back.

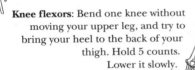

Plantar flexors: Slowly rise to your tiptoes; then slowly return. If this is too easy, rise on one leg with the other bent at the knee. Hold 5 counts.

Knee flexors: Bend one knee without moving your upper leg, and try to bring your heel to the back of your thigh. Hold 5 counts. Lower it slowly.

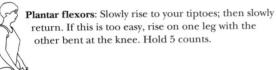

Hip flexors: Bring your knee as close to your chest as possible without bending at the waist. Hold 5 counts. Lower it slowly.

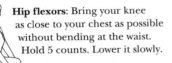

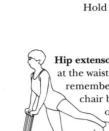

Hip abductors: Without bending your knee or waist, move one leg straight out to the side, keeping the toes pointed forward. Hold 5 counts. Lower slowly.

Hip extensors: Bend forward at the waist about 45 degrees — remember to hold onto the chair back — and lift one leg straight out behind you. Lift it as high as possible without bending your knee or moving your upper body. Lower slowly.

Exercises adapted from the May 1995 issue of the *Harvard Women's Health Watch.* © 1995 President and Fellows of Harvard University, p. 9.[37]

Follow-up

Phone Numbers

Nurse: _____ Phone: _____

Physician: _____ Phone: _____

Physical Therapist: _____ Phone: _____

Support/Exercise Group: _____ Phone: _____

National Lymphedema Network: (800) 541-3259

Comments

Patient's Signature: _____ Date: _____

Nurse's Signature: _____ Date: _____

Source: Kalinowski BH: Lymphedema, in Yarbro CH, Frogge MH, Goodman M (eds): *Cancer Symptom Management* (ed 2). Boston: Jones and Bartlett, 1999. © Jones and Bartlett Publishers.

Mild Lymphedema

Patient Name: _____

Symptom and Description   You have mild swelling of your hand or arm (foot/leg), sometimes called lymphedema. This swelling may happen anytime after lymph node surgery. The swelling may stay, it may come and go, or it may disappear. Because you have had lymph nodes removed, your body's ability to move lymph fluid has been changed. You may have noticed some swelling right after surgery. This was normal, and it decreased after the tissues healed. Now you are noticing mild swelling in your limb. What causes this to happen is unclear. Infection in the hand or arm (foot/leg) can cause swelling, as can having had radiation to the area where the lymph nodes were removed.

Learning Needs   You will learn to notice and report (even if small) any signs of infection or swelling in your extremity on the side of your surgery. (Extremity means hand, arm, foot, or leg.)

Management

1. Contact your doctor or nurse to check any swelling so that a cause (infection, trauma, etc.) can be determined and correct treatment prescribed.

2. Report any changes in your extremity (such as tightness of clothing or rings, numbness, pain, etc.).

3. Report any signs of infection. The signs are as follows:
   - Redness or warmth
   - Red streaks going up or down the limb
   - Pain or soreness that is in one area or that came on suddenly
   - Swelling in your hand/arm or foot/leg (on the side where you had surgery)

4. The following measures can be used:
   - Exercise: Gentle stretching and strengthening exercises (see exercise sheet). Do these 2 times a day.
   - Prevent injury to extremity, prevent infection, and keep skin soft and free of cracks with a good lotion.
   - Elevate extremity as often as possible, but at least 3 to 4 times a day for 20 minutes.
   - Gently massage extremity to "push" fluid from extremity toward your body (can be done by self or partner).
   - Obtain a compression sleeve or stocking. This can be ready made or custom fitted. You will need a prescription for this, and it should be covered by insurance. It should be fitted by a professional fitter when the limb is not swollen. It will provide pressure to help lymphatic drainage. Wear the sleeve or stocking during the day, especially when working or exercising. Do not wear the sleeve at night.

Follow-up   Your nurse will measure your limbs on both sides and compare the measurements. These measurements will be kept in your chart, and your progress will be monitored by how these measurements change and by your report of how you feel. It is important to tell us of any problems or questions you have, and to let us know if things have changed before your next scheduled appointment.

Date of next appointment: _____

Phone Numbers

Nurse: _____ Phone: _____

Physician: _____ Phone: _____

Support/Exercise Group: _____ Phone: _____

National Lymphedema Network: (800) 541-3259

Comments

Patient's Signature: _____ Date: _____

Nurse's Signature: _____ Date: _____

Source: Kalinowski BH: Lymphedema, in Yarbro CH, Frogge MH, Goodman M (eds): *Cancer Symptom Management* (ed 2). Sudbury: Jones and Bartlett, 1999. © Jones and Bartlett Publishers.

Moderate Lymphedema

Patient Name: _____

Symptom and Description   You have moderate swelling of your hand or arm (foot/leg), sometimes called lymphedema. This swelling may happen anytime after lymph node surgery—as soon as the first year or many years later. This swelling may stay, it may come and go, or it may disappear. Because you have had lymph nodes removed, your body's ability to move lymph fluid has been changed. New lymph channels have developed to help replace what has been removed. You may have noticed some swelling right after surgery. This was normal, and it decreased after the tissues healed and the fluid was reabsorbed. Now you are noticing swelling in your extremity (hand, wrist, arm, leg, or foot). What causes this to happen is unclear. Infection can cause swelling, as can having had radiation to the area where the lymph nodes were removed.

Learning Needs   You will learn to notice and report (even if small) any signs of infection or swelling in your hand/arm or foot/leg on the side of your surgery.

Management

1. Report any signs of infection. The signs are as follows:
   - Red streaks going up or down the limb
   - Pain or soreness that is in one area or that came on suddenly
   - Swelling in your hand/arm or foot/leg (on the side where you had surgery)

2. Report any changes in your extremity (such as tightness of clothing or rings, numbness, pain, etc.).

3. Exercise: Gentle motion, stretching, and strengthening exercises (see exercise sheet). Do these 2 times a day.

4. Prevent injury to the extremity, prevent infection, and keep skin soft and free of cracks with a good lotion.

5. Elevate the extremity as much as possible, but at least 3 to 4 times a day for 20 minutes.

6. Gently massage the extremity to "push" fluid from extremity toward your body (can be done by self or partner).

7. Obtain a compression sleeve or stocking. This can be ready made or custom fitted. You will need a prescription for this, and it should be covered by insurance. It should be fitted by a professional fitter when the limb is not swollen. It will provide compression to help lymphatic drainage. Wear the sleeve or stocking during the day, especially when working or exercising.

8. Discuss the possibility of having a physical therapist evaluate your swollen limb, show you some massage exercises, and evaluate your range of motion and strength in the swollen limb.

(continued)

9. Discuss the possibility of using a compression pump at home on a daily basis. The pump will allow you to have longer, more frequent massages to the swollen limb than your therapist or your partner is able to do. You will need to wear the compression sleeve or stocking during the day when you are not pumping. Do not wear the sleeve or stocking at night.

Follow-up   Your nurse will measure your limbs on both sides and compare the measurements. These measurements will be kept in your chart, and your progress will be monitored by how these measurements change and by your report of how you feel. It is important to tell us of any problems or questions you have, and to let us know if things have changed or not changed before your next scheduled appointment.

Date of next appointment: _____

Phone Numbers

Nurse: _____ Phone: _____

Physician: _____ Phone: _____

Physical Therapist: _____ Phone: _____

Pump Nurse/Technician: _____ Phone: _____

Support/Exercise Group: _____ Phone: _____

National Lymphedema Network: (800) 541-3259

Comments

Patient's Signature: _____ Date: _____

Nurse's Signature: _____ Date: _____

Source: Kalinowski BH: Lymphedema, in Yarbro CH, Frogge MH, Goodman M (eds): *Cancer Symptom Management* (ed 2). Sudbury: Jones and Bartlett, 1999. © Jones and Bartlett Publishers.

Severe Lymphedema

Patient Name: _____

Symptom and Description   You have swelling of your extremity (hand/arm, foot/leg), sometimes called lymphedema. This swelling may happen anytime after lymph node surgery, as soon as the first year or many years later. This swelling may stay, it may come and go, or it may disappear. The skin of your extremity may be tight and shiny, or it may look rough and brownish in color. Because you have had lymph nodes under your arm or your groin removed and/or radiated, your body's ability to move lymph fluid has been changed. New lymph channels have developed to help replace what has been removed. You may have noticed some swelling right after surgery. This was normal, and it decreased after the tissues healed and the fluid was reabsorbed. Now you are noticing swelling in your limb. What causes this to happen is unclear. Infection in the extremity has been shown to cause some of the cases of swelling, as has radiation to the area where the lymph nodes were removed.

Learning Needs   You will learn to recognize and report (even if small) any signs of infection and swelling in your hand/arm or foot/leg on the side of your surgery.

Management

1. Report any signs of infection. The signs are as follows:
   - Red streaks going up or down the limb
   - Pain or soreness that is in one area or that came on suddenly
   - Swelling in your hand/arm or foot/leg (on the side where you had surgery)
2. Report any changes in your extremity (such as tightness of clothing or rings, numbness, pain, etc.).
3. Exercise: Gentle motion, stretching, and strengthening exercises (see exercise sheet). Do these 2 times a day.
4. Prevent injury to the extremity, prevent infection, and keep skin soft and free of cracks with a good lotion.
5. Elevate the extremity as much as possible, but at least 3 to 4 times a day for 20 minutes. Use pillows to elevate your extremity when you sleep at night. A wedge pillow may be helpful.
6. If this is comfortable for you, gently massage the extremity to "push" fluid from extremity toward your body (can be done by self or partner).
7. Obtain a compression sleeve or stocking. This can be ready made or custom fitted. You will need a prescription for this, and it should be covered by insurance. It should be fitted by a professional fitter when the limb is at its lowest point of swelling. This garment will provide compression to help lymphatic drainage. Wear the sleeve or stocking during the day, especially when working or exercising.

8. Discuss the possibility of having a physical therapist evaluate your swollen limb, show you some massage techniques, and evaluate your range of motion and strength in the swollen limb.

9. Discuss the possibility of using a compression pump at home on a daily basis. The pump will allow you to have longer, more frequent massages to the swollen limb than your therapist or your partner is able to do. You will need to wear the compression sleeve or stocking during the day when you are not pumping. Do not wear the sleeve or stocking at night.

10. Discuss how to manage your pain with your physician and nurse. They will discuss which medication may be used, positioning techniques, wearing a sling to support the extremity, as well as other measures to reduce pain.

Follow-up   Your nurse will measure your limbs on both sides and compare the measurements. These measurements will be kept in your chart, and your progress will be monitored by how these measurements change and by your report of how you feel. It is important to tell us of any problems or questions you have, and to let us know if things have changed or not changed before your next scheduled appointment.

Date of next appointment: _____

Phone Numbers

Nurse: _____ Phone: _____

Physician: _____ Phone: _____

Physical Therapist: _____ Phone: _____

Pump Nurse/Technician: _____ Phone: _____

Support/Exercise Group: _____ Phone: _____

National Lymphedema Network: (800) 541-3259

Comments

Patient's Signature: _____ Date: _____

Nurse's Signature: _____ Date: _____

Source: Kalinowski BH: Lymphedema, in Yarbro CH, Frogge MH, Goodman M (eds): *Cancer Symptom Management* (ed 2). Sudbury: Jones and Bartlett, 1999. © Jones and Bartlett Publishers.

PART VI

SYMPTOMS OF DISTURBANCES
IN ELIMINATION

CHAPTER 26

Bladder Disturbances

Donna L. Berry, RN, PhD, AOCN

The Problem of Bladder Disturbances in Cancer

Disturbances of the bladder that are associated with cancer symptoms, treatment side effects, or disease sequelae can be categorized into three basic groups of human responses: pathophysiologic responses, sensory or experiential responses, and behavioral responses. Table 26-1 depicts the three groups of responses and respective symptoms. To establish clarity of terms as used in this chapter, symptom definitions are provided in Table 26-2.

A bladder disturbance in a person with cancer most likely will be composed of a set of symptoms involving more than one type of response. For example, an individual with an *Escherichia coli* infection of the bladder may experience the sensations of dysuria and urgency (sensory responses) and report urinary frequency (behavioral response). As with most cancer symptomatology, the complexity of human responses creates challenges for both self-care and management by the healthcare provider.

Incidence in Cancer

When a person with cancer presents with a disturbance of the bladder, the situation is most often related to one of the following four typical scenarios. First, an individual with carcinoma of the bladder is at risk for hematuria and irritative bladder symptoms (dysuria, urgency, fre-

quency). *Hematuria,* either gross or microscopic blood in the urine, is the hallmark manifestation of bladder cancer and is described as the presenting symptom by 75% to 85% of individuals with superficial bladder cancer.[1] Irritative bladder symptoms (IBSs) are present at diagnosis in about 20% of cases;[2,3] however, these symptoms are more common as a side effect of intravesical therapy for superficial bladder cancer. Drug-induced cystitis associated with intravesical chemotherapy has been reported in up to 49% of cases,[4,5] and irritative bladder symptoms have been reported to occur in 60% to 91% of those receiving intravesical bacillus Calmette-Guérin (BCG).[5,6] Intravesical BCG is usually given once a week for a total of six treatments. IBSs are known to occur most frequently in the third through the sixth week of BCG therapy.[7]

A second scenario involving bladder disturbances in persons with cancer is that of a *lower urinary tract infection* (UTI). The incidence of bacteriuria ($>10^5$ colony-forming units/mL) is highest in the elderly, the age group also most likely to develop cancer.[5] In adults over 65 years of age, bacteriuria is found in 20% of women and 10% of men. Common bacteria include *E. coli, Enterobacter,* and *Staphylococcus* species.[9] Immunosuppressed individuals are at additional risk for infections of the bladder, often allowing the growth of normally less virulent organisms such as fungi and *Gardnerella vaginalis.* Individuals receiving or recuperating from cancer therapy are at risk if catheterized. Forty percent of all nosocomial infections are catheter-associated UTIs.[8]

A third typical bladder disturbance scenario, manifested in men with cancer, is that of voiding dysfunction associated with *prostate cancer.* Prostate cancer constituted close to one-third of all malignancies in men diagnosed

TABLE 26-1 Human Responses and Bladder Symptoms

Response	Symptoms
Pathophysiologic	Hematuria; lower urinary tract infection; radiation or drug-induced cystitis; hemorrhagic cystitis; outflow obstruction; sphincter incompetence
Sensory/experiential	Dysuria; urgency; bladder pain
Behavioral	Frequency; voiding dysfunction

in 1998.[10] Most men with localized disease are asymptomatic or present with bladder outlet obstruction and bladder irritability. The man may experience overflow urinary incontinence.[11] Radical prostatectomy is the most common treatment for localized carcinoma of the prostate. However, 1 year after a prostatectomy, one-third to about one-half of the men will not be fully continent.[12] When treatment for prostate cancer includes either external beam radiation therapy to the pelvic region or radioactive implants to the prostate, radiation cystitis is a common side effect, ranging from mild to severe.[13,14]

Finally, functional urinary incontinence associated with *neurologic deficits,* or altered dexterity and mobility, is observed in some individuals with cancer. Cognitive dysfunction caused by metabolic derangements, chemotherapy, or radiation therapy side effects can impair toileting behaviors of the affected individual. Peripheral neuropathy, occurring in 10% to 20% of persons treated for cancer, can impair both dexterity and mobility, making voiding behaviors much more difficult.[15] Urinary incontinence, with pain and leg weakness are symptoms of spinal cord compression.[16]

Clearly the four scenarios described above are not inclusive of all individuals with bladder disturbances related to cancer; however, they are typical of the bladder disturbances frequently encountered by clinical oncology nurses. In addition, many patients, particularly the elderly, have multiple illnesses and may have bladder disturbances unrelated to their malignant processes.

Etiology and Pathophysiology

The etiology and pathophysiology of bladder disturbances associated with cancer can be discussed either as problems of the bladder urothelium or as problems of the neuromuscular function of the bladder. The mucosal lining of the bladder consists of five to seven layers of transitional epithelial cells (Figure 26-1). The mucosa overlies the collagenous lamina propria containing blood vessels, lymphatic vessels, and nerves. Below that, the lamina muscularis is organized in bundles of smooth muscle.[13] The perivesical tissue covers the bladder organ.[17]

Bladder Cancer

Malignant growth confined to the transitional epithelium and the lamina propria makes up about 80% of all diagnosed bladder cancers.[18] These superficial bladder tumors and carcinoma in situ disrupt the mucosal integrity and can infiltrate the lamina propria, causing bleeding and irritation. The less common, invasive tumors manifest the same type of symptoms but more severe discomfort.

TABLE 26-2 Bladder Disturbance Symptom Definitions

Symptom	Definition
Hematuria	Blood in the urine: can be microscopic or visible to eye alone as pink-tinged or red urine, with or without clots
Dysuria	Painful and/or burning sensations during urination
Frequency	Voiding more often than every 2 hours; daytime frequency is sometimes described as *diurnal* frequency; *nocturia* is used to describe nighttime voiding more than once if under 65 years of age and more than twice if over 65 years of age
Urgency	Compelling feeling of the need to urinate as soon as possible
Irritative bladder symptoms	A symptom index generally including dysuria, urgency, and frequency
Cystitis	Inflammation of the bladder epithelium
Hemorrhagic cystitis	An often sudden onset of hematuria combined with bladder pain and irritative bladder symptoms
Urinary outflow obstruction	An impediment near the bladder neck that can create urinary retention and overflow incontinence; usually prostate tumor in the oncology setting
Sphincter incompetence	A common complication of radical prostatectomy due to the necessary distortion of the urethrovesical junction

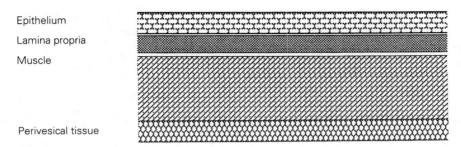

Epithelium
Lamina propria
Muscle
Perivesical tissue

FIGURE 26-1 Graphic depiction of the tissue layers of the bladder.

Bladder Infection

The bladder epithelium undergoes inflammatory change when colonized with infectious agents. Polymorphonucleocytes (PMNs) infiltrate the mucosa, while edema develops within the cellular matrix and the lamina, causing irritability.[13] Muscle irritability and painful bladder spasms may result in urge incontinence, dysuria, urgency, and frequency.[19] A very similar mechanism ensues when BCG is administered intravesically for treatment of superficial bladder cancer. Although the BCG is an attenuated form of the bacillus, the bladder epithelium reacts with an inflammatory sequence of events that ultimately leads to tumor elimination and delay of recurrence.[20] The individual receiving the treatment can experience the irritative bladder symptoms of dysuria, frequency, and urgency and pain localized to the lower pelvic region.

Chemotherapy-Induced Cystitis

Hemorrhagic cystitis is a complication associated with ifosfamide and cyclophosphamide, cytotoxic alkylating agents used in a variety of malignancies. Patients will report a sudden onset of dysuria and hematuria, which less commonly is massive and intractable. The damage to the epithelium is most likely caused by the metabolic breakdown products of cyclophosphamide and includes mucosal ulcerations, vascular telangiectasia, severe edema, and hemorrhage within the lamina propria.[13] Fortunately, this drug-induced hemorrhage is less common than in the past, due to the development and use of the agent mesna which, when administered with ifosfamide or cyclophosphamide, protects the urothelium.[21]

Intravesical cytotoxic chemotherapy such as mitomycin has been used for treatment of transitional cell carcinoma of the bladder. The local irritative effects of the agent are those of a chemical cystitis, similar to that of an infectious inflammation but without the evidence of bacteriuria.[4]

Radiation Injury

Individuals receiving radiation therapy to the pelvic area can experience radiation cystitis that is time- and dose-dependent. It is manifested as acute cystitis approximately 4 to 6 weeks after initiation of treatment; late reactions also have been reported years after therapy. Histologically, the bladder epithelium becomes transiently hyperemic, followed by extensive vascular dilation, stromal edema, and focal ulcerations.[13]

Voiding Dysfunction

There are many types of voiding dysfunction. The following etiologies are those that may frequently be encountered by oncology nurses.

Many patients with cancer are taking narcotics for pain relief. Reduced bladder muscle contractility and subsequent urinary retention can be side effects of the narcotic.[19]

Overflow incontinence or bladder outflow obstruction can occur in a man with carcinoma of the prostate. As seen in Figure 26-2, the prostate surrounds the urethra as it exits from the bladder through the bladder neck. A

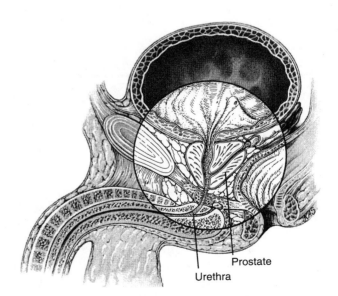

Prostate
Urethra

FIGURE 26-2 Anatomic relationships of the male bladder—sagittal section. (Courtesy of Merck Sharp & Dohme, Westport, PA, 1993.)

tumor may cause narrowing of the urethra or disruption of normal urinary sphincter function. The obstruction leads to hypertrophy and instability of the detrusor muscle, which normally empties the bladder by contracting. Urinary retention results despite intravesical pressures that may be relatively high. The bladder then spontaneously releases urine and the man experiences incontinence, including dribbling, frequent urination, and nocturia. Concomitant UTI is common because of the higher residual volumes and may result in sensations of dysuria and urgency.[22]

A common postoperative complication of radical prostatectomy is urinary incontinence. Because of the excision of the prostate plus the portion of the urethra located within the prostate, the bladder neck must be surgically repaired and reconnected to the remaining urethra during the prostatectomy procedure. Given the disruption in normal urinary anatomy and voiding function, the patient wears a urinary catheter for several weeks after the operation and then begins to regain urinary continence. The necessity of removing prostate tissue with tumor-free margins often results in partial resection of the tissues of the urinary sphincter mechanism and, consequently, stress incontinence.[23]

Spinal Cord Injury

Injury to the spinal cord due to bony metastasis or direct tumor extension can lead to detrusor paralysis and associated sphincter weakness. The detrusor muscle, which normally contracts during bladder emptying, lies flaccid allowing the bladder to overfill, and ultimately stress incontinence occurs.[22] Detrusor hyperreflexia can also occur during the bladder-filling phase, limiting the storage capabilities of the bladder.

Assessment

Measurement Tools

Voiding diary

A written record of voiding activity will be helpful in assessment and evaluation of treatment for bladder disturbances, particularly for individuals experiencing incontinence. The diary is most useful if kept simple and easy to complete. The record can be kept for a few days before a diagnostic evaluation or for certain times within a treatment period. The simplest of diaries documents only the pattern of voiding. For a more complicated diary, additional information can be added regarding fluid intake, urgency, and even dysuria.

American Urological Association Symptom Index

In 1992 members and consultants of the American Urological Association (AUA) reported the development and validation of a symptom index for benign prostatic hyperplasia (BPH).[24] The index discriminates between patients likely to have BPH and those without urologic problems; however, it does not distinguish between men and women with urinary dysfunction.[25,26] In other words, the concepts and symptoms measured in the index are not specific to BPH. The index is recommended for use in following and monitoring urinary symptomatology before and over the course of treatment for obstruction.[27] The AUA Symptom Index contains both obstructive symptom items (hesitancy, incomplete emptying, intermittency, and weak stream) and irritative symptom items (frequency, urgency, and nocturia). Note that dysuria is not included. This symptom was eliminated during instrument testing because dysuria had a low correlation with a global "bother score" in the male test sample. The investigators also stated that clinicians generally believe that dysuria is less specific to BPH.[24]

The AUA Symptom Index (Figure 26-3) could be useful for monitoring symptomatology for those individuals receiving treatment for prostate cancer. However, the omission of dysuria negates its use for assessment in patients with cancer of the bladder and those with UTIs.

Irritative bladder symptoms

Although a validated instrument has not been developed to self-report irritative bladder symptoms, many oncology research and clinical centers utilize the Common Toxicity Criteria developed at the National Cancer Institute or, as in the Southwest Oncology Group, an extension of these criteria.[28] Clarification is needed on the use of such a scale. For example, the difference between a grade 2 dysuria and a grade 3 dysuria is the presence of a positive response to phenazopyridine. Certainly some individuals use treatment strategies for their dysuria other than phenazopyridine, rendering this scale inappropriate to measure dysuria in these individuals.

The Boyarsky scoring system[29] and the Maine Medical Assessment Program (MMAP)[27] both include dysuria as an irritative bladder symptom but are clinician-scored, introducing possible problems with face-to-face disclosure of symptoms and bias in interpretation, plus requiring a trained observer. Additionally, the tools do not address hematuria, minimizing their appropriateness in an oncology setting.

Physical Assessment

Physical examination of the lower urinary tract is indicated when there is a complaint of a bladder disturbance and entails evaluation of the abdomen and the external genita-

Question	Not at All	Less Than 1 Time in 5	Less than Half the Time	About Half the Time	More than Half the Time	Almost Always
1. During the last month or so, how often have you had a sensation of not emptying your bladder completely after you finished urinating?	0	1	2	3	4	5
2. During the last month or so, how often have you had to urinate again less than 2 hours after you finished urinating?	0	1	2	3	4	5
3. During the last month or so, how often have you found you stopped and started again after several times when you urinated?	0	1	2	3	4	5
4. During the last month or so, how often have you found it difficult to postpone urination?	0	1	2	3	4	5
5. During the last month or so, how often have you had a weak urinary stream?	0	1	2	3	4	5
6. During the last month or so, how often have you had to push or strain to begin urination?	0	1	2	3	4	5
7. During the last month or so, how many times did you most typically get up to urinate from the time you went to bed at night until the time you got up in the morning?	None	1 Time	2 Times	3 Times	4 Times	5 or More Times
	0	1	2	3	4	5
AUA symptom score = sum of questions 1 to 7.						

FIGURE 26-3   AUA Symptom Index. (Source: Barry MJ, Fowler FJ, O'Leary MP, et al: The American Urological Association Symptom Index for benign prostatic hyperplasia. *J Urol* 148:1555, 1992.[24]) Reprinted with permission.

lia. Ask the individual to empty the bladder before the examination and to recline in a comfortable supine position. The bladder can then be inspected, palpated, and percussed for signs of distension. Observation of a central protrusion, tympany on percussion, and resistance to light palpation, all in the suprapubic area, are indications of a distended or retentive bladder. Urinary tract infection or a mass can also produce resistance to palpation.[30]

Inspect the perineal skin for integrity in both men and women, noting rashes or excoriations that can be caused by urinary leakage. The penis, including the glans penis and meatus, should be inspected for inflammation. In an uncircumcised man, the glans is normally moist and pink. Inspect the perineum, vulvar area, and meatus of a woman as she reclines in a lithotomy position. The labia minora should be soft and nontender. Rashes or excoriations on the labia and vaginal opening may indicate vaginitis or UTI. The urethral meatus appears as a rosette or an ovoid slit that lies in the midline or sometimes within the vagina.[30]

Certain aspects of a general physical examination are pertinent to evaluation of a bladder disturbance. Some physical findings significant to carcinoma of the bladder include pallor and edema of the lower extremities, indicating impaired circulation related to a possible mass. Systemic findings, such as fever and chills, anorexia, weight loss, and malaise, are important to note when identifying an infection that has colonized the kidneys or has become systemic and when evaluating disease progression.

Diagnostic Evaluation

All diagnostic evaluations begin with a health history. After ascertaining what has brought the individual to

the practice setting, focus the historic interview on more specific inquiries relevant to the lower urinary system and related systems (Table 26-3).

A variety of diagnostic procedures are available and indicated for the various bladder disturbances. Most common are the cystourethroscopy (also referred to as *cystoscopy*) and urodynamic testing. Table 26-4 lists several genitourinary diagnostic procedures and relevant information.

Degrees of Toxicity

The severity of selected bladder disturbances has been quantified in the AUA Symptom Index (refer to Figure 26-3) and in assessment guides such as that of Boyarsky and colleagues.[29] Generally the more frequent the disturbance, the more severe the symptom and the higher the score on the tool. The Southwest Oncology Group[28] has included factors such as type of treatment required to ascertain severity. For example, a grade 2 urinary retention is one for which catheterization is required for voiding. Hematuria is graded for amount, ranging from microscopic to gross hematuria plus clots to most severe, requiring a transfusion. Although widely used, this type of grading has only face validity.

Symptom Management

Prevention

For the individual receiving therapy for carcinoma of the bladder, prevention should focus on minimizing

TABLE 26-3 Health History Questions for a Complaint of an Altered Voiding Pattern

---

Chief Complaint: Altered Voiding Pattern (Incontinence/Retention/Dysuria)

Voiding patterns
How often does the patient urinate during the day and night?
How long can the patient wait comfortably between urinating?
How long can urination be postponed before the need to urinate is urgent?
Does involuntary loss of urine occur during coughing, sneezing, changing positions, or during physical exercise?
Is there a sense of urgency before loss of urine? Is the involuntary loss of urine continuous or intermittent, before or after urinating or both? Are pads worn, and how often do they become saturated or changed? Are any other urinary devices worn or used?
Does the patient have difficulty starting the stream of urine? Is the stream weak or involuntarily interrupted? Is there incontinence or other urinary symptoms during sexual activity?

Urologic history
Does the patient describe sensations of discomfort or burning before, during, or after urination, and where it is felt, in the bladder or urethra?
Has the patient been evaluated and treated for urinary tract infection(s)?
Were there any congenital urinary disorders?
Has the patient been evaluated and treated for kidney or bladder stones, or genitourinary tumors?
Has the patient noticed any urine color or odor changes?

Related system disorders
Are there any previously diagnosed neurologic conditions such as Parkinson's disease, multiple sclerosis, spinal cord injury or malignant metastasis, diabetes, or stroke?
Does the patient have any changes in normal bowel patterns?
Are there indications of sexual dysfunction?
If a woman, is she premenopausal or postmenopausal?

Medications affecting continence[30]
Is the patient taking any antispasmodics, antidepressants, or narcotics (agents that decrease detrusor contractility)?
Is the patient taking any cholinergics (agents that increase detrusor contractility)?
Is the patient taking any alpha-blockers or skeletal muscle relaxants (agents that reduce sphincter resistance)?
Is the patient taking any alpha-sympathomimetics (agents that increase sphincter resistance)?

Surgical history
Has the patient had any genitourinary procedures, abdominopelvic surgery, or spinal surgery?

---

irritative bladder symptoms related to intravesical therapy. The goal of prevention is to minimize conditions known to enhance bladder inflammation, primarily acidic, concentrated urine. Pretreatment fluid restriction should be avoided unless the individual has difficulty retaining the intravesical treatment agent for the prescribed duration. Oral fluids should be increased as tolerated after the intravesical retention of the treatment agent. Acidic foods and fluids should be eliminated or minimized in the diet.

Prevention of lower UTIs is particularly important in those individuals with cancer who are immunocompromised. Urinary catheterization should be avoided whenever possible. When urinary catheterization is necessary, strict aseptic technique must be followed during the procedure and meticulous catheter care implemented if the catheter is indwelling. Urinary retention must be minimized to reduce risk of a UTI.

Urinary voiding dysfunction in the person with cancer is often the result of the disease process or the surgical intervention and not highly amenable to prevention. However, careful monitoring of the individual can enable early detection of a problem and prevent further compli-

cations. For example, someone receiving vincristine may begin to exhibit peripheral neuropathies in the extremities and subsequently exhibit urinary retention.[31] Notation of the phenomenon and cessation of vincristine may prevent further progression of the neuropathy.

Therapeutic Approaches

Hematuria

Mild hematuria is commonly associated with carcinoma of the bladder and sometimes with drug-induced inflammation of the urothelium; however, it is generally tolerated without special treatment. Individuals receiving therapy for superficial bladder tumors should be informed that mild hematuria (pink-tinged urine) is not cause for alarm, but that any increase in the amount of blood should be reported to their nurse or doctor. More severe, gross hematuria and hemorrhagic cystitis are managed by bladder irrigation with saline and, as needed, with red cell transfusions to counteract blood loss. For refractory bleeding, surgical intervention may be re-

TABLE 26-4   Selected Genitourinary Procedures

Procedure/Test	Selected Indications	Contraindications	Nursing Care
Intravenous pyelogram/urogram (IVP/IVU)	Recurrent or febrile UTI Hematuria Abdominal/pelvis mass Urinary system tumor Obstruction	Allergy to either iodine-bound contrast material or iodine-based cleansing solution Allergy to shellfish	Preparation includes catharsis and dehydration Monitor for hypersensitivity reactions, renal output
Computed tomography (CT scan)	Abdominal/pelvic mass Genitourinary tumor detection and staging	Allergy to iodine-bound contrast material	Monitor for hypersensitivity reactions
Magnetic resonance imaging (MRI)	Abdominal/pelvic mass Genitourinary tumor detection and staging	Pacemaker History of aneurysm surgery with clips	Teaching of procedure Removal of metal objects from patient
Urodynamic testing (cystometrics)	Urinary incontinence Bladder outlet obstruction Neuropathic bladder Urinary retention	Current UTI Acute, debilitating illness limiting mobility	Teaching of procedure preparation and aftercare Increase fluids and abstain from voiding 1–4 hours prior to test Prophylactic antibiotics Monitor for discomfort, treat with increased fluids and warm bath
Cystourethroscopy	Recurrent or febrile UTI Obstruction of bladder outlet Urethral or bladder fistula Incontinence Hematuria	Current UTI	Antibiotics for bacteriuria Monitor for frank bleeding/clots, signs of systemic infection

quired, including cystotomy and urinary diversion with cystectomy in life-threatening cases.[21]

Irritative bladder symptoms (IBSs)

Dysuria, daytime frequency, nocturia, and urgency are sensory and behavioral symptoms often associated with intravesical therapy of superficial bladder cancer and with lower urinary tract infections.[13] The goals of symptom management in IBSs are to eliminate the sensations of pain, burning, or urgency and to return altered patterns of urinary elimination to a premorbid state.

Medical interventions usually include analgesic and antiinfective medications. Phenazopyridine provides urinary-specific analgesia in some individuals. The use of an antiinfective agent with BCG-induced cystitis is controversial. Some clinicians prescribe isoniazid in individuals who have severe IBSs, and others reserve the medication of these symptoms for instances when they are coupled with systemic symptoms such as fever.[4,6] Antibiotic therapy for bacterial bladder infections is based on the result of a urine culture and sensitivity. Trimethoprim/sulfamethoxazole given orally twice a day provides cost-effective coverage for most UTIs. The quinolones, such as ciprofloxacin, offer an effective but more costly alternative when sulfa allergies, patient preferences, or past failures are important.[9] Table 26-5 lists

nursing interventions appropriate for sensory and behavioral IBSs.

Voiding dysfunction

Bladder outlet obstruction can be caused by direct prostate tumor extension and pressure. Prompt surgical resection is indicated when urinary retention is manifest as a symptom and also because of the metastatic potential of the disease. In addition, radical prostatectomy often results in urinary incontinence due to sphincter incompetence.[23] Nursing care focuses on interventions to minimize postoperative complications and enhance continence (Table 26-6).

Functional urinary incontinence is managed based on the etiology of the dysfunction. For those individuals with impaired cognitive functioning due to brain tumor enlargement or metastasis, nursing interventions focus on developing and instituting a toileting program based on habitual patterns along with a behavioral modification program to encourage toileting behaviors.[30] However, the intensity of such a patient/family teaching program must be determined by the prognosis and general functional status of the impaired individual.

There will be occasions when continued incontinence necessitates a long-term indwelling catheter. Patients who are dependent on institutionalized care or who are expe-

TABLE 26-5 Nursing Interventions for Sensory and Behavioral Irritative Bladder Symptoms

Nursing Diagnosis	Nursing Intervention
Alterations in patterns of urinary elimination related to radiation or drug-induced inflammation or UTI	Encourage superhydration of 2500 mL/day (unless contraindicated for cardiac or other reasons). Administer analgesic and/or antibiotic agents or teach self-administration. Administer intravenous fluids as directed when a patient cannot tolerate oral fluids.
Sensations of pain/discomfort related to drug-induced inflammation or UTI	Encourage oral intake of low-acid, caffeine-free fluids. Administer prescribed urinary analgesics or teach self-administration. Encourage the individual to take warm baths in waist-level water.[30] Provide or teach application of warm, moist heat to lower back as needed. Teach the individual to report the location, intensity, quality, and pattern of their discomfort or pain.

TABLE 26-6 Nursing Interventions for Alterations in Tissue Perfusion and Urinary Elimination after Prostatectomy

Nursing Diagnosis	Nursing Intervention
Altered tissue perfusion related to surgical resection of the prostate	Monitor the indwelling catheter and urine for clots and excessive blood; pink-tinged urine is expected. If the catheter becomes dislodged, notify the physician immediately without attempting to replace it. Administer anticholinergic medications and monitor adequate bladder drainage. Monitor hemoglobin/hematocrit and vital signs. Maintain the patient on a low-residue diet and administer stool softeners.
Altered patterns of urinary elimination related to surgical resection of the prostate	Monitor the indwelling catheter for signs of occlusion and bladder distension. Administer anticholinergic or antispasmodic medications. Advise the patient that some dribbling incontinence may occur after the catheter is removed. Teach the patient to perform pelvic muscle exercises after the catheter has been removed. Teach the patient to monitor incontinence, begin a scheduled voiding program, and refer to continence specialist if incontinence persists over 3 months.[33] Teach the patient the principles of skin care: regular washing, complete drying, use of a moisture barrier, and urinary collection device.

riencing serious skin care problems, patients with a short life expectancy, and those with a chronically painful condition may prefer, or may be asked to comply with, the placement of an indwelling urinary catheter.[32] Home care involves maintaining the patency of the catheter and drainage system, along with minimizing bacterial colonization of the bag or catheter and subsequent UTI.[30] Appendix 26A contains a self-care guide for urinary catheter care.

Dexterity and mobility impaired by peripheral neuropathy can be counteracted by helping the individual obtain clothing that is easily removed. Physical or occupational therapy may be indicated.

Evaluation of Therapeutic Approaches

As discussed earlier, there is no fully validated instrument available for assessment of bladder disturbances in the oncology setting. The Southwest Oncology Group toxicity criteria[28] addresses the relevant disturbances and could be used in a clinical oncology setting to monitor individuals' responses to symptom management; however, the scale is not intended for self-report or self-monitoring. The addition of a voiding diary to clinician grading of symptoms will enhance the quality and completeness of data collected for use in evaluating the efficacy of symptom management.

The outcomes listed in Table 26-7 are goals of nursing care and interventions. Outcome criteria are included for comparison with patient data in evaluating whether the outcome has been achieved.

Educational Tools and Resources

Table 26-8 is a clinical nursing guide to be used as a quick reference to selected common medications prescribed in the urologic oncology setting. Self-care guides for catheter care (Appendix 26A), IBSs (Appendix 26B), and urinary incontinence (Appendix 26C) are provided to facilitate patient education efforts. A bladder diary is included (Appendix 26D). Table 26-9 lists resources available to nurses who manage bladder disturbances in the oncology setting and to patients with bladder disturbance symptoms.

TABLE 26-7 Outcomes of Symptom Management for Bladder Disturbances

Outcome	Outcome Criteria
Dysuria/pain has been reduced	Subjective reports of relief from dysuria, bladder pain
Urgency has dissipated	Voiding patterns have returned to normal, no subjective reports of urgent sensations
Frequency has returned to premorbid patterns	Voiding is no more often than every 2 hours during the day, no more than once per night for patients <65 years of age, and no more than twice per night for patients >65 years of age[30]
UTI has been resolved or avoided	Urine culture reveals no bacterial colonies
Hematuria is absent	Urine is not pink or red and is without clots; high-power microscopic urinalysis reveals 5 or fewer red cells per high-power field
Spontaneous voiding results in complete bladder emptying	Postvoid residual volume is less than 25% of total bladder capacity[30]
Urinary continence is regained	No reports or evidence of leakage or dribbling; perineal skin is intact without rashes or lesions

TABLE 26-8 Selected Common Medications Prescribed in the Urologic Oncology Setting

Agent	Indications	Dosage	Precautions	Side Effects	Nursing
Phenazopyridine: an azo dye with local anesthesia of the urinary mucosa	Relief of urinary tract irritation due to infection, catheterization, endoscopy, and other urinary tract procedures	200 mg PO tid after meals	Not for use with impaired renal function or severe hepatitis	Infrequent except with prolonged or high-dose use: nausea, hemolytic anemia, headache, vertigo	Take with food. Increase oral fluids to 2500 mL per day. Avoid driving or hazardous activities until individual response is known. Inform patient that urine turns orange-red, can stain clothing, interferes with urine tests based on color reactions
Sulfamethoxazole/trimethoprim: inhibits bacterial growth and reproduction of a wide range of bacteria	UTI of both gram-negative and gram-positive bacteria, including *E. coli*	160–800 mg PO q12h	Allergy to sulfa drugs. Caution with concomitant asthma, blood dyscrasias, impaired renal or hepatic function, urinary obstruction	Allergic reactions, drowsiness, confusion, dizziness, nausea/vomiting, stomatitis, diarrhea, bone marrow suppression, jaundice, fever	Increase oral fluids to 2500 mL per day. Antacids decrease absorption. Warn about potential side effects, avoid driving until individual response is known
Ciprofloxacin: one of the quinolones, antibiotics that inhibit DNA replication, causing bacterial death	UTI due to various bacteria, particularly effective against *Pseudomonas*	250–500 mg PO bid	Use by children and pregnant or nursing mothers is not recommended. Caution with CNS disorders or impaired renal or hepatic function	Allergic reactions, headache, dizziness, anorexia, restlessness, hypertension, nausea/vomiting, diarrhea, back and joint pain, hematuria, dyspnea, reduces caffeine clearance	Take on an empty stomach. Do not administer with antacids or oral iron

(continued)

TABLE 26-8 (continued)

Agent	Indications	Dosage	Precautions	Side Effects	Nursing
Nitrofurantoin	Treatment and prevention of UTI	50–100 mg PO qid, for acute infection	Not safe in pregnant women at term and in newborns Do not use in those with significant renal impairment	Allergic reactions, dizziness, drowsiness, headache, peripheral neuropathy, bone marrow suppression, nausea/vomiting, dyspnea, cough	Urine may turn dark yellow to brown Avoid concomitant antacids Take with food or milk to minimize GI disturbance Dilute oral suspension and do not crush tablets, to avoid staining teeth
Anticholinergics/ antispasmodics/ spasmolytics, e.g., oxybutynin, flavoxate; a group of agents that relax smooth muscle in the bladder	Instability incontinence, bladder spasms	Varies	Caution in those with impaired renal or hepatic function, cardiac disease, hypertension, reflux esophagitis, BPH, chronic lung disease	Allergic reactions, confusion, drowsiness, headache, nervousness, dysrhythmias, dry mouth, GI hypomotility, urinary hesitancy/urgency, impotence, blurred vision, decreased sweating	Administer on an empty stomach 1 hour before meals Avoid driving or hazardous activities until individual response is known Teach about dry mouth and orthostatic hypotension effects; avoid overheating

TABLE 26-9 Resources for Patients with Bladder Disturbances

Professional Specialty Groups

Society of Urologic Nurses and Associates, Inc.
East Holly Avenue, Box 56
Pitman, NJ 08071-0056
(609) 256-2335
e-mail: suna@mail.ajj.com

Wound Ostomy and Continence Nurses
1550 S. Coast Highway, Suite #201
Laguna Beach, CA 92651
(888) 224-WOCN
e-mail: membership@wocn.org

Educational and Support Services

American Foundation for Urologic Disease
1128 North Charles Street
Baltimore, MD 21201
(410) 468-1800
e-mail: admin@afud.org

Conclusion

Disturbances of the bladder are common symptoms for many individuals with cancer that if left unchecked or mismanaged can create much misery and dramatic changes in daily routines. Irritative bladder symptoms associated with bladder cancer intravesical therapy, bladder infections, or radiation therapy are treated with pharmacologic agents, comfort measures, and fluid and diet manipulations. Voiding dysfunction, particularly incontinence after radical prostatectomy, is often a challenge to manage. Pelvic muscle exercises and a scheduled voiding program will facilitate continence in many individuals. Participation of the patient and caregivers in the implementation of self-care prevention strategies and therapeutics is essential to comprehensive management of bladder disturbances.

References

1. Droller, MJ: Clinical presentation, investigation, and staging of bladder cancer, in Raghavan D, Scher HI, Leibel SA, Lange PH (eds): *Principles and Practice of Genitourinary Oncology*. Philadelphia: Lippincott-Raven, 1997, pp. 249–259
2. Duldulao KE, Diokno AC, Mitchell B. Value of urinary cytology in women presenting with urge incontinence and/or irritative voiding symptoms. *J Urol* 157:113–116, 1997
3. Francis RR: Carcinoma of the bladder. *J Urol* 85:552–556, 1961
4. Batts CN: Adjuvant intravesical therapy for superficial bladder cancer. *Ann Pharmacother* 26:1270–1276, 1992
5. Lamm DL, Blumenstein BA, Crawford ED, et al: A random-

ized trial of intravesical doxorubicin and immunotherapy with bacillus Calmette-Guérin for transitional-cell carcinoma of the bladder. *N Engl J Med* 325:1205–1209, 1991

6. Lamm DL, van der Meijden APM, Morales A, et al: Incidence and treatment of complications of bacillus Calmette-Guérin intravesical therapy in superficial bladder cancer. *J Urol* 147: 596–600, 1992

7. Berry DL, Blumenstein BA, Magyary D, et al: Patterns of toxicities associated with BCG intravesical therapy. *Int J Urol* 3:98–100, 1996

8. Sant GR, Meares EM: Urinary tract infections, in Sant GR (ed): *Pathophysiologic Principles of Urology.* Boston: Blackwell Science, 1994, pp. 271–297

9. Sobel JD, Kay D: Urinary tract infections, in Mandell GL, Bennett JE, Dolin R (eds): *Douglas and Bennett's Principles and Practice of Infectious Diseases* (ed 4). New York: Churchill Livingstone, 1995, pp. 662–690

10. Landis SH, Murray T, Bolden S, Wingo PA: Cancer statistics, 1998. *CA Cancer J Clin* 48:6–29, 1998

11. Flanigan RC, Shankey TV: The natural history of human prostate cancer, in Raghavan D, Scher HI, Leibel SA, Lange PH (eds): *Principles and Practice of Genitourinary Oncology.* Philadelphia: Lippincott-Raven, 1997, pp. 443–450

12. Mettlin CJ, Murphy GP, Sylvester J, et al: Results of hospital cancer registry surveys by the American College of Surgeons. *Cancer* 80:1875–1881, 1997

13. Petersen RO: *Urologic Pathology* (ed 2). Philadelphia: Lippincott, 1992

14. Wallner K: Prostate brachytherapy, in Raghavan D, Scher HI, Leibel SA, Lange PH (eds): *Principles and Practice of Genitourinary Oncology.* Philadelphia: Lippincott-Raven, 1997, pp. 526–533

15. Gilbert MR, Yasko JM: Neurotoxicities, in Kirkwood JM, Lotze MT, Yasko JM (eds): *Current Cancer Therapeutics.* Philadelphia: Current Medicine, 1994, pp. 284–288

16. Peterson R: Nursing intervention for early detection of spinal cord compressions in patients with cancer. *Cancer Nurs* 16:113–116, 1993

17. Woodruff MW, Oberheim WS, Marden HE: Neoplasms of the genitourinary system, in Lapides J (ed): *Fundamentals of Urology.* Philadelphia: Saunders, 1976, pp. 396–444

18. Herr HW, Lamm DL, Denis L: Management of superficial bladder cancer, in Raghavan D, Scher HI, Leibel SA, Lange PH (eds): *Principles and Practice of Genitourinary Oncology.* Philadelphia: Lippincott-Raven, 1997, pp. 273–280

19. Gray M, Burns SM: Continence management. *Crit Care Nurs Clin North Am* 8:29–38, 1996

20. Ratliff TL, Lattime EC, Williams RD: Immunology of bladder cancer, in Raghavan D, Scher HI, Leibel SA, Lange PH (eds): *Principles and Practice of Genitourinary Oncology.* Philadelphia: Lippincott-Raven, 1997, pp. 239–248

21. Garnick MB: Renal and metabolic complications, in Kirkwood JM, Lotze MT, Yasko JM (eds): *Current Cancer Therapeutics.* Philadelphia: Current Medicine, 1994, pp. 264–269

22. Harrison SC, Abrams P: Bladder function, in Sant GR (ed): *Pathophysiologic Principles of Urology.* Boston: Blackwell Science, 1994, pp. 93–121

23. Harris JL: Treatment of postprostatectomy urinary incontinence with behavioral methods. *Clin Nurse Spec* 11:159–166, 1997

24. Barry MJ, Fowler FJ, O'Leary MP, et al: The American Urological Association Symptom Index for benign prostatic hyperplasia. *J Urol* 148:1549–1557, 1992

25. Chancellor MB, Rivas DA: The American Urological Association Symptom Index for women with voiding symptoms: Lack of index specificity for benign prostate hyperplasia. *J Urol* 150:1706–1709, 1993

26. Chai TC, Belville WD, McGuire EJ, et al: Specificity of the American Urological Association Symptom Index: Comparison of unselected and selected samples of both sexes. *J Urol* 150:1710–1713, 1993

27. Barry MJ, Fowler FJ, O'Leary MP, et al: Correlation of the American Urological Association Symptom Index with self-administered versions of the Madsen-Iversen, Boyarsky, and Maine Medical Assessment Program symptom indexes. *J Urol* 148:1558–1563, 1992

28. Greene S, Weiss GR: Southwest Oncology Group standard response criteria, endpoint definitions and toxicity criteria. *Invest New Drugs* 10:239–253, 1992

29. Boyarsky S, Jones G, Paulson DF, et al: A new look at bladder neck obstruction by the Food and Drug Administration regulations: Guidelines for investigation of benign prostatic hypertrophy. *Trans Am Assoc Genito-Urin Surg* 68:29–32, 1977

30. Gray, M: *Genitourinary Disorders.* St. Louis: Mosby-Yearbook, 1992

31. Resnick NM: Urinary incontinence in the older woman, in Kursh ED, McGuire EJ (eds): *Female Urology.* Philadelphia: Lippincott, 1994, pp. 475–494

32. Brechtelsbauer DA: Care of an indwelling catheter. *Postgrad Med* 92:127–132, 1992

33. Wyman JF: Managing urinary incontinence with bladder training: A case study. *J ET Nurs* 20:121–126, 1993

Indwelling Urinary Catheter Care

Patient Name: _____

Symptom and Description   An indwelling urinary catheter is a tube that continuously drains urine from your bladder into a collection bag. Some persons need a catheter after certain surgeries. Others may have a catheter placed because it is too difficult or impossible to use the bathroom or because urine leakage cannot be controlled.

Learning Needs   You can help the catheter work safely by preventing blockage and infection of the catheter.

Management

Equipment

- Wash your hands with soap and water before and after handling the catheter, tubing, or bag.
- Use a leg bag during the day and the larger bedside bag at night or if you will be resting in bed more than 2 hours. Any drainage bag must be kept below the level of the bladder. Hang the larger bag on the bed or place it on a low stool. Do not lay the bag on the floor. Check the tubing for kinks that might stop the flow of urine.
- Empty the leg bag at least every 2 hours and the bedside bag at least every morning. After emptying, clean the end of the drainage tube with a cotton ball and povidone-iodine (Betadine) or 70% alcohol.
- When you change from the one type of drainage bag to the other, follow these directions to clean the bag that is not being used. If you are not using both a leg bag and a bedside bag, change or clean the drainage bag about once a week.
  1. Rinse the bag with cold water; wash with warm, soapy water; and rinse very well with cold, clear water.
  2. Then fill the bag with a solution of one part vinegar to four parts water and soak for 30 minutes.
  3. Empty the bag and let it air dry.
- If your indwelling catheter is permanent, talk with your nurse about using bleach to disinfect the bags.
- Store any green or blue protection caps in a container of 70% alcohol.

Drinking fluids

- It is important to keep your bladder flushed with plenty of fluids. Drink at least 2 quarts of water (64 ounces or 8 cups—or about 2 liters) each day.

(continued) 501

- Ask your doctor or nurse about drinking more or taking drinks that will make your urine more acid. If you are not at risk for irritative bladder symptoms, you may be able to avoid problems with bladder infections by drinking certain juices.

Hygiene and washing yourself

- You may take a shower or any kind of bath with the catheter in place. Also wash the genital area with a soapy washcloth and dry well twice a day.
- *Women* should wipe the length of the catheter with the washcloth, starting where the catheter enters the body. Then wipe the genital area from front to back, starting where the catheter enters the body, cleaning the folds around the vagina as well.
- *Men* should wipe the length of the catheter with the washcloth, starting where the catheter enters the body. Uncircumcised men should pull back the foreskin and wash the end of the penis. Then wash the penis, scrotum, and groin areas.

Follow-up   Talk to your doctor or nurse about bacteria and infections related to the catheter. People with an indwelling catheter often have some bacteria in their urine. An actual urinary tract infection occurs when enough bacteria grow to cause symptoms, such as fever or blood in the urine. Call your doctor or nurse right away if you notice any of these symptoms:

- Low back pain or stomach pain
- Cloudy, bad-smelling urine
- Material (sediment) in the urine
- Blood in the urine
- Fever or chills

Phone Numbers

Nurse: _____ Phone: _____

Physician: _____ Phone: _____

Other: _____ Phone: _____

Comments

Patient's Signature: _____ Date: _____

Nurse's Signature: _____ Date: _____

Source: Berry DL: Bladder disturbances, in Yarbro CH, Frogge MH, Goodman M (eds): *Cancer Symptom Management* (ed 2). Sudbury: Jones and Bartlett, 1999. © Jones and Bartlett Publishers.

Irritative Bladder Symptoms (IBSs)

Patient Name: _____

Symptom and Description   IBSs include three related symptoms that often occur together.

- *Dysuria* is an unpleasant sensation of pain, discomfort, or burning that occurs during urination.
- *Urgency* is when it feels like you have to urinate right away or immediately, even sometimes if your bladder is not full.
- *Frequency* is having to urinate more frequently than what is normal for you, generally more often than every 2 hours during the day.

People who are receiving treatment for cancer, or who have certain urinary tests that require insertion of an instrument or catheter into their bladder, are sometimes at risk for IBSs and bladder infections. If you have irritative bladder symptoms your doctor or nurse will want to conduct other tests to determine whether there is an infection in your bladder. People who are receiving treatment for bladder cancer through a catheter directly into their bladder are also at risk for IBSs. This would occur after the treatments for a few hours (but it can last up to several days), due to the effect of the treatment drug on the lining of the bladder. This IBS side effect usually begins after the second or third treatment.

Learning Needs   You can help prevent IBSs from occurring or from worsening and you can help treat the symptoms when they do occur by learning to:

- Specifically tell your doctor and nurse about your discomfort and symptoms
- Take certain medications
- Use warmth
- Modify what you drink and eat

Prevention   Although some IBSs may happen in certain people, you may be able to prevent IBSs by:

- Drinking plenty of liquids. Try to drink at least 2 quarts (almost 2 liters) of water every day.
- Avoiding fluids with caffeine and acid fluids (this includes most juices). Water is best!
- Not delaying if you feel the need to urinate.

Management

1. Once you've experienced IBSs, you should notify your doctor or nurse as soon as possible, describing:

   - Where the discomfort is
   - How bad it is

- What it feels like
- How long it lasts
- How often you feel the need to urinate
- How often you actually are urinating
- Whether your urine is pink or red

Your doctor or nurse may give you a bladder diary to record how often you urinate and how much you are drinking.

2. You must take any medication that is prescribed to treat a bladder infection or treat the discomfort.

3. Continue to drink a lot of nonacid and noncaffeinated fluids, increasing the amount to 2½ quarts (80 ounces or 10 cups) each day while the symptoms last.

4. Take warm baths in water up to your waist to reduce bladder pain, and use warm, moist heat for any low back pain you feel.

Follow-up   Call your physician or nurse as soon as irritative bladder symptoms begin and if you have a new fever along with the IBSs. Bring with you any record of urination and fluids you have consumed when you see your doctor or nurse. When your IBSs get better, you can return to your normal level of drinking fluids, but it should remain at least 2 quarts (almost 2 liters) per day (64 ounces or 8 cups).

Phone Numbers

Nurse: _____ Phone: _____

Physician: _____ Phone: _____

Other: _____ Phone: _____

Comments

Patient's Signature: _____ Date: _____

Nurse's Signature: _____ Date: _____

Source: Berry DL: Bladder disturbances, in Yarbro CH, Frogge MH, Goodman M (eds): *Cancer Symptom Management* (ed 2). Sudbury: Jones and Bartlett, 1999. © Jones and Bartlett Publishers.

Urinary Incontinence

Patient Name: _____

Symptom and Description   A person who cannot control the flow of urine has urinary incontinence. This loss of bladder control can involve a little leakage of urine when a person sneezes or coughs, or a total lack of control over urination. Urinary incontinence commonly occurs for several months after surgery, such as removal of the prostate, because of the surgery in the area of the bladder. Temporary incontinence can also occur with urinary tract infections and irritations.

Learning Needs   You can help manage incontinence when it occurs by learning to:

- Keep track of the times that you urinate and/or are incontinent
- Perform certain exercises
- Take good care of your skin
- Take certain medications

Prevention   It is common to experience some loss of bladder control after surgeries such as removal of the prostate, but you can help to prevent its continuation by participating in its management.

Management

- Keep track of when you urinate by completing a "bladder diary" (included).
- Try to urinate according to a schedule. If you have been leaking or urinating every hour or more, then try to urinate only once every 60 minutes. If you have been leaking or urinating every half hour, then try to urinate only once every 30 minutes. Keep on that schedule even if you don't feel the urge to urinate.
- When you have been able to urinate at that schedule without leaking in between, then increase the time interval between attempts to urinate, by 30 minutes at a time. If you feel an urgent need to urinate in between the scheduled times, try relaxation or distraction (for instance, balance your checkbook!) and the urgency may go away for a while.
- Practice pelvic muscle exercises taught to you by your nurse or doctor.
- Keep the skin around your genital area, groin, buttocks, and upper thigh clean and as dry as possible. Wash with soap and water to remove urine. Your nurse can help you select a moisture barrier to protect your skin, if needed. Change wet clothing or bedding immediately. Wear loose clothing. Wear adult briefs with pads or absorbent pads to help absorb urine and keep your skin dry.
- Call your nurse if your skin becomes reddened or irritated.
- Take any medications prescribed to relax your bladder muscles.

(continued) 505

Follow-up   Bring any record of urination and leakage with you when you see your doctor or nurse. Extending the time intervals between urination can eventually get you back to "normal" or to a point at which you are satisfied with your urinary control. Many institutions have incontinence clinics with specialists who treat urinary incontinence of all types. Your nurse or doctor may refer you to these services.

Phone Numbers

Nurse: _____ Phone: _____

Physician: _____ Phone: _____

Other: _____ Phone: _____

Comments

Patient's Signature: _____ Date: _____

Nurse's Signature: _____ Date: _____

Source: Berry DL: Bladder disturbances, in Yarbro CH, Frogge MH, Goodman M (eds): *Cancer Symptom Management* (ed 2). Sudbury: Jones and Bartlett, 1999. © Jones and Bartlett Publishers.

Bladder Diary

Patient Name: _____ Date: _____

Physician: _____ Phone: _____

Nurse: _____ Phone: _____

Your nurse or doctor will tell you what information is to be included on this bladder diary form and how many days to keep the diary. Write down the time of day, including AM or PM, in the column labeled *Time*. Place a checkmark in the *Urinated* column when you urinate on purpose. Place a checkmark in the *Leakage* column when you leak or pass urine by accident. Write down the approximate amount of fluid you *drink*. (Use ounces or cups or whatever measurement of volume you are most familiar with.) Don't forget to write down the time for each event—drinking, urinating, or leaking. In the *Comments* column, add symptoms your nurse or doctor may ask you to describe or notes that will help you remember what happened. If you have questions about how to complete the diary, call your nurse or doctor.

Time	Urinated	Leakage	Fluid Amount Taken In	Comments

Source: Berry DL: Bladder disturbances, in Yarbro CH, Frogge MH, Goodman M (eds): *Cancer Symptom Management* (ed 2). Sudbury: Jones and Bartlett, 1999. © Jones and Bartlett Publishers.

CHAPTER 27

Constipation

Carol P. Curtiss, RN, MSN, OCN®

The Problem of Constipation in Cancer

Constipation is difficult to define precisely because of the varying perceptions of normal and abnormal bowel habits and patterns of elimination. A common definition of a normal pattern of bowel elimination is the "regular and easy passage of a formed stool at least three times per week and no more than three times a day."[1-3] Constipation frequently is defined as the passage of hard, dry stools with excessive straining and a decrease in the frequency of defecation.[1,2,4,5] A more workable definition includes those individuals who report an inability to expel stool (even if it is soft) or a decrease in usual frequency (even if it remains in the so-called normal range).[6]

Incidence in Cancer

Constipation is the most common chronic digestive problem reported in the United States, accounting for 2.5 million visits to health providers each year.[7,8] However, only a few studies have reported the incidence of constipation in individuals with cancer.[1,9] Clinically, constipation is a common problem for patients with cancer, especially in advanced stages, and its occurrence has been reported in 40% of individuals with cancer referred to a palliative

care service.[10] It is the most common side effect from opioid therapy,[11-13] and it is also a potential problem in individuals receiving neurotoxic chemotherapeutic agents, antidepressants, tranquilizers, and muscle relaxants.[14] Although constipation is recognized as a common clinical problem, additional research is needed to validate the incidence and appropriate management of constipation in individuals with cancer.

Impact on Quality of Life

Failure to anticipate and adequately manage constipation is an unnecessary cause of discomfort and pain, and one that affects quality of life for individuals with cancer. Constipation causes both physical and emotional distress, and influences a person's overall sense of well-being. This frequently occurring and distressing symptom, however, is often overlooked in individuals with cancer.[1,9] Signs and symptoms that affect activities of daily living and quality of life include pain, abdominal fullness or distention, flatus, cramping, anorexia, straining at defecation, a sense of fullness or pressure in the rectal area, a feeling of incomplete emptying, a change in size, consistency, and frequency of stool, dull headache, and lassitude.[15-17]

Individuals with cancer-related pain, including severe pain, often discontinue opioid medications for pain relief because of poorly managed constipation.[11,13] A well-planned preventive bowel management program improves quality of life both directly and indirectly.

Etiology

Constipation in the person with cancer often has multiple etiologies. It can be a presenting symptom of cancer, a side effect of therapy, the result of tumor progression, or may be unrelated to cancer or therapy. Constipation is classified as primary (simple), secondary to pathologic organic conditions, or iatrogenic.[9]

Primary Causes of Constipation

Primary or simple causes of constipation in individuals with cancer include decreases in dietary intake of fluid and fiber, decreases in mobility and exercise, bed rest, and changes in usual patterns of elimination and bowel routine. Lack of privacy and comfort during defecation may also contribute to constipation by inducing the individual to ignore the urge to defecate and to change normal bowel routines.

Numerous factors can cause a decrease in dietary intake of fluids and fiber and thereby increase the risk of constipation in individuals with cancer. These factors include anorexia, dysphagia, mouth sores, taste changes, early satiety, poorly controlled nausea and vomiting, fatigue, depression, poorly controlled pain, and a tumor that affects intake and digestion. Decreases in mobility and exercise and changes in toileting routines may be caused by fatigue, physical limitations of illness and therapy, pain, alterations in patterns of elimination caused by hospital or health care setting schedules, and the use of bedpans rather than commodes or toilets. Stress, depression, or mental confusion may also contribute to constipation. Underlying conditions such as hemorrhoids or fissures exacerbate the problem.

Constipation Related to Cancer and Cancer Therapy

Constipation may also be caused by mechanical pressure on the bowel, compression of nerves that innervate the bowel, or metabolic changes due to cancer. Mechanical causes of constipation include obstruction or compression of the lumen of the bowel by tumor, pressure from the presence of ascites, and interrupted neural transmission due to nerve involvement or cord compression from tumor. Metabolic changes causing constipation include dehydration, hypokalemia, and hypercalcemia.

Numerous drugs increase the risk of constipation, including chemotherapeutic agents (vincristine and vinblastine[18]), 5HT$_3$ antagonist antiemetics, opioid therapy, anticholinergic preparations, phenothiazines, calcium- and aluminum-based antacids, antidepressants, diuretics, iron and calcium supplements, tranquilizers, and some medications to induce sleep.[16] Preexisting laxative dependence and other underlying diseases will further increase risks of constipation.

Constipation sometimes is induced intentionally for individuals receiving brachytherapy for gynecologic cancers. A low-residue diet and antidiarrheal agents are prescribed to prevent bowel movements while an implant is in place. Normal bowel activity may not return for several days after completion of therapy, but increasing dietary fiber is usually sufficient to treat this side effect of therapy.[19]

Pathophysiology

Normal Bowel Function

Normal bowel function requires gastrointestinal motility, mucosal transport, and intact reflexes for defecation. The colon mixes and propels its contents through the bowel and absorbs water and electrolytes from stool by segmental and propulsive movements.[15,20] Segmental movements churn and mix food, exposing colonic contents to the intestinal mucosa where fluid and electrolytes are absorbed. Propulsive movements, or peristalsis, drive colonic contents forward through the colon.[15,16,21] Strong peristaltic waves occur one to four times daily in response to mechanical stretching of the bowel and/or neural stimuli.[16,22] In normal individuals with normal eating habits, the strongest peristaltic waves usually occur at breakfast.[16]

The urge to defecate is initiated when a mass of feces is felt in the rectum. The process is a coordinated reflex of sacral nerve segments S-3, S-4, and S-5, and is initiated by stimulation of stretch receptors located in the anus. Contraction of abdominal muscles to increase intraabdominal pressure also facilitates bowel emptying. The urge to defecate can be a weak, easily ignored reflex, and repeated failure to respond to this urge can lead to constipation.

Regular bowel function is dependent on normal peristalsis, sensory awareness of rectal filling, motor control of the anal sphincter, adequate rectal capacity, compliance with the urge to defecate, and a physical environment conducive to comfortable defecation.[22] Changes in any of these functions can cause constipation.

Alterations in Peristalsis

Peristalsis is stimulated by the presence of a fecal mass adequate to stretch the bowel wall. When peristalsis slows or becomes sluggish, it takes longer for stool to move through the colon and more fluid than normal is reabsorbed, resulting in a hard, dry stool. Factors that decrease peristalsis include insufficient intake of dietary bulk and fluids, lack of mobility, stress, and depression.[22] Metabolic alterations such as hypercalcemia also may cause constipation. Elevated extracellular calcium present with hypercalcemia decreases the contraction of smooth muscles, leading to slowed gastrointestinal motility and delayed gastric emptying.[2]

Opioid analgesics *decrease peristalsis* by acting directly on receptor sites in the gut as well as in the central nervous system.[15,23,24] Although the exact mechanism of action is unclear, the degree of constipation caused by opioids is dose dependent and becomes more severe as analgesic doses are increased to relieve pain.[2,11,12,15]

Decreased Sensory Awareness of Rectal Filling

Sensory awareness is dependent on intact neural pathways between the anorectum and the brain and is also affected by the individual's level of consciousness.[22] Spinal cord compression, spinal lesions, tumor involvement of nerve pathways to and from the colon and rectum, and neurotoxicity from medications such as vincristine and vinblastine inhibit transmission of impulses controlling bowel function[2,18] and contribute to constipation. The presence of brain metastasis, sedation, loss of consciousness, and confusion are additional factors affecting sensory awareness of the need to defecate.

Changes in Motor Control of the Anal Sphincter and Rectal Capacity

Sphincter control is necessary to maintain fecal continence and to regularly empty the rectum. The internal sphincter is normally contracted and is controlled by the autonomic nervous system.[22] When the rectal wall is distended by stool mass, the internal sphincter relaxes and permits the rectal contents to move further toward the anus. The external sphincter is a voluntary muscle and contracts to retain feces or relaxes to expel feces. The rectum must also be able to retain and store stool to function properly. Normally the rectum can accommodate approximately 300 cc of stool and gas.[22] Presence of tumor in or around the rectum, anal fissures causing pain, therapy decreasing the capacity of the rectum (e.g., surgery), fibrosis from radiation in the anorectum, and changes in innervation to the sphincters or rectum may result in constipation.

Assessment

Measurement Tools

The Constipation Assessment Scale is one of the few measurement tools for constipation that has been empirically tested for reliability and validity.[14] The tool is easy to use and provides reliable indicators of the presence and severity of constipation. It consists of eight descriptors for constipation and is based on patient self-report. Figure 27-1 illustrates the scale, which is designed at the sixth-grade reading level and takes approximately two minutes to complete. Other assessment tools include selected portions of the history and physical data described in Table 27-1 compiled in a variety of formats, including flow sheets, computer printouts, narrative notes, problem-oriented notes, and charting by exception.

Clinical Assessment

Assessment for constipation is ongoing and requires both a careful history and physical examination. Prevention and early detection of constipation is the goal, and vigilant evaluation is key to identifying risks for

Constipation Assessment Scale

Directions: Circle the appropriate number to indicate whether, during the past three days, you have had NO PROBLEM, SOME PROBLEM, or a SEVERE PROBLEM with each of the items listed.

Item	No Problem	Some Problem	Severe Problem
1. Abdominal distension or bloating	0	1	2
2. Change in amount of gas passed rectally	0	1	2
3. Less frequent bowel movements	0	1	2
4. Oozing liquid stool	0	1	2
5. Rectal fullness or pressure	0	1	2
6. Rectal pain with bowel movement	0	1	2
7. Smaller stool size	0	1	2
8. Urge but inability to pass stool	0	1	2

Patient's Name	Date

FIGURE 27-1 Constipation Assessment Scale. Instruct the patient to respond to each of the eight items by circling the one number that most closely represents their symptoms. Add up the score. The range is between 0 (no constipation) and 16 (the most severe constipation). If the individual indicates a problem with item 4 (oozing liquid stool), consider the possibility of impaction. As the score increases, the aggressiveness of the bowel management program should also increase based on individual response. (Source: Printed with permission. Copyright Susan C. McMillan, 1989.)

TABLE 27-1 Evaluation of Constipation—History and Physical Assessment

Assessment Data	Individual Characteristics
History	
Usual pattern of elimination	• Frequency, consistency, amount • Usual routine, including time for elimination and rituals followed • Last bowel movement • Elimination aids (raised toilet seat, laxative use, etc.) • Individual's definitions of regularity and constipation • Changes since diagnosis or treatment
Previous experiences with constipation and responses	• Interventions that have worked in the past • Current or past laxative use and response to laxative therapy • Underlying conditions that increase risk for constipation
Usual and current dietary patterns	• Amounts and types of fluid daily—identify recent changes • Intake of bulk and fiber—identify recent changes • 24-hour recall of dietary intake • Changes in appetite, taste, dentition, energy
Recent changes in lifestyle	• Changes in activity, mood, increased stress, changes in mobility • Physical changes affecting defecation
Symptoms of constipation	• Flatus, bloating, cramping • Oozing stool in the presence of symptoms of constipation • Straining of defecation; difficult passage of stool; hard, dry stool • Abdominal pain, fullness, anorexia, other symptoms
Current medications	• Identify medications that increase risk of constipation • Identify laxative use
Other risk factors for constipation	• Recent and past cancer and cancer therapy • Other underlying health problems
Knowledge of individual	• Understanding of constipation and therapy for constipation
Evaluate laboratory findings	• Identify presence of thrombocytopenia or leukopenia, or metabolic conditions that cause constipation (hypercalcemia, hypokalemia)
Physical assessment	
Examine:	• Visualize abdomen for visible peristalsis, masses, distention, bulges
Palpate:	• For tenderness, decreased muscle tone, presence of palpable tumor, nodes, or stool
Percuss:	• For dullness in an otherwise tympanic area of the abdomen
Auscultate:	• For presence and character of bowel sounds
Examine:	• Rectal area (or stoma) for irritation, fissures, lesions, rashes, or scarring
Perform rectal exam:	• Evaluate external sphincter tone, rule out impaction, and evaluate hemorrhoids or presence of tumor • *Rectal exam is contraindicated in presence of leukopenia or thrombocytopenia*
Evaluate:	• Signs of systemic conditions related to hydration, overall performance status, and underlying conditions related to constipation (e.g., skin turgor) • Assess lower-extremity strength, sensation, and reflexes for possible spinal cord compression.

constipation in the person with cancer. History and physical assessment data are shown in Table 27-1. Evaluation should include:

1. Usual and recent patterns of elimination
2. Previous experiences with constipation and responses to specific therapy
3. Usual and current dietary patterns
4. Recent changes in lifestyle
5. Current symptoms of constipation
6. Current medications
7. Recent and past extent of cancer and cancer therapy
8. The individual's understanding of constipation and interventions to prevent and treat the symptom
9. An evaluation of laboratory findings for contributing causes of constipation
10. A thorough physical assessment

Symptom Management

Prevention

Identifying persons at risk is the key to prevention, as monitoring bowel function and preventing constipation are much easier than treating constipation once it occurs. A prevention program for individuals who may have problems with constipation consists of increasing dietary fiber and fluid intake along with an increase in exercise.

Foods rich in dietary fiber include whole-grain cereals and breads, legumes, root vegetables, fruits with seeds and skins (especially prunes, figs, and applesauce), nuts, peanut butter, and popcorn. However, for individuals with cancer-related constipation, increasing dietary fluid and fiber are frequently poorly tolerated and insufficient to manage the problem. Cancer patients often experience a decrease in appetite, fatigue, and other symptoms and have difficulty increasing fluids and tolerating dietary bulk and fiber. Adequate intake of nutrients has a higher priority.

Exercise within the limits of individual tolerance, including abdominal isometric exercises, also helps maintain normal bowel function. However, increases in mobility and exercise may be impaired by fatigue, advanced disease, poor pain control, fractures due to bone metastasis, or decreased endurance.

The addition of daily stool softeners and peristaltic stimulators to both soften and propel feces through the colon is often needed, especially for persons receiving opioid therapy. An individualized plan for opioid-induced constipation should include increasing the dosage of laxative as the dosage of opioid increases over time. Offering choices for specific products and regimens for maintaining bowel function will help ensure an acceptable

plan. The patient or caregiver should be instructed to monitor elimination daily, with the goal of having a soft bowel movement once a day, or less often if consistent with the person's usual pattern of elimination.

Therapeutic Approaches

Management of constipation includes a program that provides a regular schedule for toileting, privacy, comfort, regular exercises to strengthen and tone abdominal muscles, and routine reminders to respond to the urge to defecate.[23,25] As mentioned earlier, increases in dietary bulk, fluids, and exercise as tolerated will help promote regular bowel function. Table 27-2 lists several "natural" dietary remedies used to promote regular bowel function. Severe or refractory constipation is treated with the use of regularly administered laxatives (not prn), and if defecation does not occur, the laxatives are aggressively increased. Enemas are reserved for symptoms that do not respond to regular laxative therapy and dietary interven-

TABLE 27-2   Natural or Home Preparations to Manage Nonrefractory Constipation

Option #1
1 part bran
2 parts of prune juice
3 parts applesauce
Mix all ingredients together. Begin with ⅛ to ¼ cup (30 to 60 mL) one to two times daily. Increase or decrease as needed to regulate bowel function.
Option #2
1 ounce (28 g) of senna leaves (available at natural food and health stores)
1 quart (about 1 liter) of water
1 pound (.5 kg) of prunes
Boil senna leaves gently in the 1 quart of water. Strain off the leaves and simmer liquid with 1 pound of prunes until all or most of the liquid has been absorbed. Eat 1 to 3 prunes every second or third night to regulate bowel function.
Senna leaves may also be used as tea leaves with water to make senna tea. Drink as needed to regulate bowel function.
Option #3
1 pound raisins (.5 kg)
1 pound currants
1 pound prunes
1 pound figs
1 pound dates
One 28-ounce container of prune concentrate (about .83 liter). Put fruit through a food processor or grinder. Mix with prune concentrate (mixture will be very thick). Store in airtight container in refrigerator. Begin with 2 tablespoons (30 mL) daily and increase or decrease to regulate bowel function.

Data from references 3, 26, 27 and personal communication with J. Milton.

tions. Use of a bowel management protocol will facilitate consistent prevention and management of constipation. Table 27-3 describes a basic bowel management protocol to prevent constipation in patients with cancer. Figure 27-2 describes a bowel management program for those patients receiving opioid therapy and others who are at risk for refractory constipation.

Fecal Impaction

Failure to manage bowel function adequately can result in fecal impaction.[28,29] Large amounts of hard, dry feces accumulate in the rectum and cannot be eliminated normally.[18] As stool continues to collect, seepage of soft stool around the impaction may present as diarrhea. Other symptoms include rectal discomfort, lower abdominal pain, tenesmus, back pain, or urinary dysfunction. If the impaction continues, nausea and vomiting, hypotension, confusion, respiratory and circulatory compromise, and death may occur. Assessment and physical examination are similar to those for constipation, with the possible addition of a flat and upright abdominal x-ray film to rule out impaction above the rectum. Rectal exam reveals large amounts of hard stool in the rectum, unless the impaction is higher in the sigmoid. Once an impaction is recognized, the goal of therapy is to soften the stool and lubricate the bowel to remove the impaction. A glycerin suppository (placed between the rectal mucosa and the stool), oil retention or hypertonic phosphate enemas, or nonstimulating laxatives may be helpful. Laxatives that increase peristalsis or cause cramping are contraindicated until the impaction is removed and stool is able to pass through the bowel.

Manual disimpaction should be performed only after using a topical anesthetic[29] and water-soluble lubricant[3] to promote comfort. Premedication with supplemental opioids and/or benzodiazepam anxiolytics should be considered to reduce the physical and psychological pain of the procedure.[2] Gloves are required for disimpaction. Care providers with long or sharp fingernails should not perform disimpaction because of the risk of trauma and tears to the anal and rectal mucosa. After the mass is lubricated and softened, a rectal exam is performed using a single finger lubricated with 5% lidocaine ointment. After several minutes the sphincter relaxes, and a second finger is inserted. The two fingers are gently and slowly moved apart, dilating the anal sphincter. The two fingers are used to gently "slice apart" the impacted mass. Removing small pieces one at a time is less uncomfortable for the individual than attempting to remove large portions of the mass. After most of the fecal material is removed, follow with cleansing enemas. An aggressive, well-monitored bowel management program is then instituted to prevent recurrence of impaction.[30] Disimpaction is contraindicated in patients who are thrombocytopenic or leukopenic. The best treatment of impaction is prevention.

Laxative Use and Selection

The goal of laxative therapy is to promote normal elimination patterns and prevent constipation and impaction.

TABLE 27-3 Basic Bowel Management Protocol for Patients with Cancer

Goal	Assessment	Interventions
Prevention of constipation: The individual will pass stool without report of straining and maintain individual normal bowel frequency per assessment parameters.	Establish and document normal bowel pattern and habits. Assess risks for constipation—effects of tumor, therapy, medications, underlying problems, environment, diet, exercise, mobility Assess lab values for presence of leukopenia, thrombocytopenia, metabolic changes Perform physical assessment of abdomen, rectum Assess individual's understanding of interventions to prevent constipation	Monitor bowel patterns daily Document risk factors Document results of assessments Begin teaching plan Teach methods to increase dietary bulk to 5–10 g daily as tolerated Teach methods to increase fluid intake to 8 glasses of fluid daily as tolerated Plan regular exercise as tolerated; increase mobility if possible, incorporate isometric abdominal exercises and range-of-motion exercises if unable to ambulate Provide a warm or hot drink 30 minutes before usual time of defecation Provide privacy and comfort around usual defecation schedule (use toilet, commode, foot stool, etc. to promote normal position for defecation)

Data from references 15, 21, 23, 26.

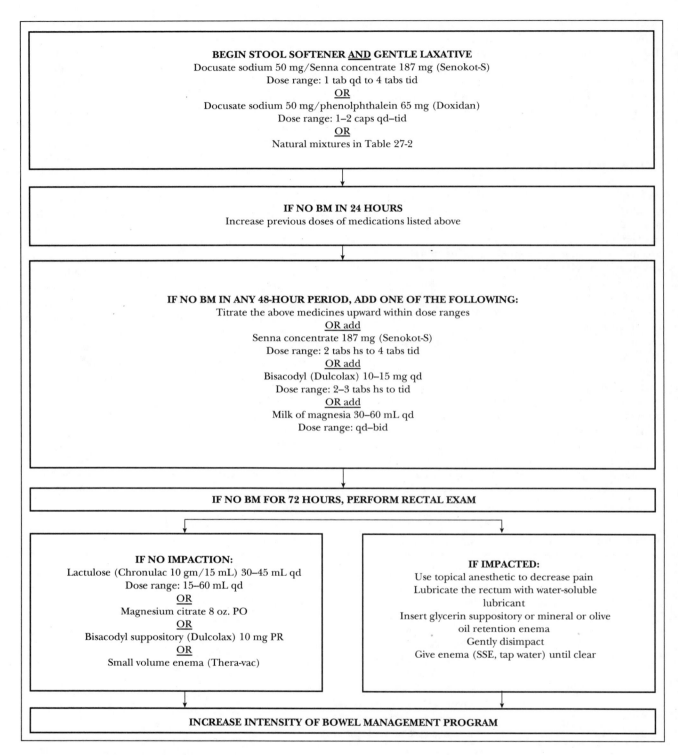

FIGURE 27-2 Prophylactic bowel management program for patients receiving opioid therapy and patients at risk for refractory constipation.

The effects of laxatives are dose related, beginning with a softener effect, then a laxative effect; high doses act as cathartics.[9] A laxative regimen titrated to individual need promotes regular bowel function without swings from constipation to diarrhea.[2]

Laxatives may be divided into the following groups:

(1) bulk producers, (2) lubricants and emollients, (3) saline laxatives, (4) osmotic laxatives, (5) detergent laxatives, (6) stimulants, and (7) suppositories and enemas. Table 27-4 lists common laxatives. All oral laxatives are *contraindicated with suspected or actual intestinal obstruction*, due to the risk of bowel perforation by increasing peristalsis in the presence of obstruction.[4]

Bulk laxatives are natural or synthetic polysaccharides or cellulose that increase peristalsis by causing water to be retained in the stool, increasing the size and weight of stool.[2,4] Bulk laxatives are of limited use for severe constipation and in individuals who are unable to tolerate at least 3000 cc (3 liters) of fluid per day.[2,4,21,22] In addition, people with anorexia, early satiety, fluid restrictions, food aversions, and other alterations in nutrition that decrease appetite need to place a priority on adequate intake of nutrients rather than increasing fluid intake as required by bulk laxatives.

Lubricants coat and soften the stool and decrease friction as the stool moves through the colon.[31] Excessive doses can lead to rectal seepage and perianal irritation. Long-term use can cause malabsorption of fat-soluble vitamins, making lubricants of limited use in a prophylactic bowel management program.

Saline laxatives contain magnesium or sulfate ions and act by drawing water into the gut, thereby altering stool consistency, distending the bowel, and increasing peristalsis.[4,16,21] They act in both the small and large intestines. This class of laxatives is of little use in a daily preventive program and is most often used for acute evacuation of the bowel.

Osmotic laxatives include lactulose and sorbitol. Lactulose, the most commonly used osmotic laxative, is a synthetic disaccharide that passes to the colon undigested. Bacteria in the colon metabolize lactulose, increasing osmotic pressure in the colon and increasing water in the stool. Lactulose also lowers serum ammonia levels and reduces colon pH.[4] Sorbitol is relatively inexpensive compared to lactulose, and comparably effective.[7]

Detergent laxatives have a direct action on the intestines, reduce surface tension, and allow water and fats to penetrate into dry stool.[2,4,16] They also decrease electrolyte and water absorption from the colon.

Stimulant laxatives act directly on the colon to stimulate motility and are activated by bacterial degradation in the intestines. Two major groups include diphenylmethanes and anthraquinones. These laxatives are the most commonly used medications in a prophylactic plan for the management of opioid-induced constipation in patients with cancer.

The use of oral naloxone to reverse opioid-induced constipation has been reported and continues to be evaluated. Treatment may begin with 4 mg oral naloxone daily and may be titrated to a maximum of 12 mg. Dosing intervals of 6 hours or longer should be used if multiple daily doses are required.[32] For patients taking morphine, the dose of naloxone may also be calculated as 20% of the 24-hour morphine dose and further titrated to effect.[33] All persons on this regimen must be monitored for signs of systemic opioid withdrawal and accompanying increases in pain. Dose reduction or increased intervals of dosing of naloxone will prevent this complication. However, oral naloxone is an expensive alternative to other medications to treat constipation.

Suppositories stimulate the intestinal nerve plexus and cause rectal emptying.[22] They are frequently used in individuals with cancer as a second step when oral laxatives are not effective in producing stool within 2 days. Enemas are not indicated for long-term bowel management in patients with cancer-related constipation,[2,22,34,35] but they may be indicated to cleanse the bowel after disimpaction. The enema fluid determines the mechanism of action. Tap water and normal saline act by increasing fluid volume and bulk in the colon. Vegetable oils and lubricants lubricate and soften. Soap acts as an irritant. Properly administered, enemas cleanse only the distal colon. Enemas and suppositories are contraindicated in individuals with neutropenia or thrombocytopenia, due the increased risk of perirectal abscesses and bleeding from rectal manipulation.

Evaluation of Therapeutic Approaches

Care of the person with cancer is guided and evaluated by the Outcome Standards for Oncology Nursing Practice.[35] The outcome standard for comfort states that the patient/significant others identify and manage factors that influence comfort. The standard for nutrition measures the ability of the patient/significant others to manage nutrition and hydration, which facilitate optimal health and comfort in the presence of disease and treatment. The outcome standard for elimination states that the patient/significant others manage alterations in elimination that are consistent with activities of daily living.

Documentation tools used by healthcare providers to record response to therapy may include a flow sheet, diary, check-off list, problem-oriented notes, or narrative documentation. Frequency of bowel function, consistency of stool, ease of passage of stool, and individual self-report of comfort are outcome measures. The person's ability to comply with dietary interventions and laxative therapy and their level of understanding of the potential and actual causes of constipation should also be documented.

Patient documentation includes the Constipation Assessment Tool described in Figure 27-1, diaries describing bowel patterns and frequency, dietary and activity recall, medication lists, and additional comments to report to healthcare providers.

Educational Tools

Tables and figures in this chapter can be used as educational tools for nurses. Assessment and physical

TABLE 27-4   Medications Used to Manage Constipation

Preparation	Action/Onset	Special Considerations	Contraindications
Bulk-Forming Laxatives Methylcellulose Psyllium Mucilloids Malt soup extracts Carboxymethylcellulose	Increase peristalsis by causing water retention in the stool. Increase size and weight of stool. Onset is from 12h to several days.	Must be accompanied by a full (8 oz) glass of water. Daily fluid intake must be increased to at least 3 liters. Failure to increase fluids decreases efficacy and may cause intestinal or esophageal obstruction.	Not appropriate for person with fluid restrictions, or for those unable to drink increased volume of fluid. Should not be used with suspected or actual bowel obstruction. Psyllium is not recommended for individuals taking salicylates, nitrofurantoin, digoxin.[4] Psyllium decreases the action of these medications.
Lubricants Mineral oil Liquid petrolatum	Coat and soften stool and decrease friction as stool moves through the colon. Onset is between 24 and 48h.[2–4,21]	Chronic use can result in rectal seepage and malabsorption of oil-soluble vitamins and medications.[4] Systemic absorption of mineral oil is increased when taken with docusate.	May cause aspiration pneumonia in persons with reflux, dysphagia, or confusion.[2,4,16,21] Do not administer at bedtime or to debilitated patients. Also contraindicated in pregnant women and persons on anticoagulant therapy. Mineral oil decreases the availability of vitamin K and thus alters coagulation.
Saline laxatives Magnesium citrate Sodium biphosphate Magnesium hydroxide	Draws water into the gut and increases water absorption into the stool. Alters stool consistency, increasing weight of stool, distending the bowel, and increasing peristalsis. Onset is dose dependent. High doses produce watery stool within 1–2h. Lower doses produce semifluid stool in 6–12h.	Of little to no use in prevention of constipation. Primary use is in the acute evacuation of the bowel.	Magnesium-containing laxatives should not be used with aluminum-containing antacids. Sodium salts should not be used in individuals with cardiac or renal disease, hypertension, or edema.
Osmotic laxatives Lactulose Sorbitol	Bacteria in the colon metabolize osmotic laxatives, increasing osmotic pressure and water retention in the stool. Lactulose also lowers serum ammonia levels and decreases colon pH.	Sweet taste of products may be unpalatable to persons with anorexia, taste changes, or nausea. Excessive amounts will result in watery diarrhea. Lactulose is more expensive than most laxatives.	Not appropriate for individuals with acute abdomen, fecal impaction, or obstruction.
Detergent laxatives Docusate Docusate sodium Docusate potassium	Act directly on the colon to reduce surface tension and allow water and fats to penetrate the stool.[2,4,16] Decrease electrolyte and water absorption from the colon. Onset is 12–24h with oral preparations. 2–15 min with rectal preparations.	Docusate increases systemic absorption of mineral oil and danthron. Enteric coated medications such as docusate must be taken whole for correct absorption. Do not split, crush, chew, or alter. Of little value in a prophylactic bowel management program for long-term constipation. Appropriate for short-term use when straining is to be avoided.	Daily use of docusate sodium and oxyphenisatin acetate for more than 8 months may produce chronic active liver disease, including jaundice.[4]

continued

TABLE 27-4   (continued)

Preparation	Action/Onset	Special Considerations	Contraindications

Stimulant laxatives
Diphenylmethanes
  Phenothalein
  Bisacodyl
 	
Anthraquinones
  Senna products
  Casanthrol
  Cascara
  Danthron
	Act directly on the colon to stimulate motility via local irritation and stimulation of intramural nerve plexus.[4]
	
	Activated by bacterial degradation in the intestines.
	
	Onset: Diphenylmethanes
	6–10h PO
	15–60 min rectally
	
	Onset: Anthraquinones
	6–12h PO
	May require up to 24h
	15–60 min rectally
		Often the mainstay of a prophylactic bowel management program for opioid-induced constipation.
		
		May cause cramping.
		
		Prolonged use results in loss of normal bowel function and dependence.
		
		Some products may tint urine pink or red
			Avoid bisacodyl within 1h of using antacids, milk, or cimetidine (tablet dissolves prematurely).
			
			Phenothalein and bisacodyl are not effective in the presence of biliary obstruction (must be excreted in the bile to be effective).
			
			Avoid bisacodyl with actual or suspected ulcerative lesions of the colon.

Suppositories Glycerin Bisacodyl Senna Phenothalein	Stimulate intestinal plexus and cause rectal emptying due to local irritation.[22] Glycerin exerts an osmotic effect. Onset is within 15 min to 1h.	Suppositories must be placed between the rectal mucosa and the stool to be effective. If placed in stool, suppository will not dissolve properly. Rectal irritation may occur with repeated use.	Rectal manipulation, including the use of suppositories and enemas, is contraindicated in individuals with neutropenia, thrombocytopenia, or rectal fissures.

examination are keys to adequate bowel management. Knowledge of physiology, risk factors, and medications to treat constipation assist the nurse in planning an effective prevention program to facilitate regular bowel function.

The Self-Care Guide in Appendix 27A provides a tool for teaching patients about preventing and managing constipation. Teaching begins as soon as the patient is identified as being at risk for constipation and continues throughout treatment. The guide must be individualized to patient need and changed as the risk for constipation increases and decreases. Although a standardized approach can serve as a guide, individualized interventions based on patient need will improve outcome.

Conclusion

Constipation is an uncomfortable, distressing symptom that often accompanies cancer, cancer therapy, and interventions to manage cancer pain. Prevention of constipation is always the goal. Bowel management programs must be instituted early for people at risk for constipation. Effective bowel management plans include active or passive exercise, fluids and foods high in fiber, a comfortable routine and environment, and the aggressive use of medications that both soften stool and increase peristalsis. The aggressiveness of the bowel management plan increases as risk factors increase. Nurses must be aware of the risk factors for constipation in people with cancer and must act quickly to prevent and control constipation. Individual patient teaching and ongoing reinforcement of the

bowel management plan helps ensure early recognition of constipation, promotes regular bowel function, and contributes to patient comfort.

References

1. McShane RE, McLane AM: Constipation—Consensual and empirical validation. *Nurs Clin North Am* 20:801–808, 1985
2. Levy MH: Constipation and diarrhea in cancer patients. *The Cancer Bulletin* 43:412–422, 1991
3. Beverley L, Travis I: Constipation: Proposed natural laxative mixtures. *J Gerontol Nurs* 18:5–12, 1992
4. National Cancer Institute: *Constipation, Impaction and Bowel Obstruction.* CancerFax PDQ Supportive Care/Screening Information. #208/03510:1–13, December 1, 1993
5. Gross J: Functional alterations—Bowel, in Gross J, Johnson BJ (eds): *Handbook of Oncology Nursing* (ed 2). Sudbury: Jones and Bartlett, 1994, pp. 517–528
6. Castle SC: Constipation: Endemic in the elderly? *Med Clin North Am* 73:1497–1509, 1989
7. Lederle FA, Busch D, Mattox KM, et al: Cost-effective treatment of constipation in the elderly: A randomized double-blind comparison of sorbitol and lactulose. *Am J Med* 89:597–601, 1990
8. Goldfinger SE: Constipation: The hard facts. *Harvard Health Letter* 16:1–4, 1991
9. Wright PS, Thomas SL: Constipation and diarrhea: The neglected symptoms. *Semin Oncol Nurs* 11:289–297, 1995
10. Curtis EB, Krach R, Walsh TD: Common symptoms in patients with advanced cancer. *J Pain Symptom Manage* 7:25–29, 1991

11. Walsh TD: Prevention of opioid side effects. *J Pain Symptom Manage* 5:362–367, 1990

12. Jacox A, Carr DB, Payne R, et al: *Management of Cancer Pain. Clinical Practice Guideline No. 9.* AHCPR Publication No. 94-0592. Rockville, MD: Agency for Health Care Policy and Research, U.S. Department of Health and Human Services, March 1994

13. Hill CS: *Guidelines for the Treatment of Cancer Pain: Final Report of the Texas Cancer Council's Workgroup on Pain Control in Cancer Patients.* Houston, TX: Texas Cancer Council, 1991

14. McMillan SC, Williams FA: Validity and reliability of the Constipation Assessment Scale. *Cancer Nurs* 12:183–188, 1989

15. Cameron JC: Constipation related to narcotic therapy—A protocol for nurses and patients. *Cancer Nurs* 15:372–377, 1992

16. Curry CE: Laxative products, in American Pharmaceutical Association: *Handbook of Nonprescription Drugs* (ed 8). Washington, DC: American Pharmaceutical Association, 1986, pp. 75–97

17. Basch A: Changes in elimination. *Semin Oncol Nurs* 3: 287–292, 1987

18. Bisanz A: Managing bowel elimination problems in patients with cancer. *Oncol Nurs Forum* 24:679–688, 1997

19. Dunne-Daly C: Principles of brachytherapy, in Dow KH, Bucholtz JD, Iwamoto RR, et al. (eds): *Nursing Care in Radiation Oncology* (ed 2). Philadelphia: Saunders, 1997, pp. 21–35

20. Moriarty KJ, Irving MH: Constipation. *BMJ* 303:1237–1240, 1992

21. Yakabowich M: Prescribe with care: The role of laxatives in the treatment of constipation. *J Gerontol Nurs* 16:4–11, 1990

22. Doughty D: Maintaining normal bowel function in the patient with cancer. *J ET Nurs* 18:90–94, 1991

23. Haylock PJ: Home care for the person with cancer. *Home Health-care Nurs* 11:16–28, 1993

24. Portenoy RK, Coyle N: Controversies in the long term management of analgesic therapy in patients with advanced cancer. *J Pain Symptom Manage* 5:307–319, 1990

25. Petrosino B, Landrum B, Hackbarth A: Elimination, in Daeffler RJ, Petrosino B (eds): *Manual of Oncology Nursing Practice: Nursing Diagnosis and Care.* Rockville, MD: Aspen, 1990, pp. 157–164

26. Brown MK, Everett I: Gentler bowel fitness with fiber. *Geriatric Nurs* 11:26–27, 1990

27. Kovach T: Managing geriatric chronic constipation. *Home Health-care Nurs* 10:57–58, 1992

28. McCaffery M, Beebe A: Managing your patients' adverse reactions to narcotics. *Nursing 89* 10:166–168, 1989

29. Glare P, Lickiss JN: Unrecognized constipation in patients with advanced cancer: A recipe for therapeutic disaster. *J Pain Symptom Manage* 7:369–371, 1992

30. Culhane B: Constipation, in Yasko JM (ed): *Nursing Management of Symptoms Associated with Chemotherapy.* Columbus, OH: Adria Labs, 1986, pp. 41–43

31. Canty SL: Constipation as a side effect of opioids. *Oncol Nurs Forum* 21:739–745, 1994

32. Culpepper-Morgan JA, Intrurrisi CE, Portenoy RK, et al: Treatment of opioid-induced constipation with oral naloxone: A pilot study. *Clin Pharmacol Ther* 52:90–95, 1992

33. Sykes NP: An investigation of the ability of oral naloxone to correct opioid-related constipation in patients with advanced cancer. *Palliat Med* 10:135–144, 1996

34. Kuck AW, Ricciardi E: Alterations in elimination, in Itano JK, Taoka KN (eds): *Oncology Nursing Society Core Curriculum for Oncology Nursing* (ed 3). Philadelphia: Saunders, 1998, pp. 259–278

35. American Nurses Association, Oncology Nursing Society: *Statement on the Scope and Standards of Oncology Nursing Practice.* Washington, DC: American Nurses Association, 1996

Constipation

Patient Name: _____

Symptom and Description   Constipation means being unable to move your bowels, having to push harder to move your bowels, or moving them less often than usual. Bowel movements will be small, dry, and hard. Constipation happens when you get less exercise, or when you eat and drink less than usual. Some medicines cause constipation. Constipation can cause pain and discomfort. Keeping your bowel routine regular and your bowel movements easy to pass is important. Your bowels should move every day with little or no strain.

You are at risk for constipation if you have a

- Decrease in the amount you eat and drink each day
- Decrease in your activity or exercise
- Medication that causes constipation
- Cancer that causes pressure on your bowel or changes in the way your bowel works

Learning Needs   You need to know how to prevent constipation and, if constipation happens, to manage it before it gets severe. You are at risk for constipation because of:

1. _____
2. _____
3. _____
4. _____

You should call _____ if you have not moved your bowels in _____.

Write down when you move your bowels and if there are changes in your normal bowel movements. Have the notes with you when you call or come for care. Try to prevent constipation by following the directions given next.

Prevention   You can help prevent constipation if you:
- Drink at least _____ glasses of fluid each day.
- Eat foods that are high in dietary fiber, especially _____ _____
- Exercise daily. If you are unable to increase your exercise, tighten and relax the muscles in your abdomen and move your legs often while sitting or in bed.
- Take medications as instructed to prevent constipation.
- Try to move your bowels at your usual times. Many people find that after breakfast is a good time to try to have a bowel movement.

(continued)

- Avoid using the bedpan if possible. A natural position on the toilet or on a commode is best.
- Tell your doctor or nurse about things that have worked for you in the past to prevent constipation.

Management   You can treat mild constipation by following the steps just listed in prevention. When your bowels have not moved for _____ or if you are at risk for severe constipation, you will need to use medications to help your bowels move regularly.

1. *Using medications to prevent constipation:* Preventing and managing constipation are easy when you work together with your healthcare provider. You may need to increase or decrease doses of medicine to achieve easy and regular bowel movements. Please follow these directions carefully, and feel free to call to ask questions or to let us know if your bowels are not regular.

2. *Goal:* To have a bowel movement every _____ day(s)

   - Take _____ at bedtime.
   - If you do not have a bowel movement in the morning, take _____ after breakfast.
   - If you do not have a bowel movement by evening, take _____ at bedtime.
   - If you do not have a bowel movement by the following morning, take _____ after breakfast.

3. If your bowels have not moved in 48 hours, call your doctor or nurse.
   - Add _____ after breakfast, while continuing to take _____ as above.

4. Once you begin to have regular bowel movements, use the morning and evening doses of medicines you were taking when you had a bowel movement as your regular dose of medicine for your bowels.

5. If you are unsure of what to do, please call.

Follow-up   If you are having trouble with your bowel movements, call your doctor or nurse. Be ready to tell them the following:

1. When you last had a bowel movement
   - Was it normal in size, color, and firmness?
   - Was it difficult to pass?
   - Have you had diarrhea?

2. The amount and kinds of fluid and food you are eating and drinking

3. The names and amounts of medicine you are taking for your bowels

4. Any changes in your health

5. Any new medications or treatments since your last visit

6. What you are doing to manage your bowels on your own

It is important to call your doctor or nurse if your pain medications are increased, so your bowel management plan can be checked.

If you need help in learning about foods that help prevent constipation, call the nutritionist.

Phone Numbers

Nurse: _____ Phone: _____

Physician: _____ Phone: _____

Nutritionist: _____ Phone: _____

Comments

Patient's Signature: _____ Date: _____

Nurse's Signature: _____ Date: _____

Source: Curtiss CP: Constipation, in Yarbro CH, Frogge MH, Goodman M (eds): *Cancer Symptom Management* (ed 2). Sudbury: Jones and Bartlett, 1999. © Jones and Bartlett Publishers.

CHAPTER 28

Diarrhea

Carole Hennessy Martz, RN, MS, OCN®

The Problem of Diarrhea in Cancer

Diarrhea, seen as an alteration in normal elimination, is a complex problem. The word diarrhea is derived from the Greek terms *dia* (through) and *rhein* (to flow). The description of diarrhea is very subjective. The definition of what constitutes diarrhea varies even among experts. In addition, diarrhea may be classified as acute or chronic and may result from any one of several abnormalities in bowel function. Consequently, a thorough patient evaluation is required to determine its cause and to recommend appropriate treatment strategies.

Most clinicians define diarrhea as an abnormal increase in stool liquid and frequency. Stools with a daily weight greater than 200 g, containing 70% to 90% water, and with a frequency greater than two to three per day are generally considered diagnostic.[1-3] Consistency may be a more reliable indicator of diarrhea than frequency, as most clinicians can agree that loose or watery stools are abnormal. Associated symptoms include abdominal pain, cramping, urge to defecate, perineal discomfort, and fecal incontinence.[2,4,5]

Concerns over bowel elimination are frequent in the healthy population. Healthcare personnel often view these concerns as exaggerated and out of proportion to the problems being addressed. However, for persons diagnosed with or receiving treatment for cancer, the onset of diarrhea should prompt immediate attention in order to prevent or minimize potentially life-threatening complications.

Incidence in Cancer

The incidence of diarrhea in the cancer care setting is not precisely known but is certainly less than that of constipation.[4] Variations in acuteness may account in part for the lack of incidence data. Many individuals with minor or short-term diarrhea never seek treatment.[5] It is estimated that nearly 10% of persons with advanced cancer will experience this problem.[1,4]

Impact on Quality of Life

Quality of life can be seriously affected by diarrhea, even in its mild, self-limiting form well known to most of us. Diarrhea can result in significant physical and emotional distress if left untreated; the social and emotional costs can be great. Persons experiencing uncontrolled diarrhea are at high risk for fluid depletion, electrolyte imbalance, skin excoriation, and even death. The emotional distress over fear of incontinence or soiling of clothing and bed linens can cause individuals to avoid leaving the home, and result in lost wages and social isolation. Frequent nocturnal defecation can lead to increased fatigue from interrupted sleep. Some individuals with chronic diarrhea alter their lifestyle and dietary behaviors to help compensate for the unpredictable nature of their bowel movements. Others restrict involvement in sports, fear sexual intimacy, or fear eating in unfamiliar surroundings.[6]

Etiology and Pathophysiology

Persons diagnosed with cancer present to their healthcare provider with varied personal and medical histories. As a result, it is important that any individual reporting the onset of diarrhea be fully evaluated as to the significance of the change in their bowel habits. A careful medical, surgical, dietary, medication, travel, and sexual history can frequently elicit valuable clues to the cause of the diarrhea.[5,7]

The most common causes of acute diarrhea (lasting less than 2 weeks but greater than 48 hours), exclusive of cancer or cancer treatment–related causes, are listed in Table 28-1. Because persons with cancer do not live in a vacuum, these causes may need to be considered. Individuals at increased risk for acute infectious diarrhea include children under the age of 5 in day-care environments, travelers, campers, immunocompromised persons, individuals with HIV disease or AIDS, overseas military personnel, and those persons being cared for in chronic care facilities.[6,8]

For diarrhea lasting over 2 months—chronic diarrhea—a firm diagnosis of etiology may be more difficult

to ascertain and may involve more intensive diagnostic testing.[4] Some of the causes of chronic diarrhea are listed in Table 28-2. Cancer or its treatment is implicated as a direct or indirect cause in several of the conditions described in this table.

The gastrointestinal (GI) tract facilitates the digestion and absorption of nutrients, and the collection and elimination of wastes. The upper (mouth, esophagus, stomach, and small bowel) digestive system's function is the digestion of food. Most electrolytes and water present in the gut are absorbed in the small intestine due to the large surface area afforded by the villi. In addition, iron, calcium, folate, fats, proteins, carbohydrates, and sugars are absorbed in the proximal small bowel. The lower (colon, rectum) digestive system's function is to absorb fluid and electrolytes, synthesize vitamins, and propel wastes from the body.[1,3]

The gut is a system that comprises a complex network of coordinated muscle and nerve activity. The presence of food in the stomach initiates this activity and associated gastric, pancreatic, and biliary secretions. Within a few hours the stomach contents are passed into the small intestine, where most nutrients and fluid are absorbed. Six to 9 hours later, the residue enters the colon for final water and electrolyte removal. The colon muscles contract, usually stimulated by the ingestion of food or by stress and activity. Once the formed stool passes into the rectum the urge to defecate occurs. Associated muscle activities involved in the passage of the stool include contraction of the diaphragm against a closed glottis, tensing of the abdominal muscles, and relaxation of the pelvic floor. Given this multifaceted scenario of events, it is easy to see that disruption of any of these pathways might lead to alterations in bowel elimination even in a healthy individual.[1,4]

A basic understanding of the pathophysiologic causes of diarrhea in the cancer care setting is necessary in order to recommend appropriate treatment. Individuals with

TABLE 28-1 Common Causes of Acute Diarrhea

Infection
Viral, bacterial, protozoan, parasitic, fungal, "food poisoning"
Drug reactions
NSAIDs, antibiotics, antacids, antihypertensives, digitalis, colchicine, lactulose, laxatives, potassium supplements, propranolol, quinidine, alcohol, opiate withdrawal, theophylline, misoprostol, gold, aldomet, metoclopramide
Dietary alterations
Lactose intolerance, formula feedings, dietetic products (sorbitol, mannitol), caffeine, diet colas, high-fiber or high-fat diet
Heavy metal poisoning (acute)
Toxic shock syndrome
Inflammatory bowel disease
Ulcerative colitis, Crohn's disease
Diverticulitis
Gastroenteritis
Pseudomembranous colitis
Intestinal ischemia
Arterial embolus or thrombosis, venous thrombosis, mesenteric ischemia, bowel strangulation
Fecal impaction

Data from references 2, 6.

TABLE 28-2 Common Causes of Chronic Diarrhea

Infections (particularly AIDS)
Inflammatory bowel diseases
Incontinence (diabetes, anorectal surgery, errant episiotomy)
Irritable bowel syndrome
Lactose intolerance
Food allergies
Laxative abuse
Diabetes, hyperthyroidism, hypoadrenalism, pheochromocytoma
Neoplasms (intestinal cancers, neuroendocrine tumors)
Malabsorption syndromes
Idiopathic secretory diarrhea
Surgeries (gastrectomy, vagotomy, cholecystectomy, intestinal resection)
Diverticulitis
Parasitic and fungal infections

Data from references 2–5, 9.

cancer may experience diarrhea as a direct result of cancer treatment or as an indirect result of changes in dietary intake, infectious disorders, hormonal imbalances, digestive and absorptive disorders, inflammatory processes, and pharmacologic manipulation.[4,10] There are four basic mechanisms of diarrhea: (1) osmotic, (2) secretory, (3) hypermotile, and (4) exudative. Management of diarrhea may require a combination of disease-specific and non-specific interventions.[4,5,10]

Osmotic diarrhea results from the presence in the gut lumen of unusual amounts of poorly absorbable, osmotically active solutes (usually carbohydrates). The major clinical hallmark of osmotic diarrhea is that the diarrhea usually stops when the patient fasts or stops ingestion of the poorly absorbable solute.[2,4-6]

Secretory diarrhea results from intestinal ion secretion or inhibition of normal active ion absorption. There are four main causes of this type of diarrhea: congenital defects in ion absorptive processes; intestinal resection; diffuse mucosal disease, in which the epithelial cells are destroyed or reduced in number or function; and abnormal mediators, which result in changes in intracellular contents. Examples include neuro-hormonal-paracrine agents, inflammatory cell products, bacterial enterotoxins, laxatives, fatty acids, and bile acids. Because this type of diarrhea is not related to the ingestion of food, it usually persists during a 48- to 72-hour fast or may continue at a reduced rate.[2,4-6]

Deranged intestinal motility can result in *hypermotile* or *hypomotile* states that can induce diarrhea. Motility problems are suspected when other mechanisms such as osmotic and secretory diarrhea have been excluded. Motility disorders frequently are difficult to prove either clinically or experimentally.[2,4-6]

Sites of bowel inflammation can also cause *exudative* diarrhea. Disruption of the integrity of the intestinal mucosa due to inflammation and ulceration may result in the discharge of mucus, serum proteins, and blood into the bowel lumen, promoting the development of diarrhea.[2,4-6]

Some of the more common causes of diarrhea related to cancer or its treatment can be found in Table 28-3. The list is quite extensive. The most common cause of diarrhea in the cancer population is related to constipation or its management. Overflow diarrhea secondary to narcotic-induced constipation is frequent and should be assessed before therapy in those persons receiving narcotic analgesics.[4,10]

Cancer can cause diarrhea directly through partial bowel obstruction, fistula formation, and hypersecretion. Obstructions usually present with signs of both obstruction and diarrhea. Fistulas may cause diarrhea both from the effects of irritation and hypermotility and from the osmotic influence of undigested food items deposited in the gut. Secretory diarrheas secondary to tumor frequently are difficult to diagnose and require intensive treatment because of the large volume of fluid lost.[2,4,7]

TABLE 28-3 Diarrhea Related to Cancer or Its Treatment

Cancer
Enterocolic fistulas
Partial bowel obstruction
Villous adenoma*
Endocrine-secreting tumors (gastrin, calcitonin, vasoactive intestinal protein, prostaglandins)*

Cancer Related
Fecal impaction
Anxiety
Steatorrhea
Melena
Opiate withdrawal

Cancer Therapy
Chemotherapy
  5-Fluorouracil (especially combined with leucovorin)
  Methotrexate
  Actinomycin D
  Doxorubicin
  Daunorubicin
  Thioguanine
  Hydroxyurea
  Nitrosoureas
  Irinotecan
Hormonal therapy
  Diethylstilbestrol
  Flutamide
Biotherapy
  Interferon
  Interleukin-2
Radiation therapy
  Enteritis
  Malabsorption
Surgery
  Gastrectomy
  Pancreatectomy
  Blind loop syndrome
  Ileal resection
  Palliative bypass
  Anorectal surgeries

* Rare.
Data from references 2–4, 12–16.

Diarrhea can occur indirectly secondary to hemorrhage within the bowel, resulting in an osmotic laxative effect. In addition, incomplete digestion of fat in the small intestine can occur secondary to biliary or pancreatic obstruction or surgical manipulation, leading to hyperosmolality diarrhea.[1-3]

Lactose intolerance can either be an inherited characteristic or result from intestinal damage secondary to repeated infections, chemotherapy, biotherapy, and radiation therapy damage to the bowel mucosa.[9,11] Regardless of the cause, insufficient lactase results in an osmotic diarrhea that is temporally related to the ingestion of dairy products.

The treatment of malignant disease frequently affects the GI tract and can cause diarrhea and contribute to anorexia, malnutrition, and cachexia. The rapidly dividing cells of the GI crypt epithelium are sensitive to the toxicity of a variety of cancer treatments. The irritation that develops can make the bowel mucosa more susceptible to bacterial overgrowth and can cause malabsorption of vitamin B_{12} and bile salts. The toxicity of chemotherapy may result in the need for dose modification and changes in the schedule of drugs and combined modality treatments. Chemotherapy, biotherapy, and hormonal drugs most commonly associated with diarrhea are included in Table 28-3. One of the newer chemotherapeutic drugs, irinotecan, a topoisomerase I inhibitor, causes two distinct forms of diarrhea—early onset cholinergic and late onset—that require different management strategies. Left untreated severe fluid and electrolyte imbalances can occur.[15] When any of these drugs are used in conjunction with radiation, the cytotoxic effects may be increased and toxicities enhanced.[4,12–15,17,18]

Radiation therapy can result in both acute and chronic diarrhea if the intestines are included within the treatment field. Toxicity is usually dependent on the total dose, dose rate, location, and volume of bowel irradiated. Individuals at greater risk for radiation enteritis are those with fixed pelvic small bowel loops from previous surgery or inflammatory disease, previous cholecystectomy, and those individuals with small vessel disease secondary to diabetes mellitus, hypertension, and generalized atherosclerosis. It usually occurs when a dose between 1500 cGy and 3000 cGy is reached. In the acute phase, with doses of 400 to 800 cGy, hypermotility of the bowels may occur as the crypt epithelial cells are damaged, resulting in a loss in absorptive surface area. The incidence of serious injury rises sharply with doses above 5000 cGy as the tissue radiation tolerance is reached. Diarrhea is usually more severe in the presence of lactose malabsorption.[19–23] Some studies have suggested that an increase in prostaglandin E synthesis secondary to radiation injury can result in decreased intestinal transit time.[22]

Late bowel effects from previous radiotherapy can result in chronic ischemic enteritis many months or years after treatments are completed. Chronic radiation enteritis results from vascular damage within the bowel wall. Ischemic changes may lead to fistula formation, ulceration, obstruction, abscess formation, stricture with bacterial overgrowth, perforation, and chronic bleeding.[23] Functional changes include malabsorption, narrowing of the bowel lumen predisposing to obstruction, and changes that may result in fibrosis and ischemia of the intestine. Again, these side effects seem to be more common in individuals with the risk factors previously mentioned, and they occur in 5% to 15% of all patients treated with lower abdominal/pelvic irradiation. However, late bowel effects do not appear to have any direct relationship to the extent of acute toxicity the patient experienced during treatment.[24] Surgical resection of the damaged bowel is sometimes necessary.

Patients receiving allogeneic bone marrow transplants (BMTs) following high-dose chemotherapy and total body irradiation usually develop diarrhea within the first week posttransplant. This diarrhea usually resolves within 15 days after the treatment was given. In mismatched BMT recipients, acute graft-versus-host disease (GVHD) may occur, resulting in diarrhea that is green, watery, and voluminous, within 7 days posttransplant. This condition is thought to be a response in which the grafted donor T lymphocytes recognize disparate non-HLA (human leukocyte antigen) host cell antigens and initiate cytotoxic injury directed at host tissue. The volume of diarrhea can range from less than 500 mL to over 1500 mL in severe cases. Stools are initially negative for blood. If the GVHD progresses it can lead to mucosal sloughing and cause stools to become heme positive.[25]

Cancer surgeries may also result in the development of diarrhea. Diarrhea may occur temporarily in the immediate postoperative period or in a chronic form. Following gastrectomy, individuals may experience both osmotic and hypermotility diarrhea associated with dumping syndrome.[1–4] Regional total pancreatectomy, involving both lymphatic interruption and surgical intestinal sympathectomy denervation, may cause diarrhea by loss of the tonic inhibitory effects of the sympathetic nerves. Postprocedure-induced fat malabsorption may also occur, leading to osmotic steatorrhea.[3,26]

Intestinal blind loop syndrome following bowel resections can result in bacterial overgrowth and malabsorptive diarrhea. The level of malabsorption depends on what portion of the bowel is resected as well as the length of the resection. Ileal resection causes diarrhea through disruption of the enterohepatic circulation of bile salts, which then feed directly into the colon, resulting in a direct bowel-stimulant effect. Bowel-shortening surgeries can also result in decreased fluid reabsorption by reducing intestinal mucosal contact and transit time, and they may decrease the absorption of electrolytes and/or bile salts. This effect, called the *short bowel syndrome*, generally occurs when more than 200 cm of bowel is resected.[1,4,27,28]

Many symptom control methods used in cancer therapy can result in diarrhea. Laxative therapy for persons receiving narcotics is a frequent cause. In addition, certain magnesium-containing antacids and nonsteroidal anti-inflammatory drugs (NSAIDs) commonly used for symptom control may cause diarrhea as a side effect.[1,4,10]

A multitude of antibiotics have been implicated in the development of diarrhea. Diarrhea as a result of antibiotic therapy occurs through direct stimulation of the bowel and subsequent alteration in normal bowel flora. Large bowel irritation from bacterial infection leads to the secretion of large amounts of water, electrolytes, and mucus as a protective mechanism, causing dilution of the irritating factors and rapid movement of feces to the anus. The typical course of antibiotic-induced diarrhea is benign and self-limiting. However, in both immunocompromised and healthy persons, some antibiotics may cause the development of pseudomembranous enterocolitis. This type of enterocolitis is almost always caused by an overgrowth of toxic strains of *Clostridium difficile*. Left untreated, *C. difficile* infection can lead to severe diarrhea, hypovolemia, dilation of the colon from toxic megacolon, perforation, hemorrhage, and even death. Persons at risk include those who have received antibiotics within the past 6 weeks and those who have recently received chemotherapeutic drugs.[29,30] Antibiotics and chemotherapeutic agents most frequently associated with the development of *C. difficile* infections are listed in Table 28-4. Most of the antibiotics listed are broad-spectrum antibiotics that have activity against anaerobic organisms.[29,30]

In addition to the preceding etiologies, diarrhea in individuals receiving total or supplemental enteral feedings must be mentioned. The type of diarrhea seen in these individuals is usually osmotic in nature but may be caused by bacterial contamination of the formula, or by lactose intolerance when formulas containing milk products are used. Accelerated delivery rates and concurrent hypoalbuminemia have also been implicated as promoting the development of diarrhea, but these ideas have been disputed.[31,32] Clearly these feedings play an important role in maintaining the patient's weight when a progressive inability to maintain oral intake occurs or when the patient's physical state prevents oral intake for a prolonged period of time. Concurrent use of antibiotics and elixir-type medications may also affect the development of diarrhea in association with tube feedings.[31,32]

TABLE 28-4 Drugs Associated with Development of *Clostridium difficile* Infections

Antibiotics
Ampicillin or amoxicillin
Cephalosporins
Clindamycin
Penicillins
Antineoplastics
Antimetabolites (e.g., methotrexate, 5-FU)
Alkylating agents (e.g., cyclophosphamide)
Antibiotics (e.g., doxorubicin)

Data from references 29, 30.

Assessment

Patients receiving treatment for cancer should undergo periodic physical exams that include vital sign and weight measurements combined with thorough medical, medication, travel, sexual, surgical, and dietary histories. A determination of normal bowel routines should always be considered during the patient's initial evaluation. Changes in bowel movements, occurrence of diarrhea, and any precipitating events should be determined. Determination of the physical location of diarrhea can be facilitated by eliciting certain clues as reviewed in Table 28-5. Specific questioning concerning the presence or absence of fecal incontinence is important, as few persons volunteer such information.

Individuals receiving cancer treatment and considered at risk for developing diarrhea should be advised at each visit of the importance of reporting the onset of any new symptom, particularly diarrhea. Patients at high risk for the development of diarrhea should be instructed about what measures should be taken to prevent or ameliorate the severity of this symptom.

For those persons already experiencing diarrhea, the severity can be rated in a number of ways. Many research studies grade the symptom according to severity or resultant lifestyle alterations. Examples of two grading mechanisms are provided in Table 28-6.[33] Most protocols rate diarrhea on a scale of 1 to 4, with 4 denoting increased toxicity. Note the variability in rating severity. In order for all team members to report the same information, a consensus should be reached on which grading scale is to be used.

The pattern and characteristics of diarrhea are important to determine to assist in identification of cause. Whether the patient is intolerant of foods containing dairy products, is undergoing a stressful period, or is taking narcotic analgesics are important pieces of information to collect. Subtly seek out signs of anxiety and high levels of stress that could be related to the development of new diarrhea. However, the nurse should not assume

TABLE 28-5 Clues to the Source Location of Diarrhea

Clues	Small Bowel/Proximal Colon	Left Colon or Rectum
Volume	Large	Small, with frequent urge to defecate and passage of small quantities of feces or passage of flatus and mucus
Stools	Watery, soupy, greasy, and/or foul smelling; without blood; containing undigested food	Mushy or jellylike and may be mixed with visible pus or blood; dark colored; rarely foul smelling
Pain location	Periumbilical or localized to the right lower quadrant	Hypogastrium, right or left lower quadrant, or sacral region
Characteristic	Intermittent, cramping, and accompanied by audible borborygmi	Gripping or aching, often accompanied by tenesmus; sometimes continuous but usually relieved by having a bowel movement, taking an enema, or passage of flatus

Data from reference 2.

TABLE 28-6 Diarrhea Toxicity Criteria

Grade	NCI	NSABP
Grade 1	Transient, <2 days	2–3 stools/24h
Grade 2	Tolerable, but >2 days	4–8 stools/24h
Grade 3	Intolerable, requires treatment	7–8 stools/24h, severe
Grade 4	Intractable	10+ stools/24h, bloody, support required

NCI = National Cancer Institute; NSABP = National Surgical Adjuvant Bowel and Breast Project.

Data from reference 33.

that stress is the only cause. Most persons who develop diarrhea secondary to stress have probably done so all their lives and will relate this to you. The healthcare provider should also not forget to assess for more obvious causes of diarrhea such as recent antibiotic, antacid, or laxative use and recent cancer treatment.

A clear description of the stools being passed is essential, as some persons report having diarrhea when in fact it is their stool frequency, not stool liquidity, that has increased. The passage of bloody stool suggests inflammation, infection, or neoplasm. The passage of pus or exudate in the stool also may indicate inflammation or infection. Mushy stools that are frothy or contain oil are suggestive of malabsorption. Classic carbohydrate malabsorption is characterized by the onset of cramping within 30 minutes of ingestion followed by diarrhea 1 to 2 hours later. Intermittent constipation and diarrhea can signal irritable bowel syndrome, especially if the stools look like pellets in the constipation phase. If bowel changes are intermittent, the nurse should suspect the possibility of diabetic autonomic neuropathy or colon cancer. In addition, the nurse must remember to ask whether the person has a problem with fecal incontinence, as this may be an indication of anal sphincter dysfunction—especially when associated with nocturnal soiling—secondary to disease or treatment. A history of fistula or abscess is suggestive of Crohn's disease. Reports of diarrhea in persons with a desire to lose weight are suggestive of laxative or diuretic abuse.[4]

The severity of diarrhea can also be assessed clinically by observing for signs of dehydration, such as dry mucous membranes, poor skin turgor, sunken eyes, tachycardia, orthostatic blood pressure changes, and fluctuations in mental status. Weight losses of 1% to 2% in a week are considered significant.[10] Adequacy of fluid intake can be determined by asking the individual about the size of glasses used to consume liquids and how many were drunk the previous day. The person with diarrhea should also be asked to describe the color, quantity, and frequency of their urine output to assist in determining the level of fluid depletion. The presence or absence of fever should also be assessed to determine whether infectious diarrhea should be considered as a potential etiology.

Bowel sounds should be auscultated and perianal skin assessed. A physical exam should include assessment for abdominal masses, abdominal bruits, lymphedema, goiter, gaseous abdominal ascites, hepatosplenomegaly, and perianal fistulas.[4,16]

Diagnostic Evaluation

The intensity of the workup for the cause of diarrhea will vary according to the physical status of the individual. Associated symptoms also should be evaluated as previously described. For patients whose diarrhea is not controlled by conservative measures (addressed in the next section) after a trial of 2 to 3 days, random stool analyses, including smears for pus, blood, fat, enteric pathogens, ova and parasites, *C. difficile* toxin, and culture and sensitivity, may be performed as directed by the physician or per standing protocol. These specimens must be kept refrigerated until the time of inspection by the laboratory.[2,8] Some gastroenterologists recommend first analyzing for the presence of fecal leukocytes. Depending on the clinical status of the individual, blood work including CBC, serum electrolytes, and blood chemistries may need to be evaluated.[2,4]

If an inflammatory process is suspected, upper and lower GI endoscopies, biopsies, and/or barium radiography may be indicated. In rare instances, for patients with large-volume diarrhea, a 24-hour urine collection for 5-hydroxyindoleacetic acid or serum analyses for vasoactive intestinal protein (VIP), gastrin, and calcitonin may be ordered. Some tumors that have been shown to secrete these peptides include medullary carcinoma of the thyroid, carcinoid tumors, and some bronchogenic tumors.[2,34,35]

Extended GI investigations for chronic diarrhea of unknown origin include breath tests to evaluate lactose, bile acid and carbohydrate absorption, small intestine biopsy, intestinal angiograms, and vitamin B_{12} analysis. Some causes of diarrhea outside the cancer care setting may never be totally explained and only symptomatic management can be recommended.[2,5,21]

Symptom Management

Prevention

Prevention of diarrhea associated with cancer or its treatment is variable. Prompt management of diarrhea is often of greater importance to minimize toxicity and associated side effects.

Modern radiation therapy incorporates careful treatment planning to avoid harmful doses of radiation to areas of normal bowel, through the use of computer-generated dose calculations. In addition, methods to displace the small bowel out of the treatment field, such as treating the patient with a full bladder and treating the patient prone, may reduce the incidence of diarrhea. When radiation therapy is to follow surgery, mesh inserted during surgery to prop the small bowel out of the treatment field is sometimes used.[11]

Minimization of diarrheal severity when secondary to acute radiation irritation is possible through the implementation of a low-residue diet at treatment initiation. In addition, avoidance of GI irritants can prevent or delay the amount or severity of subsequent diarrhea. Suggested low-residue dietary modifications are reviewed in Table 28-7. In general, foods individuals are advised to limit include those high in roughage, fried or highly seasoned foods, uncooked fruits and vegetables, rich desserts, and any that have caused GI irritation or gas in the past.

In addition, persons are advised to refrain from using medications that may cause diarrhea as a side effect (as reviewed earlier in Table 28-2) whenever this is medically feasible.[36,37]

One study suggests that oral sucralfate administered during radiation therapy over the intestines may result in less frequent diarrhea by preventing radiation-induced bowel damage or by protecting the damaged mucosa from exposure to stool bile acid irritants. The authors contend that use of this medication reduced the incidence of both early and late (>12 months) bowel reactions. Widespread use of this regimen is not common.[38]

Other preventive measures currently being investigated include the use of medications such as aspirin to suppress prostaglandins and the neutralization of pancre-

TABLE 28-7   Low-Residue Dietary Guidelines by Food Group

Foods Allowed	Foods to Avoid
Breads and cereals:	
Breads: enriched white, Vienna, French, light rye without seeds, melba toast, zwieback, corn	Breads: whole grains such as whole wheat, sprouted wheat, bran, breads with seeds or nuts such as poppy, sesame, rye, nut breads
Muffins: plain muffins, corn muffins, plain pancakes, and waffles	Muffins: made with nuts or seeds, fruit skins, or whole grains such as whole wheat or bran
Cereals: refined cereals such as oatmeal, buckwheat, cream of wheat or rice, corn flakes, Rice Krispies, Rice Chex, Cheerios, etc.	Cereals: bran cereals, whole grain, fiber, cereals with nuts
Pasta/rice: white rice, brown rice, enriched noodles, macaroni, spaghetti, most pastas	Pasta/rice: wild rice, whole-wheat noodles
Fresh fruit/frozen fruit	
Banana	All except banana
Canned fruit	
Applesauce, apricots, cherries, peaches, pears, pineapple, mandarin oranges, orange/grapefruit sections, jellies	Berries, grapes, berry pie filling, jams and preserves
Dried fruits	
None	AVOID ALL
Fruit/vegetable juices	
Fruit juices without pulp (except prune), vegetable juices without pulp, citrus juices in moderation	Prune juice, large quantities of citrus juices
Fresh vegetables/frozen vegetables	
NO UNCOOKED VEGETABLES; well-cooked green beans, beets, squash, pumpkin, white/red potatoes without skin, sweet potatoes without skin, carrots, spinach, asparagus, strained tomatoes, celery, mushrooms	ALL FRESH RAW VEGETABLES, cooked onions, cabbage, brussels sprouts, broccoli, green peppers, corn, cauliflower, dried beans/peas/lentils, turnips, rutabagas, vegetables cooked in cream sauce, potato skins, french fries, eggplant
Canned vegetables	
Green beans, peas, beets, squash, pumpkin, tomato sauce, tomato paste, tomato purée, potatoes, sweet potatoes, spinach, carrots, asparagus, strained tomatoes, mushrooms	Onions, cabbage, corn, brussels sprouts, dried beans/peas/lentils, olives, pickles
Fats	
Margarine, sour cream, butter, gravy, mayonnaise, dressing, and bacon, sparingly	Large amounts of added mayonnaise, margarine, gravies, and dressings
Beverages	
Water, weak or decaffeinated tea, ginger ale, 7-up or clear soft drinks, decaffeinated colas, Gatorade, sport drinks	Regular coffee and tea, decaffeinated sodas, alcohol (beer, wine, liquor, mixed drinks)

TABLE 28-7 *(continued)*

Foods Allowed	Foods to Avoid
Miscellaneous	
All herbs and spices, such as parsley, oregano, salt, catsup, soy sauce, and vinegar	Hot pepper, black or white pepper used in large quantities, popcorn, potato chips
Meat/Other Protein	
Stewed, boiled, baked, barbecued, well-trimmed, low-fat meats	Fried meats, fatty meats, cured meats, cold cuts, poultry skin
Nonfried eggs	Fried eggs
Low-fat cottage cheese, cream cheese, processed skim-milk cheese, part-skim mozzarella and ricotta, farmer cheese, string cheese, parmesan, and any other cheese with 5 g of fat or less per serving (read the label)	High-fat cheeses (natural cheese)
	Lima beans, peas, all dried legumes
Soups	
Broth-based soups with allowed foods, cream-based soups made with low-fat milk with allowed foods (e.g., chicken noodle, cream of asparagus soup made with low-fat milk)	Broth-based soups made with foods to avoid, cream-based soups made with whole milk or made with foods to avoid (e.g., French onion, cream of broccoli)
Desserts	
Popsicles, sherbet, water ice, jello, angel food cake, vanilla wafers, ginger snaps, plain cake, hard candy, jelly beans, pudding made with low-fat milk, arrowroot cookies, frozen yogurt, ice milk, low-fat frozen desserts, honey, jelly, syrup	Rich desserts, pies, frosting made with fat and whole milk, coconut, candied fruits
Milk	
2 cups or the equivalent per day of skim milk, low-fat milk, powdered milk, buttermilk, evaporated milk, skim-milk or low-fat yogurt, low-fat chocolate milk, ice milk, frozen yogurt, low-fat frozen desserts	All other milk beverages or products

Data from references 36, 37.

atic secretions. Use of radioprotectant drugs and elemental diets during radiation therapy is also under investigation.[39]

The institution of a low-lactose diet in individuals with temporary lactose intolerance may prevent, reduce, or control diarrhea in some patients receiving cancer therapy. Examples of permitted and restricted foods in such a diet are listed in Table 28-8. The use of lactase enzyme or drops may also be of assistance. Because complete avoidance of lactose is nearly impossible, individuals should be encouraged to read food ingredient labels closely. Fermented milk products may be easier to digest than whole milk products and their use should be encouraged. Examples of such products include buttermilk, sour cream, and yogurt.[9,36,37]

Diarrhea associated with fecal impaction secondary to narcotic analgesic use can be prevented by the implementation of a bowel management program at the start of narcotic analgesics intake. Laxatives/stool softeners for management of constipation must be titrated carefully. Nonspecific measures such as increased activity, fluid intake, and dietary fiber are usually not successful in preventing constipation in these individuals. To avoid diarrhea, the nurse must remember to advise reduction

in these laxatives concurrently with the gradual withdrawal of narcotics once pain relief is achieved.[4,16]

Diarrhea associated with the administration of chemotherapeutic drugs usually cannot be prevented, but prompt intervention can reduce the severity and adverse consequences. An exception is the early onset (cholinergic) diarrhea seen with the administration of irinotecan. It can sometimes be prevented with the administration of intravenous or subcutaneous atropine during infusion.[15]

Diarrhea associated with acute GVHD following allogeneic BMT can sometimes be prevented with immunosuppressive prophylaxis. Some institutions deplete donor marrow T cells before marrow is infused through agglutination immunoabsorption columns and treatment with anti-T-cell monoclonal antibodies. Most patients also receive immunosuppressive drugs the day prior to and several months after BMT using methotrexate, cyclosporin A, corticosteroids, antithymocyte globulin (ATG), or a combination of these drugs. Even with prophylaxis, GVHD will still occur in 30% to 50% of HLA-identical recipients.[25]

The incidence of diarrhea associated with *C. difficile* infections can be reduced by the judicious use of antibiotics in the cancer-care setting. Some researchers propose

TABLE 28-8 Low-Lactose Dietary Guidelines by Food Group

Foods Allowed	Foods to Avoid
Beverages	
Water, lactose-free carbonated beverages, fruit-flavored drinks, fruit punches, lemonade, limeade, non-dairy-product drinks, decaffeinated coffee or tea	Artificial fruit drinks containing lactose; all beverages made with milk and milk products with the exception of buttermilk or yogurt
Bread	
All	None
Cereals	
Any cooked or dry cereal not containing lactose	Instant hot cereals, high-protein cereals, all cereals with added milk or lactose
Flours	
All	None
Cheeses	
Fermented cheeses (cheddar and any cheese aged with bacteria)	All others
Desserts	
Fruit ices, gelatins, angel food cake, desserts made with non-dairy products, buttermilk, or sour cream	Ice cream, puddings, and other desserts containing milk or milk products
Eggs	
All except eggs prepared with milk or milk products	Creamed, scrambled, omelets, or other eggs prepared with milk
Fats	
Margarine not containing milk solids; vegetable oils, mayonnaise, shortening	All others, including cream, half-and-half, table and whipping cream, butter
Fruits and Fruit Ices	
All fresh, canned, or frozen fruit juices; fruits not processed with lactose	Any canned or frozen fruits and fruit juices processed with lactose
Meat, Poultry, Fish, Legumes, Nuts	
Any except those specifically excluded	Creamed or breaded fish, poultry, meat; cold cuts, hot dogs, liver, sausage, or other processed meats containing milk or lactose; gravies made with milk
Milk and Milk Products	
Fermented milk products, such as acidophilus milk, buttermilk, yogurt, and sour cream	All milk and milk products except fermented milk products
Potatoes, Rice, Pasta	
White or sweet potatoes, macaroni, noodles, spaghetti, or other pasta, rice	Any prepared with milk, such as creamed or scalloped, and commercial potato products containing dried milk
Soups	
Broth-based soups	Cream soups, chowders, commercially prepared soups that contain milk or milk products
Sweets	
Honey, jams, preserves, syrups, molasses	Candy containing lactose, milk, or cocoa; butterscotch candies, caramels, chocolates
Vegetables	
All vegetables except those prepared with milk	Any prepared with milk, such as creamed or scalloped, or any processed vegetables containing lactose
Miscellaneous	
Catsup, chili sauce, horseradish, olives, pickles, vinegar, gravies prepared without milk, mustard, all herbs and spices, peanut butter, unbuttered popcorn	Chocolate, cocoa, milk gravies, cream sauces, chewing gum, instant coffee, powdered soft drinks, artificial juices containing milk or lactose

ATTENTION: READ ALL FOOD LABELS CAREFULLY.

Data from references 36, 37.

the use of biotherapeutic agents such as microorganisms that have antagonistic activity toward pathogens in vivo to prevent antibiotic-associated diarrhea. Use of such products as *Saccharomyces boulardii* and *Lactobacillus acidophilus* in the management in immunocompromised persons has not been fully evaluated.[40] Because of the high risk for nosocomially acquired infections in the cancer patient population, healthcare workers should be vigilant about good hand-washing techniques. Nurses should keep a high index of suspicion for *C. difficile* infections in any patient presenting with profuse or bloody diarrhea associated with fever.[41–43]

Some studies have shown that the use of elemental diets and total parenteral nutrition (TPN) during radiation and chemotherapy may actually prevent bowel damage and subsequent alterations in bowel elimination, although this is controversial. The proposed mechanism of action appears to be related to a decrease in GI secretions, resulting in the protection of intestinal villi from erosion. Because of the high rate of complications associated with TPN, particularly increased infections when administered concurrently with chemotherapy, and the unpalatable taste of presently marketed elemental diets, use of these modalities to prevent diarrhea secondary to cancer treatment has not been widespread.[44–46]

Prevention of tube feeding–associated diarrhea includes the use of psyllium or pectin added to the formula, use of lactose-free and fiber-containing products, prevention of bacterial contamination of formulas during patient preparation, administration of feedings continuously, and diluting medications with water. Use of standard formulas does not generally cause diarrhea in normal individuals. Hence, other factors may be at work when diarrhea occurs in a patient using supplemental formulas (e.g., concurrent antibiotic and antacid use, the use of sorbitol-containing elixir medications).[6,32,47,48]

Therapeutic Approaches

The goals of therapy to control diarrhea are to maintain fluid and electrolyte balance, to maintain nutritional homeostasis, to prevent medical complications, and to maximize the quality of life of the individual. A variety of measures may need to be used to successfully accomplish these goals.

Because overflow diarrhea is common in patients treated with narcotics, the first intervention in these individuals should be a gentle rectal exam. If an impaction is felt, it is advisable to consider administering an anxiolytic or pain medication before disimpaction in order to minimize discomfort. In addition, it is helpful to first administer an oil retention enema or glycerin suppository to lubricate and soften the stool. The nurse should determine whether the patient's platelet and leukocyte counts are adequate before performing this procedure. Following disimpaction, the individual should be started on a bowel care regimen to prevent recurrence.[4,10,16]

Patients who develop diarrhea when pain medications are being withdrawn or being tapered may be experiencing a symptom of opiate withdrawal. This diarrhea can be managed by resuming the narcotic therapy at one-fourth of the previous daily dose and then gradually tapering off the medication over the following 2 to 3 days.[4,16]

Patients who experience persistent diarrhea while being treated with radiation and/or chemotherapy may benefit from a trial lactose-free or low-lactose diet. Temporary lactose intolerance is not uncommon in these individuals, and resumption of a normal diet once treatment-related side effects have ceased is sometimes possible. Dietary consultation can be of great benefit in maintaining adequate calcium intake because foods high in lactose are usually major sources of calcium. Sometimes reducing intestinal exposure to lactose by dividing the total dose of lactose-containing foods into small portions during the day may increase lactose tolerance. Lactase enzyme drops added to milk can significantly reduce the presence of lactose in these products. The use of lactase enzyme tablets with meals can also increase the tolerance of lactose-containing nonliquid foods. Close reading of food labels is essential to identify foods containing hidden sources of lactose such as whey, curd, and caseinate. Consultation with a pharmacist can also help determine which medications might contain lactose.[16,36,48]

Management of diarrhea secondary to bowel resection varies by the location and extent of resection. Most individuals are supported by total parenteral nutrition when extensive small bowel resections and colon resections are performed. TPN may need to be continued indefinitely. Those individuals who ultimately manage to absorb adequate amounts of nutrients may still experience large fluid losses and require supplemental oral rehydration formulas or TPN. Nutritional deficiencies may require replacement therapy such as vitamin B_{12} injections, vitamin K injections, multivitamins, and calcium supplements. Remarkably, adaptation of the bowel may occur after weeks, months, or years, and allow resumption of normal dietary intake.[9]

Diarrhea, regardless of its cause, can result in significant fluid loss if replacement liquids are not provided. Hundreds of trials worldwide have demonstrated the effectiveness of glucose-electrolyte solutions in the treatment of all types of diarrhea that result in mild to severe dehydration. These solutions, though rarely used in the adult cancer treatment experience, can potentially prevent the need for costly intravenous fluid infusions and hospitalizations. However, concurrent anorexia and nausea may render the patient with cancer unable to consume adequate quantities of rehydration fluids.[6,8,49]

Diarrheal fluid is high in sodium, potassium, and bicarbonate. The use of oral rehydration formulas is based on the principle that carbohydrate absorption (especially glucose) in the small bowel facilitates sodium and water reabsorption from the intestinal lumen into the intravascular compartment.[50] Examples of commercial rehydration formulas include Ricelyte (Mead Johnson

Nutritionals, Evansville, IN), and Pedialyte (Ross Laboratories, Columbus, OH). Sport drinks that claim to replenish fluid and electrolyte loss during exercise may be used for fluid repletion but will have little effect on increased stool consistency and may actually increase diarrhea in some individuals due to the drink's high osmolality.[51] The only true contraindications to rehydration therapy are the presence of intractable vomiting, ileus, and severe fluid deficit with toxicity.[8,49]

Similarly, early and appropriate feeding with a diet high in staple grains (especially rice) and other lactose-free foods can significantly reduce stool volume and the duration of diarrhea.[6,37,49] A listing of foods suitable to recommend for dietary management of diarrhea can be found in Table 28-9. Some people with cancer become increasingly sensitive to previously well-tolerated stimulants such as prune juice and coffee.[4]

A number of antidiarrheal medications have shown efficacy in controlling cancer-related diarrhea not managed by dietary manipulation alone. Even in those situations in which dietary changes have not totally prevented diarrhea, continuation of these modifications may aid in its eventual management. Medications found to significantly affect the frequency of diarrhea in cancer-care situations are mostly opiate derivatives. Commonly used absorbents (e.g., pectin, aluminum hydrophilic building agents) and adsorbents (e.g., kaolin, charcoal) usually have low palatability and limited efficacy in most cancer-induced diarrhea.[4,16]

The most commonly used medications, loperamide HCl (Imodium-AD, McNeil Consumer Products Co., Fort Washington, PA), atropine sulfate and diphenoxylate HCl (Lomotil, G. D. Searle & Co., Chicago, IL), and codeine phosphate, work by binding to the smooth muscle of the bowel, thereby slowing down intestinal motility and increasing fluid absorption. Octreotide acetate (Sandostatin, Sandoz, Basle, Switzerland), used as second-line therapy, is thought to inhibit the secretion of certain gut hormones and regulate intestinal water and electrolyte transport in large-volume diarrhea. A comparison of these medications is found in Table 28-10.

TABLE 28-9 Dietary Guidelines for Controlling Diarrhea

Decrease roughage in diet.
Eat foods high in pectin (bananas, grated apples, applesauce).
Eat boiled white rice, cream of rice cereal, and tapioca.
Avoid fried or highly seasoned foods.
Avoid rich desserts.
Eat foods at room temperature.
Eat smaller, more frequent meals.
Increase fluid intake to 6 to 8 glasses of liquid daily (water, broth, cranberry juice, apple juice, pear juice, Gatorade, ginger ale, nectars).
Refrain from alcohol and caffeinated drinks.
If diarrhea is worse after drinking milk, speak to dietitian.

Data from references 36, 37, 48.

Over-the-counter Imodium-AD has been shown to decrease small intestine transit time, is metabolized on first pass by the liver, does not easily cross the blood-brain barrier, and increases bile absorption. Unlike codeine and Lomotil, it has no central opioid activity when administered at normal therapeutic doses. Most persons with acute or chronic diarrhea can be controlled with 2 to 4 mg of Imodium-AD (1–2 capsules) once or twice daily. Its use is not recommended in children under the age of 12. Despite Imodium's higher cost compared with codeine phosphate, its easy accessibility and sometimes superior control of symptoms with fewer side effects makes it the logical first-line choice in the treatment of noninfectious diarrhea.[52,53] And indeed, Imodium-AD is the drug of choice in late onset (after 24 hours) diarrhea associated with the administration of irinotecan. It is prescribed in higher than standard doses—4 mg PO at onset of diarrhea, followed by 2 mg PO every 4 hours until diarrhea-free for 12 hours. Nighttime dosing is 4 mg PO every 4 hours.[54,55]

Both Lomotil and codeine are associated with more central nervous system side effects, such as dizziness, nausea/vomiting, and blurred vision. In larger doses. Lomotil (40–60 mg) can produce euphoria, respiratory depression, and coma. Lomotil is also not recommended for use in children under the age of 12 and those patients with advanced liver disease. However, Lomotil may be superior in managing diarrhea secondary to intermittent bowel obstruction.[16,52,53]

Codeine is very constipating and yet can give prompt relief for diarrhea, as well as for cough and pain in those individuals experiencing such complex problems. In patients with painful cramping associated with diarrhea, the use of anticholinergics such as atropine sulfate, scopolamine, or belladonna may be indicated. Side effects include dry mouth, blurred vision, and urinary hesitance. In refractory diarrhea, tincture of opium may be used or added to the regimen. Occasionally a combination of antidiarrheals is needed, and it may be associated with increased sedation.[4,16]

Sandostatin is the drug of choice for patients with high-volume diarrhea or those with known endocrine or secretory disorders that do not respond to the more commonly prescribed antidiarrheal medications described above. Such conditions include high-dose chemotherapy GVHD, endocrine tumors, carcinoid tumors, AIDS, and high-output ileostomy and jejunal and ileal resections. In some cases pancreatic enzymes should be coadministered. Side effects include pain at the injection site, nausea, and headaches. Pain at the injection site may be reduced by handwarming before injection or by using a smaller volume of more concentrated octreotide solution. Long-term use is associated with an increased prevalence of gallbladder sludge and gallstones. (Baseline and periodic gallbladder ultrasounds may be useful.) Dose reductions are suggested once adequate symptom control is achieved for 2 to 3 weeks to a maintenance level.[4,27,54]

None of the drugs just mentioned are recommended

TABLE 28-10 Common Antidiarrheal Medications Used in the Cancer Setting

Drug	Dosage	Side Effects	Contraindications
Imodium-AD (loperamide HCl)	Two 2-mg capsules PO initially up to a maximum of 8 per day Higher doses for irinotecan-induced diarrhea*	Constipation, abdominal cramps, gastric upset, dry mouth, skin rash, headache	Age <12 Infectious diarrhea
Lomotil (atropine sulfate/diphenoxylate HCl)	One to two tablets PO 3–4 times a day, up to a maximum of 8 tablets per day	Sedation, dizziness, dry mouth, drowsiness, rash, urine retention, blurred vision, depression	Age <12 Infectious diarrhea Advanced liver disease
Codeine phosphate	30–60 mg PO q4–6h prn	Constipation, nausea, sedation, clouded sensorium, low BP, dry mouth, urine retention, respiratory depression	Avoid use with other sedatives, hypnotics, narcotics, or MAO inhibitors or alcohol Use with caution in persons with head injury, hepatic or renal disease, chronic obstructive pulmonary disease, bronchial asthma, infectious diarrhea
Sandostatin (octreotide acetate)	50–500 μg SQ or 50–300 IV, 1–3 times daily Maximum titrated dosage up to 3600 μg/day	Nausea, pain at injection site, abdominal cramps, cholelithiasis, glucose imbalance, change in thyroid function	Infectious diarrhea Hyperinsulinemia

* See text for exception in use for irinotecan-induced diarrhea.
Data from references 4, 6, 16, 17, 20, 27, 52, 54–56.

for use in individuals with fevers and bloody or profuse diarrhea suggestive of an infectious or inflammatory process. Antidiarrheal agents may slow the elimination of the causative pathogen from the GI system and make symptoms persist longer. However, the withholding of antidiarrheals is controversial.[56] Individuals with fever and diarrhea should have stool cultures evaluated and empiric antibiotics should be started, particularly if *C. difficile* infection is suspected. All other antibiotics should be discontinued if possible. Antibiotics effective against this enterotoxin include oral and intravenous metronidazole and vancomycin. Oral metronidazole is the treatment of choice because of its low cost and ease of administration. Patients should be placed on enteric precautions and all stool-contaminated surfaces should be cleansed with sporicidal germicides. Recurrence or relapse is not uncommon. Under these circumstances, stools should be recultured before reinitiation of treatment.[30,43]

Patient and family education is essential to the management of cancer-related diarrhea. There will be some instances in which diarrhea will not be well managed by the measures just discussed. For individuals receiving outpatient follow-up, prompt reporting of situations requiring immediate attention must be emphasized with each visit. These patients will need to know to report a temperature of 100.5°F (38°C) or greater, the onset of inability to drink or hold down liquids, dizziness, decreased urine output, and other signs of dehydration. Providing healthcare contact numbers for during and after hours is essential. Occasionally intravenous infusions

will be required to prevent or manage serious fluid depletion. The outpatient should be advised to continue the use of antidiarrheal medications, to maintain oral rehydration, and to eat foods that help firm stools if this is appropriate. Depending on the patient's clinical status, additional studies may be required. Several Self-Care Guides are provided in the Appendixes that could be given to patients experiencing diarrhea secondary to cancer treatment.

Patients experiencing fecal incontinence can be instructed on how to improve anal sphincter tone with success in many instances. They should be instructed to tighten their buttocks muscles as if holding back a bowel movement, hold for 5 to 10 seconds, and relax for 10 seconds between repetitions. These exercises should be repeated ten times, four times daily.[16]

The condition of the perianal and perineal skin should not be overlooked in the person experiencing diarrhea. Liquid stools can be very caustic and result in excoriation of the skin. Cleansing of the skin and anus after each bowel movement is recommended, using a mild soap and water, or baby wipes. The skin should be patted dry and if possible allowed to air periodically if skin breakdown is present. Sitz baths utilizing tepid water several times a day may help to reduce discomfort, particularly if hemorrhoids are a problem. The use of a skin barrier product such as petroleum jelly or other moisture barrier product is often beneficial. Rectal pouches may be necessary to promote skin integrity in cases of severe diarrhea or persistent fecal incontinence. If the patient is currently receiving radiation, he or she should be gently reminded to take care not to wash off the treatment field markings and to check with the radiation staff before application of any skin care products.[10,16,48]

Evaluation of Therapeutic Approaches

The most accurate means of evaluating the effectiveness of antidiarrheal therapies is to look for a reduction in the number and liquidity of stools daily, as well as a reduction in or stabilization of antidiarrheal medications used. For those individuals in whom soiling has been a problem, progression of episodes of fecal incontinence should also be noted. A tool such as the one in Appendix 28A can be used to monitor the effectiveness of self-care measures.

Heather et al.[31] devised a tool to evaluate the effectiveness of adding psyllium to tube feedings in an effort to control diarrhea. They measured stool consistency by recording for 24 hours the numbers denoting each stool's consistency. The stools were rated in the following manner: 1 = clear, watery; 2 = creamy liquid; 3 = loose, mushy, semiformed; 4 = soft, formed; 5 = normal, formed; and 6 = hard. These ratings were summed daily

and weekly, and then divided by the number of days for which data were available to give a mean stool consistency score for the study period. A similar tool could be developed for use in a variety of settings to measure the effectiveness of interventions.

Educational Tools and Resources

Many cancer care units and outpatient departments have developed patient self-care sheets to guide individuals in the control of diarrhea. Some of these may be as simple as instructing the patient in when it is important to contact the physician about a particular side effect and including contact numbers. Nurses in office settings may use pharmaceutical company–provided materials that address symptom management. Radiation therapy departments frequently use both symptom and dietary management sheets to enhance self-care behaviors in patients at risk for diarrhea.

Dodd[57] requests that individuals experiencing side effects from cancer treatment keep a self-care behavior log

TABLE 28-11   Clinical Nursing Guide for Diarrhea

Clinical Situation	Therapeutic Approach
Frequent loose stools with concurrent narcotic analgesic use?	Check for fecal impaction. If present and blood counts are stable, gently disimpact following use of an oil retention enema; consider premedication for pain and/or anxiety. Institute preventive bowel care regimen.
Diarrhea associated with recent tapering or abrupt discontinuation of narcotic analgesics?	May indicate opiate withdrawal. Resume narcotic therapy at one-fourth previous daily dose and then taper off gradually over next 2 to 3 days. Recommended low-dose loperamide or other antidiarrheal over-the-counter medication.
Loose stools, <4 days' duration, not at high risk for infectious diarrhea?	Recommend loperamide HCl (Imodium-AD). Encourage oral rehydration and eating foods high in pectin. Avoid foods high in fat and roughage.
Loose stools related to the ingestion of milk products?	Trial low-lactose diet. Consult with dietitian. Suggest use of lactase enzyme drops or tablets. Instruct to read food labels carefully.
Loose or watery nonbloody stools, moderately controlled with standard antidiarrheals, lasting longer than 4 days' duration, no fever?	Obtain order for stool analysis. Institute/continue oral rehydration, feeding with low-residue foods, foods high in pectin, low in roughage. Continue use of antidiarrheals.
Fever and watery and/or mucus/bloody stools, high risk for infectious diarrhea, not controlled by antidiarrheal medications in past 48 hours?	Obtain order for stool analysis if not already done. Obtain order for oral or IV metronidazole or vancomycin if *C. difficile* infection suspected. Stop other antibiotics and antidiarrheals if possible. Assess for signs of dehydration. Encourage oral rehydration, use of foods high in pectin, low in roughage and fat. Determine need for IV hydration.
Watery stools, no fever, negative cultures, and not controlled by 3-day use of antidiarrheals?	Recommend trial of octreotide acetate SQ or IV. Continue oral rehydration and diet alterations or initiate IV hydration if indicated. Further GI workup may be needed.
Loose stools associated with recent chemotherapy, biotherapy, and/or abdominal, pelvic, or lower spine irradiation?	Institute low-residue diet and use of loperamide. Encourage oral rehydration. Be alert for signs of dehydration.
Loose stools not controlled with standard antidiarrheal medications and associated with nausea, vomiting, ileus, and signs of severe dehydration?	Obtain order for IV hydration and stool cultures if not already done.

rating the severity of the side effect and its resultant distress, using a visual analogue scale. In addressing symptom management strategies, she suggests that the individual document the actions taken to control these side effects and who provided the suggested action. Documentation of self-care measures used by the individual experiencing diarrhea is a good way to determine the effectiveness of teaching provided and whether an individual has reviewed the education materials provided.

Examples of several etiology-specific diarrhea self-care sheets are included in Appendixes 28B through 28E, which cover management of radiation- and chemotherapy/biotherapy-induced diarrhea, chronic diarrhea, and chronic diarrhea caused by lactose intolerance. Table 28-11 provides a diarrhea clinical nursing guide to assist nurses in determining the proper therapeutic approach given different clinical situations.

Conclusion

The overall management of diarrhea requires a joint effort among the healthcare team, the patient, and the family. Without a concerted effort, diarrhea and its concomitant concerns can easily become monumental problems. Chronic diarrhea frequently results in significant lifestyle changes as individuals learn to cope with the sometimes unpredictable nature of their bowel elimination. Open communication is important, and acceptance of coping behaviors, if constructive, is likewise important. For individuals struggling to cope, coaching and guidance on how to manage this chronic condition while retaining a sense of dignity is of prime importance.

References

1. Mercadante S: Diarrhea in terminally ill patients: Pathophysiology and treatment. *J Pain Symptom Manage* 10:298–309, 1995
2. Fine KD, Krejs GJ, Fordtran JS: Diarrhea, in Scharschmidt BF, Feldman M (eds): *Gastrointestinal Disease* (ed 5) vol 2. Philadelphia: Saunders, 1993, pp. 1043–1072
3. Phillips SF: Diarrhea: A current view of the pathophysiology. *Prog Gastroenterol* 63:495–518, 1972
4. Levy MH: Constipation and diarrhea in cancer patients. *Cancer Bull* 43:412–422, 1991
5. Branski D, Lerner A, Lebenthal E: Chronic diarrhea and malabsorption. *Pediatr Gastroenterol* 43:307–331, 1996
6. Wadle KR: Diarrhea. *Nurs Clin North Am* 25:901–908, 1990
7. Fujita S, Kusunoki M, Shoji Y, et al: Quality of life after total proctocolectomy and ileal J-pouch-anal anastomosis. *Dis Colon Rectum* 35:1030–1039, 1992
8. Cheney CP, Wong RK: Acute infectious diarrhea. *Med Clin North Am* 77:1169–1198, 1993
9. Klein S, Jeejeebhow KN: Long-term nutritional management of patients with maldigestion and malabsorption, in Scharschmidt BF, Feldman M (eds): *Gastrointestinal Disease* (ed 5) vol 2. Philadelphia: Saunders, 1993, pp. 2048–2062
10. Grant M, Ropka ME: Alterations in nutrition, in Baird SB, McCorkle R, Grant M (eds): *Cancer Nursing*. Philadelphia: Saunders, 1991, pp. 717–741
11. McCarthy CP: Altered patterns of elimination, in Dow KH, Hilderley LJ (eds): *Nursing Care in Radiation Oncology*. Philadelphia: Saunders, 1992, pp. 126–148
12. Mitchell EP: Gastrointestinal toxicity of chemotherapeutic agents. *Semin Oncol* 19:566–579, 1992
13. Cummings BJ: Concomitant radiotherapy and chemotherapy for anal cancer. *Semin Oncol* 19:102–108, 1992
14. Rahman R, Bernstein Z, Vaickus L, et al: Unusual gastrointestinal complications of IL-2 therapy. *J Immunother* 10:221–225, 1991
15. Berg D: Irinotecan hydrochloride: Drug profile and nursing implications of a topoisomerase I inhibitor in patients with advanced colorectal cancer. *Oncol Nurs Forum* 25:535–543, 1998
16. Bisanz A: Managing bowel elimination problems in patients with cancer. *Oncol Nurs Forum* 24:679–686, 1997
17. Petrelli NJ, Rodriguez-Bigas M, Rustum Y, et al: Bowel rest, intravenous hydration, and continuous high-dose infusion of octreotide acetate for the treatment of chemotherapy-induced diarrhea in patients with colorectal carcinoma. *Cancer* 72:1543–1546, 1993
18. Vokes E, Weichselbaum R: Concomitant chemoradiotherapy: Rationale and clinical experience in patients with solid tumors. *J Clin Oncol* 8:911–934, 1990
19. Fernandez-Banares F, Villa S, Esteve M, et al: Acute effects of abdominopelvic irradiation on the orocecal transit time: Its relation to clinical symptoms, and bile salt and lactose malabsorption. *Am J Gastroenterol* 86:1771–1777, 1991
20. Yeoh EK, Horowitz M, Russo A, et al: Gastrointestinal function in chronic radiation enteritis—Effects of loperamide-N-oxide. *Gut* 34:476–482, 1993
21. Danialsson A, Nyhlin H, Persson H, et al: Chronic diarrhea after radiotherapy for gynaecological cancer: Occurrence and aetiology. *Gut* 32:1180–1187, 1991
22. Mennie AT, Dalley VM, Dinneen LC, et al: Treatment of radiation-induced gastrointestinal distress with acetylsalicylate. *Lancet* 2:942–943, 1975
23. Kinsella TJ, Bloomer WD: Tolerance of the intestine to radiation therapy. *Surg Gynecol Obstet* 151:273–284, 1980
24. Fenner MN, Sheehan P, Nanavati PJ, et al: Chronic radiation enteritis: A community hospital experience. *J Surg Oncol* 41:246–249, 1989
25. Wujcik D, Ballard B, Camp-Sorrell D: Selected complications of allogeneic bone marrow transplantation. *Semin Oncol Nurs* 10:28–41, 1994
26. Dresler CM, Fortner JG, McDermott K, et al: Metabolic consequences of regional total pancreatectomy. *Ann Surg* 214:131–140, 1991
27. Sharkey MF, Kadden MK, Stabile BE: Severe post-hemicolectomy diarrhea: Evaluation and treatment with SMS 201-995. *Gastroenterology* 99:1144–1148, 1990
28. Westergaard J, Spady DK: Short bowel syndrome, in Scharschmidt BF, Feldman M (eds): *Gastrointestinal Disease* (ed 5) vol 2. Philadelphia: Saunders, 1993, pp. 1249–1257
29. Bartlett JG: *Clostridium difficile:* Clinical considerations. *Rev Infect Dis* 12(suppl 2):243–251, 1990

30. Anand A, Glatt AE: *Clostridium difficile* infection associated with antineoplastic chemotherapy: A review. *Clin Infect Dis* 17:109–113, 1993

31. Heather DJ, Howell L, Montana M, et al: Effect of a bulk-forming cathartic on diarrhea in tube-fed patients. *Heart Lung* 20:409–413, 1991

32. Burns PE, Jairath N: Diarrhea and the patient receiving enteral feedings: A multifactorial problem. *J Wound Ostomy Continence Nurs* 21:257–263, 1994

33. National Cancer Institute, Division of Cancer Treatment, Cancer Therapy Evaluation Program. *Investigator's Handbook: A Manual for Participants in Clinical Trials of Investigational Agents Sponsored by the Division of Cancer Treatment.* Rockville, MD: National Cancer Institute, October 1993

34. McArthur KE, Anderson DS, Durbin TE, et al: Clonidine and lindamidine to inhibit watery diarrhea in a patient with lung cancer. *Ann Intern Med* 92:323–325, 1982

35. Gordon P, Comi RJ, Maton PN, et al: NIH Conference: Somatostatin and somatostatin analogue (SMS 201-995) in treating hormone-secreting tumors of the pituitary and gastrointestinal tract and non-neoplastic diseases of the gut. *Ann Intern Med* 110:35–50, 1989

36. U.S. Department of Health and Human Services: *Eating Hints* (Publication No. 91-2079). Bethesda, MD: National Institutes of Health, 1990

37. U.S. Department of Health and Human Services: *Radiation Therapy and You* (Publication No. 92-2227). Bethesda, MD: National Institutes of Health, 1992

38. Henriksson R, Franzen L, Littbrand B: Effects of sucralfate on acute and late bowel discomfort following radiotherapy of pelvic cancer. *J Clin Oncol* 10:969–975, 1992

39. Ito H, Meistrich ML, Barkley TH, et al: Protection of acute and late radiation damage of the gastrointestinal tract by WR-2721. *Int J Radiat Oncol Biol Phys* 12:211, 1986

40. Elmer GW, Surawicz CM, McFarland LV: Biotherapeutic agents: A neglected modality for the treatment and prevention of selected intestinal and vaginal infections. *JAMA* 275:870–876, 1996

41. Cudmore MA, Silva J Jr, Fekety R, et al: *Clostridium difficile* colitis associated with cancer chemotherapy. *Arch Intern Med* 142:333–335, 1982

42. Nolan NPM, Kelly CP, Humphreys JFH, et al: An epidemic of pseudomembranous colitis: Importance of person-to-person spread. *Gut* 28:1467–1473, 1987

43. Bartlett JG: Pseudomembranous enterocolitis and antibiotic-associated colitis, in Scharschmidt BF, Feldman M (eds): *Gastrointestinal Disease* (ed 5) vol 2. Philadelphia: Saunders, 1993, pp. 1174–1189

44. McArdle AH, Wittnich C, Greeman CR, et al: Elemental diet as prophylaxis against radiation injury. *Arch Surg* 120:1026–1032, 1985

45. Copeland EM III: Intravenous hyperalimentation and chemotherapy: An update. *J Parenter Enteral Nutr* 6:236–239, 1982

46. Pezner R, Archambeau JO: Critical evaluation of the role of nutritional support for radiation therapy patients. *Cancer* 55:263–267, 1985

47. Edes ET, Walk BE, Austin TL: Diarrhea in tube-fed patients: Feeding formula not necessarily the cause. *Am J Med* 88:94, 1990

48. Fruto LV: Current concepts: Management of diarrhea in acute care. *J Wound Ostomy Continence Nurs* 21:199–205, 1994

49. Snyder JD: Oral therapy for diarrhea. *Hosp Pract* 26:86–88, 1991

50. Klein S, Fleming CR: Enteral and parenteral nutrition, in Scharschmidt BF, Feldman M (eds): *Gastrointestinal Disease* (ed 5) vol 2. Philadelphia: Saunders, 1993, pp. 2062–2096

51. Weizman Z: Cola drinks and rehydration in acute diarrhea. *N Engl J Med* 315:768, 1986

52. Palmer KR, Corbett CL, Holdsworth CD: Double-blind cross-over study comparing loperamide, codeine, and diphenoxylate in the treatment of chronic diarrhea. *Gastroenterology* 79:1272–1275, 1980

53. Ericsson CD, Johnson PC: Safety and efficacy of loperamide. *Am J Med* 88(suppl 6A):10S–14S, 1990

54. Harris AG, O'Dorisio EA, Woltering LB, et al: Consensus statement: Octreotide dose titration in secretory diarrhea. *Dig Dis Sci* 40:1464–1473, 1995

55. A complete product profile Camptosar irinotecan HCl injection. Kalamazoo, MI: Pharmacia & Upjohn, Inc., 1997

56. Petrelli NJ, Rodriguez-Bigas M, Rustum Y, et al: Bowel rest, intravenous hydration, and continuous high-dose infusion of octreotide acetate for the treatment of chemotherapy-induced diarrhea in patients with colorectal carcinoma. *Cancer* 72:1543–1546, 1993

57. Dodd MJ: *Managing the Side Effects of Chemotherapy and Radiation.* New York, Prentice Hall, 1991

Weekly Bowel Movement Recording Sheet

Patient Name: _____

Date								Total
Number of stools per day								
Character* (see code below)								
Soiling episodes per day								
Amount of medication used per day								
Comments (e.g., diet change, anxiety, new medication)								

*Stool Character
1 = hard, formed
2 = soft, formed
3 = loose
4 = watery
5 = bloody

Source: Martz CH: Diarrhea, in Yarbro CH, Frogge MH, Goodman M (eds): *Cancer Symptoms Management* (ed 2). Sudbury: Jones and Bartlett, 1999. © Jones and Bartlett Publishers.

Diarrhea from Radiation Therapy

Patient Name: _____

Symptom and Description   Diarrhea is defined as more than two loose or watery stools per day. It can be caused by radiation over your bowels. Diarrhea may be worse if you are also receiving chemotherapy.

Learning Needs   These loose or watery stools may start 2 weeks after your treatments begin. If left untreated, diarrhea can result in weakness, weight loss, skin soreness, and poor nutrition. You need to learn strategies for controlling diarrhea, and you need to learn when you should get in touch with your nurse or doctor.

Prevention   Eating a low-residue diet may help to reduce the number of loose stools per day.

Management

- Avoid eating foods high in fiber, fatty foods, rich desserts, and other foods that increase bowel activity such as hot peppers, drinks with caffeine, and alcohol.
- Use Imodium, an over-the-counter medicine for loose stools, as directed:

  _____

- Follow low-residue food list provided by nutritional services or dietitian.
- Increase your intake of liquids to six 8-ounce glasses (about 1.4 liters) per day (unless told not to do so by your doctor).

Follow-up   Let your doctor or nurse know if these measures do not control your diarrhea. In addition, you should let them know if:

- You have bloody or hard stools
- You have a temperature of 100.5°F (38°C) or greater
- You are unable to keep down liquids
- You become dizzy
- You notice your urine becoming dark yellow in color, more concentrated

Phone Numbers

Nurse: _____ Phone: _____

Physician: _____ Phone: _____

Dietitian/Nutritional Service: _____ Phone: _____

Comments

Patient's Signature: _____ Date: _____

Nurse's Signature: _____ Date: _____

Source: Martz CH: Diarrhea, in Yarbro CH, Frogge MH, Goodman M (eds): *Cancer Symptom Management* (ed 2). Sudbury: Jones and Bartlett, 1999. © Jones and Bartlett Publishers.

Diarrhea from Chemotherapy/Biotherapy

Patient Name: _____

Symptom and Description   Diarrhea is defined as more than two loose or watery stools per day. It can be caused by your cancer treatments. Diarrhea may be worse if you are also receiving radiation treatments over your abdomen.

Learning Needs   Loose or watery stools may start a few days after your treatments. If left untreated, diarrhea can result in weakness, weight loss, skin soreness, and poor nutrition. You need to learn strategies for controlling diarrhea, and you need to learn when you should get in touch with your nurse or your doctor.

Prevention   Eating a low-residue diet may help to reduce the number of loose stools per day.

Management

- Avoid eating foods high in fiber, fatty foods, rich desserts, and other foods that increase bowel activity such as hot peppers, drinks with caffeine, and alcohol.
- Use Imodium-AD, an over-the counter medicine for loose stools, as directed: use Lomotil as directed: _____ ; or use Sandostatin as directed: _____ .
- Follow low-residue food list provided by nutritional services or dietitian.
- Increase your intake of liquids to six 8-ounce glasses (about 1.4 liters) a day (unless told not to do so by your doctor).

Follow-up   Let your doctor or nurse know if these measures do not control your diarrhea, or if

- You develop a temperature of over 100.5°F (38°C)
- You have hard or bloody stools
- You are not able to keep down liquids
- You notice your urine becoming dark yellow in color
- You become dizzy

Phone Numbers

Nurse: _____ Phone: _____

Physician: _____ Phone: _____

Dietitian/Nutritional Service: _____ Phone: _____

Comments

Patient's Signature: _____ Date: _____

Nurse's Signature: _____ Date: _____

Source: Martz CH: Diarrhea, in Yarbro CH, Frogge MH, Goodman M (eds): *Cancer Symptom Management* (ed 2). Sudbury: Jones and Bartlett, 1999. © Jones and Bartlett Publishers.

Chronic Diarrhea

Patient Name: _____

Symptom and Description   Chronic diarrhea is defined as loose or watery stools, more than two per day, that last longer than 2 months. Chronic loose stools can occur as a result of your cancer treatments.

Learning Needs   Loose watery stools, if left untreated, can result in weakness, weight loss, skin soreness, and poor nutrition. You need to learn strategies for controlling diarrhea, and you need to learn when you should get in touch with your nurse or doctor.

Management

- Follow the low-residue diet food list provided by nutritional services or dietitian.
- In general, avoid foods high in fiber, fatty foods, rich desserts, and other foods that increase bowel movements or gas such as hot peppers, drinks with caffeine, and alcohol.
- Keep a list of foods that cause you more problems and try to avoid them.
- Use Imodium-AD, 1 to 2 tablets twice a day; *or* use Sandostatin as directed: _____ .
- If diarrhea occurs after meals, schedule your meals to allow enough time to move your bowels before planned activities.
- Increase your intake of liquids to six 8-ounce glasses (about 1.4 liters) per day (unless told not to do so by your doctor).

Follow-up   You should have less diarrhea if you follow these tips. If you do not, let your doctor or nurse know. More tests may need to be done. In addition, let them know if:

- You develop a temperature of over 100.5°F (38°C)
- You are not able to keep down liquids
- You become dizzy
- You notice your urine becoming dark yellow in color
- You have bloody stools
- You develop right upper abdominal pain (if taking Sandostatin).

Phone Numbers

Nurse: _____ Phone: _____

Physician: _____ Phone: _____

Dietitian/Nutritional Service: _____ Phone: _____

Comments

Patient's Signature: _____ Date: _____

Nurse's Signature: _____ Date: _____

Source: Martz CH: Diarrhea, in Yarbro CH, Frogge MH, Goodman M (eds): *Cancer Symptom Management* (ed 2). Sudbury: Jones and Bartlett, 1999. © Jones and Bartlett Publishers.

Chronic Diarrhea Due to Lactose Intolerance

Patient Name: _____

Symptom and Description This kind of diarrhea is more than two loose stools, per day, that have persisted for longer than 2 months, and is related to eating foods that contain lactose (a substance found in milk products).

Learning Needs Lactose intolerance may be inherited or may occur due to your cancer treatments. Being unable to digest foods with lactose in them can result in poor nutrition.

Prevention Use commercially available lactase enzyme tablets or drops when you plan to eat foods that contain lactose or drink milk.

Management

- Follow low-lactose diet provided by nutritional services or dietitian.
- Read food labels carefully to find out what foods contain lactose.
- When eating foods that contain lactose, space them over the course of the day to encourage tolerance.
- Use Imodium-AD, an over-the-counter medicine for diarrhea, as directed on the label, to control stools not controlled by diet.
- Increase your intake of non-milk-product liquids to replace fluids lost with loose stools.

Follow-up If you continue to have more than two loose stools per day after using these measures, let your doctor or nurse know. In addition, let them know if:

- You develop a temperature of 100.5°F (38°C) or greater
- You are unable to keep down liquids
- You become dizzy
- You notice your urine becoming dark yellow in color
- You have bloody stools

Phone Numbers

Nurse: _____ Phone: _____

Physician: _____ Phone: _____

Dietitian/Nutritional Service: _____ Phone: _____

Comments

Patient's Signature: _____ Date: _____

Nurse's Signature: _____ Date: _____

Source: Martz CH: Diarrhea, in Yarbro CH, Frogge MH, Goodman M (eds): *Cancer Symptom Management* (ed 2). Sudbury: Jones and Bartlett, 1999. © Jones and Bartlett Publishers.

PART VII

Symptoms of Alterations in Coping

CHAPTER 29

Altered Sexual Health

Deborah Watkins Bruner, RN, MSN

Ryan R. Iwamoto, RN, MN, CS

The Problem of Altered Sexual Health in Cancer

Estimates of sexual dysfunction after cancer treatments range from 10% to 90% depending on the site.[1] Cancer and cancer therapies alter sexual function in a multitude of ways. Although sporadic studies have documented the impact some cancer therapies have on sexual function, much research is still needed. Unlike other outcomes such as morbidity, mortality, and even quality of life, sexual outcomes and interventions have been comparatively neglected in the literature.

Research into interventions to maintain or improve sexual function after cancer therapies is vital for preserving quality of life and is an integral part of total or holistic cancer management. Nursing has long embraced the philosophy of holistic care and yet ignored including the promotion of sexual health as a routine part of our practice. "Sexual health means the ability to enjoy sexual activity and exercise that ability free of negative feelings (i.e., fear or guilt) that inhibit sexual response."[2]

General Problems

Cancer and its therapies affect the physical, psychological, and social ability of the patient to maintain sexual health. Debilitating physical symptoms such as fatigue, nausea, anorexia, and pain can greatly diminish sexual desire.

Surgical procedures resulting in amputation, organ removal or translocation, changes in patterns of elimination, hormonal manipulation/ablation, or vascular, muscular, or neurologic impairments have an impact on body image, libido, fertility, and sexual performance. Cancer and its therapies may cause depression and anxiety in some cancer patients, including anxiety due to fear of death, mutilation, or loss of functioning. Depression and anxiety can interfere with sexual desire, arousal, and ability to achieve orgasm. The diagnosis and treatment of cancer also intrude on social relationships and leisure functioning, resulting in diminished intimacy and altered sexual self-concept and gender identity.[3] Hospitalization or symptoms that prohibit role functioning (e.g., mother, father, wife, husband) can also diminish a person's culturally ingrained sexual self-concept.[4]

Site-Specific Problems

Breast

Women treated with modified radical mastectomy have identified problems with sexual functioning in the range of 25%, including loss of desire, decreased frequency of intercourse, and diminished sexual excitement.[5] A recent study of women treated with either lumpectomy or mastectomy and either chemotherapy or radiation therapy found that although 90% of the women continued sexual activity, the majority experienced a reduction in the quality of their sex lives. Sixty-four percent of the women reported an absence of sexual desire, 38%

dyspareunia, 44% frigidity, and 42% lubrication problems.[6] Several studies have reported a more positive sexual outcome for women treated with lumpectomy and radiation therapy as opposed to mastectomy in terms of body image, comfort with nudity, and frequency of intercourse.[7,8] However, at least one study documented statistical differences favoring mastectomy versus breast conserving therapy in the areas of sexual interest and average sexual severity scores.[9]

Other issues that women treated for breast cancer face include weight gain and alopecia. Both have an impact on body image. If treated with chemotherapy, the patient may experience irregular menstrual periods or even early menopause, including the potential for hot flashes, insomnia, irritability, depression, vaginal dryness, dyspareunia, infertility, osteoporosis, and myocardial infarction.

Gynecologic

The woman treated for a gynecologic malignancy faces a 50% or greater chance of sexual dysfunction due to a potential threefold assault on her sexual being: body image, sexual functioning, and fertility.[10] Radical vulvectomy is a particularly mutilating surgical procedure that includes removal of the clitoris, labia, and distal third of the vagina, and bilateral inguinal lymph node dissection with or without pelvic node dissection. The approximation of the surgical edges causes tension, which may interfere with range of motion for the most common positioning for sexual intercourse. Wound dehiscence is a complication in well over 50% of cases and can leave a disfiguring scar. Inguinal lymphadenectomy predisposes patients to leg edema, ranging from a mild +1 pitting edema to elephantiasis, in up to 69% of cases,[11] which can be devastating to body image. Fortunately, the increased use of wide local excision, now commonly used for early-stage vulvar cancer, eliminates the need for extensive lymph node dissection, although it still frequently involves removal of the clitoris. Clitoridectomy does not necessarily preclude orgasm, although the clitoris may be necessary for orgasm in women who masturbate for their sexual release.[12]

Women who have surgical manipulation or intracavitary radiation implants for vulvar cancer, cervical cancer, or endometrial cancer may be left with a shortened vagina. Dyspareunia may occur with deep penile penetration. Hysterectomy, frequently a part of the surgical treatment for cervical, endometrial, and ovarian cancers, may also interfere with the sexual response cycle. The absence of rhythmic contractions of the uterus may inhibit or prevent orgasm. Oophorectomy or ovarian ablation due to radiation or chemotherapy potentiates dyspareunia due to vaginal dryness and thinning of the vaginal lining. In fact, 33% to 46% of women undergoing hysterectomy with oophorectomy for both benign and malignant tumors reported a decreased sexual response postsurgery.[13] With this multifaceted assault on a woman's

sexuality, it is not surprising that one study found that 77% of those treated for cervical cancer and 50% of those treated for endometrial cancer, versus only 16% of those treated with hysterectomy for benign disease, described their sex lives as being rather to severely negative. The women treated for cancer rated the following factors as negatively affecting their sexual life: vaginal dryness, reduced desire, reduced ability to have an orgasm, less joy in sex, and negative genital sensations during arousal or intercourse.[14]

Women undergoing total pelvic exenteration face a serious challenge to both their physical recovery and their emotional coping. The operation includes removal of bladder, rectosigmoid, vagina, uterus, adnexa, and pelvic lymph nodes. In select cases, the surgery may be limited to either anterior exenteration with removal of the bladder and preservation of the rectosigmoid or posterior exenteration with removal of the rectosigmoid and preservation of the bladder.[15]

Infertility is, of course, a major concern for many patients being treated for gynecologic and other malignancies but is beyond the scope of this chapter. For further information the reader is referred to other resources.[16–18]

Male genital cancers

Prostate cancer, the most common diagnosed cancer in men, and its relationship to sexual functioning have been the subject of a great deal of research. Prostate cancer is most common in men 65 years of age or older. Distinguishing diagnosis-related dysfunction from age-related dysfunction is somewhat difficult, as it is estimated that "8% of men at age 50 years, 20% of men at age 60 years and 80% of men at age 80 years fail to have adequate erections."[12]

Treatment of early-stage prostate cancer commonly involves surgery or radiation therapy. Diagnostic transurethral resection of the prostate (TURP) commonly causes retrograde ejaculation. Biopsy alone carries a 20% to 30% risk of erectile dysfunction,[19] while radical prostatectomy, modified prostatectomy, and external-beam radiation therapy carry a risk of erectile failure in 90%, 75%, and 30% of patients, respectively.[20–22] Based on preliminary studies, two comparatively minimally invasive therapies for localized prostate cancer, interstitial radiation implants and cryosurgical ablation, carry a 45% and 90% risk of impotence, respectively.[23] As noted, most studies of sexual function after prostate cancer therapy focus on potency, but one rare study on orgasm after radical prostatectomy documented a 50% weakening of the orgasm sensation. More disturbing was the report that 64% of patients had involuntary loss of urine at orgasm, causing more than half to avoid sexual contact with their partner.[24]

Endocrine manipulation is the treatment of choice for patients with metastatic prostate cancer or extensive regional spread. Therapy may consist of bilateral orchiectomy, estrogen therapy, or both. Erectile dysfunction for orchiectomy alone has been estimated at 47%, for estrogen alone 22%, and for combined therapy 73%.[25] In addition to erectile dysfunction associated with endocrine therapy, other sexual sequelae include diminished libido and phallic atrophy. Body image is a concern also for men treated with estrogen who experience gynecomastia.

Testicular and penile cancers are far less common than prostate cancer but frequently cause grave concern about sexual health when they do occur. Testicular cancer occurs in young males, whose body image is often devastated by the removal of usually one or sometimes both of their testes. Radical inguinal orchiectomy and lymphadenectomy, which includes removal of the testis, epididymis, portion of the vas deferens and the regional lymphatics, interferes with ejaculation, orgasm, and libido, particularly when bilateral.[26,27] Penile cancer may require partial or total penectomy. Patients will probably be little comforted to hear that although infrequent, there have been reports of orgasm via scrotal and perineal stimulation.[28]

Bladder

There is little documentation of the sexual disruptions for either males or females caused by the diagnosis and treatment of bladder cancer. Early-stage therapy, which usually consists of transurethral resection with or without intravesical chemotherapy, is thought to have a mild, transient effect on sexual functioning. Suprapubic and urethral pain and dyspareunia are possible.[29] Radical cystectomy or external-beam radiation therapy is used in the treatment of invasive bladder cancer. One study reported that more than 90% of men treated with radical cystectomy experienced impotence.[30] Lacking research, it is assumed that women undergoing radical cystectomy experience posttreatment outcomes similar to those having anterior exenteration with only partial vaginectomy. Dyspareunia may occur and sexual excitement and orgasm may thus be impaired due to difficult penetration.[31]

Colorectal cancer

Surgical resection of the tumor with pelvic lymphadenectomy with or without chemotherapy is the most common treatment for colorectal cancer. Early-stage disease that may be treated with removal of the rectum only may interfere with orgasmic potential, although erectile dysfunction is less common.[32] The more extensive the surgery, the higher the reported incidence of sexual dysfunctions, at least in males, on whom more research has been done than on females. A study of 60 men who were sexually active pretreatment and who received either high anterior resection, low anterior resection, or abdominoperineal resection found the latter group to have the highest percentage of sexual problems. Sixty-five percent

became sexually inactive, 50% were unable to ejaculate, and 45% reported erectile dysfunction.[33]

Surgery that includes formation of an ostomy leaves many patients with unique stoma-related sexual concerns. Body image can become an obsessive concern to those acutely aware of their stool collecting visibly in a pouch under their clothing. Fear of embarrassing public and intimate moments due to ostomy appearance, sounds, odors, and leakage can cause the person to feel unattractive and to have diminished libido. Fear of rejection can cause stress in relationships and have a negative impact on self-concept.

Other cancers

Cancers that do not directly affect sexual organs may have no less an impact on sexual self-image. Head and neck cancers may be treated with disfiguring surgery affecting body image. Radiation therapy used in the treatment of head and neck cancers may cause permanent xerostomia, affecting comfort and libido and impairing the ability for oral sexual contact. A recent study of 55 patients treated for head and neck cancer reported 78% to have problems with sexual functioning, including fantasy, arousal, behavior, orgasm, drive, and satisfaction.[34] Sarcomas often require amputation of a limb, which is an obvious assault on body image. Limb-sparing radiation therapy has been used to treat sarcomas with the assumption it would provide improved quality of life. A now-classic study by Sugarbaker et al.[35] was unable to substantiate this assumption and found that sexual functioning of individuals who participated in the limb-sparing treatment group was indeed worse. Lung cancer, the number one cause of cancer deaths, with its symptomatic correlates of fatigue and respiratory impairment, has a negative influence on sexual desire and functioning. Similarly, patients with Hodgkin's disease report decreased energy and sexual desire.[36]

Impact on Quality of Life

A recent study sought to document the long-term effects of cancer treatment and consequences of cure on quality of life (QOL). The researchers used a battery of QOL instruments tested for reliability and validity. They concluded that "cancer survivors enjoy QOL similar to their neighbors" in all but one aspect of daily life: sexual functioning. "Despite using multiple measures of QOL, sexual dysfunction as determined by Goldberg's Clinical Interview Schedule was the only symptomatic long-term sequela of cancer treatment in index [cancer] cases compared to neighborhood controls." The study cites premature menopause as the most commonly reported abnormality in females and performance dysfunctions as the most commonly reported abnormality in males treated for cancer.[37]

Etiology

Cancer therapy most often requires a multimodality approach including any combination of surgery, chemotherapy, radiation therapy, hormonal therapy, and immunotherapy. These treatments not only cause a change in sexual functioning but can be psychologically intimidating.[38] Patients have many misconceptions about how cancer therapy can alter their sexual functioning. For example, Lancaster[39] interviewed 50 women treated with radiation therapy for gynecologic cancers and reported, "Ignorance was the most striking [feature]: the women were neither prepared for the treatment nor subsequent side effects. . . . Some subjects chose to avoid sexual contact altogether, others elected to preserve the marriage by resorting to various strategies." The fear of total loss of sexual functioning is the excuse used by many to avoid seeking definitive therapy. And, in fact, Singer et al.[40] found in a sample of men with localized prostate cancer that some were willing to choose a treatment with somewhat shortened survival in order to preserve sexual potency. A knowledge of how cancer therapies affect sexual functioning is needed by healthcare providers in order to prepare patients psychologically and assist their coping with sexual problems, to prevent problems when possible, and to treat sexual dysfunction when necessary.

Surgery

Surgical treatment for cancer can affect sexual functioning by impairing the vascular supply or the innervation to pelvic organs, by amputation of pelvic organs, or by reducing the circulating hormone levels. In the male, such treatments can cause impotence, dry ejaculation, retrograde ejaculation, and diminished intensity of orgasms. In the female, surgery can cause premature menopause, dyspareunia, diminished vaginal lubrication, diminished or lost orgasmic ability, and decreased libido. Both men and women may experience negative body image as well as infertility.

There has been an increasing trend toward developing cancer surgeries that are less radical, disfiguring, or debilitating and to add surgical procedures or combined therapies that may help prevent or repair damage. Breast surgery has evolved from radical mastectomy to modified radical mastectomy with reconstruction to, in appropriate cases, lumpectomy with radiation therapy. Much research has been done on the psychological effects of these procedures, and although there are some conflicting reports, breast preservation has predominantly provided higher satisfaction among both female patients and their significant others.[8,41,42] Radical vulvectomies have given way to wide local excision when possible. And for men, Walsh[22] has pioneered a nerve-sparing radical prostatectomy procedure that, he reports, preserves potency in 70% of men versus 10% with traditional radical prostatectomy. Unfortunately, reports of potency preservation after nerve-sparing prostatectomy in a recent prospective cohort study showed much less favorable results: only 21% potency.[21] Surgery for rectal cancer has also improved with an autonomic nerve-preserving operation. One study found potency to be preserved in 86% of men younger than 60 years of age and in 67% of men older than 60 years of age, with 87% of men retaining their ability to achieve orgasm. The same study found 85% of women treated with this nerve-sparing surgery to experience arousal with vaginal lubrication and 91% to maintain the ability to achieve orgasm.[43]

Chemotherapy

Systemic effects of chemotherapy can affect body image, sexual functioning, and fertility. Side effects include fatigue and nausea and vomiting that diminish libido and cause alterations of body image, along with hair loss, weight changes, pallor, and dry skin. Mucositis can interfere with kissing and oral sex. Immunosuppression may require a temporary break from intercourse, particularly in women, to prevent infection.

A study of 50 women who had surgery plus either chemotherapy or radiation therapy found the greatest decrement in sexual function in the women treated with chemotherapy (26%) versus radiation therapy (6%).[6]

Gonadal tissue is especially sensitive to alkylating agents. These agents can cause ovarian ablation in women and germinal aplasia and azoospermia in men. Dnistrian et al.[44] documented the similarity in hormonal levels of women treated with the alkylating agent–containing regimen CMF (cyclophoshamide, methotrexate, and 5-fluorouracil) for breast cancer, women who had oophorectomy, and postmenopausal women. Men treated for Hodgkin's disease with MOPP (mechlorethamine/nitrogen mustard, vincristine, prednisone, and procarbazine) have an 80% or greater chance of azoospermia and testicular atrophy with elevated follicle-stimulating hormone levels.[45]

Radiation Therapy

During treatment with external beam radiation therapy in combination with lumpectomy for breast cancer, women have an estimated 75% disruption in sexual activity,[46] probably due to inflammation and desquamation of the skin and to fatigue, both temporary side effects of therapy. After therapy, there are conflicting reports of the impact on body image and desire in women treated with breast conservation therapy.[5,9]

Up to 79% of women treated with external beam and intracavitary radiation therapy for cervical cancer have reported sexual impairments.[47] This can in part be related to the denuding of the vaginal epithelium, narrowing and obliteration of the small vessels, and circumferential fibrosis of the perivaginal tissue, all of which contribute to vaginal stenosis. Vaginal stenosis following intracavitary implants has been reported in 72% to 88% of women studied.[48,49] Vaginal stenosis has also been documented in women treated with implants for endometrial cancer.[50] It also occurs in some women treated with external-beam radiation therapy for rectal cancer. In addition to vaginal stenosis, women treated with brachytherapy for cervical cancer report dyspareunia (31%–79%), vaginal dryness (74%), lack of desire (58%), and decreased coital frequency.[47,50]

Radiation can cause loss of ovarian function and sterility at relatively low doses. This has been of major concern for young girls treated for Hodgkin's disease. Surgical relocation, called oophoropexy, can assist in ovarian preservation during abdominopelvic irradiation. The ovaries are displaced laterally or centrally during surgery and then shielded during radiation therapy. Reports of these patients resuming normal menstruation have been variable.[51,52]

Radiation therapy can decrease a man's ability to have voluntary erections, even though desire and sexual sensations are still present. Although radiation therapy does not damage the corporal nerves, it accelerates atherosclerotic disease, which in time interferes with the arterial blood supply of the penis and results in impotence. Studies have demonstrated that men who are potent and sexually active prior to external-beam radiation therapy tend to maintain their potency after radiation therapy is completed.[53]

Testicular function can be impaired with a single dose of 600 cGy, causing disturbances of spermatogenesis.[54] Other side effects of radiation therapy that affect sexual function include fatigue, cystitis, diarrhea, and hair loss from the irradiated site. Total body irradiation used prior to bone marrow transplants and whole mantle irradiation with inverted Y technique can cause premature menopause with concomitant symptomatology and infertility.

Hormonal Therapy

Antiandrogenic therapies were originally used for metastatic prostate cancer to reduce plasma testosterone levels. Men with low levels of testosterone may experience lowered sexual desire, difficulty in achieving a functional erection, less pleasurable orgasm or difficulty in reaching orgasm, decreased semen production, and diminished spermatogenesis.[55] If estrogen is used, estrogen excess can cause gynecomastia, feminization, penile and testicular atrophy, and erectile dysfunction. Similar side effects can be seen when a luteinizing hormone–releasing agonist and an antiandrogen drug such as flutamide are used in combination to achieve total androgen blockade. In an effort to improve control of prostate cancer, several randomized trials are assessing the combination of antiandrogens and radiation therapy for localized disease. Conventional wisdom held that sexual function would be

the same as that postradiation once the hormones were stopped. However, a recent study contradicts this, with 55% of men treated with radiation and off hormones versus 67% of men treated with radiation alone maintaining erectile function.[56]

Immunotherapy

Little has been written regarding the effects of immunotherapy on sexual functioning; however, the fatigue experienced by patients receiving interferon and interleukins is likely to impair sexual desire.

Pathophysiology

Sexual Response Cycle

The human sexual response cycle was originally described by Masters and Johnson as a four-phase physiologic pattern that included *excitement,* characterized by female vaginal lubrication and male penile erection; *plateau,* which describes a high degree of sexual arousal that occurs prior to reaching the threshold levels required to trigger orgasm; *orgasm,* marked by rhythmic contractions of the uterus, vagina, and rectal sphincter in the female and ejaculation in the male; and *resolution,* a relaxation of the vagina and uterus in the female, and a refractory period of loss of erection in the male.[57]

Complementary to an understanding of the impact of site-specific cancers and therapies on the human sexual response cycle is the comprehension of the multifactorial nature of sexual disturbances. Schain[58] describes three major areas of sexual dysfunction: desire (interest), arousal (excitement), and orgasm (tension release). Orgasmic sexual disturbances can be a direct result of the neurovascular morbidity caused by cancer therapies as described above. Myotonia and vasocongestion are required for male and female physiologic sexual arousal, both of which can be impaired by surgery and radiation therapy. Endocrine changes due to hormonal manipulation can decrease sexual desire and arousal. Side effects associated with cancer and therapy, such as fatigue, anemia, anorexia, alopecia, pain, mucositis, and xerostomia, also affect sexual desire.

Indirect sexual impairments can result from the myriad psychological concerns associated with cancer. Coping with the diagnosis of cancer and body image changes can be difficult. Anxiety and depression play a major role in loss of desire. Other psychosocial issues related to self-esteem, such as career and employment, also affect sexual functioning. The man may see himself as less of a sexual partner if he is incapable of functioning at his previous level of activity.[59] Women may perceive themselves as less attractive or desirable.

Assessment

In order to address sexual concerns and prevent or treat sexual impairments related to cancer and therapy, healthcare professionals must be able to assess sexual health. Unfortunately, a continued lack of knowledge and conservative attitudes regarding sexual functioning by both nurses and physicians have been documented over the past several decades.[60-64]

Since a direct correlation between attitudes regarding sexuality and practice has been noted,[62] it is imperative that medical and nursing curricula incorporate teachings that improve knowledge and increase the comfort of healthcare professionals when discussing alterations in sexual function with patients.

The American Nurses Association and the Oncology Nursing Society included sexuality as one of the eleven high-incidence problem areas to be continually and systematically evaluated under their Standard I on assessment. The standard states that the oncology nurse will collect data on the effects of disease and treatment on body image and sexual functioning. The oncology nurse is also to assess the psychosocial responses of the patient and significant other to disease and treatment, as well as past and present sexual patterns and functioning.[65] To document this assessment, several measurement tools are available.

Measurement Tools

Several approaches to assessment of sexual function have been presented in the literature. Before taking a history, certain preassessment factors should be considered. The first is the demographic and diagnostic information that may influence sexuality, including gender, age, socioeconomic status, education level, cultural/ethnic background, diagnosis, treatment, concomitant medical/psychiatric problems, and medications. Second, an atmosphere conducive to enhancing respect and trust and protecting confidentiality is mandatory to successfully addressing sexual issues. Third, attention to both verbal and nonverbal communication is vital to an accurate assessment of factors influencing sexual health such as self-esteem and body image.

Several authors have suggested treading lightly in assessing sexual health by moving from less sensitive to more sensitive issues[66] or by informing the patient when you are about to ask sexual questions that some questions may be sensitive and that they may choose not to answer them.[2] It has been the authors' experience that if the sexual history is incorporated at a natural point in the overall medical history and treated matter-of-factly, patients respond in kind. If we do not pause before asking patients personal questions about how they urinate and defecate to inform them that "some of these questions

may be sensitive," we need not do so before asking if they are sexually active.

The sexual assessment included in McPhetridge's 1968 article on the nursing history is one of the most frequently cited in nursing literature.[67] Table 29-1 presents an alternative sexual assessment guide. Kolodny, Masters, and Johnson[68] took a more utilitarian approach, suggesting a purely functional assessment (Table 29-2). Andersen[69] developed a more comprehensive clinical assessment using the acronym ALARM for *a*ctivity, *l*ibido/desire, *a*rousal and orgasm, *r*esolution, *m*edical history, designed to assess both important sexual behaviors and the sexual response cycle (Table 29-3). Andersen[70] has also developed a questionnaire to assess what she terms "sexual self-schema," cognitive generalizations about sexual aspects of oneself that are derived from past experience and manifest in present experience and sexual behavior. This assessment has been used to identify women at risk for sexual dysfunction after cancer therapy.[1]

There are as many ways to take a nursing history as there are different institutions with departments of nursing to choose or develop them. In choosing or developing a method of sexual assessment to add to the history, a wide variety of tools may be desired for review. Many of the research tools developed to measure sexual function could be adapted to the clinical setting. Schiavi et al.[71] published a compendium of psychosexual assessment measures. Reviewing these research instruments allows

TABLE 29-1 General Sexual Assessment

1. Has your role as parent, spouse, or intimate friend changed since you were diagnosed with or treated for cancer?
2. Do you feel different about yourself or your body since you were diagnosed with or treated for cancer?
3. Has your sexual functioning changed (or do you think it will change) due to your diagnosis or cancer treatment? [If yes] How has it/will it change?

TABLE 29-2 Functional Sexual Assessment

1. Are you sexually active?
2. If yes, about how often?
3. Are you satisfied with your sexual activity? If no, why?
4. Do you ever have pain with intercourse?

Men Only:

5. Can you have an erection?
6. Can you keep the erection to complete intercourse?
7. Are you able to control the timing of your ejaculation?

Women Only:

8. Do you have any problems reaching orgasm?

Adapted from Kolodny R, Masters W, Johnson V, et al. *Textbook of Human Sexuality for Nurses.* Boston: Little, Brown, 1979.[68]

TABLE 29-3   ALARM: Model for the Assessment of Sexual Functioning—Sample Questions

A: Activity

Frequency of current sexual activities (e.g., intercourse, kissing, masturbation). Sample questions:

- Before the appearance of any signs/symptoms of your illness, how frequently were you engaging in intercourse (specific weekly or monthly estimate)?
- On occasions other than intercourse (or an equivalent intimate activity), do you share other forms of physical affection with your partner, such as kissing and/or hugging on a daily basis?
- In the recent past (e.g., last 6 months) have you masturbated? If so, estimate how often this has occurred (specific weekly or monthly estimate).

L: Libido/Desire

Desire for sexual activity and interest in initiating or responding to partner's initiation of sexual activity. Sample questions:

- Before the appearance of your illness, would you have described yourself as generally interested in having sex?
- In your current regular sexual relationship, who usually initiates sexual activity?
- Your current frequency for intercourse is [X] per week/month. Would you personally prefer to have intercourse more often, less often, or at the current frequency?

A: Arousal and Orgasm

Occurrence of erection/lubrication and ejaculation/vaginal contractions, accompanied by feelings of sexual excitement. Sample questions:

For men:

- When you are interested in having sexual activity, with your partner or alone, do you have any difficulty in achieving an erection? Do you feel emotionally aroused?
- If erectile difficulty: When did this problem start, how often does it occur, are there particular circumstances for its occurrence (e.g., with partner only), what do you understand to be the cause of the difficulty?
- During sexual activity, either alone or with a partner, do you have any difficulty with ejaculation, such as coming "too soon" or only after an extended period of time?
- If premature/delayed ejaculation is suggested: While it is difficult to estimate precisely, how long would you estimate that it takes on the average to ejaculate after intensive stimulation begins?

For women:

- When you are interested in engaging in sexual activity do you notice that your genitals become moist?
- If postmenopausal: Has there been any change in vaginal lubrication during sexual activity since the menopause? Are you currently taking hormonal replacement therapy?
- If arousal deficit: Do you experience any pain with intercourse? How long have you had problems with becoming aroused during sexual activity, and are there particular circumstances during which you have felt more arousal than others?
- During sexual activity, either alone or with a partner, can you experience a climax or orgasm?
- If orgasm does not occur: Are you bothered at all by the absence of orgasm?

R: Resolution

Feelings of release of tension following sexual activity and satisfaction with current sexual life. Sample questions:

- Following intercourse or masturbation, do you feel that there has been a release of sexual tension?
- On a scale from 1 (indicating that it could not be worse) to 10 (indicating that it could not be better), how would you rate your current sexual life?
- Do you have any feelings of discomfort or pain immediately after sexual activity?
- If resolution difficulty: Describe the problems you are having after sexual activity, how long they have occurred, and your understanding of their cause(s).

M: Medical History Relevant to Sexuality

Current age and history that may have caused acute or chronic disruption of sexual activity or responses:

- Medical (e.g., diabetes, hypertension)
- Psychiatric (e.g., affective disorders)
- Substance abuse (e.g., alcoholism)

ALARM = *a*ctivity, *l*ibido/desire, *a*rousal and orgasm, *r*esolution, *m*edical history.

Adapted from Andersen B: How cancer affects sexual functioning. *Oncology* 4:81–88, 1990.[69]

nurses to choose on which areas they wish to focus. For example, some instruments focus on the psychological/emotional aspects of sexuality; some focus on physical functioning, some focus on body image, and others on relationships.

Several cancer-specific sexual assessment instruments have also been developed. The Sexual Adjustment Questionnaire (SAQ) was designed to assess the impact of cancer and surgery on sexual function.[72] SAQ is a self-administered measure assessing desire, activity level, relationship, arousal, sexual techniques, and orgasm. SAQ has recently been modified by the Radiation Therapy Oncology Group (RTOG). Psychometric properties show the SAQ to be a reliable and valid tool to assess sexual function in men with prostate cancer.[73] Bransfield[74] developed a site-specific scale for assessing sexual function after treatment for gynecologic cancer. This, too, is a self-administered questionnaire, but as with SAQ, it could easily be adapted to interview format for inclusion in a nursing history. Krumm and Lamberti[75] developed a sexual behavior questionnaire for women following treatment for cervical cancer. This questionnaire also assesses the partner's sexual function. It could easily be used with any disease site and for males as well as females. Both Wilmoth[76] and Thirlaway et al.[77] have developed questionnaires to measure sexual activity/behaviors in women treated for breast cancer.

Physical Assessment

History

In addition to the specific questions on sexuality just described, a comprehensive sexual history includes an assessment of all the factors that could affect sexual functioning, including:

1. *Cancer diagnosis.* Stage, grade, treatment, expected side effects, and prognosis.

2. *Age.* There are normal physiologic changes that occur with age that affect sexual function, described in detail elsewhere.[78,79]

3. *Gender.* Males tend to suffer performance-related disorders (e.g., erectile disorder, premature ejaculation), whereas females tend to experience dysfunctions involving desire or satisfaction (e.g., inhibited sexual desire, inhibited orgasm) with performance disorders being relatively infrequent.[80]

4. *Pre-illness sexual functioning.* This has been found to be the best predictor of posttreatment functioning.

5. *Pre-illness sexual relationship(s).* Poor or dysfunctional premorbid sexual relationships are not likely to improve after cancer diagnosis or therapy. Good, healthy premorbid sexual relationships are likely to endure or even improve posttherapy despite significant sexual dysfunction related to disease and treatment.

6. *Cultural/ethnic background.* Sexual values and rules are taught to us from birth. The process, called sexual enculturation, exerts an enormous amount of social pressure to conform to accepted norms. These norms, however, vary widely among cultures.[4]

7. *Body image.* As it contributes to the larger concept of self-esteem should be assessed using verbal and nonverbal cues.

8. *Concomitant chronic illness.* May have an impact on sexual functioning due to effects on the muscular, neurologic, and/or vascular systems (e.g., diabetes, hypertension, arthritis, urologic problems).

9. *Concomitant psychological illness.* A history of psychiatric problems or sexual abuse may have an impact on sexual functioning. More commonly with cancer patients, the psychological trauma of the cancer diagnosis may cause dysfunction. Anxiety, fear of pain, amputation, death, depression, financial worries, grieving over loss of role functioning, etc., all may negatively affect sexual function.

10. *Medications.* Such as antihypertensives, antipsychotics, antidepressants, opiates, recreational drugs such as cocaine, tobacco, marijuana, sedatives, and alcohol may cause decreased libido and erectile dysfunction.[81]

Female physical

The female pelvic exam is performed with the woman in the dorsolithotomy position with her feet in stirrups. Inspection and palpation are used to determine any effects of cancer or therapy that may interfere with sexual functioning. The vulva is examined for lesions, excoriation, edema, scarring, desquamation, or hair loss. The labia are separated and the clitoris is inspected for edema, excoriation, lesions, secretions, and atrophy. The urethral opening is inspected for signs of inflammation or discharge. The vagina is spread using a speculum for inspection for lesions, inflammation, bleeding, discharge, edema, petechiae, adhesions, fistula, stenosis, and atrophy. The speculum is removed and well-lubricated gloved index and middle fingers are inserted into the vagina. If the cervix is still in place, it is located with the index finger; if not, the apex of the vagina is palpated for masses. The patient is asked to squeeze down on your fingers to assess the strength of the pubococcygeal muscle, which envelopes the penis during intercourse and contracts during orgasm. The fingers can be spread laterally to break up any adhesions caused by surgery or radiation. Vaginal tone and length are assessed. The external hand presses down on the abdomen just below the umbilicus to bring the uterus and ovaries (if present) toward the internal fingers for assessment of size, shape, mobility, tenderness, and masses.

Male genital exam

The male genital examination includes an assessment of inflammatory, endocrinologic, neurologic, traumatic, neoplastic, vascular, or congenital disorders associated with problems of erection or ejaculation.

The penis and scrotum are inspected for lesions and areas of discoloration. The entire length of the penis is palpated for lesions and areas of plaque formation and masses. Retract the foreskin, if present, to examine the glans penis for signs of infection or other lesions. Inspect the urethral meatus for any signs of discharge.

The scrotum is inspected and the testicles palpated for masses, swelling, and areas of increased tenderness. The epididymis and spermatic cord containing the vas deferens are palpated.

The rectal area is inspected after the genitalia in both males and females. Again, effects of cancer and therapies are assessed when appropriate. The skin is inspected for lesions, edema, excoriation, desquamation, fistula, bleeding, and mucus discharge. The rectum is palpated for lesions and muscle tone. The importance of rectal functioning in many sexual relationships, particularly male homosexual relationships, should not be undervalued.

Diagnostic evaluation

Aside from patient interviews and a scattering of patient self-reports, there has been little advancement over the years in diagnostic evaluation of sexual function. For obvious reasons, scientific techniques and sophisticated equipment are difficult to apply to the evaluation of sexual health. The equipment and environment used by Masters and Johnson in the 1950s and 1960s to measure sexual response are not available or even commonly acceptable for use in routine examinations. Equipment, called the *photoplethysmograph,* does exist to quantify sexual excitement; however, it is not without technical difficulties.[82]

Several investigators have attempted to measure the effects of intracavitary radiation therapy on the vagina by assessing vaginal length. Most of this research has used rudimentary measures such as finger length[49] to assess stenosis. Bruner et al.[50] were the first to report using a modified vaginal dilator calibrated in centimeters to measure vaginal length. Other measures of radiation effect on the vaginal mucosa have included vaginal smears and punch biopsy to assess epithelial changes and estrogen effect.[83]

Possibly because the penis is an external sexual organ and easier to assess or because clinical research trials have focused disproportionately on males, there are a variety of physiologic techniques available to assess erectile dysfunction. Rigiscans are conducted to determine the extent of erectile dysfunction and are especially helpful to differentiate psychogenic from organic etiologies. A cuff is placed around the shaft of the penis at bedtime in a sleep laboratory. During the night the occurrence, duration, and extent of penile erections are monitored and recorded.

A simpler technique to determine the man's ability to have erections is to securely place a length of postage stamps around the circumference of the shaft of the penis before the man goes to bed at night. If in the morning the stamps are separated, it may indicate that the man had an erection during the night.

In certain patients, a variety of radiologic studies such as sonography and angiography may also be conducted to evaluate the vascular and neurologic components of the erection.[84]

Although not a direct measure of sexual function, hormone levels can be checked to determine the impact of certain cancer treatments that cause ovarian ablation in women and decreased estrogen and testosterone suppression in men.

Degrees of Toxicity

In addition to being given a pelvic exam and some method of assessing vaginal stenosis, women are questioned regarding pain or bleeding with intercourse, and whether they have sufficient vaginal lubrication for intercourse. Men are questioned as to the degree of impotence. Does he awaken in the morning with an erection? Is he able to have voluntary erections? What is the quality of the erection? How firm is the erection? How long does it last?

Symptom Management

Prevention

The most effective means of managing sexual morbidity in patients treated for cancer is prevention. Any technique that spares or minimizes damage to sexual organs or body image, such as lumpectomy for breast cancer or nerve-sparing prostatectomies, is helpful in maintaining sexual health.

Preparing the patient prior to therapy for the impact cancer treatment may have on sexual function should be part of the informed consent and decision-making process. One of the most commonly cited methods of prevention and intervention for sexual morbidity is the P-LI-SS-IT Model developed by Annon,[85] which stands for *p*ermission, *li*mited *i*nformation, *s*pecific *s*uggestions, and *i*ntensive *t*herapy. Table 29-4 describes this four-step process that is designed not only to diagnose and counsel the patient, but to lead the healthcare professional through an increasingly specialized sequence of activities that can be gauged to their own level of comfort and expertise with the topic. Shipes and Lehr[86] estimate that about 70% of sexual problems related to cancer therapy can be managed using the first three levels of this mode. Approximately 30% of patients will require intensive therapy.

The P-LI-SS-IT model can assist in dealing with con-

TABLE 29-4   P-LI-SS-IT Model

Permission
Permission to have or not have sexual thoughts, feelings, or concerns begins at initial consultation. It is up to the oncology health-care professional to initiate the discussion of sexual matters related to diagnosis and therapy. If the health professional does not provide a safe and open environment for sexual discussion, it is unlikely that the patient will broach the topic.

Limited Information
Specific, factual information about the impact therapy will have on sexual function should be part of the treatment decision-making process (e.g., impotence rate after treatment for prostate cancer). It should dispel myths about cancer or therapy (e.g., breast cancer is not caused by too much fondling, sex will not infect the partner with cancer, sex after radiation therapy will not cause the partner to become radioactive, etc.). This information should also begin with a general statement about available treatments for sexual dysfunctions that will be discussed in detail as therapy continues and as the next level of the model is reached.

Specific Suggestions
A sexual history is necessary before providing specific suggestions. It is necessary to know if the sexual dysfunction the patient faces is related to sexual organ dysfunction, changes in body image, treatment-related side effects or relationship discord. Once the problem(s) are diagnosed, concrete methods of dealing with them should be presented in language the patient can understand. This level of the model requires a comfort and knowledge of sexuality beyond cursory medical jargon that would suffice in the first two levels. It also requires an armamentarium of approaches that includes teaching new sexual behaviors, new options for sexual expression, improved communications skills, and medical and surgical interventions.

Intensive Therapy
When the patient's sexual dysfunction is severe, prolonged, existed before cancer diagnosis or treatment, or is related to marital problems, intensive therapy is required. The patient should also be referred for more intensive therapy when sexual counseling is beyond the knowledge or comfort level of the healthcare professional. It has been estimated that only about 30% of cancer patients would require referrals at this level of the P-LI-SS-IT Model.

cerns directly or indirectly related to sexuality. Suggestions for preventing some of the major side effects of therapy from severely altering sexual desire, activity, or body image follow.

1. *Depression or anxiety.* Antidepressants may be useful but some can interfere with erectile function; consult with a pharmacist.

2. *Fatigue.* Napping prior to sexual activity as well as avoiding heavy meals and alcohol can be helpful. Sexual positions can be suggested that require minimal effort, such as the side-lying position during sexual activity (see Figure 29-1A and 29-1F).

3. *Pain.* Timing of medication is important prior to sexual activity. The goal is to provide pain control without drowsiness. Relaxation techniques, warm baths or soaks, and massage may decrease pain and, when done as a couple, can be a sensual opportunity for foreplay.

4. *Nausea.* Medicating prior to sexual activity is suggested. A light meal or crackers prior to activity may be helpful. Usual accoutrements of sexual activity such as perfumes, colognes, and scented candles may have to be avoided if smells cause nausea.

5. *Secretions.* Patients with tracheostomies should suction or otherwise clear the tracheostomy prior to sexual activity; heavy breathing could cause mucus production. If a concern remains about secretions, a thin gauze can be placed over the tracheostomy to allow ventilation but prevent overflow. Positions for sexual activity that minimize fear of expectorating on their partner can be suggested (Figure 29-1H). The stoma should be cleaned and

the tracheostomy pad and ribbon changed to enhance appearance.

6. *Elimination.* Ostomies should be emptied prior to sexual activity. Deodorizers are available if odors are a concern. Pouch covers are also available to shield the bag's contents. (see Figures 29-1C, 1G, 1J for positions involving ostomy bags). For women with dwelling urinary catheters, penile penetration is possible (see Figure 29-1F). The tube should be cleansed with mild soap and water to remove all secretions; the catheter can be bent upward and taped to the abdomen. For men with indwelling urinary catheters, intercourse is more challenging but possible. Again, the catheter should be washed with warm soap and water to remove secretions. The catheter can be bent back along the penis and taped to the abdomen. A well-lubricated condom is placed over the penis and catheter, and intercourse can be achieved.

Therapeutic Approaches

Interventions for sexual dysfunctions related to therapy can be psychological, behavioral, medical, or surgical.

Psychological

Psychological intervention includes investigating and dealing with fears, anxieties, and depression related to diagnosis and therapy. It includes exploring personal, interpersonal, and intrapersonal concerns and conflicts. Patients with histories of sexual abuse or marital problems should be referred to a professional counselor or psychologist.

Behavioral

Behavioral interventions include enhancing communication between partners and creating a sensual environment or "setting the mood" with whatever appeals to the couple—candlelight, wine, massage, bathing together, sensual or erotic clothing, erotic pictures, movies, etc. It includes exploring alternative forms of sexual expression such as touching, caressing, and finding new erogenous zones (e.g., neck, inner thighs, buttocks, feet). Suggestions could include trying new sexual positions (Figure 29-1) or trying sexual activities such as oro-genital sex or mutual masturbation. Anal intercourse is an alternative technique requiring education about the use of lubricants and gentle dilation. Use of mechanical devices such as vibrators can help maintain sexual gratification if the male patient is impotent and the female partner desires vaginal penetration or the homosexual partner desires anal penetration.

Behavioral interventions also address activities that maintain a positive body image, such as good hygiene, perfumes, colognes, and wigs (with wig tape to hold the piece in place during sexual activity). Cosmetic and prosthetic techniques and devices are available to camouflage treatment-related defects. Breast prosthetics can now be fashioned to match both the shape and color of the existing breast. Adhesives can hold the prosthesis in place so bras or nightgowns can be removed during sexual activity if desired.

Medical

Medical interventions include drug therapy and medical devices that maintain sexual function. Pharmacologic interventions include hormone replacement therapy for women who have experienced ovarian ablation and vasoactive agents for men who have lost erectile function. Hormone replacement therapy has been controversial after breast or endometrial cancer, although several clinical trials are studying the risk-benefit outcomes in certain of these populations. Excluding patients with a history of thrombophlebitis, women treated for cervical cancer should be encouraged to take estrogen replacement therapy (ERT). Aside from the cardiovascular and bone-density benefits, ERT has been reported to prevent atrophic vaginitis and dyspareunia, maintain libido, improve sense of well-being, and prevent postmenopausal depression.[87,88] Estrogen can be administered orally, transdermally, or intravaginally. Progesterone is added to prevent endometrial cancer when the uterus is intact but may not be necessary after hysterectomy or uterine irradiation. Hormone replacement therapy is addressed in detail in Chapter 8, Menopausal Symptoms.

Pharmacologic and nonpharmacologic interventions are available that can restore voluntary erectile function for sexual intercourse. Vasoactive agents such as papaverine and phentolamine mesylate cause temporary vasodilation and vasocongestion within the spongy tissue of the penis by reducing the resistance of the arteriolar and cavernosal smooth muscle tissue.[89] This leads to an increased arterial inflow and subsequent venous trapping and filling of the corpus cavernosum, resulting in penile erection.

The medication is injected into the lateral aspect of the shaft of the penis. A good-quality erection usually develops within 8 to 10 minutes and can last 30 to 90 minutes. Orgasm and ejaculation are not adversely affected. Penile pain and bruising can occur, however. With long-term use, scar tissue and plaques can form along the shaft of the penis and result in its disfigurement. Therefore, the patient is instructed to use the medication no more than twice a week. Another adverse effect of this drug therapy is priapism (prolonged erections). The patient is instructed to seek medical attention to have the blood drained if the erection lasts longer than 4 hours.

Systemic effects of these vasoactive agents include syncope, flushing, and hypotension. They are contraindicated for patients with unstable cardiac disease, sickle-cell disease, hypotension, transient ischemic attacks, or significant penile venous incompetence.

It may be difficult for the man to learn to give himself an injection into his penis. Patient education is crucial for this intervention to be successful. The self-care guide addressing this procedure may be helpful (see Appendix 29A). Close follow-up and monitoring of the patient for the proper use and administration of the medication are important.

Newer techniques of administering pharmacologic therapies for erectile dysfunction are gaining popularity. Urethral insertion of a gel pellet of prostaglandin E1 allows for mucosal absorption of the medication into the corpora cavernosum (Figure 29-2). Within 5 to 10 minutes, an erection is achieved.[90] An oral medication, sildenafil, is also available. Sildenafil is a 5-phosphodiesterase inhibitor that acts specifically on the penis. The pill is taken 1 hour prior to intercourse, and with stimulation erections can be achieved and last up to 1 hour.

Medical devices that help maintain sexual function include vaginal dilators for women and vacuum devices for men. Women at risk for vaginal stenosis are directed to have something dilate the vagina at least three times per week, be it a penis or a dilator, although there is to date no scientific research to support this practice. Patient instructions for use of a vaginal dilator are provided in the self-care guide to vaginal stenosis (Appendix 29B). Instructions for vaginal lubrication are provided in the self-care guide to vaginal dryness (Appendix 29C).

Vacuum devices are the least invasive and least expensive technique for achieving erections.[91] A hollow tube is placed around the flaccid penis and vacuum is applied,

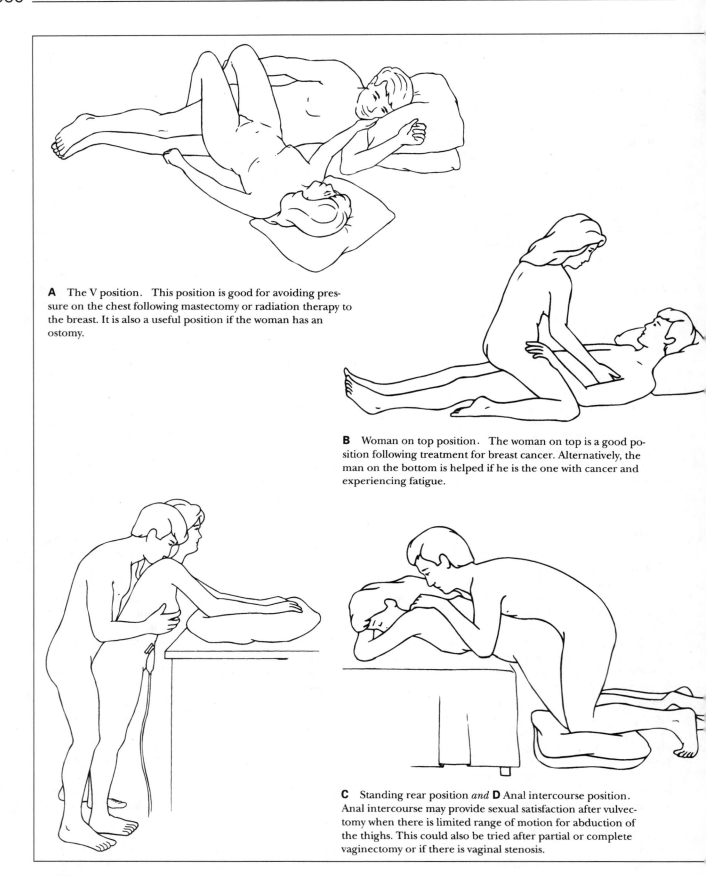

A The V position. This position is good for avoiding pressure on the chest following mastectomy or radiation therapy to the breast. It is also a useful position if the woman has an ostomy.

B Woman on top position. The woman on top is a good position following treatment for breast cancer. Alternatively, the man on the bottom is helped if he is the one with cancer and experiencing fatigue.

C Standing rear position *and* **D** Anal intercourse position. Anal intercourse may provide sexual satisfaction after vulvectomy when there is limited range of motion for abduction of the thighs. This could also be tried after partial or complete vaginectomy or if there is vaginal stenosis.

FIGURE 29-1A–J Sexual positions to aid sexual adjustment after cancer therapy.

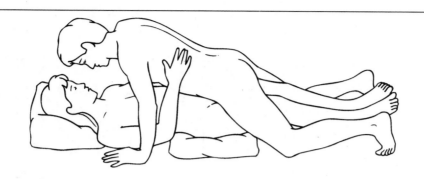

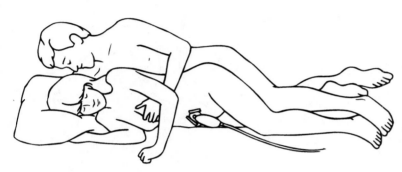

E Adducted thigh position *and* **F** Side-lying position. If the vagina has been surgically shortened or if range of motion is limited due to vulvectomy or bone metastasis to hips or thighs, these positions may facilitate sexual intercourse. Lubrication of the adducted thighs in (E) creates the sensation of extended vaginal length and prevents deep penile thrusting. Vaginal rear entry in (F) accomplishes the same thing. This position is particularly useful for the woman with an indwelling Foley catheter that can be placed anteriorly or taped up on the abdomen.

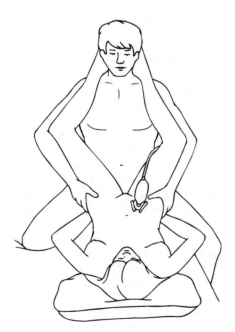

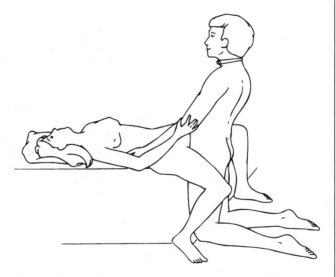

G The diamond position. This position does not require breast, chest, or abdominal pressure on the woman if any of these areas are being treated for cancer. This is an alternative position for the woman with an ostomy.

H Kneeling position. For men with a tracheotomy this upright position minimizes fear of mucus hitting their partner. It also allows for maximum chest expansion if he is uncomfortable or feels short of breath with pressure on his chest.

FIGURE 29-1A–J (*continued*)

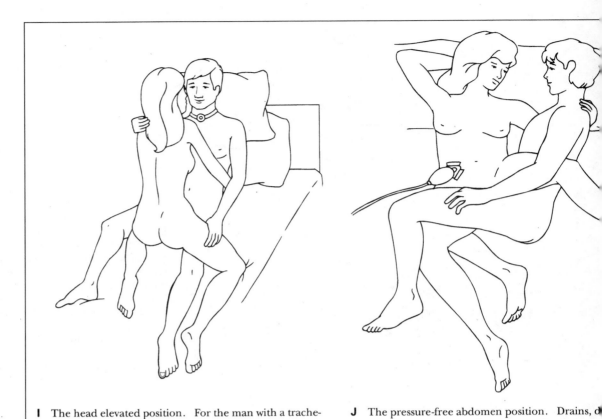

I The head elevated position. For the man with a tracheotomy fearing shortness of breath while lying down, this position is helpful. It is also good if the man is experiencing fatigue.

J The pressure-free abdomen position. Drains, d catheters, or ostomies can be accommodated using position.

FIGURE 29-1A–J (*continued*)

creating a negative pressure (see Figure 29D-1 in Appendix 29D). Blood flows into the penis, filling the corpora cavernosa, and when an erection is achieved, an elastic constriction band is placed around the base of the penis to preserve the rigidity of the penis to allow sexual intercourse. The constriction may be maintained for up to 30 minutes. The vacuum device may be used daily (see self-care guide Appendix 29D). With excessive use, penile injury with ecchymosis can occur.

Some patients find the vacuum device cumbersome and time-consuming. It may be especially awkward for a single individual who is not involved in a long-term relationship. Because the penis is not erect proximal to the constriction band, the penis exhibits a "hinge" effect. Some decreased sensation in the penis also is possible because of the constriction band. In addition, blocked or retrograde ejaculation occurs because the ejaculate is trapped in the proximal urethra due to the constriction band.

No matter the method, one study found that men who used erectile aids at least 50% of the time after either radical or nerve-sparing prostatectomy had statistically significant improvements, over those who did not use the aids, in the areas of frequency of sexual activity, erection, orgasm, desire, and satisfaction.[92]

Surgical

Surgical interventions to minimize the s cancer therapies create include breast re vaginal reconstruction, and penile implan construction is most common performed implants placed underneath the subcutan pectoral fascia. Other implants, such as salir investigation, but the dual role of the Silas mains popular, as it can serve as both a tiss and implant requiring one less surgery. O the Silastic implant can be injected over tim the size until the affected breast is symme unaffected breast. The transverse rectus abd ocutaneous (TRAM) flap technique, re using the rectus abdominal muscle, has attention. The popularity of this procedure double cosmetic effect. A football-shaped inc below the umbilicus and the muscle flap is under the skin to the affected breast. T mound is contoured to match the symmetr fected breast and the removal of the rectu muscle serves as a "tummy tuck." The surger 5 hours, and as expected, recovery is lon standard breast reconstruction. A less comm

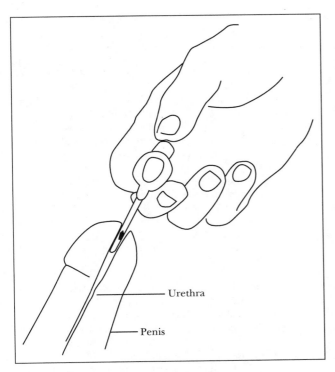

FIGURE 29-2 Insertion of prostaglandin E1 pellet with applicator.

involves swinging a flap of the latissimus dorsi muscle around to the chest and creating a breast mound.

Nipple reconstruction for any of the three methods is usually done at a later date about 3 months after reconstruction. When using the Silastic implant, one technique for nipple creation is overexpanding the breast slightly, removing some of the fluid, and using a pursestring-like technique to form a raised nipple. Tattooing is then used to match the pigment of the unaffected nipple. Other methods of nipple development include using skin from the labia, inner thigh, inner arm, ear lobe, or toe.

Vaginal reconstruction may be required following complete or partial vaginectomy performed as part of pelvic exenteration for recurrent cervical cancer, rectal cancer, or for the relatively rare vaginal cancer. Tissue from the inner thigh, the gracilis muscle, is used to create a neovagina. Cosmetic and functional results are quite good. Dilation is required for the remainder of the woman's life to maintain patency, and lubricants may be required for easier penile penetration.

Although the procedure for vaginal reconstruction was first described in 1976 with the assumption that it would improve sexual adjustment after pelvic exenteration, it took 20 years before anyone actually tested this assumption. In what appears to be the only study on the subject, 52.5% of 40 women who underwent vaginal reconstruction with a mean follow-up of 6 years resumed sexual activity. The most frequently cited sexual adjustment problems were self-consciousness about ostomy, dis-

comfort being seen in the nude by partner, vaginal dryness, and vaginal discharge.[93]

Three types of penile prostheses are available: malleable (semirigid), semiinflatable, and fully inflatable prostheses. The malleable prosthesis is convenient and easy to use (see self-care guide Appendix 29E). Two solid silicone rods are placed into the corpora cavernosa. These rods are firm enough to allow sexual intercourse but leave the patient with a permanent erection. The erection is sometimes difficult to conceal but may be positioned up against the abdomen and secured with elastic briefs when the person is not engaging in sexual intercourse.

The semiinflatable prosthesis consists of two cylinders, each with its own pump and reservoir, which are placed into the corpora cavernosa. The patient pumps behind the glans penis several times to move the fluid from the reservoirs and into the two cylinders to create an erection at the site of inflation. Deflation is accomplished by holding the penis downward for 10 seconds and then releasing the penis. This allows the fluid to return to the reservoir. The advantage of the semiinflatable prosthesis is that full erections are possible with no permanent erection. However, although the penis is more concealable, it never becomes totally flaccid. There is also no increase in the girth of the penis (see self-care guide Appendix 29G).

The fully inflatable prosthesis consists of three parts: a spheric reservoir containing saline, two cylinders, and a pump with a release valve (see Figure 29G-1 in self-care guide Appendix 29G). The reservoir is implanted in the lower abdomen in the prevesicle space between the pubic bone and the bladder, under the rectus muscle. The cylinders are placed in the corpora cavernosa and the pump is placed in the scrotal sac. To operate, the pump is squeezed to move the fluid from the reservoir to the cylinders in the penis to produce an erection. By pressing the release valve on the pump, the fluid returns to the reservoir and the penis becomes flaccid (see self-care guide Appendix 29G). The fully inflatable prosthesis produces more natural erections, with an increased girth of the penis, and also allows for total flaccidity. However, manual dexterity is needed for the patient or partner to operate the pump skillfully.

A recent study of 50 men who underwent immediate placement of a penile prothesis while undergoing radical prostatectomy reported a 96% return to sexual intercourse (versus 10% to 20% normally reported after the same surgery without the prosthesis). No apparent increase in surgical morbidity was noted, however, 8% required surgical revisions for mechanical failure of the prosthesis.[94]

Educational Tools and Resources

Symptom management as outlined above may require referrals to surgeons, gynecologists, or urologists. Patients requiring intervention at the intensive therapy level of the P-LI-SS-IT model also need to be referred to appropriate medical professionals such as social workers, psychologists, psychiatrists, or sex therapists. It is best to have an updated list of resources on hand before taking the sexual history. Your institution may have some of these resources available; if not, the American Association of Sex Educators, Counselors and Therapists, Chicago, Illinois, publishes a nationwide directory.

Many of the cancer support groups, such as the American Cancer Society programs "I Can Cope" and "Look Good, Feel Better" and the national prostate support program "US TOO," deal with issues of body image and sexuality. The American Cancer Society has also published two excellent patient booklets, one for men and one for women with cancer, entitled *Sexuality and Cancer.*

Conclusion

Alteration in sexual functioning has for too long been the orphan nursing diagnosis. We know it exists but most of us choose to ignore it because of fear and lack of information. Adopting the practice of sexual assessment and incorporating sexual interventions into our practice is the only way to overcome this fear. Sexual health should be as much a routine concern of our caring for the patient with cancer as are the patient's physical and mental health.

References

1. Andersen BL, Woods X, Cryanowski J: Sexual self-schema as a possible predictor of sexual problems following cancer treatment. *Can J Hum Sexuality* 3:165–170, 1994
2. Nevidjon B: Sexuality, in McIntire S, Cioppa A (eds): *Sexuality.* New York: Wiley, 1984, p. 258
3. Woods N: Toward a holistic perspective of human sexuality: Alterations in sexual health and nursing diagnosis. *Holistic Nurs Pract* 1:1–11, 1987
4. Brink P: Cultural aspects of sexuality. *Holistic Nurs Pract* 1:12–20, 1987
5. Schover L: The impact of breast cancer on sexuality, body image. *CA Cancer J Clin* 41:112–120, 1991
6. Barni S, Mondin R: Sexual dysfunction in treated breast cancer patients. *Ann Oncol* 8:149–153, 1997
7. Poulsen B, Graversen HP, Beckmann J, Blichert-Toft M: A comparative study of post-operative psychosocial function in women with primary operable breast cancer randomized to breast conservation therapy or mastectomy. *Eur J Surg Oncol* 23:327–334, 1997
8. Fallowfield L, Hall A: Psychosocial and sexual impact of diagnosis and treatment of breast cancer. *Br Med Bull* 47:388–399, 1991
9. Gilbar O, Ungar L, Fried G, et al: Living with mastectomy and breast conservation treatment: Who suffers more? *Support Care Cancer* 5:322–326, 1997
10. Anderson BL, Woods XA, Copeland LJ: Sexual self-schema and sexual morbidity among gynecologic cancer survivors. *J Consult Clin Psychol* 65:221–229, 1997
11. Podratz KC, Symmonds RE, Taylor WF: Carcinoma of the vulva: Analysis of treatment failures. *Am J Obstet Gynecol* 143:814–817, 1982
12. Glasgow M, Halfin V, Althausen A: Sexual response and cancer. *CA Cancer J Clin* 37:322–333, 1987
13. Zussman L, Zussman S, Sunley R, et al: Sexual response after hysterectomy-oophorectomy: Recent studies and reconsideration of psychogenesis. *Am J Obstet Gynecol* 140:725–729, 1981
14. Lalos O, Lalos A: Urinary, climacteric and sexual symptoms one year after treatment of endometrial cancer. *Eur J Gynecol Oncol* 17:128–136, 1996
15. DiSaia P, Creasman WT: *Clinical Gynecologic Oncology* (ed 3). St. Louis: Mosby, 1984
16. Howard G: Fertility following cancer therapy. *Clin Oncol* 3:283–287, 1991
17. Kaempfer S, Wiley F, Hoffman D: Fertility considerations and procreative alternatives in cancer care. *Semin Oncol Nurs* 1:25–34, 1985
18. Kaempfer S, Major D: Fertility considerations in the gynecologic oncology patient. *Oncol Nurs Forum* 13:23–27, 1986
19. Madorsky M, Ashmalla M, Schussler I, et al: Post-prostatectomy impotence. *J Urol* 115:401–404, 1976
20. Herr H: Quality of life in prostate cancer patients. *CA Cancer J Clin* 47:207–217, 1997
21. Talcott JA, Ricker P, Clark JA, et al: Patient-reported symptoms after primary therapy for early prostate cancer: Results of a prospective cohort study. *J Clin Oncol* 16:275–283, 1998
22. Walsh P, Mostwin J: Radical prostatectomy and cystoprostatectomy with preservation of potency: Results using a new nerve-sparing technique. *Br J Urol* 56:694–697, 1984
23. Chai DC, Broderick GA, Malloy TR, et al: Erectile dysfunction following minimally invasive treatments for prostate cancer. *Urology* 48:100–104, 1996
24. Koeman M, Van Driel MF, Weijmar Schultz WCM, et al: Orgasm after radical prostatectomy. *Br J Urol* 77:861–864, 1996
25. Ellis W, Grayhack J: Sexual function in aging males after orchiectomy and estrogen therapy. *J Urol* 89:895–899, 1963
26. Schover L, vonEschenbach A: Sexual and marital counseling with men treated for testicular cancer. *J Sex Marital Ther* 10:29–40, 1984
27. Narayan P, Lange P, Fraley E: Ejaculation and fertility after extended retroperitoneal lymph node dissection for testicular cancer. *J Urol* 127:685–688, 1982
28. Bracken B: Cancer of the testis, penis, and urethra: The impact of therapy on sexual function, in vonEschenbach A, Rodriquez D (eds): *Cancer of the Testis, Penis, and Urethra: The Impact of Therapy on Sexual Function.* Boston: Hall, 1981
29. Bachers E: Sexual dysfunction and genitourinary cancer. *Semin Oncol Nurs* 1:18–24, 1985
30. Schrover LR, Evans RB, vonEschenbach AL: Sexual rehabilitation and male radical cystectomy. *J Urol* 136:1015–1017, 1986
31. Anderson B: Sexual functioning morbidity among cancer survivors. *Cancer* 55:1835–1842, 1985
32. Zenico T, Neri W, Zoli M, et al: Sexual dysfunction after excision of the rectum. *Acta Urol Belg* 57:213–216, 1989
33. Koukouras D, Spiliotis J, Scopa C, et al: Radical consequence in the sexuality of male patients operated for colorectal carcinoma. *Eur J Surg Oncol* 17:285–288, 1991

34. Monga U, Tan G, Osterman HJ, et al: Sexuality in head and neck cancer patients. *Arch Phys Med Rehabil* 78:292–304, 1997

35. Sugarbaker P, Barofsky I, Rosenberg S, et al: Quality of life assessment of patients in extremity sarcoma clinical trials. *Surgery* 91:17–23, 1982

36. Cella D, Tross S: Psychological adjustment to survival from Hodgkin's disease. *J Consult Clin Psychol* 54:616–620, 1986

37. Olweny C, Tuttner C, Rofe P: Long-term effects of cancer treatment and consequences of cure: Cancer survivors enjoy quality of life similar to their neighbours. *Eur J Cancer Clin Oncol* 29A:826–830, 1993

38. Heinrich-Rynning T: Prostatic cancer treatments and their effects on sexual functioning. *Oncol Nurs Forum* 14:37–41, 1987

39. Lancaster J: Women's experiences of gynecological cancer treated with radiation. *Curationis* 16:37–42, 1993

40. Singer P, Tasch E, Stocking S, et al: Sex or survival: Trade-offs between quality and quantity of life. *J Clin Oncol* 9:328–334, 1991

41. Aaronson N, Bartelink H, vanDongen J, et al: Evaluation of breast-conserving therapy: Clinical, methodological and psychosocial perspectives. *Eur J Surg Oncol* 14:133–140, 1988

42. Holmberg L, Omne-Ponten M, Burns T, et al: Psychosocial adjustment after mastectomy and breast-conserving treatment. *Cancer* 64:969–974, 1989

43. Havenga K, Enker W, McDermott K, et al: Male and female sexual and urinary function after total mesorectal excision with autonomic nerve preservation for carcinoma of the rectum. *J Am Coll Surg* 182:495–502, 1996

44. Dnistrian A, Schwartz M, Fracchia A, et al: Endocrine consequences of CMF adjuvant therapy in premenopausal and postmenopausal breast cancer patients. *Cancer* 51:803–809, 1983

45. Sherins R, DeVita V: Effects of drug treatment of lymphoma on male reproductive capacity. *Ann Intern Med* 79:216–220, 1973

46. Frank D, Dornbush R, Webster S, et al: Mastectomy and sexual behavior: A pilot study. *Sexuality Disability* 1:16–26, 1978

47. Grigsby PW, Russell A, Bruner DW, et al: Late injury of cancer therapy on the female reproductive tract. *Int J Radiat Oncol Biol Phys* 31:1281–1299, 1995

48. Seibel M, Graves W, Freeman M: Carcinoma of the cervix and sexual function. *Obstet Gynecol* 55:484–487, 1980

49. Vasicka A, Popovich, Brausch C: Post radiation course of patients with cervical carcinoma. *Obstet Gynecol* 11:403–414, 1958

50. Bruner DW, Lanciano R, Keegan M, et al: Vaginal stenosis and sexual function following intracavitary radiation for the treatment of cervical and endometrial carcinoma. *Int J Radiat Oncol Biol Phys* 27:825–830, 1993

51. Ray G, Trueblood H, Enright L, et al: Oophoropexy: A means of preserving ovarian function following pelvic megavoltage radiotherapy for Hodgkin's disease. *Radiology* 96:175–180, 1970

52. Thomas P, Winstanly D, Peckham M, et al: Reproductive and endocrine function in patients with Hodgkin's disease: Effects of oophoropexy and irradiation. *Br J Cancer* 33:226–231, 1976

53. Banker FL: The preservation of potency after external beam irradiation for prostate cancer. *Int J Radiat Oncol Biol Phys* 15:219–220, 1988

54. Rowley M, Leach D, Warner G, et al: Effect of graded doses of ionizing radiation on the human testes. *Radiat Res* 59:665–678, 1974

55. Smith D, Babaian R: The effects of treatment for cancer on male fertility and sexuality. *Cancer Nurs* 15:2711–2715, 1992

56. Bruner DW, Hanlon A, Nicolaou N, Hanks H: Sexual function after radiotherapy I androgen deprivation for clinically localized prostate cancer in younger men (age 50–65). *Oncol Nurs Forum* 24:327, 1997

57. Kolodny R, Masters W, Johnson V: *Textbook of Sexual Medicine.* Boston: Little, Brown, 1979

58. Schain W: Sexual Problems of Patients with Cancer, in DeVita V, Hellman S, Rosenberg S (eds): *Sexual Problems of Patients with Cancer.* Philadelphia: Lippincott, 1982, pp. 278–291

59. Rosen R, Leiblum S: Treatment of male erectile disorder: Current options and dilemmas. *Sex Marital Ther* 8:5–7, 1993

60. Lief H, Payne T: Sexuality—Knowledge and attitudes. *Am J Nurs* 75:2026–2029, 1975

61. Fisher S, Levin D: The sexual knowledge and attitudes of professional nurses caring for oncology patients. *Cancer Nurs* 6:55–61, 1983

62. Wilson M, Williams H: Oncology nurses' attitudes and behaviors related to sexuality of patients with cancer. *Oncol Nurs Forum* 15:49–53, 1988

63. Pauly I: Influence of training and attitudes on sexual counseling in medical practice. *Med Aspects Human Sex* 6:84–117, 1972

64. Driscoll C, Coblel R, Caplan R: The sexual practices, attitudes and knowledge of family physicians. *Fam Pract Res J* 1:200–210, 1982

65. American Nurses Association and Oncology Nursing Society: *Statement on the Scope and Standards of Oncology Nursing Practice.* Washington, DC: American Nurses Publishing, 1996

66. Lamb M, Woods N: Sexuality and the cancer patient. *Cancer Nurs* 4:137–144, 1981

67. McPhetridge LM: Nursing history: One means to personalize care. *Am J Nurs* 68:73–74, 1968

68. Kolodny R, Masters W, Johnson V, et al: *Textbook of Human Sexuality for Nurses.* Boston: Little, Brown, 1979

69. Andersen B: How cancer affects sexual functioning. *Oncology* 4:81–88, 1990

70. Andersen BL, Cryanowski JM: Women's sexual self-schema. *J Pers Soc Psychol* 67:1079–1100, 1994

71. Schiavi R, Derogatis L, Kuriansky J, et al: Development of the sexual adjustment questionnaire. *J Sex Marital Ther* 5:169–224, 1979

72. Waterhouse J, Metcalfe M: Development of the sexual adjustment questionnaire. *Oncol Nurs Forum* 13:53–59, 1986

73. Bruner D, Scott C, McGowan D, et al: Validation of the Sexual Adjustment Questionnaire (SAQ) in prostate cancer patients enrolled in RTOG studies 9020 and 9408. Abstract. ASTRO, Phoenix AZ, 1998

74. Bransfield D, Horiot J, Nadib A: Development of a scale for assessing sexual function after treatment for gynecologic cancer. *J Psychosoc Oncol* 2:3–19, 1984

75. Krumm S, Lamberti J: Changes in sexual behavior following radiation therapy for cervical cancer. *J Psychosom Obstet Gynecol* 14:51–63, 1993

76. Wilmoth MC, Townsend C: A comparison of the effects of lumpectomy versus mastectomy on sexual behaviors. *Cancer Pract* 3:279–285, 1995

77. Thirlaway K, Fallowfield L, Cuzick J: The sexual activity questionnaire: A measure of woman's sexual functioning. *Quality Life Res* 5:81–90, 1996

78. Frank-Stromborg M: Sexuality and the elderly cancer patient. *Semin Oncol Nurs* 1:49–55, 1985

79. Shell J, Smith C: Sexuality and the older person with cancer. *Oncol Nurs Forum* 21:553–558, 1994

80. Derogatis L: Article review: How cancer affects sexual functioning. *Oncology* 4:92–93, 1990

81. Wilson B: The effect of drugs on male sexual function and fertility. *Nurs Pract* 16:12–24, 1991

82. Beck J, Sakheim D, Borlow D: Operating characteristics of the vaginal photoplethysmograph: Some implications for its use. *Arch Sexual Behav* 12:43–58, 1983

83. Pitkin R, Bradbury J: The effect of topical estrogen on irradiated vaginal epithelium. *Am J Obstet Gynecol* 92:175–182, 1965

84. Rosen MP, Schwartz AN, Levine FJ, et al: Radiologic assessment of impotence: Angiography, sonography, cavernosography, and scintigraphy. *AJR Am J Roentgenol* 157:923–931, 1991

85. Annon J: *The Behavioral Treatment of Sexual Problems,* vol 1. Honolulu: Mercantile Printing, 1974

86. Shipes E, Lehr S: Sexuality and the male cancer patient. *Cancer Nurs* 3:375–381, 1982

87. Huppert L: Hormonal replacement therapy: Benefits, risks, doses. *Med Clin North Am* 71:23–38, 1987

88. Beard M, Curtis L: Libido, menopause, and estrogen replacement therapy. *Postgrad Med* 86:225–228, 1989

89. Williams L: Pharmacologic erection programs: A treatment option for erectile dysfunction. *Rehabil Nurs* 14:264–268, 1989

90. Padma-Nathan H, Hellstrom WJ, Kaiser FE, et al: Treatment of men with erectile dysfunction with transurethral alprostadil. Medical Urethral System for Erection Study Group. *N Engl J Med* 336:1–7, 1997

91. Lewis J: Nursing management for patients using external vacuum devices: A unique opportunity. *Urol Nurs* 13:80–85, 1993

92. Perez MA, Meyerowitz B, Lieskovsky G, et al: Quality of life and sexuality following radical prostatectomy in patients with prostate cancer who use or do not use erectile aids. *Urology* 50:740–746, 1997

93. Ratliff CR, Gershenson DM, Morris M, et al: Sexual adjustment of patients undergoing gracilis myocutaneous flap vaginal reconstruction in conjunction with pelvic exenteration. *Cancer* 78:2229–2235, 1996

94. Khoudary KP, DeWolf WL, Brunmy CO, et al: Immediate sexual rehabilitation by simultaneous placement of penile prosthesis in patients undergoing radical prostatectomy: Initial results in 50 patients. *Urology* 50:395–399, 1997

Self-Injection of Medication for Erections

Patient Name: _____

Description   Medication has been prescribed for you to enable you to have an erection. *This medication can be used no more than twice a week.* This medication is injected into the side of the penis when you are ready to have an erection. The erection develops in 8 to 10 minutes and can last for 30 to 90 minutes. This medication will not interfere with orgasm or ejaculation.

Learning Needs   You will learn to give yourself an injection and identify side effects of the medication. Ways to take care of those problems will be explained to you.

Procedure

1. Assemble equipment:

   - medication bottle
   - syringe and needle
   - alcohol swab

2. Wash your hands with soap and water. Dry your hands thoroughly.

3. Prepare the medication. Using the syringe and needle (30-gauge, ½ inch [13 mm]) provided you, withdraw the prescribed amount of medication into the syringe.

4. Select the site of injection along the left or right side of the penis where there are no veins, as shown in Figure 29A-1. It is important to alternate the areas where you inject the medication.

5. Wipe the site of the injection with an alcohol swab for 1 minute.

6. Grasp the penis firmly and stretch the skin taut by pulling the penis forward. You may lay the penis against the thigh.

7. Insert the entire length of the needle at a 90-degree angle, as shown in Figure 29A-2; the needle should not be leaning forward or back toward you.

8. Slowly inject the entire amount of medication into the penis.

9. Withdraw the needle and apply pressure to the injection site with a cotton ball or clean gauze for approximately 30 seconds or until the bleeding stops.

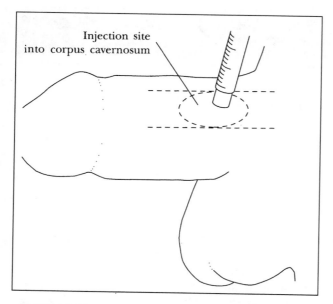

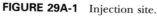

FIGURE 29A-1 Injection site.

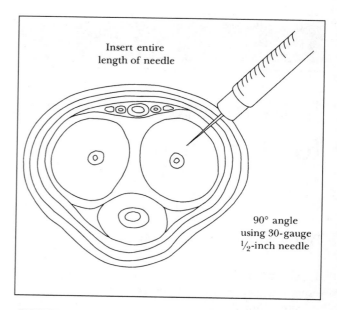

FIGURE 29A-2 Insert the needle at a 90-degree angle (cross-section view).

Management   There are some side effects that the injection of this medication can cause. You need to watch for:

- Bleeding at the site of the injection:
  Apply pressure to the injection site until the bleeding stops.

- Pain or numbness at the tip of the penis:
  This is a temporary effect that goes away in 2 to 3 minutes.

- Flushing or dizziness:
  Lie down for 5 to 10 minutes or until the symptoms subside. Call your doctor if the flushing or dizziness lasts longer than 20 minutes.

- Extreme bruising or swelling:
  Firmly compress the entire penis with your hand for 10 minutes and do not perform self-injection again until instructed by your doctor.

- Prolonged erections, lasting longer than 4 hours:
  Call your doctor or go to the emergency room of your hospital.

- Scars or areas of tenderness on the penis:
  Call your doctor for an examination.

Follow-up   Be sure you understand what to expect and what to do should problems occur. Notify your nurse and/or doctor if any of the following occurs:

- Flushing or dizziness lasting more than 20 minutes.

- Extreme bruising or swelling.

- Prolonged erection, lasting longer than 4 hours.

- Scars or areas of tenderness on the penis.

If you are unsure of any of the instructions, be sure to clarify them with your doctor or nurse.

Phone Numbers Call your doctor or nurse if you have any problems with injecting this medication.

Nurse: _____ Phone: _____

Physician: _____ Phone: _____

Other: _____ Phone: _____

Comments

Patient's Signature: _____ Date: _____

Nurse's Signature: _____ Date: _____

Source: Bruner DW, Iwamoto RR: Altered sexual health, in Yarbro CH, Frogge MH, Goodman M (eds): *Cancer Symptom Management* (ed 2). Sudbury: Jones and Bartlett, 1999. © Jones and Bartlett Publishers.

Vaginal Stenosis

Patient Name: _____

Symptom and Description   A possible late effect of radiation is a decreased supply of blood to the radiated vagina. This may lead to drier, tender, less elastic feeling in the vagina. Another possible side effect of radiation therapy is the formation of scar tissue that can lead to a shortened or closed vagina. These conditions are called vaginal *stenosis*. Regular use of a vaginal dilator may help prevent this. A vaginal dilator is a smooth plastic cylinder measuring 6 inches (15 cm) in length. Vaginal dilators come in four different sizes (diameters)—extra small, small, medium, and large.

Learning Needs   You will need to learn how to use a vaginal dilator to keep the vagina open.

Prevention   Vaginal stenosis may be prevented in two ways: by regular sexual intercourse that includes penile penetration at least three times per week, or by using a dilator with a prescribed cream or jelly. Intercourse or the use of a vaginal dilator will keep the vagina open (dilated) and the tissue more elastic. This is important as it provides more comfort during sexual activity as well as pelvic exams and allows your doctor to see the treated area better.

Procedure

1. Stand with one leg up on a stool or toilet seat as if you were inserting a tampon, or lie back in bed or in a warm tub with your knees bent and apart.

2. If your doctor has ordered estrogen cream, spread it on the rounded end of the dilator. If you are not using estrogen cream, use a water-based lubricant such as K-Y jelly. Oil-based lubricants such as Vaseline or baby oil are *not* recommended and can cause irritation that may lead to discomfort or infection. Before applying cream/jelly, warm the tube by running it under hot water so that the lubricant will be more comfortable.

3. Insert the rounded end into your vagina as far as possible using firm but gentle pressure. Using an in-and-out motion, repeat this over 10 to 15 minutes.

4. The dilator may be washed with mild soap, dried well, and stored until next use.

Follow-up

- Be sure to see your physician for regularly scheduled follow-up pelvic examinations.
- If you experience pain with penile penetration deep thrusting, notify your nurse or physician.

Phone Numbers

Nurse: _____ Phone: _____

Physician: _____ Phone: _____

Other: _____ Phone: _____

Comments

Patient's Signature: _____ Date: _____

Nurse's Signature: _____ Date: _____

Source: Bruner DW, Iwamoto RR: Altered sexual health, in Yarbro CH, Frogge MH, Goodman M (eds): *Cancer Symptom Management* (ed 2). Sudbury: Jones and Bartlett, 1999. © Jones and Bartlett Publishers.

Vaginal Dryness

Patient Name: _____

Symptom and Description   A woman's ovaries stop producing estrogen at the time of normal menopause or after some cancer therapies such as surgical removal of the ovaries, radiation therapy to the ovaries, or certain chemotherapeutic drugs that shut down the ovaries. Without estrogen the vagina becomes drier and less elastic, sexual intercourse or masturbation may become uncomfortable or even painful, and the vagina may feel irritated and become infected. Proper use of vaginal lubricants may prevent vaginal dryness and restore vaginal moisture and integrity.

Learning Needs   You will need to learn proper use of vaginal lubricants.

Management/Procedure

- Use only water-based lubricants such as K-Y jelly (Johnson & Johnson), Astroglide (Astro-Lube, Inc.), or Replens (Parke-Davis).
- Do *not* use Vaseline, baby oil, or other oil-based lubricants because they can irritate the vagina.

For intercourse or masturbation:

- Squeeze the lubricant into the vagina just before intercourse, using the applicator. (If no applicator was supplied, you may use the plastic applicator that comes with medications for yeast infections or the one you used to use for contraceptive jellies or creams, if you have one; they can be washed in warm, soapy water and reused.)
- If one application of lubricant does not seem to last during intercourse, you can keep the lubricant by the bed. Cold lubricant can be annoying, so to keep it warm, the tube may be wrapped in a heating pad or set in a warm cup of water. Warm lubricant can be sensually applied to the labia, vagina, or penis by either partner.
- Lubrin, a water-soluble vaginal suppository, can be inserted with the fingers and will melt.
- Lubricated condoms may be used on the penis or vibrator.

Follow-up   If vaginal dryness is still a problem, ask your nurse or doctor if you are a candidate for estrogen vaginal cream or estrogen replacement therapy.

Phone Numbers

Nurse: _____ Phone: _____

Physician: _____ Phone: _____

Other: _____ Phone: _____

Comments

Patient's Signature: _____ Date: _____

Nurse's Signature: _____ Date: _____

Source: Bruner DW, Iwamoto RR: Altered sexual health, in Yarbro CH, Frogge MH, Goodman M (eds): *Cancer Symptom Management* (ed 2). Sudbury: Jones and Bartlett, 1999. © Jones and Bartlett Publishers.

Use of a Vacuum Device for Erections

Patient Name: _____

Symptom and Description   A vacuum device can be used when an erection is desired. This device may be used daily.

Learning Needs   You will learn how to use the vacuum device.

Procedure

1. Assemble equipment:
   - Vacuum device with constriction band
   - Water-soluble lubricant
2. To create an erection:
   - Place a constriction band around the open end of the hollow cylinder.
   - Apply water-soluble lubricant on the penis and at the base of the penis.
   - Place the penis into the cylinder and hold the cylinder tightly against the body to create a tight seal as shown in Figure 29D-1.
   - Apply the vacuum.
   - Once the erection is attained, slip the constriction band off the lip of the cylinder and onto the base of the penis.

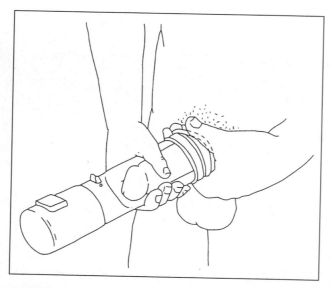

FIGURE 29D-1   Placement of external vacuum device.

- Open the pressure-release valve to allow the vacuum to release, and remove the cylinder.

3. To allow the penis to become flaccid (limp), remove the constriction band.

4. Clean the vacuum device according to the manufacturer's recommendations.

Management   Some common experiences and problems can occur with the use of the vacuum device. *The constriction band must not be left in place for more than 30 minutes.*

- Watch for bruising and swelling of the penis. Report any tenderness or pain in the penis. Report any signs of unusual swelling along the penis.
- There may not be any ejaculate because it is trapped behind the constriction band. The ejaculate will pass once the band is removed.
- There may be decreased sensation along the penis from the constriction.
- Penis may feel cold to the touch from the constriction.
- Penis will "hinge" at the base due to the constriction band.

The band should be kept off for at least 1 hour before reapplying the device.

Follow-up   Be sure you understand what to expect and what to do should problems occur. Notify your nurse and/or doctor if any of the following occurs:

- Tenderness of penis
- Unusual swelling along the penis

Phone Numbers   If you have any problem or question about the use of your vacuum device, please call your doctor or nurse.

Nurse: _____ Phone: _____

Physician: _____ Phone: _____

Other: _____ Phone: _____

Comments

Patient's Signature: _____ Date: _____

Nurse's Signature: _____ Date: _____

Source: Bruner DW, Iwamoto RR: Altered sexual health, in Yarbro CH, Frogge MH, Goodman M (eds): *Cancer Symptom Management* (ed 2). Sudbury: Jones and Bartlett, 1999. © Jones and Bartlett Publishers.

Semirigid Penile Prosthesis

Patient Name: _____

Symptom and Description   You have had a penile prosthesis implanted because you are unable to have an erection as a result of treatment. Your penile prosthesis is to be used when an erection is desired. Infections and irritation of the penis can occur with this implant.

Learning Needs   You will learn how to use and care for your prosthesis, and when and how to report signs and symptoms of infection.

Management

1. When you engage in sexual intercourse, the penis can be gently positioned for use.
2. When sexual intercourse is completed, the penis can be positioned downward or up against the abdomen.

Wearing elastic briefs can help make the penis less conspicuous.

Follow-up   Careful monitoring can prevent serious problems with the prosthesis. Report any of the following problems to your doctor or nurse:

1. Tenderness or pain in the penis
2. Discharge from the penis
3. Temperature greater than 100°F (38°C)
4. Discharge of pus from the urethra (from the opening at the end of the penis)
5. Unusual swelling along the penis
6. Signs of penile irritation, such as:
   - The skin of the penis appears translucent (you can almost see through it)
   - The implant is partly visible beneath the penile skin

Phone Numbers   If you have any problem or question about the use of your prosthesis, please call your doctor or nurse.

Nurse: _____ Phone: _____

Physician: _____ Phone: _____

Other: _____ Phone: _____

Comments

Patient's Signature: _____ Date: _____

Nurse's Signature: _____ Date: _____

Source: Bruner DW, Iwamoto RR: Altered sexual health, in Yarbro CH, Frogge MH, Goodman M (eds): *Cancer Symptom Management* (ed 2). Sudbury: Jones and Bartlett, 1999. © Jones and Bartlett Publishers.

Semiinflatable Penile Prosthesis

Patient Name: _____

Symptom and Description   You have had a penile prosthesis implanted because you are unable to have an erection as a result of treatment. Your penile prosthesis is to be used when an erection is desired. Infections and irritation of the penis can occur with this implant.

Learning Needs   You will learn how to use and care for your prosthesis, and when and how to report signs and symptoms of infection.

Procedure

1. To create an erection: Firmly squeeze and release the pump that is located behind the head of the penis several times. This moves the fluid from the reservoir to two cylinders located in the shaft of the penis.
2. To deflate the prosthesis: Hold the penis in a downward position for 10 seconds and release. This motion will cause the fluid to return to the reservoir.

Wearing elastic briefs can help make the penis less conspicuous.

Follow-up   Careful monitoring can prevent serious problems with the prosthesis. Report any of the following problems to your doctor or nurse:

1. Tenderness or pain in the penis
2. Discharge from the penis
3. Temperature greater than 100°F (38°C)
4. Discharge of pus from the urethra (from the opening at the end of the penis)
5. Unusual swelling along the penis
6. Signs of penile irritation, such as:
   - The skin of the penis appears translucent (you can almost see through it)
   - The implant may be partly visible beneath the penile skin

Phone Numbers   If you have any problem or question about the use of your prosthesis, please call your doctor or nurse.

Nurse: _____ Phone: _____

Physician: _____ Phone: _____

Other: _____ Phone: _____

Comments

Patient's Signature: _____ Date: _____

Nurse's Signature: _____ Date: _____

Source: Bruner DW, Iwamoto RR: Altered sexual health, in Yarbro CH, Frogge MH, Goodman M (eds): *Cancer Symptom Management* (ed 2). Sudbury: Jones and Bartlett, 1999. © Jones and Bartlett Publishers.

Fully Inflatable Penile Prosthesis

Patient Name: _____

Symptom and Description   You have had a penile prosthesis implanted because you are unable to have an erection as a result of treatment. Your penile prosthesis is to be used when an erection is desired. Infections and irritation of the penis can occur with this implant.

Learning Needs   You will learn how to use and care for your prosthesis, and report signs and symptoms of infection.

Procedure

1. To create an erection: The pump for the prosthesis is located in the scrotum. It is easily identified because it is rectangular in shape. Squeeze the pump several times to move the fluid from the reservoir to the cylinders located in the shaft of the penis, as pictured in Figure 29G-1.

2. To deflate the prosthesis: Locate the pump in the scrotum. Squeeze the sides of the pump to release the fluid back into the reservoir, as pictured.

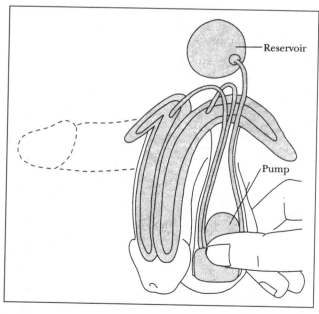

FIGURE 29G-1   Fully inflatable prosthesis. The fully inflatable prosthesis consists of three components: a reservoir placed under the rectus muscle, two cylinders placed in the corpora cavernosa, and a pump placed in the scrotal sac.

Follow-up   Careful monitoring can prevent serious problems with the prosthesis. Report any of the following problems to your doctor or nurse:

1. Tenderness or pain in the penis
2. Discharge from the penis
3. Temperature greater than 100°F (38°C)
4. Discharge of pus from the urethra (from the opening at the end of the penis)
5. Unusual swelling along the penis
6. Signs of penile irritation, such as:
   - The skin of the penis appears translucent (you can almost see through it)
   - The implant may be partly visible beneath the penile skin

Phone Numbers   If you have any problem or question about the use of your prosthesis, please call your doctor or nurse.

Nurse: _____ Phone: _____

Physician: _____ Phone: _____

Other: _____ Phone: _____

Comments

Patient's Signature: _____ Date: _____

Nurse's Signature: _____ Date: _____

Source: Bruner DW, Iwamoto RR: Altered sexual health, in Yarbro CH, Frogge MH, Goodman M (eds): *Cancer Symptom Management* (ed 2). Sudbury: Jones and Bartlett, 1999. © Jones and Bartlett Publishers.

CHAPTER 30

Anxiety

Barbara Holmes Gobel, RN, MS

The Problem of Anxiety in Cancer

The diagnosis and management of cancer can cause a number of stresses. One of the most commonly identified responses to the cancer experience, in addition to depression, is that of anxiety. Anxiety can be described as vague, uneasy, and unpleasant feelings of potential harm or distress. These feelings are accompanied by an arousal that is due to real or perceived threats to one's physical or mental well-being.

Cancer-related anxiety is considered to be a normal reaction to the diagnosis and management of a potentially life-threatening illness. One's level of anxiety can, however, impede the processing of information the nurses or physicians may share with the patient or may make a planned treatment unpleasant. This chapter contains information to assist oncology nurses in informing their patients about techniques to manage this anxiety. It also provides information on how to assess patients who are at risk for the development of anxiety or who are experiencing anxiety.

At times, levels of anxiety and distress related to cancer may exceed what is considered to be normal. Psychiatric assistance may be required in these circumstances. This chapter contains information on identifying and assessing higher levels of anxiety. Selected research and clinical instruments to measure the response of anxiety are pre-

sented. Finally, areas for future nursing research are suggested.

Incidence

The incidence and prevalence of anxiety among patients with cancer has not been objectively quantified. Researchers are attempting to determine the scope of this problem.

One of the first efforts to obtain objective data on the type and frequency of psychological problems of patients with cancer was conducted by the Psychosocial Collaborative Oncology Group.[1] This group determined the prevalence of psychiatric disorders in 215 patients with cancer at three cancer centers, using the criteria from the *Diagnostic and Statistical Manual of Mental Disorders,* Third Edition (DSM-III) classification of psychiatric disorders. Greater than half (53%) of the patients studied were found to be adjusting normally to the stresses of cancer. The others (47%) had clinically apparent psychiatric disorders. Of those patients with clinically apparent disorders, 68% had reactive anxiety and depression (adjustment disorders with depressed and/or anxious mood), 13% had major depression, 8% had an organic mental disorder, 7% had a personality disorder, and 4% had a preexisting anxiety disorder. These data demonstrate that about 90% of the psychiatric disorders identified were most likely reactions to or manifestations of disease or treatment. One of the conclusions to this study was that the majority of individuals with cancer are psychologically healthy but may experience emotional reaction to the stresses of cancer and its treatment.[2]

Etiology

Risk Factors

There are a number of risk factors that increase the potential for the development of cancer-related anxiety.

- Previous Mental Health: Anxiety disorders are the most common of the psychiatric illnesses.[3,4] Anxiety disorders affect approximately 5% of people at some point in their lifetime.[4,5]

- Serious Medical Illness: Serious medical illness may lead to stressors that may result in the symptoms of anxiety. Examples of these stressors may include fear of the unknown, fear of treatment of the illness, social isolation, loss of abilities, concerns over finances, management of complex treatments, sexual dysfunction, and the impact of the illness on family and friends.

- Age: Data suggest that elderly patients have a higher prevalence of clinically significant anxiety than younger patients. Contributing stressors in the elderly include failing physical health, loss of autonomy related to decreased physical or mental capabilities, death of friends and spouses, and age-related changes in brain function.[6]

- Gender: Females have a higher prevalence of anxiety disorders than males.[4,5]

- Unrelieved Physical Symptoms: Unrelieved symptoms such as pain or nausea or vomiting can increase the likelihood of the presence of anxiety.

- Medications: Many medications that are taken by patients with cancer may have anxiety as a side effect (Table 30-1).

Pathophysiology

The symptom of anxiety is a highly personal experience that may be affected by past feelings and situations. The level of anxiety is highly variable. Anxiety reactions can range from mild anxiety to panic. Mild anxiety reactions usually result in a heightened sensitivity to environmental stimuli. Moderate anxiety reactions can result in decreased attentiveness; the individual can be easily distracted. Physical signs of anxiety may be apparent as well, including sweating palms, restlessness, and tremulousness. Severe anxiety can distort the thought processes

TABLE 30-1 Medications That May Cause Anxiety

Classes of Medications	Examples
CNS stimulants	Caffeine, amphetamines, cocaine, ephedrine, pseudoephedrine
CNS depressant withdrawal	Barbiturates, benzodiazepines, ethanol
Psychotropics	Antipsychotics, buspirone, tricyclic antidepressants
Cardiovascular	Captopril, digitalis, enalapril
Other	Albuterol, aminophylline, interferon alfa, nonsteroidal antiinflammatories, steroids, theophylline

Data from reference 7.

and can result in the inability to make decisions and act. Panic disorders are considered when an individual exhibits severe, acute anxiety reactions associated with a variety of signs and symptoms related to anxiety. Such signs and symptoms may include dizziness, palpitations, tachycardia, and feelings of unreality.[8] According to Massie and Holland,[9] the variability in the level of distress is accounted for by three major factors: *medical factors* (site, stage of disease, medical illness such as pain); *psychological factors* (coping ability, previous coping skill, ability to modify life plans); and *social factors* (support of family, friends, and significant other).

Anxiety may be acute or chronic in nature. Acute anxiety may be related to the stress of cancer and its treatment. For example, a patient may experience acute episodes of anxiety related to upcoming chemotherapy treatments or to periods of uncontrolled pain. Chronic anxiety generally predates the cancer diagnosis, but may be exacerbated during treatment.

Anxiety can be accompanied by almost any other psychiatric illness. Depression frequently accompanies anxiety, and there is a great deal of symptom overlap with depression and anxiety. Difficulty sleeping, poor appetite, or difficulty concentrating may be key symptoms for either anxiety or depression or both. Effective treatment of anxiety, when accompanied by depression, requires management of the depression as well.

Most individuals who receive a diagnosis of cancer or learn of a recurrence of the cancer generally demonstrate what are considered to be normal responses to stress. These responses may include a period of initial shock and disbelief, followed by a time of turmoil accompanied by symptoms of anxiety and depression. Disruption of sleep and appetite may occur during this time. Ruminating about the diagnosis and fears of the future may also occur.[2] The mood of the individual is often sad or anxious, with a sense of despair and hopelessness. In the absence of a crisis, such as a cancer diagnosis, these responses may be considered pathologic. In the context of adjustment to this diagnosis, they are signs of normal and adaptive coping. This response generally diminishes over a period of a week to 10 days. Encouragement and support by family and friends during this period of time can help ensure the individual's emotional well-being. The treating physician is also in a position to help the individual by offering support, compassion, and reassurance, while detailing the facts of the medical situation. As the individual begins to gain a sense of mastery of the situation, a sense of hope will usually emerge.

Cancer-related stress resulting in anxiety may, however, continue to be appraised by some individuals as intolerable. If levels of anxiety are considered by the individual to be intolerable, or if they persist for several weeks or months, psychiatric treatment may be required.

Assessment

The State-Trait Anxiety Inventory (STAI) is the instrument used most commonly to measure the symptom of anxiety in individuals with cancer.[10] The STAI is made up of two scales: the A-State scale is a measure of state anxiety; and the A-Trait scale is a measure of trait anxiety. The A-State scale consists of 20 items on a 4-point scale (not at all, somewhat, moderately so, and very much so). The summation of the state anxiety scores indicates the subject's level of transitory anxiety "characterized by feelings of apprehension, tension, and autonomic nervous system–induced symptoms: nervousness, worry, and apprehension."[11] The A-Trait scale also consists of 20 items on a 4-point scale (almost never, sometimes, often, and almost always). The trait anxiety scores measure the subject's general level of arousal and tendency to anxiety. Scores range from 20 to 80 for each scale, a higher score representing a higher level of anxiety. There is abundant information in the literature supporting concurrent validity and discriminate validity for this tool.[12,13]

The *Diagnostic and Statistical Manual of Mental Disorders*, Fourth Edition (DSM-IV) is another tool used to classify the symptom of anxiety. This tool is used most frequently in the psychiatric setting with the purpose of defining anxiety as a psychiatric disorder. The DSM-IV classifies anxiety disorders into primary and secondary disorders. The primary disorders are classified into six types: generalized anxiety disorders (GAD), panic disorder, phobic disorders, obsessive-compulsive disorder (OCD), post-traumatic stress disorder (PTSD), and acute stress disorder. The secondary anxiety disorders include anxiety disorders due to a general medical condition, and substance abuse anxiety disorder.[7]

In most situations, individuals with cancer are not assessed with these tools unless they are part of a research program or have sought psychological or psychiatric assistance. Assessment of anxiety in daily clinical practice is different from the assessments and measurements done

for the purpose of research. The clinician at the bedside does not have easy access to sophisticated measurement tools or have the time to use them. Because of the lack of clinically useful and objective tools, clinicians use their judgment to assess the presence or absence of anxiety. Gobel and Donovan[14] proposed a practical method of screening to determine which patients are anxious or depressed or are at high risk for these symptoms. The tool currently has no data available regarding reliability and validity testing. The tool is a mini-assessment for anxiety/depression using the acronym P-SCREEN (Table 30-2). The symptoms of anxiety and depression often occur concomitantly. For this reason, most screening tools used to assess these symptoms screen for both anxiety and depression. The treatment for these two symptoms can, however, be very different. The author refers the reader to Chapter 31 for a review of the symptom of depression.

In addition to using tools to assess for anxiety, talking with the individual with cancer and reviewing the medical record may provide valuable information regarding the existence of anxiety. Opening communication by simply asking "How are you feeling?" may provide a great deal of information. For example, if the individual responds

TABLE 30-2 Mini-Assessment for Screening for Anxiety/Depression (PSCREEN)

Circle the letter(s) for all symptoms confirmed by the patient	
Psychomotor changes	
Slowed/retarded	D
Shakiness/agitation/restlessness	A
Sleep disturbances	
Difficulty falling asleep	A
Awakening 30–90 minutes early	D
Concentration decreased	A/D
Reduced pleasure	
In those things that were previously pleasurable	D
Excessive autonomic activity	
Sweating, tachycardia, tachypnea	A
Eating changes	
Nausea, lump in throat	A
Increase/decrease in eating	D
Negative mood	
Sad/blue	D
Fearful	A
Results	

3 As = High risk of anxiety. Proceed with exploration of anxiety as a problem including consultation with a psychiatric-liaison nurse, psychiatric social worker, psychologist, or psychiatrist.

3 Ds = High risk of depression. Proceed with exploration of depression as a problem including consultation with a psychiatric-liaison nurse, psychiatric social worker, psychologist, or psychiatrist.

Source: Gobel BH, Donovan MI: Depression and anxiety. *Semin Oncol Nurs* 3:267–276, 1987.[14] Reprinted with permission.

by stating that eating or sleeping are problems, the clinician can provide input into managing these problems. Anxiety may thereby be reduced through managing symptoms identified during an open dialogue. Moving from less personal questions (sleep, diet, exercise) to more personal questions (relationships, coping abilities, and the impact of the cancer diagnosis on family and friends) may help to establish a sense of trust between the individual with cancer and the clinician. Asking the individual directly whether he or she has ever been treated for anxiety, "nerves," or depression can help to determine whether the symptoms of anxiety preceded the diagnosis of cancer.

A review of the medical record includes a thorough review of medications that the individual is currently taking and when the medication was started. Many medications can induce symptoms of anxiety (see Table 30-1). The medical record or discussion with the individual may reveal certain medications that may have been discontinued, perhaps inadvertently. Sudden withdrawal of sedatives or alcohol in an individual who is physically dependent on them may precipitate withdrawal symptoms, which may incorrectly appear to be primary severe anxiety. Individuals who smoke more than two packs per day and who must stop smoking while in the hospital may also experience withdrawal symptoms, including anxiety, irritability, and restlessness.[8]

A calm, reassuring approach when communicating with the individual may help to lessen the sense of anxiety. This approach is demonstrated through both verbal and nonverbal behavior. Communication with someone with a medical illness may be enhanced by demonstrating attentive behavior and a nonjudgmental attitude. The family also needs this same empathic approach to the management of their anxiety.

Symptom Management

Psychosocial interventions for individuals with cancer are systematic efforts to influence coping behavior, primarily through educational and psychotherapeutic means. Goals of these interventions are to increase morale, self-esteem, and coping ability, thereby decreasing distress. Enhancing a sense of personal control over the cancer experience is another broad goal.[15]

It is essential that every treatment plan be individualized and based on an accurate assessment of the person with cancer. For the most part, individuals with cancer are psychologically healthy but are reacting to the stresses of cancer and its treatment. Psychiatric complications may, however, cause increased morbidity and have a significant impact on the individual's quality of life.

Various treatment interventions may be used individually or in combination with one another. These interventions include social support, counseling and support groups, cognitive-behavioral techniques, education, and pharmacologic approaches. All of these potentially anxiety-reducing interventions will be discussed.

Social Support

Cancer affects not only the individual with the disease but all members of the individual's social support system. This social system is unique to each individual. For many individuals, their primary support system is the family. Family today, however, may be unlike the traditional family of the past. Families may consist of same sex partners, grandparents raising their children's children, or others. Regardless of the composition of the family, "family-centered care" is an essential component of the comprehensive treatment of someone with anxiety. Open and honest communication with both the patient and the family, and structured time designed to enhance their communication with each other are critical to the success of any treatment plan. If appropriate, the family may be encouraged to participate in counseling or psychotherapy with the patient.

Some individuals may seek their social support outside of the family. They may look for a new social network composed of individuals facing similar problems, such as in group psychotherapy or support groups. This psychotherapeutic support provides a necessary social connection.

The presence of appropriate social support is positively correlated with better psychosocial adjustment to cancer.[16] Spiegel et al.[17] found evidence that in illness social support can actually accelerate recovery and protect against the health consequences of life stress. Other studies related to social support suggest that patients with cancer who receive social and emotional support through group therapy may actually live longer and improve the quality of their lives, compared to patients who do not have this social support.[16,18,19]

Counseling and Support Groups

Individual counseling is the most common form of therapy provided to the cancer patient with anxiety. The therapist generally provides short-term psychotherapy based on a crisis intervention model.[20] This approach offers individuals emotional support, provides information to help the individual adapt to the crisis, emphasizes past strengths, and enhances previously used successful coping methods. Pharmacologic management may be used in addition to counseling. As symptoms improve, medication can be decreased or eliminated.

There are many different types of support groups. There is no clear definition of a support group. Some groups are self-led or facilitated by a patient, and other support groups are facilitated by healthcare professionals. A number of studies suggest that the problems patients with cancer experience, such as anxiety and depression, can be reduced through participation in support groups.[21] When an individual with cancer participates in a support group composed of understanding people who have experienced or are experiencing similar problems, the individual may receive emotional and social support as well as assistance in coping with the day-to-day stresses of living with cancer. Regardless of whether support groups are self-help groups or are professionally led groups, support groups enable people to help each other.[19] Goals of support groups often include sharing, education, socializing, and affirmation.

Studies have shown that self-help or mutual help groups are a cost-effective complement to professional healthcare services.[22] A patient talking with another experienced patient may facilitate coping by providing a credible source of information. Self-help groups are often independent of medical care but can be a link between health care and the public. Most support groups have been grouped by diagnoses, though there are no data supporting the superiority of diagnosis-based homogeneous groups over heterogeneous groups.

Support groups run by health professionals are common in cancer care. Problems that arise in the course of daily living and adapting to illness are amenable to the group setting.

There are a vast array of professionally led support groups. In many communities, one may find support groups set up for specific diseases (e.g., breast cancer support groups) or for specific points along the disease trajectory (e.g., grief support groups). If a support group is not available where a patient is being treated, the local American Cancer Society office usually offers a list of local support groups. National programs designed to support cancer patients also exist. Two well-known established programs include the Y-me organization and the Candlelighters Childhood Cancer Foundation. The Y-me organization is set up to support and advocate for women with breast cancer. The Candlelighters focus on assisting families to cope with the emotional stresses of dealing with children with cancer.[23]

Of particular note are those patients who may be geographically isolated or unable to travel, yet are able to verbalize concerns and may benefit from a support group. Recent advances in telecommunications and computer technologies may help to remedy this problem. Colón[24] described the initiation of and clinical issues associated with a long-term telephone support group serving a population of cancer patients who were homebound, isolated, or otherwise unable to travel to a central location. The group uses a telephone company service that makes and maintains the calls to participants. Benefits of this type of telecommunication-based support group included connecting persons with cancer who would not otherwise be able to participate in a support group, allowing participants to remain in familiar and informal surroundings while supporting one another, maintaining privacy and possibly equalizing relationships among the group members,[25] and enhanced continuity, as the partic-

ipant may be able to continue in the group regardless of their setting of care (e.g., home, hospital, or nursing home).

Electronic networks and computer-based support systems are other examples of the usefulness of communications technology. Not only do various organizations and institutions place information on electronic networks, but some networks are set up specifically for cancer patient support. One example is an Internet group called "Caregivers and Stress."[23,26] Computer-based support systems have also been set up for breast cancer patients. Results of pilot studies on these groups have identified a positive response to this mode of support and positive emotional responses related to feelings of relief, acceptance, motivation, and understanding.[27,28]

A landmark study, as mentioned above, published by Spiegel et al.[18] supports the benefits of support groups. In this study, 86 women with metastatic breast cancer were randomly assigned either to a control group or to a support group. Both groups received conventional medical treatment. The support group met weekly for 1 year. The group provided psychological support plus training in self-hypnosis for pain control. Patients in the support group lived an average of 18 months longer than the patients in the control group ($p < 0.0001$). Spiegel et al. proposed three reasons for the study outcomes: (1) effectiveness of the medical treatment in some way was enhanced by the support received, (2) depression was decreased or alleviated by the support, thus improving patients' appetites and general nutrition, and (3) pain control obtained with self-hypnosis allowed patients to maintain a greater degree of normal activity.

Limitations of group support may impede a more widespread reliance on group intervention. Limitations include the difficulty of forming a group at exactly the time that a particular patient is in need of assistance, the greater number of counselors prepared with an individual rather than a group orientation, and the preference of many patients for privacy. (The problem regarding privacy may be averted by participation in a telephone- or computer-based support system.)[29] Problems of attendance at group meetings may occur as well, regardless of the type of support group in which the patient is participating. The number of participants in a group may fluctuate for a number of reasons, including individuals' inability to attend due to feeling ill from current treatment, other commitments on the day of the therapy, inclement weather, and potentially a lack of interest. Group dynamics will change as the size and composition of the group changes.

Spiritual counseling is another source of psychosocial support. Religious faith may be strengthened or shaken by a diagnosis of cancer. The individual diagnosed with cancer may seek spiritual counseling from a number of sources. These sources may include clergy, family, friends, significant others, social workers and nurses. It has been demonstrated in studies that nurses do not accurately assess spiritual health of patients. In a study by Highfield[30] it was also shown that patient and nurse subjects preferred different spiritual caregivers. Although the nurse may be well aware of hospital-based resources, such as chaplains, the patient may actually prefer spiritual support from a friend or others with whom they may have ongoing relationships. The full impact of these incongruencies between nurse and patient perceptions is unclear. It underscores the need to assess, treat, and refer spiritual concerns of the patient on an individual basis. These studies also highlight the need for open communication, particularly in regard to spiritual needs and concerns.

Cognitive-Behavioral Interventions

Cognitive-behavioral techniques are well suited to the treatment of anxiety because the techniques are often effective not only in symptom control, but also in restoring or enhancing a sense of self-control. The perception of having increased control over a situation may lead to decreased feelings of helplessness and hopelessness, thus promoting an improved psychological affective state (mood). Examples of cognitive-behavioral techniques include cognitive distraction or focusing, systematic desensitization, passive relaxation, progressive muscle relaxation, hypnosis, biofeedback, and music therapy (Table 30-3). Some of these techniques are primarily cognitive in nature, focusing on perceptual and thought processes, whereas other techniques focus attention on modifying patterns of behavior that facilitate coping. Techniques such as hypnosis or biofeedback use elements from both cognitive and behavioral interventions. Most often these techniques are used in combination. For example, the use of progressive muscle relaxation is frequently combined with guided or controlled imagery. When any of these techniques are used to manage anxiety concomitant with pain or nausea and vomiting, it is important that they

TABLE 30-3 Cognitive-Behavioral Techniques Used by Cancer Patients

Cognitive	Behavioral
Preparatory information	Self-monitoring
	Graded task management
Cognitive restructuring	Systematic desensitization
	Contingency management
Focusing	Modeling
Controlled mental imaging	Behavioral rehearsal
Distraction	Relaxation
Controlled attention	Passive, progressive
Mental, behavioral	Meditation
Music therapy	Music therapy
Hypnosis	Hypnosis
Biofeedback	Biofeedback

Used with permission: Breitbart W, Holland JC: Psychiatric complications of cancer, in Brain MC, Carbone PP (eds): *Current Therapy in Hematology Oncology* (ed 3). Philadelphia: Decker, 1988, p. 269.[20]

not be used as a substitute for appropriate pharmacologic management. They should be used as part of a comprehensive multimodal approach to symptom control.

Cognitive techniques

Cognitive interventions are based on how an individual interprets life events and bodily sensations. The attempt is to identify dysfunctional automatic thoughts and underlying beliefs in order to allow for a more rationale response. When individuals are facing difficult problems, such as the diagnosis and treatment of cancer, cognitive therapy may help them to see the situation from a new point of view. Life-threatening problems may continue to seem real but not overwhelming.[31] Challenging self-defeating thoughts, demonstrating the fallacies in the belief structure, stressing realistic goals, and establishing a plan that ensures incremental successes are basic cognitive strategies relevant to the treatment of anxiety in the individual with cancer. Enabling hope is another way of reinterpreting negative thought processes. The act of planning, encouraging humor, and finding a reason for living are among the underutilized techniques to develop and maintain hope.

Behavioral techniques

Behavioral techniques are aimed at modulating patterns of behavior that help individuals cope. One of the most fundamental behavioral techniques to manage anxiety is self-monitoring. When an individual is able to monitor his or her own behavior, it allows that individual to identify dysfunctional reactions and then learn to control them. For example, a woman may experience an extreme anxiety reaction every time the needle to her vascular access device needs to be changed. This person can be taught to monitor her own reaction and the outcome of that reaction. With assistance from a clinician, she may identify that her reaction is causing a delay in her care whenever the needle requires changing. She may then learn new approaches or techniques to control her reaction. It may be necessary to combine self-monitoring with other behavioral techniques. These techniques may include systematic desensitization, which diminishes reactions over time; graded task assignment, which is gradual, progressive, incremental movement toward coping; progressive muscle relaxation, self-hypnosis, meditation, and biofeedback.

Relaxation and imagery techniques

Relaxation and imagery techniques are cognitive-behavioral techniques commonly used in the management of anxiety. The use of these techniques in the treatment of anxiety is directed at attempting to achieve an antistress response, with resulting mental and physical relaxation. Specific relaxation techniques include meditation, progressive muscle relaxation, passive relaxation, and focusing attention on feelings of warmth and decreased tension in parts of the body. These techniques, as well as hypnosis, biofeedback, and music therapy, use strong elements of both the cognitive and behavioral interventions.

A mode of action postulated to explain the usefulness of the relaxation techniques involves the individual's appraisal of environmental stimuli. How one interprets various environmental stimuli determines whether or not the individual feels threatened and then is aroused to action.[32] Depending on the level of stress or anxiety, the appraisals may be realistic or distorted. When relaxation techniques are mastered, the response can neutralize the effects of the "flight or fight" physiologic response. In addition to being able to decrease one's heart, respiratory, and metabolic rates using these techniques, one can decrease skeletal muscle tension. According to Jacobson,[33] the developer of progressive relaxation, anxiety cannot exist with relaxed muscles. Thus, the individual is able to change his or her appraisal of what is perceived as a potentially threatening situation by increasing the sense of control over the situation. Consider the individual who perceives a bone marrow aspirate and biopsy procedure to be highly threatening. When even thinking about this procedure, the individual may experience feelings of anxiety as well as physiologic responses of tachypnea, tachycardia, profuse sweating, and skeletal muscle tension. To attempt to alter this individual's stress response, one could teach progressive muscle relaxation and guided imagery. It would, however, be important to teach these techniques well in advance of the next bone marrow procedure. The reason for this timing is that progressive muscle relaxation and guided imagery are skills that are learned. To become proficient, these skills require practice over time. Many people find it helpful to make audiotapes of a relaxation teaching session. Others find it helpful to listen to soothing music while practicing these skills. Depending on the degree of anxiety involved, the individual may benefit from the administration of a short-acting anxiolytic medication in addition to the use of progressive muscle relaxation and guided imagery.

Although relaxation and imagery techniques have been cited as being effective tools in the management of anxiety,[34,35] their use in clinical settings is not widespread. Limitations include time and cost. Time must be spent teaching patients these techniques. Patients must then be motivated to practice these techniques for them to be of benefit. In some settings, these techniques are taught by psychologists or psychiatrists who bill for their services. Mynchenberg and Dungan[36] developed a protocol for nurses to introduce relaxation to the anxious patient as an effective clinical strategy. Their protocol included an audio cassette recording of a 25-minute musical selection, such as Pachebel's Canon.[37] A relaxation script was dubbed over the first 15 minutes of the music. A nurse familiar with the patient presented the audiotape and coached the patient for the first session. Someone trained in relaxation techniques, or even a nurse with a calm voice, can make the relaxation audiotapes.

Relaxation techniques used primarily for symptom control are most helpful when combined with some distracting or focusing imagery. The focus of attention, such as pain, is diverted by the use of distraction or focusing. An individual may begin to relax using progressive muscle relaxation, then may add a pleasant image to focus his or her attention. Perhaps this image is a beautiful, warm, white sandy beach. The individual may use this image to "escape" to and imagine warm sand being gently poured over areas of discomfort. See Appendix 30A for a self-care guide that teaches progressive muscle relaxation and guided imagery.

Patient Education

There are numerous outcomes of patient education. Outcomes related to patient education may be patient oriented (e.g., the patient needs to understand their diagnosis, treatment options, and results related to treatment). Outcomes regarding patient education also may be provider oriented (e.g., the heathcare professional has a responsibility to ensure that a patient has an appropriate knowledge base on which to make appropriate decisions).[23] There are basically five rationales that support the need for patient education. These rationales include the patient's right to receive education, professional standards under which healthcare professionals practice, legal and accreditation requirements for various healthcare settings, and benefits to society and to healthcare organizations.[38] Regardless of the rationale for patient education, providing information in a caring and compassionate manner can promote a sense of control in a person's life. This sense of control has been shown to be significantly related to a more positive emotional response among patients.[39–42]

A nationally recognized psychoeducational program for individuals with cancer is the "I Can Cope" program based on a model developed by Judith Johnson, PhD, RN, and Pat Norby, RN. This program drew on research regarding information needs perceived by patients, and it demonstrated a reduction in the level of anxiety in individuals with cancer.[43] This structured educational program conveys facts and information helpful to the patient, not only in understanding and managing the changes the disease will cause in his or her life, but also in understanding the sensory experience. Patients receive information about what they will see, hear, feel, smell, taste, and experience. This particular educational program is a group program. The social support one receives by participating in a group intervention may be a factor in decreasing anxiety in the individual with cancer. Recently a national evaluation of the "I Can Cope" program provided data in eight areas: demographics, class format, course objectives, course content, audiovisual and instructional materials, facilitator training, and program evaluation. Participants indicated that they learned what they needed to from the course and that they were satisfied with the program's results.[44]

Preoperative teaching can influence a person's anxiety level. The literature contains inconsistent data regarding the effect of preoperative teaching on postoperative outcomes. However, studies have demonstrated a positive impact of teaching on postoperative outcomes among surgical patients.[45,46] Some of these outcomes have included a decreased length of stay in the hospital, reduced cost of hospitalization, a decrease in patient anxiety, and an increase in "customer satisfaction."[47,48]

Treatment selection for many cancers is complex. This complexity can be confusing and anxiety provoking, yet patients are expected to be active participants in their treatment decisions and rehabilitation options. When a woman is considering treatment for breast cancer, a multitude of choices must be understood. Some of these treatment decisions include whether she should have a modified radical mastectomy versus lumpectomy plus irradiation, immediate versus delayed reconstruction, preoperative versus postoperative adjuvant chemotherapy, and the specific tumor features that influence all of the options.[49] During this period of information seeking, a woman may receive information from a variety of sources. Traditional sources of information include discussions with physicians and nurses, and written materials. Patients may also access information from the American Cancer Society (ACS) and the National Cancer Institute (NCI). Patients can connect with organizations via the telephone or the computer.

As noted earlier, the ACS provides services, support programs and informational resources. The NCI provides up-to-date information to both health professionals and to the general public. One of the major resource programs established by the NCI to allow easy access to up-to-date information is the Physician Data Query (PDQ) program. Although the PDQ was initially intended for physician use, a patient component has been added in recent years. This component is called the Patient Information File (PIF). Both on-line and CD-ROM versions are available for direct access to PDQ. It can be accessed through the MEDLARS system of the National Library of Medicine. A newer electronic service, CancerNet, allows access to PDQ and some other information services, free to users with access to Internet E-mail (cancernet@icicb.nci.nih.gov).[50]

Some authors suggest the need to determine whether patients have actually understood the information given to them regarding treatment options. Ward and Griffin[51] describe an 18-item instrument to test women's knowledge of surgical treatment options for early-stage breast cancer. The instrument is called the Breast Cancer Information Test—Revised (BCIT-R). A tool such as this one may allow for identification and intervention related to knowledge deficits.

Patient education, at any point along the cancer continuum, must be individualized. This individualization is based on a number of factors: amount and type of information desired by the individual, the individual's preferred style of learning, (oral or written, group or individual), and the presence of factors that may impede learning (pain, fatigue, anxiety).

Pharmacologic Treatment of Anxiety Symptoms and Disorders

The most commonly used medications for the treatment of acute and chronic anxiety are the benzodiazepines. There are currently fifteen benzodiazepines available in the United States, and eight are marketed as antianxiety agents. The eight benzodiazepine antianxiety agents include chlordiazepoxide, diazepam, oxazepam, clorazepate, lorazepam, prazepam, alprazolam, and halazepam.[7] The short-acting benzodiazepines (alprazolam, lorazepam, and oxazepam) are generally preferred for medically ill patients. Due to their short half-life, the short-acting benzodiazepines are better tolerated by sicker individuals and cause less drug accumulation in an individual receiving other sedating medications.[52] Table 30-4 lists various pharmacologic aspects of commonly prescribed benzodiazepines.

The starting dose of benzodiazepines is based on the severity of the individual's anxiety, their medical condition, and the concurrent use of other medications (analgesics, antiemetics, antidepressants). The dose interval depends on the half-life of the drug and on the character of the underlying illness. Intermittent therapy may be used for the individual who has periodic symptoms or symptoms triggered by anxiety-producing situations, e.g., just prior to a procedure or chemotherapy treatment. Individuals whose symptoms persist may require continuous or around-the-clock treatment.[52]

The most common side effect of the benzodiazepines is sedation. Sedation is most severe in patients with impaired liver function. Other side effects include confusion, problems in visual accommodations, decreased speed of thought, and motor incoordination. These side effects are dose dependent and are reversible. Tolerance to benzodiazepine-related sedation often occurs during long-term therapy, while the anxiolytic effects continue. Benzodiazepines have additive effects if combined with other medications that have CNS depressant properties, such as the opioids. Abrupt withdrawal of benzodiazepines can lead to a withdrawal syndrome similar to alcohol withdrawal. All benzodiazepines should be tapered off slowly over periods as long as 2 to 4 months.[7,52]

Other medications used in the treatment of anxiety include the azapirones, antidepressants, beta-blockers, and antihistamines. The azapirones are a nonbenzodiazepine class of anxiolytics. The first azapirone marketed in the United States (in 1986) was buspirone (Buspar).[53] Buspirone lacks general CNS effects and has comparable efficacy to benzodiazepines in the treatment of anxiety.[54] As a group of medications, the azapirones are considered to be relatively free of the potential for abuse and depen-

TABLE 30-4 Commonly Presented Benzodiazepines in Cancer Patients

Drug (trade name)	Absorption	Half-life (h)	Usual Dose Range ≤65 yr	Maximum Recommended Dose ≥65 yr	Comments
Chlordiazepoxide (Librium)	Intermediate	5–30	15–100 mg/day	40 mg/day	Long half-life leads to accumulation of active metabolites
Diazepam (Valium, Valrelease)	Fast	20–70	2–40 mg/day	20 mg/day	Same as chlordiazepoxide; rapid oral absorption
Oxazepam (Serax)	Slow–intermediate	5–15	30–120 mg/day	60 mg/day	Short half-life reduces risk of excessive plasma accumulation
Clorazepate (Tranxene, Tranxene-SD)	Fast	30–200	15–60 mg/day	30 mg/day	Same as chlordiazepoxide
Lorazepam (Ativan)	Intermediate	10–20	2–6 mg/day	3 mg/day	
Alprazolam (Xanax)	Intermediate	10–15	0.5–6.0 mg/day	2 mg/day	

Data from reference 7.

dence. Buspirone may be considered preferable for patients who are elderly, medically ill, have mixed anxiety-depression, or who have a history of substance abuse or dependence.[54]

The antidepressants include tricyclic antidepressants (TCAs), selective serotonin reuptake inhibitors (SSRIs), and monoamine oxidase inhibitors (MAOIs). These tend to be used primarily for panic disorder and obsessive-compulsive disorder.[13] Current studies have shown that the antidepressants imipramine (Tofranil), amitriptyline (Elavil), and trazodone (Desyrel) are comparable or even superior in efficacy to benzodiazepines for the treatment of generalized anxiety disorder.[55–57] However, most patients in these studies had depressive symptoms in addition to their anxiety.

The beta-blockers are not considered to be as effective as the benzodiazepines in the management of anxiety.[57] The beta-blockers suppress sympathetic nervous system activity and autonomic symptoms; as such, they may be used in preventing performance anxiety ("stage fright").[7] Antihistamines have been used for years as an adjuvant in the treatment of anxiety and insomnia. Antihistamines have potent sedative effects, and are used as needed for insomnia. Antihistamines have significant anticholinergic effects that compound problems such as constipation, confusion, and cognitive impairment.[58]

Treatment of elderly patients with benzodiazepines

The treatment of elderly patients with benzodiazepines requires special care. With advancing age, there are changes in hepatic enzyme function that affect the metabolism of benzodiazepines. The two enzymatic pathways of hepatic benzodiazepine detoxification are microsomal oxidation and glucuronide conjugation. Although conjugation does not change appreciably with age, oxidation becomes less efficient with age.[58] The conjugated

benzodiazepines are oxazepam, lorazepam, and temazepam; all other benzodiazepines are oxidized. These medications can be used to treat anxiety but with special attention to dose, schedule, and signs of accumulation. (See Table 30-4 for a review of dosing guidelines in the elderly patient.) Many aspects of brain function are more vulnerable to the side effects of benzodiazepines with increasing age. Side effects that may be more pronounced in the elderly include depressed mood or dysregulation, memory disturbance, disorientation, excessive drowsiness, and changes in gait and balance.[58]

Evaluation of Therapeutic Approaches

There is considerable inconsistency in the reported efficacy of psychosocial interventions for individuals with cancer. It may be that subject-intervention matching is difficult within the constraints of a quasi-experimental design (randomization); yet, this matching process (subject-intervention) is the key to identifying effective outcomes. Every effort should be made to match the intervention to the style, needs, and preference of the patient. Patients often demonstrate a distinct preference for the way they prefer to receive support (group, education, individual therapy). If the support is not available in the format desired by the patient, the patient may refuse the assistance or go elsewhere to find what they need.

Conclusion

There is abundant information in the literature regarding anxiety as a response to the experience of cancer. Many studies have attempted to demonstrate the existence of anxiety at specific points along the disease trajectory. Currently, no studies clearly identify that the response of anxiety will predictably occur at any given time in the individual's illness. Yet, it is important that nurses not assume the existence or absence of the symptom of anxiety. Development of clinical assessment tools to identify the existence of anxiety as a response to cancer would enhance the clinical care of individuals with cancer. Interventions to assist the individual in coping with the illness may be more focused and more timely if assessments are based on objective data. Studies to identify when to use these tools would be beneficial to patient care as well.

Anxiety, like most responses to cancer, is highly personal and affected by past feelings and experiences. The anxiety response may be mild and time limited, or it may be prolonged and require psychiatric assistance. Regardless of the level of the response, the existence of anxiety can affect the individual's quality of life. As such, healthcare professionals need to be aware of the potential for its occurrence and have support interventions in place to assist individuals in their coping process.

Studies have demonstrated the value of a range of psychosocial interventions to provide emotional support to individuals with cancer. This range of interventions is necessary to help meet the needs of each individual. Not every setting in which individuals with cancer are treated can provide a full range of psychosocial interventions. All care settings can, however, include families in treatment planning, assist with communication between the individual with cancer and their family, provide excellent physical care with a focus on management of physical symptoms, provide educational opportunities, and incorporate many components of the cognitive-behavioral therapies into the clinical care of the individual with cancer. Staff nurses can learn and effectively incorporate music therapy and relaxation therapy with guided imagery into the nursing care and treatment plan. If a support intervention is not available in a particular setting, referrals should be made to the appropriate setting. It is essential that the treatment plan for the management of anxiety be individualized and focused on the specific needs of the person with cancer.

References

1. Derogatis LR, Morrow GR, Fetting J, et al: The prevalence of psychiatric disorders among cancer patients. *JAMA* 249:751–757, 1983
2. Massie M, Holland C: The cancer patient with pain: Psychiatric complications and their management. *J Pain Symptom Manage* 7:99–109, 1992
3. Dubovsky SL: Generalized anxiety disorder: New concepts and psychopharmacologic therapies. *J Clin Psychiatry* 51(suppl 1):3–10, 1990
4. Regier DA, Narrow WE, Rae DS, et al: The defacto U.S. mental and addictive disorders service system. Epidemiologic catchment area prospective 1-year prevalence rates of disorders and services. *Arch Gen Psychiatry* 50:85–94, 1993
5. Brown TA, Barlow DH: Comorbidity among anxiety disorders: Implications for treatment and DSM-IV. *J Consult Clin Psychol* 60:835–844, 1992
6. Markovitz PJ: Treatment of anxiety in the elderly. *J Clin Psychiatry* 54(suppl):64–68, 1993
7. Grimsley SR: Anxiety disorders, in Young LY, Koda-Kimble M (eds): *Applied Therapeutics: The Clinical Use of Drugs* (ed. 6). Vancouver, BC: Applied Therapeutics, Inc., 1995, pp. 73-1–73-31
8. Badger M: Calming the anxious patient. *Am J Nurs* 94:46–50, 1994
9. Massie M, Holland C: The cancer patient with pain: Psychiatric complications and their management. *Med Clin North Am* 71:243–258, 1987
10. American Psychiatric Association: *Diagnostic and Statistical Manual of Mental Disorders* (ed 4). Washington, DC: American Psychiatric Association, 1994
11. Clark J: Psychosocial responses of cancer patients, in Groenwald SL, Frogge MH, Goodman M, Yarbro CH (eds): *Cancer Nursing Principles and Practice* (ed 3). Sudbury: Jones and Bartlett, 1993, pp. 449–468
12. Spielberger CD, Gorush RL, Lushene RE: *Manual for the State-Trait Anxiety Inventory*. Palo Alto, CA: Consulting Psychologists Press, 1983
13. Averbach SM: Trait-state anxiety and adjustment to surgery. *Consult Clin Psychol* 40:264–271, 1983
14. Gobel BH, Donovan MI: Depression and anxiety. *Semin Oncol Nurs* 3:267–276, 1987
15. Spiegel D: Health caring. *Cancer* 74(suppl):1453–1457, 1994
16. Wellisch DK: Beyond the year 2000: The future of groups for patients with cancer. *Cancer Pract* 1:198–201, 1993
17. Spiegel D: *Living Beyond Limits: New Hope and Help for Facing Life-Threatening Illness*. New York: Times Books, 1993
18. Spiegel O, Kraemer HC, Bloom JR, Gottheil E: Effect of psychosocial treatment on survival of patients with metastatic breast cancer. *Lancet* 2:888–891, 1989
19. Cella DF, Yellen S: Cancer support groups: The state of the art. *Cancer Pract* 1:56–61, 1993
20. Barsevick AM, Much J, Sweeney C: Psychosocial responses to cancer, in Groenwald SL, Frogge MH, Goodman M, Yarbro CH (eds): *Cancer Nursing Principles and Practice* (ed 4). Sudbury: Jones and Bartlett, 1997, pp. 1393–1411
21. Bottomley A: Cancer support groups—Are they effective? *Eur J Cancer* 6:11–17, 1997
22. Ontario Medical Association Committee on Medical Care and Practice. Self-help/mutual aid groups. *Ont Med Review* August 1991
23. Padberg RM, Padberg LF: Patient education and support, in Groenwald SL, Frogge MH, Goodman M, Yarbro CH (eds): *Cancer Nursing Principles and Practice* (ed 4). Sudbury: Jones and Bartlett, 1997, pp. 1642–1665
24. Colón Y: Telephone support groups: A nontraditional approach to reaching underserved cancer patients. *Cancer Pract* 4:156–159, 1996
25. Rounds KA, Galinsky MJ, Stevens LS: Linking people with AIDS in rural communities: The telephone group. *Soc Work* 36:13–18, 1991
26. Sletten J: Computer technology in cancer patient education. Washington, DC: Cancer Patient Education Network Conference, Sept. 1995

27. Gustafson D, Wise M, McTavish F, et al: Development and pilot evaluation of a computer-based support system for women with breast cancer. *J Psychosoc Oncol* 11:69–93, 1993

28. McTavish F, Gustafson DH, Owens BH, et al: CHESS: An interactive computer system for women with breast cancer piloted with an under-served population. *Proc Ann Symp Comput Appl Med Care* 94:599–603, 1994

29. Freedhoff S: Structured cancer support groups: A valuable piece of the cancer care mosaic. *Can Oncol Nurs J* 3:6–10, 1993

30. Highfield MF: Spiritual health of oncology patients: Nurse and patient perspectives. *Cancer Nurs* 15:1–8, 1992

31. Anderson BL: Psychological interventions for cancer patients to enhance the quality of life. *J Consult Clin Psychol* 60:552–568, 1992

32. Cotanch PH, Strom S: Progressive muscle relaxation as antiemetic therapy for cancer patients. *Oncol Nurs Forum* 14:33–37, 1987

33. Jacobson E: *Anxiety and Tension Control.* Philadelphia: Lippincott, 1984

34. Gagne D, Toye RC: The effects of therapeutic touch and relaxation therapy in reducing anxiety. *Arch Psychiatr Nurs* 3:184–189, 1994

35. Beck JG, Stanley MA, Baldwin LE, et al: Comparison of cognitive therapy and relaxation training for panic disorder. *J Consult Clin Psychol* 62:818–826, 1994

36. Mynchenberg TL, Dungan JM: A relaxation protocol to reduce patient anxiety. *Dimen Crit Care Nurs* 14:78–84, 1995

37. Jeffries G (Musician): The Meditative Classic with Ocean Waves: Pachebel's Canon. Audiotape cassette. New York: The Relaxation Co., 1990

38. Fernsler JI, Cannon CA: The whys of patient education. *Semin Oncol Nurs* 7:79–86, 1991

39. Jensen AB, Madsen B, Andersen P, et al: Information for cancer patients entering a clinical trial—An evaluation of an information strategy. *Eur J Cancer* 29A:2235–2238, 1993

40. Grahn G, Danielson M: Coping with the cancer experience. II. Evaluating an education and support programme for cancer patients and their significant others. *Eur J Cancer* 45:182–187, 1996

41. Midmer D, Wilson L, Cummings S: A randomized, controlled trial of the influence of prenatal parenting education on postpartum anxiety and marital adjustment. *Fam Med* 27:200–205, 1995

42. Fawzy FI, Fawzy NW, Arndt LA, et al: Critical review of psychosocial interventions in cancer care. *Arch Gen Psychiatry* 52:100–113, 1995

43. Johnson J: The effects of a patient education course on persons with a chronic illness. *Cancer Nurs* 5:117–123, 1982

44. McMillan SC, Tittle MB, Hill D: A systematic evaluation of the "I Can Cope" program using a national sample. *Oncol Nurs Forum* 20:455–461, 1993

45. Cupples SA: Effects of timing and reinforcement of preoperative education on knowledge and recovery of patients having coronary artery bypass graft surgery. *Heart Lung* 20:654–660, 1991

46. Kratz A: Preoperative education preparing patients for a positive experience. *J Post Anesth Nurs* 8:270–275, 1993

47. Martucci B: One hospital's approach. *Patient Educ Update* 7:3, 1992

48. Heinen C: "Operation information" for ambulatory surgical patients. *Nurs Manage* 23:64Q–64T, 1992

49. Wainstock JM: Breast cancer: Psychosocial consequences for the patient. *Semin Oncol Nurs* 7:207–215, 1991

50. Hubbard SM, Martin NB, Thurn AL: NCI's Cancer Information Systems: Bringing medical knowledge to clinicians. *Oncology* 9:302–307, 1995

51. Ward S, Griffin J: Developing a test of knowledge of surgical options for breast cancer. *Cancer Nurs* 13:191–196, 1990

52. Shader R, Greenblatt D: Use of benzodiazepines in anxiety disorders. *N Engl J Med* 328:1398–1405, 1993

53. Gelenberg AJ: Buspirone: Seven-year update. *J Clin Psychiatry* 55:222–229, 1994

54. Rickels K: Buspirone in clinical practice. *J Clin Psychiatry* 51(suppl 9):51–54, 1990

55. Rickels K, Schweizer E: The treatment of generalized anxiety disorder in patients with depressive symptomatology. *J Clin Psychiatry* 54(suppl 1):20–23, 1993

56. Hollister LO: Clinical uses of benzodiazepines. *J Clin Psychopharmacol* 13(suppl 6):15–16, 1993

57. Rickels K: Antidepressants for the treatment of generalized anxiety disorder: A placebo-controlled comparison of imipramine, trazodone, and diazepam. *Arch Gen Psychiatry* 50:884–895, 1993

58. Stoudemire A, Moran MG: Psychopharmacologic treatment of anxiety in the medically ill elderly patient: Special considerations. *J Clin Psychiatry* 54(suppl 5):27–33, 1993

Anxiety: Progressive Muscle Relaxation and Guided Imagery

Patient Name: _____

Symptom and Description   It is common to feel stress or anxiety when you have cancer. Anxiety can be a vague or uneasy feeling of distress. There are many things that can bring on these feelings, such as trips to your doctor's office, treatments for your cancer, or fears about your cancer.

Learning Needs   There are many things that you can do to help your stress. Two things that are easy to learn are called *progressive muscle relaxation* and *guided imagery*. They may also help with pain, and nausea and vomiting.

These skills take practice. The more you practice these skills, the more helpful they are. Some people find it helpful to make a tape to listen to as they practice. A soothing tape of music may help. Many libraries have "relaxation tapes" or quiet, soothing music.

Management

Preparation

1. Find a quiet, comfortable spot to practice.
2. Sit up or lie down while you practice.
3. Have a blanket or sheet handy. Often when people are relaxed, they find they are cooler and need a light blanket.
4. Take a few minutes to think about your breathing. (You can keep your eyes open or closed.) Try to do stomach breathing. Fill your stomach as you breathe in and then breathe out. Begin to slow down, and slow your breathing down. Try to focus on your breathing.

Progressive Muscle Relaxation

1. Take in a deep breath. Hold that breath for a count of four, let it out, and begin to relax. Do this about four times. As you breathe in, think about good, soothing energy flowing in. As you breathe out, breathe out your stress and bad thoughts.
2. Allow your mind to focus on one body part at a time. Move from the top of your head all the way down to your toes.
3. Relax your head and your scalp. Repeat this two or three times.

4. Move down to your eyes. Relax your eyes and the muscles around your eyes. Squeeze your eyes tight for four counts, then relax. Notice the difference in your eyes and face when your eyes are squeezed and tense, and when they are relaxed.

5. Focus on your mouth. Relax your mouth. Allow it to go limp. . . . Move down your neck, relax your neck. . . . Relax your shoulders. . . .

6. When you get to your arms, you may relax them one at a time or both at the same time. You may even choose to relax each finger, one at a time.

7. Move all the way down to your toes using this skill.

Extra Tips (tips that may help body areas that are tense or painful)

1. As you move down your body, you may want to tighten and then relax certain body parts. This helps to show how different your body feels when it is tense and when it is relaxed. You can tense and then relax your eyes, hands, toes, mouth, and shoulders. You should get more relaxed as you move down your body. If you feel relaxed, you may not feel like doing this part past your mouth or shoulders.

2. Warm often feels good. Think about any part of your body being warmed by the sun. For example, if your right arm has pain, you can focus on this arm. Think about warm rays of sun on your arm as you relax.

3. Tense or sore muscles may feel better with the "knot" method. Think about your sore spot, such as your shoulder, as a big, tight knot. In your mind, slowly untie the knot. As you untie the knot, the sore spot becomes less and less sore. When you untie the knot all the way, you can focus on how your body is more relaxed.

4. Try the "sandbag" method for a body part that hurts. Think about the area that hurts as an empty sandbag. Slowly fill up the sandbag with warm sand. As you fill the bag, push out the hurt. Fill the bag until you can't put any more sand in it. Slowly pour out the sand. Any hurt that is left flows out with the sand. Enjoy the soothing feeling of the bag when it is again empty.

Guided Imagery

1. It is best to do this skill after you have done the progressive muscle relaxation. Once your body is relaxed, you can allow your mind to rest.

2. Before you begin, think about a special image or place. This can be a place where you have been or it can be a made-up place. Choose a relaxing place. Think about the whole scene. What does it look like? What do you hear? What do you taste or smell? Be as detailed as you like.

3. Some examples of pleasant places might include a warm, sunny beach, a sparkling lake, a walk in the woods, or a lovely snow-capped mountain.

4. Your image should be a place where you can be very relaxed. It is a place with no stress or worry. You can go to this place when you need a break.

Example of a Guided Imagery Scene

I am lying alone on a beach in the late afternoon sun. It is nice and warm, but not too hot. The water is aqua blue, with small white caps close to the shore. The sky is light blue, with a few white puffy clouds. I am lying with my feet to the water, with the sun moving to the right of me. I can feel my warm beach towel under me and warm sand on my hands and feet. I feel the soothing sun on my body. I hear seagulls flying over me. I hear sea grass swaying in the breeze behind me. I hear some children playing in the sand, but I can't hear what they are saying. The water is gently lapping on the shore, over and over and over . . .

Follow-up

1. These skills are not to be used instead of pain medicine or any other type of medicine that you need. They should be used *with* your current treatment.

2. It is okay to fall asleep during either progressive muscle relaxation or guided imagery. It does not mean that it is not working. It may mean that you need the sleep. Give yourself the rest that comes with a relaxed body and mind.

3. Progressive muscle relaxation and guided imagery take practice to help you relax. When you feel good with these skills, they may also help with pain or nausea and vomiting.

4. Talk with your doctor, nurse, or someone you trust about your stress. They may be able to give you other ideas.

Phone Numbers

Nurse: _____ Phone: _____

Physician: _____ Phone: _____

Other: _____ Phone: _____

Comments

Patient's Signature: _____ Date: _____

Nurse's Signature: _____ Date: _____

Source: Gobel BH: Anxiety, in Yarbro CH, Frogge MH, Goodman M (eds): *Cancer Symptom Management* (ed 2). Sudbury: Jones and Bartlett, 1999. © Jones and Bartlett Publishers.

CHAPTER 31

Depression

Judith Kehs Much, RN, MSN, AOCN
Andrea M. Barsevick, RN, DNSC, AOCN

The Problem of Depression in Cancer

One of the most common psychosocial problems that oncology nurses manage in their patients is depression. It is a difficult problem to manage, in part because of the difficulties inherent in diagnosing and predicting human behavior. This chapter contains information to assist oncology nurses in recognizing who is at risk for depression, how to assess the patient who is suspected of having depression, and how to manage depression and suicidal ideation.

The mood state called depression includes a broad spectrum of moods and behaviors. It is described as a feeling of gloom, emptiness, numbness, or despair. It may occur in physically healthy people, in those with a psychiatric disorder, and in those with a physical illness such as cancer. Oncology nurses recognize that depression is not a unitary phenomenon: it exists on a continuum of emotional responses ranging from minor mood changes to major depression with feelings of worthlessness and recurrent death wishes. It may be accompanied by somatic symptoms such as appetite or sleep changes and loss of energy. And some individuals may experience cognitive distortions such as viewing many events in their lives as negative and paying unrealistic attention to negative details. Regardless, every individual experiencing depressed mood requires acknowledgment and assessment by the nurse to determine whether intervention is needed.

A depressed mood is not necessarily abnormal. It is an appropriate part of an uncomplicated grief response. The distinguishing characteristic of grief is the presence of a loss. Most commonly, we think of the death of a loved one. But individuals also grieve after the loss of their health, the loss of a body part such as a breast, or a loss of functioning such as the ability to walk without pain. Grief work or mourning is an adaptive process of separating oneself from the loss and getting on with one's life.

Another common form of depressed mood seen by oncology nurses is mild, chronic depression, which is called *dysthymia* in psychiatry. It is characterized by irritability, annoyance, loss of pleasure in life, feelings of sadness, self-criticism, and self-blame. The individual may withdraw from loved ones, feel guilty in various situations, and suffer aches and pains. In many instances, this reaction is barely noticeable, but some impairment in usual functioning may be observed.

Indicators of moderate to severe depression include feelings of failure or punishment, loss of interest in people, and suicidal ideas. These symptoms are distinguished from mild depressive symptoms by their intensity, pervasiveness, persistence, and degree of interference with usual functioning. In addition to careful monitoring and intervention by the oncology nurse, referral to a psychiatric professional for further evaluation is necessary for persons with moderate to severe depression.

Incidence in Cancer

Studies of the prevalence of depression in cancer patients have had widely varying results depending on the population sampled. The highest rates of depression (45% excluding somatic criteria) have been documented for individuals with advanced disease who had low performance status indicated by a Karnofsky Performance Status score of less than 40.[1,2] Among individuals hospitalized for cancer, 25% were found to have depression.[3,4] This is about the same prevalence rate as for hospitalized persons with other diseases, suggesting that people with cancer experience depression at about the same rate as any other medical-surgical population. In a randomly accessed population of ambulatory and hospitalized persons with cancer, the prevalence rate of depression was 13%, about twice the distribution in the population at large, suggesting that there is a significant group of depressed cancer patients waiting to be recognized.[5]

Impact on Quality of Life

Research has demonstrated that depression, even at low levels, can have profound effects on quality of life including functional status. Colorectal cancer patients who have depressive symptoms before surgical treatment or 1 month after surgery are likely to have poorer functional status 3 and 6 months later than persons who reported no depressive symptoms.[6]

Depressive symptoms are also related to survival time after a cancer diagnosis. In a recent study, routine psychiatric evaluations were conducted on 100 adult patients undergoing allogeneic bone marrow transplantation for acute leukemia.[7] The findings demonstrated that depressive mood was associated with shorter duration of survival. Another investigation demonstrated that women with metastatic breast cancer who participated in a support group reported lower levels of distress, including depression, and lived an average of twice as long as women who did not have the benefit of the support group.[8]

Studies of other patient populations emphasize the impact of depressive symptoms on recovery of functioning after physical illnesses and surgical procedures. People with hip fractures who have high levels of depressive symptoms are more likely to be dependent in walking, are less likely to return to prefracture levels of physical functioning, and have the poorest physical functioning when compared with others recovering from hip fractures who had low levels of depressive symptoms.[9]

A recent, large-scale study compared outcomes for two groups of people: those reporting depressive symptoms and those with diagnosed depressive disorders.[10] The two groups were examined for the presence or absence of chronic medical conditions. The researchers found significant morbidity associated with depressive symptoms. People with both diagnosed depression and chronic medical conditions had the poorest functioning. However, people who had depressive symptoms without depressive disorders had poorer functioning than individuals with eight major chronic medical conditions alone. For example, individuals with depressive symptoms spent more time in bed than individuals with hypertension, diabetes, or arthritis who did not report depressed mood. Thus, depressive symptoms, even at low levels, are important to attend to because they may erode people's ability to function in their usual roles and activities for considerable periods of time.

Depressive symptoms can also have an economic impact. Researchers found that hospitalized medical patients who were anxious and depressed remained hospitalized 40% longer with 35% higher medical costs than nondepressed patients.[11] Depressed medical outpatients who received psychotherapy had a significant decrease in outpatient medical costs after treatment.[12]

Etiology

Risk Factors

There are a number of risk factors that increase the potential for the development of depression.

- *Age:* Overall adaptation to illness tends to be poorer in younger persons than in older persons.[13–16]
- *Health Problems:* Advanced stage of disease, relapse or progression, unrelieved symptoms, medications, and body image problems have all been associated with the development of depression.[2,17–21]
- *Previous Mental Health:* An individual or family history of depression or a history of substance abuse places the person with cancer at greater risk of depression.[2,22]
- *Disease Recurrence:* Times of treatment failure and recurrence of disease increase one's vulnerability to depression.[17,23,24]
- *Medications:* Many classes of the medications commonly prescribed for cancer patients can have depression as a side effect (Table 31-1).
- *Unrelieved Symptoms:* The presence of unrelieved symptoms, particularly pain, puts people at risk for depression.

Pathophysiology

The past few decades of research suggest that mood disturbances have multiple etiologies that involve the interaction of biological and psychosocial causes.[25]

TABLE 31-1 Classes of Medications That May Have Depressive Side Effects

Analgesics	Cytotoxics
Anticonvulsants	Hormones
Antihistamines	Immunosuppressive agents
Antihypertensives	
Antiinflammatory agents	Sedatives
	Steroids
Antimicrobials	Stimulants
Antineoplastics	Tranquilizers
Antiparkinsonian agents	

Data from references 17 and 35.

- Genetic factors make some people more susceptible to the development of depression.
- Developmental events or losses may sensitize an individual to stressors resulting in negative thinking and learned helplessness as coping strategies.
- Physiologic stressors, including drugs, endocrine or nutritional disturbances, or infections, can induce biochemical changes that precipitate depression.
- Psychosocial stressors can overwhelm coping mechanisms.

One or more of these factors can cause disturbances in neurotransmission as well as disturbances in mood, arousal, motivation, and psychomotor function. This integrative multicausal model provides guidance in assessing patient behavior holistically. There is increasing evidence that mood disturbances are associated with biochemical changes in the brain.[26] Norepinephrine and serotonin are neurotransmitters located in the nerve cells of the brain that have been most often implicated in depression. Drugs that are typically used to treat depression influence the regulation of these transmitters. Currently studies also suggest that there is dysregulation of the limbic-hypothalamic-pituitary-adrenal (LHPA) axis.

Assessment

Barriers to Recognition and Treatment

Acknowledgment of depression in those with cancer is difficult for both clinicians and patients, in part because of several myths that set up barriers to diagnosis and treatment.[17] The first of these is that depression is to be expected in cancer patients. This myth is not supported by empirical data. Cancer patients are no more likely to develop depression than other medical-surgical patients. The implication that cancer patients do not need treatment for their depression because it is a "normal" occurrence is equally false. People with cancer who also suffer from depression are as likely to benefit from its treatment as any other individual.

Another myth is that there is not enough time to deal with patients' psychosocial problems. However, minimal time and psychosocial skill are needed to conduct a brief assessment and make a referral. Clinicians can also provide empathy and support in the course of their regular work with patients.

Lack of cooperation by the patient is another barrier that may be incorrectly interpreted as laziness, manipulation, attention-seeking, or noncompliance. Symptoms of depression include low energy, lack of interest, and negativism. These behaviors are to be recognized as signs of depression that can be treated rather than a lack of compliance.

Another myth is that suicide is a logical choice for all cancer patients. While there currently is national debate about the rights of persons with debilitating, painful diseases to end their lives, clinicians have a professional obligation to ensure that correctable problems such as depression, unmanaged pain, or unrelieved symptoms are dealt with.

Both clinicians and patients have to deal with these barriers. In addition, patients may need to deal with embarrassment about being depressed, their desire not to "bother" a busy physician or nurse, or their fear of being stigmatized by acknowledging it. Clinicians face the additional barrier that symptoms used to diagnose depression in the general population may be less reliable for cancer patients because somatic symptoms in cancer patients could signal depression *or* the effects of illness or treatment. If clinicians ignore these somatic signs, they run the risk of missing patients who are depressed; if they include these signs, they run the risk of overdiagnosing.[17] To make a formal diagnosis of major depression, the most severe form of depression, *Diagnostic and Statistical Manual of Mental Disorders*–IV of the American Psychiatric Association[27] requires that dysphoric mood and at least four other symptoms of depression must be present for at least 2 weeks (Table 31-2). A less severe form of depression called dysthymia may also be diagnosed if fewer symptoms are experienced but they persist for a longer period of time (at least 2 years). The classic picture of the individual with *dysthymia* includes introversion, brooding, inability to enjoy oneself, and preoccupation with personal inadequacy.[28]

Recognition of depression in cancer patients is hampered by the presence of physical symptoms that can mimic as well as cover up depressive symptoms. Consider the major somatic signs of depression: changes in appetite or sleep patterns, fatigue, and decreased ability to concentrate. These may result from depression, the cancer, or cancer treatment. Because of lack of clarity about the origin of these symptoms, oncology professionals are forced to rely more on the presence of psychological symptoms in determining the existence of depression. These include mood indicators (sadness, gloom, loss of pleasure, guilt, low self-esteem, and suicidal thoughts)

TABLE 31-2   Major Depressive Episode

A major depressive episode is defined as:
1. Depressed mood or loss of interest or pleasure for at least 2 weeks;
2. At least five of the following symptoms during the same 2-week period:
   a. Significant weight loss or weight gain when not dieting;
   b. Sleep disturbance (especially early morning awakening);
   c. Psychomotor agitation or retardation;
   d. Fatigue or loss of energy;
   e. Feelings of worthlessness or excessive inappropriate guilt;
   f. Diminished ability to think or concentrate, or indecisiveness;
   g. Recurrent thoughts of death, recurrent suicidal ideation, suicidal plan, or suicidal attempt.

American Psychiatric Association: *Diagnostic and Statistical Manual of Mental Disorders* (ed 4). Washington, DC: American Psychiatric Association, 1994.[27] Reprinted with permission.

and the intensity and longevity of these moods, as well as the degree to which they affect usual functioning.

Indicators of Depression in Individuals with Cancer

An initial assessment of depression is based on the presence of typical signs and symptoms. The best indicator is depressed mood. Other psychological signs include loss of pleasure, feelings of punishment or failure, irritability, or suicidal ideation. Somatic signs may also be present including sleep disturbance (especially early morning wakening), appetite or weight changes, fatigue or loss of energy, and diminished ability to think or concentrate. Because cancer and its treatment can cause these symptoms, they need to be reviewed carefully to determine whether they are related to depression. For example, the nurse could ask, "Did you have difficulty sleeping before you began adjuvant treatment? Was it about the same time you began feeling sad?"

The initial assessment also includes a judgment about the severity of the depression. Every individual with cancer experiences times of disappointment and sadness related to their condition. The nurse must judge whether this episode is of sufficient severity or persistence to require additional intervention. Some indicators that could assist the nurse in making this judgment include:

- The individual has been feeling low for more than a week.
- Reaction seems out of proportion to the stressor.
- Family/friends report current mood is out of character.
- The individual reports persistent difficulty concentrating on tasks.

A more thorough assessment must be conducted if the nurse determines that the depression is severe or persistent enough to require special attention. This assessment, based on the multicausal model, includes a review of genetic vulnerability and stressors. Gathering this information enables the nurse to provide specific comprehensive information to the mental healthcare provider about the individual's depression.

Measurement

Because the clinical signs of depression in physically ill people may be ambiguous, the administration of a depressive symptom scale could be a useful adjunct in identifying the presence and degree of depression. It is also known that clinicians perceive the affective state of their patients differently than the patients themselves do. Generally professionals overestimate the amount of depression and anxiety experienced by those in their care.[2,29] The use of an objective measurement tool could help prevent this overestimation. Many assessment tools are available, and they range from visual analogue scales[30] to lengthy and comprehensive tests. The clinician should investigate any tool that he or she plans to use, paying particular attention to applicability to patient population being tested, what the tool will be testing, in what populations it has been shown to be valid and reliable, ease of administration, and responder burden.

The following tools have established reliability and validity in the medically ill population, have minimal responder burden, and can be administered in virtually any care setting.

The Beck Depression Inventory (BDI)

The Beck Depression Inventory is one of the oldest and most widely used scales.[31] Quick and easy to administer, this 21-question self-report measure takes approximately 10 minutes to complete. The BDI has norms and cutoff scores indicating clinically diagnosable depression, and has been shown to have validity in screening for depression in medically ill individuals.[32]

The Geriatric Depression Scale (GDS)

The Geriatric Depression Scale is designed specifically for rating depression in the elderly. Like the BDI, it has norms and cutoff scores indicating clinically diagnosable depression. A 30-question self-report scale, the GDS takes about 5 minutes to complete (Figure 31-1). The scale contains no items measuring somatic symptoms that could confound patient responses in a medically ill population, making it very attractive for use in elderly individuals with cancer. The GDS has also been shown to be valid and reliable.[34,35]

Choose the best answer for how you felt over the past week.

1. Are you basically satisfied with your life?   Yes   No
2. Have you dropped many of your activities?   Yes   No
3. Do you feel that your life is empty?   Yes   No
4. Do you often get bored?   Yes   No
5. Are you hopeful about the future?   Yes   No
6. Are you bothered by thoughts you can't get out of your head?   Yes   No
7. Are you in good spirits most of the time?   Yes   No
8. Are you afraid that something bad is going to happen to you?   Yes   No
9. Do you feel happy most of the time?   Yes   No
10. Do you often feel helpless?   Yes   No
11. Do you often get restless and fidgety?   Yes   No
12. Do you prefer to stay at home, rather than go out and do new things?   Yes   No
13. Do you frequently worry about the future?   Yes   No
14. Do you feel you have more problems with memory than most?   Yes   No
15. Do you think it is wonderful to be alive?   Yes   No
16. Do you often feel downhearted and blue?   Yes   No
17. Do you feel pretty worthless the way you are now?   Yes   No
18. Do you worry a lot about the past?   Yes   No
19. Do you find life very exciting?   Yes   No
20. Is it hard for you to get started on new projects?   Yes   No
21. Do you feel full of energy?   Yes   No
22. Do you feel that your situation is hopeless?   Yes   No
23. Do you think that most people are better off than you are?   Yes   No
24. Do you frequently get upset over little things?   Yes   No
25. Do you frequently feel like crying?   Yes   No
26. Do you have trouble concentrating?   Yes   No
27. Do you enjoy getting up in the morning?   Yes   No
28. Do you prefer to avoid social gatherings?   Yes   No
29. Is it easy for you to make a decision?   Yes   No
30. Is your mind as clear as it used to be?   Yes   No

FIGURE 31-1 Geriatric Depression Scale. (From Yesavage J, Brink TL: Development and validation of a geriatric depression screening scale: A preliminary report. *J Psychiatr Res* 17:37–49, 1983.[33] Elsevier Science Ltd., Pergamon Imprint, Oxford, England. Reprinted with permission.)

Assessment of Suicide Potential

Assessment of suicidal ideation can lead to early detection of those at risk, allowing time for appropriate consultation and intervention.

General risk factors for suicide

Depressed mood Feelings of sadness, hopelessness, gloom, or loss of pleasure are present in 50% of all individuals who attempt or commit suicide. Therefore, identification and treatment of those with underlying depression can substantially reduce the risk of suicide.[25,36]

Preexisting psychopathology Personality disorders with self-destructive behaviors, major depression, bipolar disorder, psychosis, and alcohol or substance abuse increase the risk of suicide.

Individual or family history An individual's risk substantially increases if that person has made an attempt at suicide at least twice in the past. There is also suspected (but not proven) to be a genetic or biochemical vulnerability to suicide,[36] possibly related to serotonin level, which would also herald other signs such as depressed mood.

Drug or alcohol abuse The current abuse of drugs or alcohol places the individual at increased risk of suicide.

Specific suicide plan The degree of suicidal risk increases as the plan becomes more specific and the means for carrying it out become more available. For example, if an individual tells you that he or she plans to die by gunshot wound to the head, yet there is no access to a firearm, the ability to carry out successful suicide is decreased. If the individual states that he or she "wants it to be over," but is unable to provide you with any specific plan, the risk is decreased. If, however, the individual states that he or she can no longer "stand the pain" and goes on to mention the purchase of 30 days' worth of pain medication, the potential for suicide is high. Finally, the risk of suicide increases if the individual refuses a *no suicide contract*, which is, in effect, a promise by the individual not to harm himself or herself intentionally for a specific period of time.

Risk factors for suicide that are specific to cancer patients

Disease site Suicidal risk is highest among persons with head and neck, gastrointestinal, and lung cancers. The explanation for this is not known. It may have to do with multiple stressors, including disfigurement from radical surgery, and the associated smoking and drinking that could reflect limited coping skills.[37]

Prognosis Those with advanced illness and poor prognosis are more likely to commit suicide, even if their physical capacity is reduced or limited.[37] Often this is a time of difficult symptom management, pain, depression, fatigue, fear of dying, and loss of control.

Suboptimal pain management Poor or inadequate pain management places the individual at risk.[17,24,36] Poorly managed pain is also related to depression.[37] The presence of pain affects quality of life and sense of control and reduces one's perception of support.

Fatigue Intolerable fatigue, which is described as multidimensional, physical, emotional, financial, spiritual, and the exhaustion of psychological resources, places the individual at increased risk. Both depth and duration of fatigue influence its impact.

Delirium   Delirium is a biologically induced acute confusional state that is marked by impaired cognition and decreased ability to maintain attention. Delirium is present in at least 25% of cancer patients (all stages and types) and increases to up to 85% in terminal patients. Causes include primary or metastatic brain tumor, brain irradiation, and chemotherapy or biological therapy. Other causes include metabolic disturbances due to electrolyte imbalance, sepsis, hypoxia, polypharmacy, and age.[38] Not addressing the cause of delirium may leave the cancer patient at risk for impulsive suicidal attempts.[36]

Helplessness and loss of control   Loss of control and a sense of helplessness may be induced by functional and psychological deficits caused by cancer and its treatment.

Symptom Management

Prevention

Cancer patients need to be educated not only about their disease and its treatment, but also about the potential psychosocial hazards they face (Figure 31-2). Such preparation could reduce the impact of those problems should they develop.[39–41] Individuals and their family members should know the signs and symptoms of depression and have access to a resource list of professionals to call for assistance. They need to be taught about the milestones of the cancer experience when depression is most likely to occur, such as when there is change in body image or role function, when pain is poorly controlled, and when the person is taking certain classes of medications.

Encouragement allows individuals with cancer and their families to discuss the disease and the impact it has on family dynamics and function. Issues of loss and grieving, stress associated with the disease and treatment, coping with anger, changes in sexual function, changes in body image, role change, and work-related issues are all normal.[21–24] Opportunity for open and honest discussion can enhance adaptation. The nurse works at establishing a trusting, honest, and supportive therapeutic relationship with the individual so that information exchange is facilitated. Active listening is employed in this process. The nurse displays an understanding of the unique cultural attributes the individual and family bring to this experience, as this may influence willingness to share information, acknowledge grief, accept the disease, and cope with role changes. The nurse assesses and supports positive coping mechanisms that have been helpful to the individual in the past.

Teaching symptom management skills and stress management skills increase the individual's sense of control over his or her own destiny. Numerous authors stress the preventive aspect of these interventions.[37,39,41] The individual should be given oral and if possible written information regarding particular symptoms that are expected to occur, with concrete management interventions and guidelines related to when and how to notify professionals if the interventions are not successful.

Activity should be encouraged as well as conservation of energy during periods of fatigue, as these factors can influence mental wellness.[42] Adequate pain management is important to minimize the risk of depression and suicide.[2,13,24,36,37] Successful pain management lessens physical pain and decreases the suffering experienced by both the individual with cancer and those struggling to care for him or her. The nursing role is to evaluate the type and amount of pain medication and its scheduling, the amount of supplemental medication the patient is requiring for pain not relieved by around-the-clock medications, and what level of pain relief the patient is receiving from his or her medication.

Therapeutic Approaches

If it is determined that an individual is depressed, all medications being taken by that person should be scrutinized and if possible the medications should be stopped or changed to an equivalent medication that does not cause depression as a side effect. Because persons with cancer often obtain prescriptions from more than one provider, a review of all the medications is in order. If a psychiatric consultant is to be involved, these medications should be brought to his or her attention.

Patient and family education about pain control and all other symptoms the patient may experience is of paramount importance. Evaluation of fatigue and teaching about energy conservation are helpful. Because not all individuals have the same sleep patterns or sleep requirements, individual sleep patterns should be discussed and barriers to comfort, rest, and sleep should be eliminated. Adequate nutrition must be ensured to minimize fatigue and increase feelings of well-being, even in the individual with advanced disease.

Interventions for management of depression range from supportive and cognitive to psychotherapeutic and pharmacologic. An individual who does not experience a major depression but who expresses sadness may benefit from supportive counseling alone, by the nurse or social worker. An individual expressing suicidal ideation could require all strategies. An individual experiencing moderate depression might utilize one or all of the strategies.

Supportive interventions

The depressed patient is best managed with consistent emotional support in the context of a trusting relationship. This relationship helps in problem solving, acknowl-

TEACHING GUIDE: DEPRESSION

Learner Objective	Date started	Date completed	Comments/Signature
		Instruction	
1. Patient/family know personal risk factors for depression.			
2. Patient/family understand side effects of the medication being taken (if any).			
3. Patient/family know not to abruptly stop taking medication.			
4. Patient/family verbalize when to call professional.			
A. Acute change in self-care (physical or psychological)			
B. Suicidal ideation			
C. Inability to manage symptoms			
5. Patient/family have knowledge of resources.			
A. Personal			
B. Professional			
C. Community			

FIGURE 31-2   Teaching Guide: Depression. To be used as a guide to determine what teaching needs to be accomplished.

edges the patient's fears, and allows for control and decision making based on the individual's own unique needs. The goals of this intervention are to regain one's previous level of self-worth, correct misconceptions about the past and present, and integrate the present illness into one's self-concept.

Active listening is employed by the nurse to build trust and acceptance.[43] The nurse uses communication skills to facilitate a sense of partnership with patients. Good communication sets a stable tone and is supportive of hope.[44] Communication involves provision of support by the nurse and the identification of other psychosocial supports for the individual, such as friends, family, other patients with similar disease and good outcome, support groups, and community resources for rides, food, and financial matters. This approach emphasizes past strengths, supports past useful coping strategies, and mobilizes both internal and external resources.

Good communication can be used to build a partnership with patients and families. Exam rooms or consultation areas can provide the forum for discussion of the patient's needs and strengths. Nurses can be the catalyst for impromptu support groups in waiting areas by introducing people with similar issues or problems. Experienced nurses routinely weave these activities into bathing, ambulating, and treatment and medication administration time and only rarely need to create separate "support time."

Supportive interventions can be provided in a group format as well as individually. Support groups typically focus on shared problems and concerns, and the group is used to provide peer support and emotional encouragement.[45] Research has demonstrated that support groups result in sustained improvement in depression, anxiety, and psychosocial functioning.[45]

Cognitive interventions

Negative thought patterns or distortions of thought can trigger or exacerbate depression. Cognitive intervention focuses on increasing patient awareness of this negative focus, identifying the sequence of thoughts that led to the distorted conclusion, and learning new strategies to stop this type of thinking while substituting more positive thoughts.[17] Nurses often incorporate these strategies into their daily practice by "reframing" negative thoughts in a more positive light. For example, an individual with neutropenia requiring a treatment delay could react by complaining that the white count is "always too low" and that treatments are "never" delivered on time. The nurse can point out the reality that this is only the second time a treatment delay has been necessary and cognitively reframe the patient's comment with the observation that chemotherapy affects all fast multiplying cells, including the cancer and one's blood cells. It may be helpful also to point out the negative thought pattern and how it can reinforce and increase depressive feelings. The nurse can help the individual identify more positive, hopeful thoughts to substitute for the negative ones. In this way, the individual learns a skill to decrease depressive symptoms and to increase his or her sense of control over a problem situation. Once the individual is aware and able to identify negative thoughts, it may be helpful to ask the individual to keep a daily log of typical negative thoughts along with "good" things that have happened. In review of the log, it would be appropriate for the nurse to offer support and correct distorted perceptions.

Psychotherapy

Premorbid psychosocial problems can be exacerbated by illness. The role of psychotherapy in this context is to assist the patient and family to cope with the illness and its treatment. It is not to solve preexisting problems. Short-term psychotherapy often uses the crisis intervention model and supportive techniques. This type of intervention is practiced by clinicians experienced in the technique and may require a social work or psychiatric referral if the resources aren't available in the care area to provide the service.

Psychopharmacology

Pharmacologic treatment for depression has its basis in the biochemical theory of depression, that depression is a result of levels of circulating norepinephrine (NE) and serotonin (5-HT) within the central nervous system. Treatment usually involves at least one of a number of classes of drugs (Table 31-3). Tricyclic antidepressants (TCAs) have been the gold standard for depression until the recent emergence of selective serotonin reuptake inhibitors (SSRIs). Other drugs used to treat depression include lithium, the benzodiazepines, and monoamine oxidase inhibitors (MAOIs). Of special note in the treatment of depression are stimulants for the very depressed dying patient who does not have the luxury of waiting 4 to 6 weeks for an antidepressant effect or for individuals with motor retardation or fatigue secondary to illness.

The nurse caring for the cancer patient needs to be aware of the action and side effects of psychoactive drugs as well as potential interactions with other drugs being taken for cancer, its treatment, or its symptoms.

There are four basic principles involved in the administration of psychiatric drugs to cancer patients.[46]

- The starting dose of the drug is generally lower than that typically given to healthy individuals.
- The dosage is increased more slowly.
- The therapeutic dose may be significantly lower in cancer patients than in healthy individuals.
- Potential side effects must be monitored very carefully, as antidepressants often affect the same organs as cancer treatment drugs or the disease itself.

Patients must be instructed (and clinicians must know) that TCAs should be taken as scheduled and should not be withdrawn or stopped suddenly. To do so may risk cholinergic rebound, including nausea and vomiting, headache, diaphoresis, chills, coryza, muscle aches, and nightmares or colorful vivid dreams.

TABLE 31-3 Prototype Drugs Used in the Treatment of Depression

Class/Drug Names	Dose Range (mg/day)	Onset of Action at Therapeutic Dose	Drug Interaction*	Side Effects*	Specific Comments*
Selective Serotonin Reuptake Inhibitors (SSRIs)					
Paroxetine (Paxil)	10–50	3–10 days	Monoamine oxidase inhibitors (MAOIs)	Nausea	Caution in elderly, renal or hepatic impairment, pregnancy, lactation, history of mania, or suicidal patients.
Sertraline (Zoloft)	50–200	7 days	Cimetidine (paroxetine)	Dry mouth	Do not use concurrently with MAOI.
Fluoxetine (Prozac)	20	2–4 wk	Caution with CNS active drugs	Rash	Fluoxetine and paroxetine can cause hyponatremia.
			Hypoglycemic agents (fluoxetine)	Headache	Use with alcohol not recommended.
			Digitoxin	Nervousness	Do not stop medication suddenly.
			Oral anticoagulants	Drowsiness	Anaphylaxis has been reported (rare).
				Loss of libido	If drowsiness occurs, administer at bedtime.
				Diarrhea	
				Postural hypotension	

continued

TABLE 31-3 (continued)

Class/Drug Names	Dose Range (mg/day)	Onset of Action at Therapeutic Dose	Drug Interaction*	Side Effects*	Specific Comments*
Tricyclic Antidepressants (TCAs)					
Amitriptyline (Elavil)	25–250	4–6 wk	MAOIs	Anticholinergic: urinary retention, dry mouth, thirst, blurred vision, glaucoma, constipation, sedation, nausea and vomiting, impaired speech, trouble swallowing, tachycardia	Caution in suicidal patients, hepatic and renal dysfunction, cardiac disease, pregnancy and lactation.
Doxepin (Sinequan)	50–150	4–6 wk	Cimetidine		
Imipramine (Norpramin)	25–150	4–6 wk	Amphetamines CNS depressants		All therapeutically equal—choose on basis of side effects.
Nortriptyline (Pamelor)	50–150	4–6 wk	Thyroid medications Cardiac medications	Antihistaminic: sedation, weight gain	Must do baseline ECG—then monitor for toxicity.
Trazodone (Dyseril)	50–250	1–4 wk	Oral contraceptives	Alpha-adrenergic: hypotension	Blood levels correlate with therapeutic effect in imipramine, desipramine, and nortriptyline.
Desipramine (Norpramin)	25–150	4–6 wk	Oral anticoagulants Smoking	Cardiac: tachycardia, orthostasis, arrhythmia, delayed conduction	Much of drug is protein-bound.
				Withdrawal reaction: nausea, vomiting, headache, chills, coryza, muscle aches, nightmares, vivid colorful dreams	Toxicity increases with protein depletion. Never abruptly stop medication. Switch ONLY after adequate trial. Maintain on drugs for 12 symptom-free months. Report rapid weight gain.
Lithium					
Lithane	600–1200	Rapid	Drugs high in sodium	Dehydration	Caution in history of renal or thyroid disease.
Lithobid	Start lower dose, bid	Rapid	Aminophylline Mannitol Sodium bicarbonate Nonsteroidal anti-inflammatory agents Thiazide diuretics Phenothiazines Iodides	Hyponatremia Lithium poisoning: fine tremor, muscle weakness, then muscle twitch, ataxia, nausea, diarrhea, difficulty in concentration, somnolence, dysarthria Neuropathy Hypothyroidism Cardiac abnormalities	Monitor ECG, thyroid function, BUN, creatinine, creatine clearance. Lithium blood levels are accurate: adjust dose to get plasma levels 0.8–1.2 mEq/liter Measure plasma levels 12 hours after last dose. Monitor levels frequently in medically unstable patients. Available in liquid and tablet form. Psychiatrist referral to monitor patient status if in need of surgery.
Sympathomimetic Stimulants					
Dextroamphetamine (Dexedrine, Obetrol)	2.5–5 in AM	Rapid	MAOIs Insulin	Appetite suppression Irritability, insomnia, palpitations, tachycardia	Use controversial. Improves mood and possibly appetite in terminal patients.
Methylphenidate (Ritalin)	5–10, 8 AM & 12 noon	Rapid	Phenothiazines Urinary alkalinizers and acidifiers		Cautious use with seizures or cardiac abnormalities. Reported decrease in narcotic consumption. Can reverse sedative effects of narcotics.

TABLE 31-3 (continued)

Class/Drug Names	Dose Range (mg/day)	Onset of Action at Therapeutic Dose	Drug Interaction*	Side Effects*	Specific Comments*
Monoamine Oxidase Inhibitors (MAOIs)					
Phenelzine (Nardil)	30–60, start lower dose, bid	1–6 wk	CNS depressants Sympatho- mimetic and catecholamine- releasing drugs (including levodopa, dopamine, amphetamines, methyldopa, tryptophan, epinephrine, norepinephrine) Other MAOIs, TCAs Insulin Antihypertensives Thiazide diuretics, oral hypo- glycemics Anesthetics	Anorgasmy Impotence Hypomania Syncope Dizziness Headache Constipation Blurred vision Orthostatic hypotension Dry mouth	Instruct patient to avoid tyramine-containing foods, e.g., aged cheese, red wine, beef extract, etc. (can cause hypertensive crisis). Give patient instruction card with list of foods to avoid. Discontinue 24–48 hours prior to emergency surgery or 1–2 weeks prior to elective surgery. Do not give with meperidine. Caution in suicidal patients, hepatic or renal dysfunction, and alcohol usage. Do not stop medication abruptly. Report rapid weight gain. Teach patient over-the- counter medications may contain substances that could precipitate hypertensive crisis.
Tranylcypromine (Parnate)	20–40, start lower dose, bid	1–6 wk			
Isocarboxazid (Marplan)	20–40, start lower dose, bid	1–6 wk			
Benzodiazepines					
Alprazolam (Xanax)	0.25–1 qid, then 0.75–6 mg/day	Rapid	Cimetidine, CNS depressants, oral contraceptives Cigarettes Caffeine Diogoxin Levodopa	Sedation Confusion Motor incoordination Somnolence	Acts as both antidepressant and anxiolytic. More rapid effect than TCA. Reduces nausea and vomiting, especially anticipatory. Caution with hepatic impairment.

*Relates to entire class of drugs unless otherwise indicated.

Data from manufacturer's product information.

Patterns of response of antidepressant medi-cations   Response to antidepressant drugs is usually gradual. Individuals who experience sleep or appetite disturbance secondary to their depression might expect improvement in sleep and appetite within 2 to 7 days. Improvement in mood may lag behind 3 to 10 days in the newer class of SSRIs or 2 to 8 weeks for the TCAs. Response may be delayed even longer in the elderly debilitated individual. This makes drug selection important in those with limited life expectancy. Lessening of psychomotor retardation or agitation would be expected before mood improves.

Metabolism of antidepressant medications   It is important for the oncology nurse to understand metabolism of antidepressant medications, as this will provide clues to toxicities, dosage ranges, and length of time it might take individuals to experience therapeutic benefit. Most antidepressant medications are metabolized in the liver. Liver failure or dysfunction is a common problem secondary to cancer or its treatments and will inhibit the individual's ability to properly metabolize antidepressants, thereby reducing their efficacy. Normal metabolism of TCAs produces some substances that are cardiotoxic. These substances cannot be measured by doing routine serum levels of the drug. These metabolites are excreted through the renal system. If renal function is reduced by cancer or its treatments, the toxicity of the antidepressant medication increases.

Use of antidepressants can result in cardiac conduction abnormalities, particularly for TCAs and to a lesser degree the SSRIs. Because of this side effect, an ECG is usually obtained at baseline for those with a history of arrhythmias or cardiac disease. In individuals over age 50, a baseline ECG is generally obtained regardless of cardiac history. Because the QRS segment of the ECG is exquisitely sensitive to the cardiotoxic properties of TCAs, ECGs should be followed to measure response. Changes in the QRS interval over the baseline will necessitate either a reduction or no further increase in dosage of the TCA.

Blood levels measure both protein-bound and unbound drug. Drug bound to protein is inactive. The only exception to this is lithium, which is not protein bound, and thus lithium blood levels are an accurate indicator of drug availability. Changes in the individual's medical condition can alter the amount of active drug available. If protein becomes depleted, more unbound drug becomes available and toxicity increases.

Measuring drug blood levels can, however, indicate whether the patient is compliant in taking the drug; and in the case of imipramine, desipramine, and nortriptyline, blood level correlates with therapeutic effect.

Side effects All antidepressants are therapeutically equivalent, but it is difficult to predict which drug will be best for any individual. For individuals with cancer, prescribers generally choose an antidepressant based on three factors: (1) the nature of the depressive symptoms, (2) medical problems that could confound or be adversely affected by the side effects, and (3) the side effect profile of the drug.[46] For example, individuals having difficulty with sleep might benefit from nortriptyline because it has significant sedative properties. Conversely, individuals who may benefit from less sleep could do well on one of the SSRIs because of their stimulating effect. Side effects for antidepressants are listed in Table 31-3.

Treatment of the elderly The elderly deserve special mention in both diagnosis of depression and treatment with antidepressant. Actual signs and symptoms of depression in the elderly may vary slightly. What might appear to be a disturbance of sleep in the form of early morning wakening may actually be a need for less sleep. Loss of appetite in the elderly may be related to poorly fitting dentures and taste changes. Physiologic changes of the aging process can influence metabolism and excretion of drugs:

- Delayed stomach emptying results in delayed drug adsorption. Instruct the individual to take the medication early with orange juice to facilitate absorption.
- Loss of albumin is a common problem for the elderly, resulting in more free drug in the system and there-

fore more side effects. Dosage may need to be reduced.

- Delayed excretion may mean an increase in the time the drug is in the body. This increases the risk of cardiotoxicity.

Management of the suicidal patient

The goal of intervention with the suicidal patient is to provide effective management of illness-related problems and to create a safe therapeutic environment for the individual. The establishment of rapport is a crucial first step. The individual must be allowed to talk about his or her feelings and the suicide plan. Often, individuals contemplating suicide feel there are no options. Therefore, it is important to help them examine what other options are available to them. Referral to a psychiatrist is essential, as is the nursing assessment and risk evaluation. Results of the assessment and collaboration with the psychiatrist determine the type and degree of intervention. Symptom management is aggressive and focused. The environment must be made safe through removal of all cords, sharp objects, and other implements with which the individual could hurt himself or herself. Medication administration must be supervised, and psychiatric medication is started after psychiatric consultation. A "no harm" contract is solicited from the individual with special attention being given to the individual who will not agree to "no harm." The individual's support system is mobilized. One-to-one nursing or continuous or frequent monitoring is initiated, based on perceived risk (Table 31-4).

Not all suicides can be prevented, even with the best of planning and treatment. When the suicidal patient is treated such that the depression lifts, the individual may finally have the energy to carry out the suicide plan. A successful suicide can have damaging effects on both family and the staff who cared for the patient. Caregivers may feel guilty for having relaxed their vigilance. The family and professional care team may question their judgment and have feelings of guilt. Support groups can be helpful for family members. Breitbart[36] suggests that the professional care team may benefit from a "psychological autopsy" (p. 297) in which the case is reviewed in an attempt to understand how and why the suicide occurred. Routines can be reviewed and revised if needed, risk factors reinforced, and most importantly, feelings aired.

Referral for Further Psychiatric Evaluation

Depressed individuals should receive further psychiatric evaluation when their symptoms last longer than a week, worsen rather than improve, or interfere with the individual's ability to carry out activities of daily living or cooperate with treatment.[3]

TABLE 31-4   Fox Chase Cancer Center Nursing Department: Standard of Nursing Care—Nursing Diagnosis: Potential for Violence, Self-Directed

Definition:
A state in which an individual experiences behaviors that can be physically harmful to self.

Related Factors:
Advanced illness and poor prognosis, inadequate pain control, lack of psychosocial support, prior suicide history (family).

Defining Characteristics:
Presence of risk factors, such as:
- Presence of suicide plan
- Increasing anxiety levels
- Depression and hopelessness
- Delirium
- Preexisting psychopathology
- Prior suicide attempts
- Exhaustion
- Fatigue
- Rage/panic states
- Self-destructive behavior
- Active aggressive suicidal acts

Assessment Data:
1. Patient's understanding of illness and present symptoms and their meaning to the patient
2. Mental status
3. Psychosocial supports
4. Change in coping skills
5. Present suicide attempts
6. Need for effectiveness of psychopharmacologic agents
7. Need for one-to-one supervision

Patient Outcome	Nursing Interventions
The patient will not harm self or others. The patient will reside in a secure environment.	1. Clear patient room of items that may be harmful (i.e., razors, bell cord, metal utensils, sharp objects, belts, cords, etc.) 2. Search patient's personal effects to identify and remove potentially dangerous objects (in conjunction with Security). 3. Provide one-on-one observation/companionship if family is unable to provide same. 4. Observe body language, verbalizations, motor activity, aggressive acts, suspicion of others, delusions, hallucinations, or withdrawal q30 min, and document changes. 5. Administer medications as ordered. 6. Provide support for patient. 7. Transfer to other facility as necessary. 8. Arm restraints/posey will be used only when necessary in the opinion of the RN and when the patient will have constant monitoring.

Used with permission from Fox Chase Cancer Center, Philadelphia, PA.

Any patient expressing suicidal ideation should be assessed immediately for the degree of risk for carrying out the threat. A referral to psychiatry should be initiated for further evaluation. Different institutions may vary with regard to who assesses patients at risk for suicide. Some institutions have delegated the assessment to social workers or psychiatric nursing staff. In others, it might be handled by the nurse caring for the patient who in turn initiates the referral.

Evaluation of Therapeutic Approaches

Nursing care is by its nature an interactive process. Nurses form a partnership with patients and their families; nurses negotiate with patient and family to perform certain professional care activities, leaving other activities for the patient and family to conduct; and nurses teach patient and family the knowledge and skills needed to carry out their responsibilities. Therefore, evaluation of care includes review of both patient and family knowledge and achievement of desired clinical goals (see Figure 31-2). These goals include:

- *The individual and family have knowledge of depression sufficient to be able to participate effectively in care.* This includes knowledge of personal risk factors, signs and symptoms, and strategies to reduce risks or complications of depression. They also need to be aware of resources that are available to assist them by providing additional support or practical advice.

- *The individual reports a decrease in number and severity of depressive symptoms.* It may be helpful for the patient and family to participate in the evaluation process by keeping a record of depressive symptoms so they can track changes over time. (See Appendix 31A for a sample symptom log.)

- *The individual is able to carry out usual roles and activities without interference due to depression.* As the depression lifts, individuals should be able to resume usual functional roles and self-care activities.

- *The individual takes medication prescribed for depression in an appropriate manner.* Individuals require the same information about antidepressant medications that they need for any oncologic drug, including name, action, side effects, and when to contact a professional.

- *The individual does not express suicidal ideas or engage in suicidal behaviors.*

Educational Tools and Resources

It is important to provide the patient with written information to which he or she can refer when at home. The Self-Care Guides provided as appendixes to this chapter are one such resource. Utilizing these, patients and families have access to reminders of what side effects from medications may be seen, what characteristics of depression may be manifested, etc. These guides also provide phone numbers and names of healthcare providers with which the patients and families are already familiar (see Appendixes 31B–31E).

Additional resources include the following, which can provide books, pamphlets, and information regarding support groups:

- ACS (American Cancer Society): check local number in phone directory
- Cancer Information Service: (800) 422-6237
- Local health department or community mental health center: check phone directory for number
- National Alliance for the Mentally Ill: (800) 950-6264 (950-NAMI)
- National Depressive and Manic Depressive Association: (800) 826-3632

- National Foundation for Depressive Illness: (800) 248-4344
- National Mental Health Association: (800) 969-6642
- Department of Health and Human Services: (800) 358-9295
  Ask for Publication No. AHCPR 93-0553 "Depression Is a Treatable Illness: A Patient's Guide"
- DEPRESSION Awareness, Recognition, and Treatment (D/ART) Program: (800) 421-4211, for free publication about depression in individuals of all ages
- CANCER CARE (800) 813-4673

Conclusion

Nurses are in an ideal position to support cancer patients through the diagnostic, treatment, and supportive care phases of their experience. Symptom management is an integral part of high-quality oncology nursing care. Although depressive symptoms are less tangible than some physical symptoms, they deserve the same careful attention and management.

References

1. Bukberg J, Penman D, Holland JC: Depression in hospitalized cancer patients. *Psychosom Med* 46:199–212, 1984
2. Lynch ME: The assessment and prevalence of affective disorders in advanced cancer. *J Palliat Care* 11:10–18, 1995
3. Massie MJ: Depression, in Holland JC, Rowland JH (eds): *Handbook of Psychooncology: Psychological Care of the Patient with Cancer.* New York: Oxford University Press, 1990, pp. 283–290
4. Carroll BT, Kathol RG, Noyes R, et al: Screening for depression and anxiety in cancer patients using the hospital anxiety and depression scale. *Gen Hosp Psychiatry* 15:69–74, 1993
5. Derogatis LR, Morrow GR, Fetting J, et al: The prevalence of psychiatric disorders among cancer patients. *JAMA* 249:751–757, 1983
6. Barsevick AM, Pasacreta J, Orsi A: Psychological distress and functional status in colorectal cancer patients. *Cancer Pract* 3:105–110, 1995
7. Colon E, Callies AL, Popkin M, et al: Depressed mood and other variables related to bone marrow transplantation survival in acute leukemia. *Psychosomatics* 32:420–425, 1991
8. Spiegel D, Bloom JR, Kraemer HC, et al: Effect of psychosocial treatment on survival of patients with metastatic breast cancer. *Lancet* 2:888–891, 1989
9. Mossey JM, Knott K, Cranik R: The effects of persistent depressive symptoms on hip fracture recovery. *J Gerontol Med Sci* 45:M163–168, 1990
10. Wells KB, Stewart A, Hays RD, et al: The function and well-being of depressed patients. *JAMA* 262:914–919, 1989
11. Levenson JL, Hammer RM, Rossiter LF: Relation of psycho-

pathology in general medical inpatients to use and cost of services. *Am J Psychiatry* 147:1498–1503, 1990

12. Hellman CJ, Budd M, Borysenkso J, et al: A study of the effectiveness of two group behavioral medicine interventions for patients with psychosomatic complaints. *Behav Med* 16:165–173, 1990

13. Cassileth BR, Lusk EJ, Strouse TB, et al: Psychosocial status in chronic illness. *N Engl J Med* 311:506–511, 1984

14. Ganz PA, Schag CC, Heinrich RL: The psychosocial impact of cancer on the elderly: A comparison with younger patients. *J Am Geriatr Soc* 33:429–435, 1985

15. Roberts CS, Rossetti K, Cone D, et al: Psychosocial impact of gynecologic cancer. *J Psychosoc Oncol* 10:99–109, 1992

16. Vinokur AD, Threatt BA, Caplan RD, et al: Physical and psychosocial functioning and adjustment to breast cancer. *Cancer* 63:394–405, 1989

17. Farrington A: Cancer, emotional response, and cognitive behavioral psychotherapy. *Eur J Cancer Care* 3:175–180, 1994

18. Valente SM, Saunders JM: Evaluating depression among patients with cancer. *Cancer Pract* 2:65–71, 1994

19. Schag CA, Ganz PA, Polinsky ML, et al: Characteristics of women at risk for psychosocial distress in the year after breast cancer. *J Clin Oncol* 11:783–793, 1993

20. Waligora-Serafin B, McMahon T, Pruitt BT, et al: Relationships between emotional distress and psychosocial concerns among newly diagnosed cancer patients. *J Psychosoc Oncol* 10:57–74, 1992

21. Aass N, Fossa SD, Dahl AA, Moe TJ: Prevalence of anxiety and depression in cancer patients seen at the Norwegian Radiation Hospital. *Eur J Cancer* 33:1597–1604, 1997

22. Ell K, Nishimoto R, Morvay T, et al: A longitudinal analysis of psychological adaptation among survivors of cancer. *Cancer* 63:406–413, 1989

23. Mahon SM, Cella DF, Donovan MI: Psychosocial adjustment to recurrent cancer. *Oncol Nurs Forum* 17(suppl):47–54, 1990

24. Saunders JM, Valente SM: Cancer and suicide. *Oncol Nurs Forum* 15:575–581, 1988

25. McDaniel JS, Musselman DL, Porter MR, et al: Depression in patients with cancer: Diagnosis, biology, and treatment. *Arch Gen Psychiatry* 52:89–99, 1995

26. Kaplan HI, Sadock BJ, Grebb JA: *Synopsis of Psychiatry* (ed 7). Baltimore: Williams & Wilkins, 1994

27. American Psychiatric Association: *Diagnostic and Statistical Manual of Mental Disorders* (ed 4). Washington, DC: American Psychiatric Association, 1994

28. Burgess AW: *Psychiatric Nursing in the Hospital and the Community.* Englewood Cliffs, NJ: Prentice-Hall, 1985

29. Husted SA, Johnson JG: Oncology clients' affective states and their nurses' expectations of clients' affective states. *Cancer Nurs* 8:159–165, 1985

30. Sutherland HJ, Walker P, Till JE: The development of a method for determining oncology patients' emotional distress using linear analogue scales. *Cancer Nurs* 11:303–308, 1988

31. Beck AT, Steer RA: *Beck Depression Inventory (BDI) Manual.* San Antonio, TX: The Psychological Corporation, Harcourt Brace Jovanovich, 1987

32. Cavanaugh SV, Clark DC, Gibbons RD: Diagnosing depression in the hospitalized medically ill. *Psychosomatics* 24:809–815, 1983

33. Yesavage V, Brink TL: Development and validation of a geriatric depression screening scale: A preliminary report. *J Psychiatr Res* 17:37–49, 1983

34. Koenig HG, Meador KG, Cohen HJ, et al: Self-rated depression scales and screening for major depression in the older hospitalized patient with medical illness. J Am Geriatr Soc 36:699–706, 1988

35. Koenig HG, Meador KG, Cohen HJ, et al: Depression in elderly hospitalized patients with medical illness. *Arch Intern Med* 148:1929–1936, 1988

36. Breitbart W: Suicide, in Holland JC, Rowland JH (eds): *Handbook of Psycho-oncology: Psychological Care of the Patient with Cancer.* New York: Oxford University Press, 1990, pp. 291–299

37. Spiegel D, Sands S, Koopman C: Pain and depression in patients with cancer. *Cancer* 74:2570–2578, 1994

38. Anderson B, Holmes W: Altered mental status: An algorithm for assessment of delirium in the cancer patient, in Hubbard SM, Greene PE, Knobf MT (eds): *Current Issues in Cancer Nursing Practice Updates* 2:165–172, 1993

39. Fobair P, Hoppe RT, Bloom J, et al: Psychosocial problems among survivors of Hodgkin's disease. *J Clin Oncol* 4:805–814, 1986

40. Munkres A, Oberst MT, Hughes SH: Appraisal of illness, symptom distress, self-care burden, and mood states in patients receiving chemotherapy for initial and recurrent cancer. *Oncol Nurs Forum* 19:1201–1209, 1992

41. Oberst MT, Hughes SH, Chang AS, et al: Self-care burden, stress appraisal, and mood among persons receiving radiotherapy. *Cancer Nurs* 14:71–78, 1991

42. Owen DC: Nurses' perspectives on the meaning of hope in patients with cancer: A qualitative study. *Oncol Nurs Forum* 16:75–79, 1989

43. Herth KA: The relationship between level of hope and level of coping response and other variables in patients with cancer. *Oncol Nurs Forum* 16:67–72, 1989

44. McCabe MS: Psychological support for the patient on chemotherapy. *Oncology* 5:91–99, 1991

45. Cella DF, Yeller SB: Cancer support groups. *Cancer Pract* 1:56–61, 1993

46. Massie MJ, Lesko LM: Psychopharmacological management, in Holland JC, Rowland JH (eds): *Handbook of Psycho-oncology: Psychological Care of the Patient with Cancer.* New York: Oxford University Press, 1990, pp. 470–491

Depression

Below is a list of symptoms. Your nurse has marked the symptoms you had when you were depressed. Look at this list each week. Draw an arrow in the box if you feel worse ($\downarrow$), better ($\uparrow$), or the same (—). Also mark any new symptom you may feel. If you see by looking at the arrows that your symptoms are getting worse, call you doctor or nurse right away. If you have the wish to hurt yourself, call your doctor or nurse right away. Be sure to bring this sheet to each clinic visit.

Patient Name: _____

Symptoms	Baseline	1	2	3	4	5	6	7
Eating								
Able to think								
Get angry								
Want to be left alone								
I don't take care of myself								
Crying								
Sadness								
I wish I were dead								
I can't do anything right								
Bad thoughts								
Can't sleep								
Sleep too much								
Other (list)								

Source: Much JK, Barsevick AM: Depression, in Yarbro CH, Frogge MH, Goodman M (eds): *Cancer Symptom Management* (ed 2). Sudbury: Jones and Bartlett, 1999. © Jones and Bartlett Publishers.

Depression

Patient Name: _____

Description Many people who have cancer become depressed. Symptoms of depression are varied. You may have felt this way for a week or more. You may not be able to cope with your daily activities or your cancer. You may be feeling at least one of the following:

- Not worth anything
- Low in spirits
- Not enough sleep
- Less appetite
- Grouchy
- Loss of pleasure in life
- Wanting to be left alone
- Sadness, crying
- Sleeping too much
- More appetite
- Negative thoughts
- Increased anger
- Feeling no good
- Self-blame or self-criticism (I can't do anything right.)
- Death thoughts

Some of these symptoms are because of your cancer and its treatment, but you may also be depressed.

Many things can contribute to the development of depression. These include family history, many losses, many types of medications, and stress.

Learning Needs You and your loved ones need to know:

- How to recognize depression
- Why depression may be happening to you
- Things you can do to help yourself

Ask yourself the following questions:

1. Have you felt "low" for more than a week?
2. Have you felt grouchier than normal?
3. Have you reacted more strongly to situations or not reacted at all?
4. Have you cried a lot?
5. Have you had difficulty concentrating or sticking to tasks?
6. Do your loved ones think you are behaving differently?
7. Have you had chronic pain that is not relieved by medication?

Management   You can do the following to deal with depression:

- Make a list of all the medications you take. Show this to your doctor or nurse. Some medicines may have to be stopped.
- Ask your doctor or nurse what side effects can be caused by the cancer and its treatment. Learn as much as you can to help to manage those side effects.
- Ask your doctor or nurse for help managing the side effects.
- Get plenty of rest, and exercise when you feel you have the energy.
- Eat a balanced diet. Do not try to lose weight at this time. Foods should be good for you and have lots of nutrition. Ask your nurse or dietitian for help if you are having problems with eating.
- You are not alone. Depression in cancer is common. It does not mean you are weak. Talk about how you are feeling with your doctor or nurse.
- Avoid alcohol. It can make you depressed.
- If medications have been ordered for you for depression, take them as directed. Let your doctor or nurse know of any side effects you may be experiencing.

Follow-up

1. As your depression goes away, you should experience:
   - Better sleep patterns
   - A decrease in grouchiness
   - Better focus on tasks
   - Ability to withstand stresses without overreacting
   - Ability to think positively
   - An improvement in mood
   - Enjoyment in living
2. Treatment of depression is not quick. It may take weeks to months to notice improvement. Continue to take your medication.
3. Depression may come back. But knowing what it feels like, you will be able to recognize it.

Phone Numbers

Nurse: _____ Phone: _____

Physician: _____ Phone: _____

Other: _____ Phone: _____

National Alliance for the Mentally Ill: (800) 950-6264 (950-NAMI)

National Depressive and Manic Depressive Association: (800) 826-3632

National Foundation for Depressive Illness, Inc.: (800) 248-4344

National Mental Health Association: (800) 969-6642

Comments

Patient's Signature: _____ Date: _____

Nurse's Signature: _____ Date: _____

Source: Much JK, Barsevick AM: Depression, in Yarbro CH, Frogge MH, Goodman M (eds): *Cancer Symptom Management* (ed 2). Sudbury: Jones and Bartlett, 1999. © Jones and Bartlett Publishers.

Avoiding Dizziness When Standing

Patient Name: _____

Symptom and Description   Do you feel dizzy when you stand up too fast?. This is called *postural hypotension*. It can be caused by your medication for depression. You may start to feel dizzy a few days after starting your medication. You need to know what to do if this happens, so you don't fall.

Learning Needs   Is your blood pressure usually low? Ask your doctor or nurse about this. Taking your pills for depression can make your blood pressure lower. If you are older, you are more likely to feel dizzy when taking your pills for depression. You must get up slowly from bed. Sit for a minute or two before standing or walking. Don't change position quickly.

Management

- Get up slowly.
- Sit on the edge of the bed or couch for a few minutes before standing.
- Stand slowly. Do not walk until the dizzy feeling goes away.
- If the dizzy feeling does not go away, get help when you get up.

Follow-up   Check if you have the following:

_____ Dizziness
_____ Light-headedness when getting up
_____ Light-headedness going from sitting to standing
_____ Light-headedness going from lying to sitting
_____ Light-headedness during sudden changes in position.

If the dizzy feeling does not go away:

- Call your doctor or nurse.
- Write down what helped and what didn't.
- Write down when the dizzy feeling happens and what makes it worse.

Your doctor or nurse needs to know about any problem you have with your drugs so they can change your prescription.

Phone Numbers

Nurse: _____ Phone: _____

Physician: _____ Phone: _____

Other: _____ Phone: _____

Comments

Patient's Signature: _____ Date: _____

Nurse's Signature: _____ Date: _____

Source: Much JK, Barsevick AM: Depression, in Yarbro CH, Frogge MH, Goodman M (eds): *Cancer Symptom Management* (ed 2). Sudbury: Jones and Bartlett, 1999. © Jones and Bartlett Publishers.

Hypertension (High Blood Pressure)

Patient Name: _____

Symptom and Description   You are taking a pill for depression called a monoamine oxidase inhibitor. While you are taking this pill, you must not eat or drink certain foods and beverages. These foods and drinks contain something called *tyramine*, which can make your blood pressure go up very quickly. This is called a *hypertensive crisis*. This is a serious, sometimes life-threatening increase in your blood pressure. You might experience severe headache, your heart pounding wildly, stiff neck, chest pain, sweating, nausea, vomiting, and blackouts.

You will need to be careful as long as you are taking this pill and until the effects of the drug have left your body—for at least 2 weeks *after* taking the last pills.

Learning Needs   There are foods, drinks, and medications you cannot take with your antidepression drug. You must be careful to avoid the following foods and drinks:

- Aged cheese
- Aged, over-ripe, fermented foods
- Beef and chicken liver
- Beer
- Broad beans
- Caffeinated drinks
- Canned figs
- Chocolate
- Pickled herring
- Preserved sausages
- Sour cream
- Soy sauce
- Wine (especially red)
- Yeast products
- Yogurt

Prevention   You can safely take your pills by not eating the foods on the list. Call your doctor, nurse, or dietitian if you are unsure. Some people try small amounts of some of the foods on the list and have little problem, but we cannot tell if you can safely try these foods. All of the foods listed can cause high blood pressure in people, and there is no easy way to know if they are safe for you as an individual. If you want to try some of these foods, please call your doctor or nurse first.

(continued)

There are other drugs that can interact with your pills, including:

- Over-the-counter cold medicines
- Amphetamines (stimulants)
- Epinephrine, norepinephrine
- Tricyclic antidepressants
- High blood pressure pills
- Drugs for diabetes
- Amipaque (contrast dye used for some CT scans)
- Diet pills
- Methyldopa, levodopa, dopamine
- Alcohol
- Certain narcotics
- Water pills (thiazide diuretics)
- Antabuse

You should read the labels on any drug you buy over-the-counter to see what it contains. If you're not sure whether it is safe for you, call your doctor or nurse.

Management   Be careful to explain to any other doctor or nurse you may need to see that you are taking a monoamine oxidase inhibitor, and that you are aware that you need to be very careful about taking other medications with this drug. Feel free to call the doctor or nurse who ordered the pills if someone else wants you to take other drugs. Not all doctors and nurses know about the drugs that can cause you problems.

- Carry a card in your wallet explaining the medication you are taking.
- Be sure the card has the list of foods and drugs you can't take.
- Show this to any doctor or nurse who is caring for you.
- Let your family or friends know that it is in your wallet in case of emergency.

Follow-up   Before you leave the office, your doctor or nurse will review this information with you. You will be asked to show that you understand the information. You will be given a small card to carry in your wallet containing information about the drugs you are taking and the foods and drugs to avoid. A loved one or other person whom you identify as significant will also be given this information so that they will be able to help you in an emergency situation.

Remember that you can avoid this increase in blood pressure. Also remember that you can still safely enjoy many other foods that you have always enjoyed.

Call your doctor, nurse, or pharmacist if you have any questions. Call immediately if you have any of these symptoms:

- Nausea/vomiting that won't go away
- Severe or frequent headaches
- Rapid heart rate
- Stiff or sore neck
- Chest pain
- A lot of sweating

If you can't reach your doctor or nurse by phone to tell them about how you are feeling, immediately go to your nearest emergency room.

Phone Numbers

Nurse: _____ Phone: _____

Physician: _____ Phone: _____

Other: _____ Phone: _____

Comments

Patient's Signature: _____ Date: _____

Nurse's Signature: _____ Date: _____

Source: Much JK, Barsevick AM: Depression, in Yarbro CH, Frogge MH, Goodman M (eds): *Cancer Symptom Management* (ed 2). Sudbury: Jones and Bartlett, 1999. © Jones and Bartlett Publishers.

(continued)

Taking Antidepressant Medications

Patient Name: _____

Symptoms and Description   You have been asked to take drugs for your feelings of depression.

Learning Needs   To take antidepressant drugs safely, you will need some information.

Management   Here is information to help you safely take your pills.

- Don't drink alcohol with antidepressant medication. Alcohol may make you more depressed and keep your pills from working.

- If you have taken your pills for a long time (months) and you feel it is "not working anymore," contact your doctor or nurse, because you may need to have your dosage increased.

- Do not suddenly stop taking your pills. You will need the help of your doctor or nurse. Stopping suddenly can make you feel nauseated, dizzy, and unable to sleep. It can also give you a headache, the "blahs," nightmares, and return of depressive symptoms.

- Antidepressant pills can take a long time to work. Depending on the medication, it can take 2 to 8 weeks at the right level for you for the antidepressant effects to be felt. Most people first sleep better, then are less grouchy, and then have a better mood. You will still have the same kinds of "troubles" or concerns you felt before starting the medication, but now those same troubles are not as overwhelming. Remember, it takes a long time for the medications to work. You may feel the temptation to stop taking the drugs. Continue to take the drugs even if the symptoms of depression have not changed. Keep in close contact with your physician or nurse.

- Be careful when first taking your medication and driving a car or dangerous machinery. Sometimes antidepressants can make you sleepy or dizzy. Contact your physician or nurse if side effects affect your usual activities. Your dosage or medication may need to be changed.

- Antidepressant medication may cause your mouth to be dry. You can help this by taking frequent sips of water, sucking on hard candies, chewing on sugarless gum, and doing good routine oral care.

- Antidepressants can sometimes cause headaches. If you are not currently receiving chemotherapy, you can take some non-aspirin pain reliever for the headache. If the headaches continue or are not relieved by the pain reliever, or if you are undergoing chemotherapy, contact your physician or nurse to discuss what else you can do.

- Antidepressants can cause either diarrhea or constipation. If you have hard stools, increase the amount of fruits, vegetables, and fiber in your diet. If you have diarrhea, decrease the amount of fruits, vegetables, and fiber in your diet. If your changes in diet don't work, call your physician or nurse for suggestions before taking over-the-counter medications.
- You may have nausea when you first start to take your antidepressants. Many times the nausea will decrease in a few days. You may find that you need to adjust when and how you take your medication, such as with food, after food, or before food. If the nausea continues, contact your physician or nurse.

Follow-up   Call your physician or nurse immediately if the following occur:

- Vomiting that won't stop
- Unable to continue with usual activities
- Illness that makes you stop taking your medication
- Extreme anxiety or unable to sit down
- Can't pass your urine

Phone Numbers

Nurse: _____ Phone: _____

Physician: _____ Phone: _____

Other: _____ Phone: _____

Comments

Patient's Signature: _____ Date: _____

Nurse's Signature: _____ Date: _____

Source: Much JK, Barsevick AM: Depression, in Yarbro CH, Frogge MH, Goodman M (eds): *Cancer Symptom Management* (ed 2). Sudbury: Jones and Bartlett, 1999. © Jones and Bartlett Publishers.

CHAPTER 32

Grief

Virginia Bourne, RN, MSN

Margaret Hansen Frogge, RN, MS

The Problem of Grief in Cancer

Grief is a natural and expected reaction to any loss. "Loss is a state of being deprived of or being without something one has had."[1] Grief can ensue from a divorce, separation, and even loss of a valued piece of property such as a favorite sweater, desk, or fishing rod. Grief can occur when a job is lost, a friend moves away, a child goes off to school, or over the loss of health, independence, or the ability to care for oneself, as may happen in chronic illness.

The diagnosis of cancer has a deep impact on the person with cancer and their family. There can be feelings of loneliness, despair, and uncertainty. A person being treated for cancer may experience many losses, such as loss of energy; loss of a body part or function; loss of a positive attitude, pride, or self-esteem; loss of a job, possessions, role, position in the family; loss of control— all these can trigger a grief reaction. The most intense grief follows the loss of a loved one through death.

It is imperative that we grieve when we experience a loss. Suppressed grief, if left unheeded, may be debilitating for the rest of the survivor's life.[2]

"Grief is a process of psychological, social, and somatic reactions to a loss."[3] The intensity and longevity of grief hinge on how important the lost person, ability, or body part was in one's daily life. If what was lost was seldom seen or used, grief may occur only periodically at those particular times that bring the loss to mind. If that which was lost has been part of a person's daily existence, he or she will grieve more intensely and longer.

Some losses may not be recognized by others, but this does not invalidate a person's grief. Just as people may grieve over a variety of losses, they grieve in a variety of ways. There is no *one* way to grieve. There is no *one* time-table for grief. Grief is a highly individualized process of adaptation. People do not get *over* grief, rather they get *through* it and adapt or adjust. Some people may adjust to a loss, but grieve indefinitely. Wolfeldt[4] believes "we never get over our grief, but become reconciled to it."

Etiology

There are numerous causes for grief in the individual diagnosed with cancer. Living with cancer may entail rigorous diagnostic procedures, multiple treatment modalities, constant surveillance, uncertainty, and many real or perceived losses: loss of control of one's body and health, loss of self-esteem, and a change in one's role in the family structure, all due to the side effects of treatment, including loss of hair, energy, and mobility.

As a result of these changes and losses, the person with cancer may be less able to function at work or fulfill his or her role in the family. Income may decline and threaten plans for the future. With certain types of cancer, the treatment may result in disfigurement. The person with cancer may lose sleep because of anxiety or as a side effect of medication. Many chemotherapeutic drugs cause alopecia, which for many people is devastating. For women with cancer of the breast, a mastectomy, wedge resection, or lumpectomy may be a source of grief due to the loss of a body part and may be a threat to sexuality. Even if the body part removed or altered is not visible to the public, this loss can trigger an acute grief reaction. Men undergoing treatment for prostate cancer may suffer impotence and incontinence. This loss of control of physical ability may produce a profound effect and result in an acute grief reaction.

The loss of certainty, the threat to one's future plans, and sense of well-being are all common causes of grief and sorrow in persons with cancer and their loved ones. Chronic sorrow has been described as a common response to living with cancer.[5] The grief reactions resulting from a diagnosis of cancer can be significant.

Grief can also be experienced *before* any losses have occurred. This is called *anticipatory grief,* and it produces the same symptoms of acute grief and requires similar interventions but occurs in anticipation of the loss as well as after the loss. It is important when counseling patients with cancer that the patients be aware of the possible side effects of a particular drug, test, or treatment to reduce unnecessary distress.

Pathophysiology: The Grief Process

The symptoms and reactions commonly experienced by a grieving person range in scope and intensity. The physiologic and psychological reactions to grief vary greatly from person to person. The critical point to emphasize with grieving individuals and their families is that reactions to a loss are important expressions of grief. It can be helpful to review the typical reactions to grief with the individual who is experiencing a loss. This review can reassure the person that they are normal and healthy.[6]

Psychological Reactions

1. *Loss of interest* in things one used to enjoy such as reading, knitting, listening to music, watching television, or jogging. The individual with cancer may find it difficult to stay interested in a project due to sadness, worry, or preoccupation with health status.

2. *Inability to concentrate.* People who are grieving find they must read a paragraph again and again because they simply cannot concentrate on the words; or when asked about a program they are watching on television, they will be unable to describe what the program entails.

3. *Intense preoccupation* with thoughts of what has been lost. The person with cancer may be trying to recall how it felt to be healthy and independent.

4. *Feelings of helplessness*—experienced by both patient and loved ones.

5. *Feelings of guilt.* All the "I should haves" and "If onlys" may be expressed, such as, "If only I had gone to the doctor sooner," or "I should have quit smoking." The patient may look for things that they did or didn't do that could have caused the disease. The family of a patient with cancer may assume guilt for not being more supportive, or not encouraging their loved one to get treatment soon enough.

6. *Feelings of unreality.* "It just can't be true." "It just couldn't have happened."

7. *Feelings of anger.* The bereaved may be angry at God, the medical profession, the hospital, the nurses; the anger then can trigger a guilt reaction. The patient may be angry because he or she lived a healthy lifestyle yet became ill. In contrast, the family may feel anger because the patient did not lead a healthy lifestyle.

8. *Intense need to speak* about the last few days or hours around the time of the loss, either at the time of diagnosis or death, or whenever the loss occurred.

9. *Feelings of losing one's mind* because the grieving person may hear, feel, smell, or sense the presence of a deceased loved one. This is a common phenomenon and grieving people need to be reassured. Elderly widowers often speak of hearing their spouse call them during the night. Parents who have lost a child may hear the child crying. One mother whose teenager died suddenly said at certain times of the day she could smell her daughter's perfume. Although these occurrences are not repeated often, they can be frightening for those who have experienced the loss of a loved one.

Physiologic Reactions

1. *Tightness in the throat.* The feeling a person may have when watching a sad movie or hearing a beautiful poem, which occurs because the person is trying not to cry. It is that "choked-up" feeling.

2. *Feeling short of breath,* sighing often. This unconscious reaction has no pathophysiologic basis. It may be a manifestation of stress.

3. *Empty feeling* in the abdomen—not hunger, just empty.

4. *Loss of appetite.* The majority of grieving people lose weight, but a few eat more and gain weight.

5. *Decrease in physical strength.* One woman complained because she was finding it difficult to lift the laundry basket when she was grieving. A young man who had recently experienced the death of his grandfather could not jog his usual 5 miles and stated, "I just don't have the strength."

6. *Decrease in energy levels.* One young mother who worked full time and cared for the house and children found she barely had the energy to go to work now that she was grieving. The person with cancer undergoing treatment will experience weakness and a decrease of energy, both as a result of the treatment and as a result of grief over the many losses that have occurred.

7. *Disturbances in sleep patterns.* Grieving people often find it difficult to get to sleep, and if they do, they will wake up in a few hours and be unable to get back to sleep. Another often-heard complaint is "Even if I manage to sleep all night, I'm still tired."

8. *Accident proneness* may be a consequence of sleeplessness and preoccupation with thoughts of the loss. Grieving people may find an increased tendency to drop things, bump into walls.

9. *Tears are often present,* but not everyone can cry in public. Some people cry alone at night, in the shower, or in the company of a select group. Others can cry anytime with anyone. Crying is a very personal event.

10. *Feeling cold.* Many grieving people complain that they simply can't get warm.

11. *Assuming the symptoms of the deceased.* On occasion, grieving people will assume symptoms similar to those experienced by the ill or deceased person. If the deceased died of a brain tumor, the bereaved may have headaches. If the symptoms are severe or persist, insist that the person see a physician.

12. *Weakening of the immune system.* It is known that stress can reduce the body's ability to ward of illness. Grief is a stressful situation. Considering that the person is not sleeping or eating properly and is under a great deal of stress, a grieving person can be more prone to infections and bleeding problems.

The intensity of these reactions may differ for different people, as well as in the same person at different times. Variations are common. The grief process can be viewed as a journey. The grieving person may find it difficult to come back up once down in the valley of grief, or may feel guilty if not down all the time. As adaptation progresses, the griever will spend more time feeling good and less time in the valley.

Tasks, Responses, and Stages in Grief

Different authors present different views related to the journey through the grief process. The following three views are presented to acquaint the reader with some of the classic theories. The studies conducted on grief over the past century concur that grief does not follow an exact course, that people grieve in their own way and at their own time. The grieving individual will move back and forth through the various tasks, responses, and stages.

Studies done more recently have supported the original work done by Worden, Engel, and Lindeman.

Worden[7] describes four tasks of grief:

1. Accepting the reality of the loss
2. Working through the pain of grief
3. Adjusting to an environment in which the lost is missing
4. Emotionally relocating the loss and moving on with life

Engel[8] writes of responses in grief:

1. Shock and disbelief
2. Developing awareness of the loss
3. Restitution—the work of mourning

Lindeman[9] identifies three stages of grief:

1. Shock and disbelief
2. Acute mourning
3. Resolution of the grief process

The outcomes of the individual's response to grief can be adaptive or maladaptive. Pathologic grief is usually prolonged and characterized by a few classic responses: intrusion, denial, and dysfunctional adaptation.[10] *Intrusion* describes a pathologic grief state in which the grieving person inappropriately idealizes the memories of the lost person or body part or function. The loss takes on a distorted level of importance or is elevated to an unrealistic level. *Denial* occurs when there is no acknowledgement of the loss or there are behaviors manifesting the denial. A classic example of pathologic denial is when the grieving person continues to launder clothes, prepare meals, and purchase items for the deceased person. *Maladaptation* or dysfunctional grief can range from slight to severe. Symptoms of maladaptation are prolonged and create dysfunction in one's life. Symptoms include failure to work, excessive fatigue, and severe weight loss.

Cultural Variations

Some cultures have definite rituals surrounding grief. For example, in Orthodox Judaism, the time from death to burial, the position of the body, and the behavior of the mourner are all part of the funeral ritual. The Laotian communities need to be present, dress the dying, and assist with final preparation of the body. This is important to the grieving process in this culture. Nurses must be sensitive to important rituals that may be present in certain cultures.

Distinction Between Grief and Depression

There is often confusion between grief and depression. Mild depression is a natural reaction to a loss; however, abnormal depression differs in its severity and symptoms. Table 32-1 describes some of the differences between depression and grieving.[11] Depression may require professional intervention if it occurs over a prolonged period. Some clinicians recommend that additional help be provided as soon as signs of depression develop.

Assessment

An initial nursing assessment includes questions related to recent losses in the life of the patient. The following questions might be asked:

- Have you suffered any recent loss?
- How has this loss affected your daily life?
- What have you done in the past that has helped with a loss?
- Do you have a support system?
- What are you doing now to help yourself cope with this loss?

Researchers have attempted to quantify variables that would place a person at high risk for difficult or prolonged bereavement. These high risk individuals may need professional assistance with bereavement. Factors that place an individual in the high risk category include[12]:

- Lack of health insurance
- Limited or no financial resources
- Age greater than 50 years
- Lack of family support
- Expressed feelings of hopelessness
- Prolonged anger
- Lack of self-control
- Lack of self-esteem

Figure 32-1 outlines a nursing care plan that identifies contributing factors, expected outcomes, and nursing interventions.

Symptom Management

Prevention

Grief should not be prevented, but rather facilitated. The goals of bereavement interventions are the facilitation of the grieving process and the prevention or alleviation of detrimental consequences of grief.[9] Many grieving people are told to "carry on," "keep busy," "keep your chin up." Many people are not aware of the need to grieve and must be given permission to express feelings in a safe environment.

TABLE 32-1 Key Differences Between Grief and Depression

Issue	Grieving	Depression
Loss	There is a recognized loss.	A specific loss may or may *not* be identified.
Cognitive schemas	Focus is on the loss. Preoccupation with the deceased, the implications of the loss experiences, and the future.	Focus is on the self. Persistent, distorted, and negative perceptions of self.
Dreams, fantasies, and imagery	Vivid, clear dreams, sometimes of the loss and which the dreamer finds comforting.	Negative fantasy or imagery that contributes to negative thinking and to an intensified physical response.
Physical	Modulated physical response: the body is allowed to collapse and the person admits exhaustion. Moderate weight change/exercise.	Unmodulated physical response: bodily damage and increased vulnerability to illness through extended lack of sleep, anorexia/weight gain, or unnecessary physical risk.
Spiritual	A connection felt to something beyond the self, e.g., a belief in God; a continued dialogue with anger, rage, allows challenges to previously held beliefs.	Especially a year or more past a loss, a persistent failure to find meaning, focus on "why me" and unfairness of the loss—no answers to questions.
Emotional states	Variable: shifts in mood from anger to sadness to more normal states in the same day.	Fixed: withdrawal, despair, reports feeling immobilized or stuck; difficult to "read" emotionally.
Responses	Responds to warmth and pressure, reassurance.	Responds to promises and urging *or* unresponsive.
Pleasure	Variable restriction of pleasure.	Persistent restriction of pleasure.
Attachment behavior	Feels reassured by the presence of close friends or someone who will listen to their story.	Loss of connection with self and with others.

From Schneider, John M. *Finding My Way: Healing and Transformation Through Loss.* Colfax, WI, 1994, p. 381.[11] Reprinted with permission of author.

NURSING DIAGNOSIS: Grief re:

Date started

Date Resolved

Initial

Initials

DC/Date Initial

CONTRIBUTING FACTORS:

Start Date | Freq. | NURSING INTERVENTIONS

- Loss of life expectancy or physical ability or change in body image—other

DEFINING CHARACTERISTICS:

- Crying—teary
- Sad countenance
- Speaking of loss
- Expressing inability to concentrate
- Expressing feelings of anger
- Expressing feelings of guilt
- Reports decrease in interests
- Reports loss of faith
- Reports anger toward God
- Reports difficulty with religious activities
- Reports changes in appetite
- Reports decrease in energy
- Reports feeling of lump in the throat
- Reports frequent sighing
- Expressed need to speak of loss

NURSING INTERVENTIONS

- establish trusting relationship
- allow for privacy
- assist to verbalize fears/concerns
- legitimize feelings
- utilize active listening skills
- utilize therapeutic touch
- educate about grief process
- convey sense of availability
- give information on community support groups
- assist to develop realistic goals
- consult with clinical nurse specialist, chaplain, MSW as needed
- assess whether grief is increased by feelings of helplessness, loss of control, or lack of knowledge
- determine impact on qualify of life and assist with priority setting

ASSESSMENT:

EXPECTED OUTCOMES:

Target Date

- Pt/S.O. identify support network
- Pt/S.O. adapt/adjust to loss and the impact on their life
- Pt/S.O. verbalize understanding of grief process
- Pt/S.O. seek out support

Init/Sign: _____ Init/Sign: _____

Init/Sign: _____ Init/Sign: _____

FIGURE 32-1 Nursing Diagnoses Care Plan Kardex. Pt = patient S.O. = significant other (Reprinted with permission from St. Luke's Medical Center, Milwaukee, Wisconsin.)

Giving people information about grief and permission to grieve is a way to facilitate grief. Teach information related to reactions to a loss. This will legitimize the person's feelings. Unexpressed grief can result in symptoms such as migraine headaches, rashes, asthma attacks, and other symptoms associated with stress. Educating people about the feelings inherent in grief and loss can facilitate healthy grieving.

Therapeutic Approaches

Presence

The presence of someone who cares is healing. A grief shared is a grief diminished. To be helpful to grieving people, a person need only be accepting and available, rather than have "the right words," for it is impossible to know what the right words are. In fact, one must be careful to avoid inappropriate statements that wound rather than heal. For example, telling a grieving person that you know exactly how they feel may be hurtful and inaccurate. No one knows how another person feels about a loss, even if two people have had a similar loss. The meaning one attaches to a loss is very individual. Telling parents that they are lucky to have other children, an elderly widow that she was lucky to be married so long, or any griever that it is a blessing now that the deceased is at peace—all these negate their pain. If the bereaved make these statements, however, supporting them in their belief is helpful. Being present, silently and in a supportive manner, is helpful to a grieving person.

Listening

Grieving people may need to talk about their loss. They need the opportunity to express their feelings of anger, guilt, helplessness, pain, and despair. They need a willing listener. They will want to share memories, good and bad. They need the freedom to cry or laugh without being judged. It is a myth to think that talking about the loss causes sadness. Grieving people are already sad.

Touch

It is believed that touch is the greatest of our senses. Meaningful touch can be understood at a very early age and even when one is too ill, depressed, or sedated to understand spoken words. Touch is eloquent; it says "I care," "I'm not afraid," and "I want to help." Those who are grieving are often unable to respond to the spoken word but will understand the meaning of a hand on their shoulder, a hug, or a pat on the back. For the elderly, many of their principal touchers and affection givers are dead, and they are in need of a simple hug. Touch is usually received as positive if it is appropriate to the situation and therefore does not communicate a negative message. A meaningful touch can imply caring, concern,

tenderness, awareness, and availability.[13] Touch can lessen discomfort and loneliness and afford healing.[14]

Anticipatory guidance

People who are grieving often make wrong decisions and need someone to guide them. Encourage those who are grieving to ask friends, family, or trusted associates to assist in decision making. Encourage grieving people to wait for several months to make major changes in their lives, as grief may affect their judgment. Because they are having difficulty sleeping and concentrating, stress the need to care for their physical health by eating properly, getting enough exercise, and postponing any elective procedures, as their immune system may be weak due to grief. Do what you can to be sure well-meaning friends and relatives do not hurry the bereaved to make critical decisions.

Denial

Sometimes it is beneficial to forget or deny. Denial is good for the short haul and individuals with cancer may try to forget their loss. When one sleeps at night one rests the body; and if one can forget for a time, one rests one's emotions as well. The person with cancer may attempt to resume normal activities in order to, at least for a time, forget; and as long as it does not interfere with individual treatment or safety, it can be beneficial.

If possible, physicians will schedule treatments around an important day in patients' lives to enable them to join in the festivities. This can be very beneficial for the emotional well-being of the patient and family. Important days may be a family gathering, a fishing trip, an anniversary, whatever the individual deems important. Reality sets in again very quickly for a grieving person, and this respite is remembered and talked about when times are hard.

Support groups

Many grieving people benefit by joining a support group. Many find comfort and acceptance in the company of those experiencing a similar illness. One need not make excuses for feelings or tears; the members of the group lend credibility and acceptance to both. Often other members of the group can give advice about particular problems. This advice is well received for it comes from someone going through a similar experience. Availability, locations, times, and types of support groups can be learned via local telephone books, local American Cancer Society offices, local churches, or other community organizations. It is helpful if times and locations are written down and given to someone who is grieving, for too often the bereaved individual does not have the energy or ability to get this information on his or her own.

Helping grieving people means being present during this painful period in their lives, listening to what they need to say, touching them meaningfully, and providing them some anticipatory guidance.

Grief following a sudden death

Although uncommon, there are times when an individual is diagnosed with cancer and dies suddenly. Individuals suffering the loss of a loved one through sudden death will experience shock and disbelief. They are cast into an unfamiliar world with little or no warning. There has been no time for final words, no rehearsal of "what if," no thoughts of how it would be when. . . . "The sudden death of a loved one can be viewed as a disaster, an unexpected event that has widespread effects."[15] Interventions to assist these survivors are similar to those for an anticipated death. The individuals may need to verbalize their feelings, have answers to their questions, have time to prepare themselves to view the body, have their immediate needs met, and be allowed unrestricted expression of their grief. They may also need sensitive assistance in making decisions.

Evaluation

It is difficult to evaluate whether interventions are helpful to the grieving individual, because grief has no specific timetable and is difficult to measure. The symptoms of grief will wax and wane. If, however, the patient expresses relief after sharing their feelings, if they are interested in joining a support group, if they more easily speak about their loss, sleep better, have more energy, and find their appetite has improved, they are moving through the grief process.

It is important that the patient understand that the feelings of loss may return again and again on their way through the grief process; but as time and grief work go on, they will eventually adjust and accommodate to the loss.

Education and Resources

Appendix 32A provides a self-care guide to assist individuals who are grieving. Some other resources are:

- *Taking Time*—booklet available from local American Cancer Society offices.
- *When Someone in Your Family Has Cancer*—booklet for children, available from local American Cancer Society offices.
- National Cancer Institute—the Cancer Information Network online at: www.cancernetwork.com

Support groups:

- Living with Cancer
- I Can Cope
- Make Today Count

Grief support groups—times, locations from:

- Local American Cancer Society office
- Local telephone book
- Social service department in hospital or clinic
- Local churches

Conclusion

When we have lost someone or something, we must grieve. Grief cannot be accelerated or avoided. Some people may want us to repress the emotions of grief. In some cultures and eras, a stoic philosophy has encouraged grievers to exhibit self-control. Being able to express emotions and feelings is a pathway through the grief process. Nurses can assist grieving people through this process by giving them permission to express the feelings and emotions inherent in grief and by stressing that grief is a normal, healthy reaction to a loss.

References

1. Peretz D: Development, object-relationships, and loss, in Schoenberg B, Carr AC, Peetz D, Kutscher AH (eds): *Loss and Grief: Psychological Management in Medical Practice.* New York: Columbia University Press, 1971, pp. 3–19
2. Staudacher C: *Men and Grief.* Oakland, CA: New Harbinger, 1991
3. Rando TA: *Grief, Dying and Death.* Champaign, IL: Research Press, 1984
4. Wolfeldt AD: Resolution versus reconciliation: The importance of semantics. *Thanatos* Winter:11–13, 1987
5. Eakes GG: Chronic sorrow: A response to living with cancer. *Oncol Nurs Forum* 20:1327–1334, 1993
6. Abrahm JL, Cooley M, Ricacho L: Efficacy of an educational bereavement program for families of veterans with cancer. *J Cancer Educ* 10:208–212, 1995
7. Worden WJ: *Grief Counseling and Grief Therapy: A Handbook for the Mental Health Practitioner* (ed 2). New York: Springer, 1991
8. Engel GL: Grief and grieving. *Am J Nurs* 64:93–98, 1964
9. Lindeman E: Symptomatology and management of acute grief. *Am J Psychiatry* 101:141–148, 1944
10. Horowitz MJ, Bonanno GA, Holen A: Pathologic grief: Diagnosis and explanation. *Psychosom Med* 55:260–273, 1993
11. Schneider JM: *Finding My Way: Healing and Transformation Through Loss.* Colfax, WI: 1994, p. 381
12. Robinson LA, Nuamah IF, Lev EL, et al: A prospective longitudinal investigation of spousal bereavement examining Parkes and Weiss' bereavement risk index. *J Palliat Care* 11:5–13, 1995
13. Montagu A: *Touching: The Human Significance of Skin.* New York: Columbia University Press, 1971
14. Colgrove M, Bloomfield HH, McWilliams P: *How to Survive the Loss of a Love.* Los Angeles: Prelude, 1991
15. Shneidman E: *Voices of Death.* New York: Harper & Row, 1980

Grief and Loss

Patient Name: _____

Symptom and Description   Since your loss, you may feel sad, lonely, fearful, angry, guilty, or you may have difficulty enjoying things. You may find it hard to talk to anyone about your loss. You are grieving—feeling the effects of a loss. It is normal and healthy for you to feel these things.

Learning Needs   There are some things you can do to make yourself feel better. First, you need to know that these feelings are normal and most people feel some of these things when they have had a loss:

- Loss of interest in things you used to enjoy
- Not able to concentrate
- Thinking a lot about your loss
- Feeling helpless
- Keeping to yourself
- Feeling guilty
- Anger
- Talking a lot about your loss
- Feeling like you are losing your mind
- Tight feeling in your throat
- Feeling like you can't breathe
- Empty feeling in your stomach
- No appetite
- Tired, lack of energy
- Cry easily

Management   Here are some of the things you can do to help yourself:

- Talk to your nurse, doctor, clergy, or friends
- Cry with someone or cry alone
- Join a support group—get times and dates from your nurse
- Talk to someone who has had a similar loss
- Get help from family or friends when making a decision
- Read about grief
- Pray or meditate
- Write down how you feel
- Go for walks
- Listen to music

(continued) 625

Follow-up   It is normal to grieve when you have lost someone or something. This includes loss of health, energy, strength, job, hair, or body parts. Talking to someone about your feelings can help. Please tell your nurse if you need help.

Phone Numbers

Nurse: _____ Phone: _____

Physician: _____ Phone: _____

Office/Hospital: _____ Phone: _____

Comments

Patient's Signature: _____ Date: _____

Nurse's Signature: _____ Date: _____

Source: Bourne V, Frogge MH: Grief, in Yarbro CH, Frogge MH, Goodman M (eds): *Cancer Symptom Management* (ed 2). Sudbury: Jones and Bartlett, 1999. © Jones and Bartlett Publishers.

CHAPTER 33

Saying Good-Bye

Michelle Goodman, RN, MS

The Problem of Saying Good-Bye

Too often and for many reasons, incurable patients traverse the cancer trajectory without much hint of what to expect. It may be because no one wants to say for sure what lies ahead, or because the patients make it clear that they do not want to know that a cure is not possible or that life will soon end. The person feels well for now, so why dwell on the inevitable? The problem with this approach is that when the time comes to make final decisions or to say good-bye, the patients are not well enough to perform these final acts as fully as they might have had they known sooner. There may be a sudden rush to make critical decisions that the individual is now too weak to make.

Consider a situation that happens often: As the patient labors to breathe and begins to die, a family member, not knowing what else to do, calls emergency 911. Suddenly the person is being rushed to the nearest emergency room where life-saving measures will begin. If the family and caregivers are prepared and the patient's wishes are known, this would be an unlikely scenario.

The argument is made that no one can say definitively when a person will die. Troubling is the fact that when a diagnosis of incurable cancer is given, patient and family tend to think in terms of years, not weeks or months. As healthcare professionals, we must be honest without destroying hope. Our challenge is to help the patient and family redefine hope, to express what is realistic and tangible. We cannot halt the course of nature, but we can help provide a better quality of death. A quality death cannot happen in an emergency room with the family expecting medical personnel to use all of medicine's life-sustaining abilities and machines to thwart the inevitable, at the same time unintentionally robbing their loved one of a peaceful, even painless death.

Too often, discussions regarding end of life are confined to textbooks and symposia and do not occur with patients and their families. Referrals to hospice care commonly occur within days or weeks of death and are often made primarily for necessary equipment (e.g., hospital bed or oxygen) and for pain control, that is, at a time when it is too late for the patient and family to benefit from all that hospice care can provide. All members of the cancer care team need to recognize that when cure is not possible, our responsibilities as caregivers are centered on quality of life. We need to ensure that a person's quality of death is given as much consideration as any treatment decision.

As nurses, we recognize points of transition in a patient's illness, where we can help patients and their families acknowledge that the disease is progressing and that there is not as much time left as they might think. This chapter describes ways in which the nurse can help patients begin to think more about end-of-life issues, how they want to be remembered, and how they want to say good-bye.

This chapter also demonstrates how the nurse-physician team can facilitate a timely referral to home care and a smooth transition to hospice care, if desired by the patient. It is not uncommon for patients to say good-bye, knowing they will not return to the ambulatory care

627

center/physician office, either because they have become too weak for treatment or because there is no suitable treatment. While all involved caregivers usually understand this departure, often appropriate referrals and suggestions for care in the home are not delivered to the patient in a way that invites clarification or discussion. Instead, the physician will tell patients that a "drug holiday" is recommended and that they should go home and get stronger. A hospice referral and a frank discussion concerning what the patient and family can expect is essential before the conclusion of active care in the office.

Acknowledging the end of treatment and formally saying good-bye is difficult for caregivers and family as well, especially if the patient does not initiate the discussion. Further, it is even more difficult if the physician has not communicated openly by helping the patient to understand that the disease is terminal and that death will happen soon. Unfortunately, without essential doctor-patient interactions on these subjects, there is less of a chance for the patient to make plans. This chapter addresses how the nurse can help the patient and family define what services and information they need concerning their end-of-life decisions and how, as caregivers, we might say good-bye more compassionately to our patients.

This chapter is written primarily for the oncology nurse caring for patients with cancer over an extended period of time, usually months or years. Because of the duration of this relationship between patient, family, and nurse, there exists a bond of trust, compassion, and even friendship. The nurse provides a needed link to all other medical disciplines and thus can coordinate various services to help meet the patient's needs. With sensitivity and diligence, nurses are able to identify the appropriate time to begin a dialogue about end-of-life issues with patients and their families. Discussing these issues reassures patients that when medical therapy no longer works they will not be abandoned, and that while a treatment may fail, it does not mean that they themselves have failed.

The Patients

Generally, there are four types of patients with cancer who may need assistance thinking about how to say good-bye or end-of-life issues: (1) the person who receives curative therapy over a defined time period; (2) the individual who has active, controlled disease but is temporarily in remission or suspending therapy for the time being; (3) the individual who receives treatment for control of symptoms of obvious disease; (4) the patient who is no longer undergoing active therapy and enters hospice care with less than 3 to 6 months to live.

Patients Receiving Curative Therapy

Patients who receive adjuvant therapy over weeks or months look forward to being cured of their disease and to resuming their usual activities. Still, it is not uncommon for patients who have finished treatment to want to mark this milestone in some meaningful way. Though a joyful time, finishing treatment can also be anxiety provoking—a time fraught with emotion and fear. While such patients may have established a close relationship with their nurse and doctor, understandably it may not be a relationship they wish to continue; they may feel torn. Patients will sometimes express feelings of despair and fear when finishing their adjuvant chemotherapy or radiation. While most patients usually feel relief at finally being finished with their cancer treatment, some may fear that the cancer might now grow unopposed.

Many patients say that receiving cancer treatment is one of the hardest things they have ever done. Completion of treatment may be coupled with a tremendous sense of accomplishment, but patients also may feel somewhat abandoned by their healthcare team, because they no longer need to return for weekly or monthly examinations. Reassure patients that they will continue to be monitored. Make a return appointment to the doctor for the patient, with the appropriate tests ordered, *before* the final treatment session. As well, give the patient the phone numbers of the healthcare team, and encourage he or her to call with any concerns. Mark a calendar with the 1-month anniversary of the patient's end of treatment, and follow-up with a phone call.

Recognize patients' concerns and accomplishments in a tangible way by giving them a small gift of closure such as a Survivor Kit. The Survivor Kit, designed by the nursing staff at the Rush Presbyterian St. Lukes Medical Center, Rush Cancer Institute (Chicago, IL), is shown in Table 33-1. The Survivor Kit is a yellow bag containing useful information from the National Coalition for Cancer Survivorship; a copy of *Cope*, a magazine; a T-shirt that says Carpe Diem ("seize the day") on the pocket; as well as any other information appropriate for the individual's particular disease site. Examples of disease-specific materials include a cancer survivor's pin (pink for breast cancer, clear for lung cancer, and silver for all other cancers), information about menopausal symptoms and osteoporosis for women who received chemotherapy that might trigger menopause or for women currently entering menopause, nutrition information, and an information booklet about leading a healthy life. The National Cancer Institute (NCI) booklet, "Facing Forward: A Booklet for Cancer Survivors," and *A Cancer Survivor's Almanac*, published in 1998 by the National Coalition for Cancer Survivorship, are valuable additions to the Survivor Kit.

Every effort should be made to personalize the Survivor Kit. For example, patients with head and neck cancer who have a long-term problem with xerostomia can be

TABLE 33-1 Survivor Kit

Description: The Survivor Kit is given to patients who complete their chemotherapy treatment, usually adjuvant chemotherapy for curative disease. It can also be given to patients receiving chemotherapy for more advanced disease who are in remission. The bag is bright yellow to symbolize hope. The kit can be adapted to any setting.

Contents: The contents of the bag are individualized and based on the personal needs of the patient. The idea is to be creative and hopeful. The following list includes several types of items that might be included in the Survivor Kit.

1. Guardian Angel Pin
2. Nutrition information—available from health food stores, the ACS and the NCI as well as from various pharmaceutical companies. Sometimes samples of nutritional supplements are included.
3. "Menopausal Symptoms and Management Strategies"—a self-care guide (Chapter 8) given to patients who are currently menopausal or who are menopausal due to therapy.
4. "Osteoporosis: Maintaining Healthy Bones"—a self-care guide (Chapter 8) given to men and women who are experiencing osteoporosis. Calcium supplements may be included if appropriate.
5. "Facing Forward"—NCI booklet for cancer survivors.
6. Cancer Patient's Bill of Rights—available from the National Coalition for Cancer Survivorship.
7. *A Cancer Survivor's Almanac*—available from the National Coalition for Cancer Survivorship.
8. Skin-care products—samples of skin-care products such as sunscreen are often available from pharmaceutical companies.
9. T-shirt with Carpe Diem printed on the pocket.
10. *Cope* magazine or *MAMM*—whichever is most appropriate for the patient.
11. Information on how to join the National Coalition for Cancer Survivorship.
12. "The seasons of survival: Reflections of a physician with cancer," *N Engl J Med* (July 25, 1985)
13. Cancer survivor's pin
14. Cancer support information specific to cancer type.

Funding: Funding for the Survivor Kit can come from a variety of sources, including private donations and donations from pharmaceutical companies; other funds may be available from nursing's contribution to institutional research.

ACS = American Cancer Society; NCI = National Cancer Institute.

given a water bottle or a sample of artificial saliva. Patients who have had extensive radiation therapy may have skin problems; for them, sample skin-care products are helpful. The most appreciated item in the Survivor Kit is the guardian angel pin. The primary nurse ceremoniously pins the angel on the patient, to recognize his or her accomplishment and to remind the patient that the nursing staff is always available and willing to help. Funding for the Survivor Kits can come from private donations or various nursing programs.

Patients Receiving Therapy for Control of Their Disease

These patients may work in or out of the home and do the things they want to do, with minimal limitations caused by the disease or the treatment. It may be difficult for such individuals to accept that they have metastatic disease, as most feel well and have only minor symptoms of advancing disease. Others may feel betrayed by their bodies, particularly if they received adjuvant therapy, thinking they were cured, only to have the disease recur or progress. Still others may have presented with metastatic disease, responded to therapy for a time, and now require another therapy to bring the disease under control.

Some people in the medical profession believe that patients intuitively know when their disease is no longer

curable. However, some patients believe that disease recurrence does not necessarily mean that they are incurable. For them, the recurrence means only that the first treatment did not work and that they must once again receive chemotherapy or radiation therapy. It is unreasonable for a nurse to surmise that patients know they are incurable. Patients in this situation may say, "We're going to get it this time." Professionals, on the other hand, may say that if patients want to know more about their prognosis, they will ask. Many patients do ask that but in a way that implies their desire to hear only the good news. For example, stating, "I hope this new chemo gets this cancer once and for all!" is different from asking, "Will this new treatment cure me of my cancer once and for all?"

For this patient population, it is appropriate for caregivers to support hope for controlling the disease because it is an important goal; however, we must be careful not to mislead patients into thinking that the disease will be cured. Most patients in this group eventually understand that cure is not an option. Their hope is based on thoughts of a miracle cure or something that will control the disease forever. While they understand that the disease may cause them to die, they are acutely aware that no one knows when this will occur. In other words, as long as they are not labeled "terminal," they are free to hope. Because it is too soon to broach the subject of dying, this seems reasonable.

For some patients, there may be many years of therapy, depending on the type of cancer and individual response. For this group, the process of saying good-bye may mean documenting their life experiences and experiences with cancer, establishing a legacy for children or grandchildren they may never know as adults.

Patients and their families are our best teachers. The following examples describe how some have chosen to say good-bye:

G. K. When G. K. was diagnosed with colon cancer, he received adjuvant therapy and was deemed cured. He felt his diagnosis was a wake-up call on life, and he began to live his life as if each day were his last. When he experienced a recurrence of the colon cancer, he was disappointed and somewhat fearful but not surprised. He felt that the best gift he could give his grandchildren was an appreciation of the belief that each day is a gift and that we must, whenever we can, "document time." G. K. elected to be treated. He was healthy and experienced only slight nausea and at times diarrhea from his chemotherapy. He was retired and spent as much time as possible with friends and family, especially his grandchildren. He documented this time with a handheld video camera. Later he edited the videos into movies as a way to teach those younger and as a way to live on in the minds of those he left behind. G. K. chose one movie in particular to be played at his funeral.

M. L. M. L. had a 9-year-old daughter, and she knew she would not see her grow up. M. L. was 34 when she was first diagnosed with breast cancer, and after two failed bone marrow transplants she responded to herceptin therapy for 14 months. Gradually, M. L. experienced a resurgence of the disease. Over a 4-year period, M. L. said she experienced denial, anger, and resentment but never fear or pity. She felt her husband would do okay once she was gone. Her main concern was her daughter Lisa. While she loved her husband very much, she knew she would say good-bye to him and he would understand. Saying good-bye to her daughter was going to be much harder. She thought about making videos of herself speaking to her daughter but feared they might interfere with Lisa's ability to establish a close relationship with a new stepmother should her husband remarry. She chose instead to write letters for Lisa to open at certain times. The envelopes had titles, examples of which are included here:

- *Birthday.* There was a letter for each of Lisa's birthdays for the next 10 years. Each envelope had a picture of the two of them together in the previous 10 years, in descending order. Each described what they were doing on that day and her hopes for Lisa during the coming year.
- *Graduation.* There was a letter for Lisa to open when she graduated from grade school, high school, and a letter about how to choose the right college.

- *Ordinary days and special occasions.* She had letters for Lisa to open entitled, "Open if you are sad," or "Open if you are angry." There was also one for her wedding day.

These letters were M. L.'s way of helping to ease the pain that came in knowing she would not be there while her daughter was growing up. They gave her a way of making the best of the days she had with her daughter. She gave the letters to her husband to give to her daughter at the various times, if he felt it was appropriate.

Hollis: Patients sometimes use the arts to express their feelings about their illness, what the treatments mean to them, and the anger they feel when treatments fail to work. An excellent example of one's use of the arts to express the devastating experience of breast cancer is the work of Hollis Sigler, a professional artist. In 1998, her disease spread to her bone and bone marrow, thereby affecting her ability to produce white blood cells and platelets. She became so weak that she could only paint in bed. In one painting in the collection, there are flasks of blood carried by winged hands as gifts to sustain her. In another, she painted trees with pairs of shoes for leaves signifying her fatigue and inability to do what used to be so simple such as walk, run, and dance. Another painting expresses the ever-present nature of death. Death is a black dress hovering over a room decorated with balloons. Hollis's paintings are a gift to us; they are her unique way of saying good-bye. Pictures of these paintings may be used by the cancer-care team to help prompt patients to express their feelings about the terminal nature of their illness. Her paintings and drawings can be viewed in galleries and museums around the country.

As nurses caring for patients who have controlled disease, there is a transition point where the disease begins to be more resistant and each therapeutic attempt provides less in the way of tumor response and consequently time. If patients have not begun to talk about how the news of more disease or recurrence might affect their future, it is important that you communicate your desire to help in a meaningful way if they want to talk about it.

For example: You and the doctor are looking at an x-ray of a 48-year-old woman with metastatic disease of the lung. According to the previous film, the disease is not much better following three courses of chemotherapy. The woman appears to have chemotherapy-resistant disease, and although she is being offered another combination of drugs, the outcome is not expected to produce a complete response. Her reaction when she is told that the chemotherapy is not working as well as expected and that she need to switch to something else is, "Well, this one will just have to work because I am *not* giving up!" She is crying, clearly afraid, but hopeful and trying to be brave. The nurse in this situation takes her cues from the patient. Sometimes it is best to simply ask, "Do you feel like you want to talk about it?" Or, "Have you thought about how you want to tell your family?"

While teaching about a new drug combination, there is often an opportunity to ask the patient if she has thought about how her family will respond to this new development. If there are children and depending on their ages, it may be helpful to offer literature on how to talk to them about cancer and its treatment. Most of the literature is quite good, and it stresses honesty. As time passes, the patient might wish to see a family social worker or a psycho-oncologist to discuss family issues in light of the severity of her illness. It is important for the mother to explain to the children that they did nothing wrong to make her ill; no matter what their fears, the children are not to blame.

Such conversations are difficult to initiate, especially where children are concerned. We must be sympathetic with the patient, but we also must have a well-thought plan and a specific way of helping. We are obviously there to support hope in any way we can. One way we can do this is to help the patient set realistic goals for the future.

The nursing staff at the Rush Cancer Institute in Chicago gives patients a journal to document their experiences and personal responses to treatment. Some patients use it as one might use a diary, to document how they are feeling. Others use the journal as a means to tell their story from the time they were diagnosed with cancer. They write about their response to treatment and the manner in which they and their family are able to cope. For one man, the journal became the only way for him to describe his feelings. He revealed the details of his experiences throughout his illness. Without pen and paper, he felt incapable of expressing his feelings.

Patients Who May or May Not Be Receiving Therapy for Control of Their Symptoms

This group of individuals includes those who have incurable disease and for whom the goal of therapeutic intervention is palliation of their symptoms. Some patients may be working, usually only part-time due to limitations caused by their disease. While many such patients may be receiving active therapy, it is obvious to most that they are quickly running out of treatment options and that the disease is progressing. Regardless, these individuals usually remain quite hopeful and can require considerable assistance in addressing end-of-life issues.

In the past few years, tremendous strides have been made in our understanding of end-of-life issues and the challenges faced by cancer survivors whose disease is no longer controlled and whose death is certain. Many cancer care professionals are uncomfortable and unprepared to talk to patients about the implications of a lack of response to treatment. These healthcare professionals are unable to bridge the gap between accurately in-forming the patient of his/her condition and fear that the truth may be too painful or too difficult.

In 1997, Dr. Roger Bone died from renal cell carcinoma. During the last year of his life, he became profoundly aware that within the medical community the needs of those with serious, life-threatening illnesses were not being met as well as they should be. He wrote a book entitled, *Reflections: A Guide to End-of-Life Issues for You and Your Family,* an example of how a person can write about their experiences, confronting his or her own destiny while helping others to do the same. The book is intended to help patients and their family members identify what they need to address as the end of life approaches, and how to go about getting the help they need. A well-written and useful guide, this book assists patients with questions concerning how to say good-bye. It is available through the National Kidney Cancer Foundation. (Call 800-850-9132 for more information.)

As stated earlier, we can inform the patient about disease progression without destroying hope. We can reassure them that we will continue to care for them and to manage their symptoms and that a temporary cessation of therapy or a referral to hospice care does not mean we are abandoning them. An illness progression and needs assessment tool might be useful to determine patients' level of understanding about their illness, their understanding of the control/palliative nature of therapy, and the appropriateness of any community referrals. (See Appendix 33A: Illness Progression and Needs Assessment Tool.)

Often, patients will ask questions of the nurse instead of their doctor, and they usually initiate a dialogue about the terminal nature of their illness when they are ready. Respond with sensitivity to any questions, as patients may not wish or be prepared to hear a lot of detail. For example, when a patient asks, "How long am I going to have to take this chemotherapy?" The answer is usually, "For as long as it helps you, and we hope that is a very long time." The dialogue may end there, or it may continue as the patient asks, "Do you mean I am going to have to have chemotherapy for the rest of my life?" When it seems clear that the patient is seeking information regarding the course of his or her illness and issues concerning the end of their life, do not brush it off with false assurance; rather, establish a plan to help the individual gain more information.

Asking patients if they want to discuss these issues further, possibly with their doctor, is a first step toward active information gathering aimed at increasing understanding. Help the patient prepare for a meeting with the physician, and inform the physician when such a discussion is planned because it usually takes more time than is allotted. Propose to the patient that they complete the Physician Conference Worksheet (see Appendix 33B). Be aware that the patient may decide to reject the plan at any point, and that is fine. The dialogue has begun and that is the first step.

Four-step plan to information gathering

1. Establish the appointment Begin with a scheduled appointment with the physician or delegate, with all parties aware of the visit's intent. Too often, a family member will stop the physician in the hall and confidentially ask how the patient is *really* doing. Or, the nurse may page the doctor to come speak with the patient, without adequately informing the doctor of the nature of the visit and without the patient being prepared with the appropriate family support or having important questions outlined. Often patients will have questions about advanced directives, durable power of attorney, or hospice care. If the physician knows the intent of the meeting, such information can be gathered and made available to the patient and family. If the physician does not feel the family needs to be present for this meeting and wishes to assign someone such as the nurse or resident physician to ensure the patient's needs are met, this is acceptable as long as the patient agrees.

2. Establish the intent of the meeting What does the patient want to accomplish as a result of meeting with the physician? Encourage patients to write down their questions and to share them with family members or whomever will be attending the meeting. The nurse can facilitate further dialogue by encouraging the patient to ask family members if they have any questions to add to the list.

Some may find it difficult to ask questions in such a formal setting because they are afraid of the answers or they want to protect others. As such, most patients and family members prefer to ask less specific, less pointed questions. Questions like "How's my husband doing, Doc?" are a lot different from, "Our daughter is getting married in 3 months, do you think we should move up the wedding?"

Most patients are seeking reassurance that they are doing fine. Unless both patient and family can identify and agree on the intent of the meeting, it is probably best not to schedule it. However, even in such a situation, the dialogue has begun, which is most important. Do not dwell on gaining information concerning the death and the dying process, unless the patient is ready. Instead, engage the patient and family in conversation about what additional services are available should they be needed. Answer questions honestly, and explain what can be expected over time. Provide reassurance that you will help patient when they are ready. Listening to their concerns and answering their questions are appropriate nursing actions.

3. Who should attend the meeting? A meeting without the patient is usually not appropriate. A durable power of attorney, if selected, should attend the meeting. In addition, the patient should indicate whom they wish to attend. The nurse might suggest that the patient consider inviting others who might be helpful in planning

for the future. For example, clergy, a social worker, or hospice representative. (See Appendix 33A.)

4. Document the events of the meeting Someone should be available to record the remarks and suggestions of those present at the meeting. It is a stressful time, and often important points are missed. Having questions and concerns written down beforehand and using them as the agenda for the meeting is a useful way to keep track of what is said. Once the meeting is over, the individual documenting the meeting might want to provide a written summary for those present and note where additional information might be needed and how this information might be obtained. For example, the patient may be seeking home care, a hospice referral, or information concerning alternative methods of treatment.

Planning and preparation

Informing patients about their illness enables them to ask questions, to make plans, and to prepare their families for a future without them. The time for patients to learn that their disease has progressed beyond cure is not after they have brain metastases or are confined to a wheelchair or bed. Rather, the time to inform the patient of their incurability is when the physician knows this to be true. What makes this communication difficult for both physician and patient is the fact that the patient may appear quite healthy at the time.

If patients want to create any memories for those they love, it is best for them to begin while they are still able, when they are in control and able to do what they want. Most people would not change their life from what they do every day if they knew they had a fatal illness, but this is a personal choice.

Once patients understand their situations, the nurse can help them identify future goals in a positive and constructive manner. Such a conversation might revolve around the self-care guide called, Tips on Tasks (Appendix 33C), which centers on what one needs to do to put one's affairs in order. The patient and family may be able to identify tasks that require attention and to make decisions concerning what needs to be done to help create a smooth transition when the patient dies, and to ensure that the individual's wishes are met.

The nurse can encourage the patient to let others help in any way they can. Unfortunately, as patients become progressively weaker, possibly even confined to bed, their immediate family oftentimes is becoming fatigued and less able to help. At the same time, fewer friends may be stopping by to help. Encourage family members and friends to help in any way and for as long as they are able. Often, those who want to help do not know how to help. In such instances, encourage the patient or family members to take some initiative and tell the friend exactly what they need. For example, when someone says, "If you ever need me to car pool, just let me know," say "How about Tuesdays?" instead of just saying, "Thanks,

I'll let you know." People appreciate the sincerity of such a request and will feel a part of the individual's life, just knowing that they are helping in a meaningful way. Not having a tangible way of helping can make friends feel helpless, and the patient may suffer some loneliness. Seasons Hospice Park, Inc., Ridge, IL has compiled a list of 25 practical tips individuals can use to help those facing a serious illness (see Appendix 33D).

Patients Entering Hospice Care

The opportunity for staff to say good-bye to those being referred to hospice needs to be scheduled in what might be termed a "closure interview" (see Appendix 33E). Without such an interview, saying good-bye might be nothing more than a tearful hug in the hall. Most physicians know when a referral to hospice care is appropriate, although most wait too long to make the referral. When the referral is made to hospice care, the nurse, either with the physician or following the physician's consultation, conducts the closure interview with the patient and family.

The purpose of the closure interview is to permit the patient, family, and healthcare team to express feelings about the care rendered and to identify patient needs for hospice care or care in the home. This is an opportunity for the nurse and any other members of the healthcare team to be certain the needs of the patient and family are adequately identified and that measures are taken to ensure a smooth transition to the hospice or home environment. A copy of the closure interview is then sent to the referral agency and given to the patient, along with appropriate referrals, phone numbers, and prescriptions.

Benefits of Saying Good-Bye

Dying from a chronic illness gives a person an opportunity to say good-bye, whereas death due to sudden, unforeseen events robs an individual of the opportunity to set things right or to do or say whatever is necessary. The timing of saying good-bye is a real challenge—it may be said too soon or, for some, it may be said too late. Why, then, do so many people fail to acknowledge that they are dying and not take steps to help ease the burden of those they are leaving behind?

Saying good-bye is a loving act of kindness. It puts closure on a relationship and gives people the opportunity to forgive and others the opportunity to grow. Saying good-bye allows individuals to decide how they want to be remembered and gives others permission to express their feelings, needs, and concerns regarding the person who is dying. Who better to discuss it with? This process also encourages family and friends to express their feelings, either among themselves or in the presence of the individual, about what life will be like without their loved one.

For persons who are dying, saying good-bye helps them find peace with what cannot be controlled and gives them a chance to contribute to the family's growth, even when they are no longer there. It helps individuals feel as if they have helped others in the grieving process. Saying good-bye helps the family talk about their feelings and, in turn, helps the person to express his or her feelings and fears about dying. It may also help caregivers quell those fears.

Having an opportunity to discuss feelings about dying helps patients know that they have been honest; they can therefore worry less about how the family members will react to their death. Talking openly about dying with members of the healthcare team and family members helps remove the perception that the patient is somehow being deceived or that others are not truthful.

Ideally, a person should learn that his or her time to feel healthy is limited before being impaired in any way by the illness or by the treatment. Communicating this information is difficult, because it is rarely obvious to the individual. Some will become angry; others will lose hope. Avoiding the topic or trying to protect the patient is not the right thing to do, nor it is fair. Patients must be informed of the status of their illness. Many people are stronger and braver than the medical profession and often their families perceive them to be.

While it rarely seems appropriate to say that a patient has only a finite number of months to live, it is equally unfair to withhold such information if it seems certain that the disease will likely cause incapacitation in a few months, particularly when having such information may prompt the individual to do something significantly different with that time.

For example, Susie had three children ages 3, 5, and 8 whom she cared for with the help of her husband and her mother-in-law. She had metastatic breast cancer for about 1 year, and while she was responding well to the chemotherapy, it was known that she was would eventually stop responding. The subject was not discussed with her until she was found to have brain metastases. She was receiving radiation and steroids and had become confined to a wheelchair because of bone metastases in her spine. She wanted to know what this meant now that she had brain involvement. Did it mean she wouldn't walk again? She said this was okay, as long as it meant she could live to see her children grow up. Susie died about 8 months later. It was particularly sad because had she known she was not going to be rid of the cancer, she could have made videos for her children before she became debilitated by the steroids and her disease. She was too weak and did not want her children to see her this way when the video idea was suggested. Writing was too difficult for her, and a computer was too impersonal. With the help of her mother-in-law, she was able to complete a number of family albums. She died without sufficient time to build the type of memories she wanted for her children. Without a doubt, she would have done things differently had she known sooner that her disease would be so incapacitating.

Is it reasonable for the physician to delay such conversations unless asked directly? As caregivers, we know such discussions take a lot of time, and we know that what we say will make the patient sad. Being able to offer only our good intentions and palliative measures, this is a difficult task. Sometimes we will feel ill-equipped to comfort our patients appropriately, but that should not stop us from trying.

A particularly troubling situation occurs when the patient is realistic about the situation and the limited time available, while the family or the significant other is unwilling to suspend therapy or accept hospice. Often, the family convinces the patient to accept therapy that the patient might not have elected without the urging of the family. This apparent lack of understanding may stem from the family members not being involved with the patient's routine care, doctor's visits, and the person's illness over time. Frequently, this is seen with grown children who have not seen their parent in 6 months and now want to know why nothing is being done to help him or her. In such situations, be aware of the patient's wishes and encourage him or her not to be persuaded into doing something else unless it is a personal choice. Involving family members at all levels of discussion and especially during visits to the doctor is beneficial. If the family member lives far away and is unable to visit regularly and participate in the care of the patient, ask the patient if it is all right to phone and update the family member after each visit. Family members will need extra time individually to sort through all the information, which for them will likely be overwhelming, particularly if they have not been a part of the loved one's illness until a more terminal phase.

Another common situation is the husband who is at the wife's side for every visit and every treatment but who cannot accept his wife's stopping therapy. Even though his wife is clearly exhausted and requesting a quality of life that does not include chemotherapy, he resists this option. If possible, try to assess or evaluate early on which patients or family members might respond this way. It is advisable to start patient and spouse or significant other in a support group or in counseling with a trained psycho-oncologist, to begin the anticipatory grieving process and to ensure they are as knowledgeable as they can be concerning the patient's circumstance.

Conclusion

Persons with cancer need help to begin the process of saying good-bye to those close to them and to consider what they need to do personally to put their affairs in order. Cancer care professionals need to recognize that they may need to say good-bye to patients who have finished their therapy and are essentially cured, temporarily ending therapy, or entering hospice. Whatever the phase of survival, patients leaving the care environment need to mark the event in a meaningful way. In some situations, the event may be a cause for celebration, as would be appropriate for someone who is finishing adjuvant therapy; or, the event may be sad, as the cancer can no longer be controlled and the patient must enter hospice care. As nurses and caregivers, we need to learn how to say good-bye compassionately to patients with cancer and, more importantly, to help patients begin to talk of end-of-life issues, how they want to be remembered, and how they can say good-bye to their loved ones.

Illness Progression and Needs Assessment Tool

Patient Name: _____

The purpose of this chart is to assist you, with the help of your nurse, to identify the level of your understanding of your illness and any resources and referrals you might find helpful.

Step 1 Circle the statement that best describes your understanding of your illness.

My cancer is well controlled.	I have pain.	I know my cancer is worse, but I	I understand that my cancer
I have symptoms and do not require	I am not able to eat.	have faith that I can still be cured.	cannot be cured, and I have
any referrals at this time.	I know little about my illness.		only a short time to live.

Other: _____

Step 2 Circle all of the options for assistance that you would like to discuss with your nurse and doctor.

Nutrition	Hospice	Social services	Legal help	Financial help	Alternative therapies
	Sexual counseling		Meals at home	Nurse aide at home		Equipment for my home
Support groups	Spiritual counseling	Pain management	Physical therapy	Insurance information	Handicapped parking permit
	Home oxygen	Sleep	Fatigue	Information about Advanced Directives/Living Will

Step 3 Would you like to have a discussion regarding your health with your doctor?   Yes ____   (see Physician Conference Worksheet, Appendix 33B)   No, not at this time ____

Comments _____

Patient's Signature: _____   Date: _____

Nurse's Signature: _____   Date: _____

Source: Goodman M: Saying good-bye, in Yarbro CH, Frogge MH, Goodman M (eds): *Cancer Symptom Management* (ed 2). Sudbury: Jones and Bartlett, 1999. © Jones and Bartlett Publishers.

Physician Conference Worksheet

Patient Name: _____ Appointment Date: _____ Time: _____

Physician Informed _____ by _____

Delegate Assigned _____

Intent/Goal of the meeting:

1. _____

2. _____

3. _____

Who should attend the meeting?

1. _____ Phone: _____

2. _____ Phone: _____

3. _____ Phone: _____

4. _____ Phone: _____

Questions to ask:

1. _____

Answer _____

_____

2. _____

Answer _____

_____

3. _____

Answer _____

4. _____

Answer _____

_____

Comments:

Patient's Signature: _____ Date: _____

Nurse's Signature: _____ Date: _____

Source: Goodman M: Saying good-bye, in Yarbro CH, Frogge MH, Goodman M (eds): *Cancer Symptom Management* (ed 2). Sudbury: Jones and Bartlett, 1999. © Jones and Bartlett Publishers.

Tips on Tasks: Thoughts on End-of-Life Concerns

Patient Name: _____

Description   This guide is organized around a series of tasks that may be important for you to consider as you approach the end of your life. You might want to discuss the different questions and concerns with your family members. They may have ideas and concerns they wish to discuss with you.

    As you address each area, jot down your thoughts and decisions. You may have identified someone in the family that you would like to assume responsibility for one task or another. Make a note of this, and be sure to include them in your decision making. Remember, everyone usually wants to help but does not know how to help. It is your job to tell or show them how they can be helpful. You may not have the energy to complete certain tasks, but you can still be involved.

1. Is my life insurance policy paid at least 6 months into the future?

Yes ☐

No ☐

Assign to: _____

Insurance policy location: _____

_____

2. Have I informed members of my family of my condition?

Yes ☐

No ☐

Contact: _____

_____

Action: _____

_____

Assign to: _____

3. Should I consult with a patient service organization, social worker, or lawyer?

Yes ☐

No ☐

Plan: _____

Assign to: _____

4. Should I consult with a hospice representative?

Yes ☐

No ☐

Assign to: _____

Notes: _____

5. Have I discussed current financial situation and status of bill payment with spouse or other family member?

Yes ☐

No ☐

Action: _____

_____

Assign to: _____

_____

Notes: _____

_____

_____

For medical bills, contact: _____

Accountant: _____

6. Do I need a Durable Power of Attorney?

Yes ☐

No; I have one. ☐

Name: _____

Phone: _____

Need more information: _____

Assign to: _____

7. Do I need a Living Will?

Yes ☐

No; I have one. ☐   No I do not need one. ☐

I have one but need to distribute it. ☐

Assign to: _____

8. Have I provided adequate information to my family concerning their financial planning, establishing a will, death benefits, and trust funds?

Yes ☐

No ☐

Action: _____

Assign to: _____

9. What do I want to happen the last few days of my life?

_____

_____

_____

10. Where do I want to die?

Home: _____ Hospital: _____ In-patient Hospice: _____

Comments: _____

_____

11. Are the appropriate funeral arrangements made?

No ☐   Assign to: _____

Yes ☐   Describe: _____

      Funeral home: _____

      Phone number: _____

      Contact person: _____

Cemetery: _____

      Plot purchased: No ☐   Yes ☐

      Comment: _____

      Plan: _____

_____

12. If cremation is planned, what do I want done with my ashes?

Describe: _____

Assign to: _____

13. Do I want flowers sent, or do I want contributions sent to the charity/ organization of my choosing?

Describe: _____

_____

Assign to: _____

Comments

Patient's Signature: _____ Date: _____

Nurse's Signature: _____ Date: _____

Source: Goodman M: Saying good-bye, in Yarbro CH, Frogge MH, Goodman M (eds): _Cancer Symptom and Management_ (ed 2). Sudbury: Jones and Bartlett, 1999. © Jones and Bartlett Publishers.

Practical Ways for Family and Friends to Be Helpful

Patient Name: _____

I have a serious illness and, like most people, find it hard to ask others for help. Because you asked about ways you could help me and my family, I am passing this list of ideas along. I appreciate your help and thank you in advance for all you are able to do for me and my family.

1. Don't avoid me. Be the friend, the loved one you've always been.

2. Touch me. A simple squeeze of the hand tells me you still care.

3. Call and tell me you're bringing over my favorite dish. Bring food in disposable containers so I won't worry about returning them.

4. Watch my children while I take a little time to be alone with my loved one. My children may also need a vacation from my illness.

5. Cry with me when I cry, and laugh with me when I laugh. Don't be afraid to share these emotions with me. Pain isolates. Help me reconnect with others.

6. Take me out for a pleasure trip, but know my limitations.

7. Call for my shopping list, and make a special delivery to my home.

8. Before you visit, call to let me know, but don't be afraid to visit. I need you. I can get lonely.

9. Help me celebrate holidays (and life) by decorating my hospital room or home, or by bringing me flowers or other natural treasures.

10. Help my family. Invite them out. Take them places. I am sick, but they may be suffering too. Offer to come and stay with me to give my loved ones a break.

11. Be creative. Bring me a book of reflections, taped music, a poster for my wall, cookies to share with my family and friends.

12. Let's talk about it. Maybe I need to talk about my illness. Find out by asking, "Do you feel like talking about it?"

13. Don't always feel we have to talk. Sitting quietly together is fine. Your presence confirms that I am still important and alive.

14. Can you take me and/or my children somewhere? I may need transportation to a treatment, to the store, or to my physician.

15. Help me feel good about myself.

16. Please include me in decision making. I've been robbed of so many things. Please don't deny me a chance to make decisions in my family and in my life.

17. Talk to me about the future. Tomorrow, next week, next year. Hope is so important to me.

18. Bring a positive attitude. It's catching. Help me respect reality.

19. What's in the news? Magazines, photos, newspapers, and verbal reports keep me from feeling like the world is passing me by.

20. Could you help me with some chores? During my illness, my family and I still face dirty clothes, dirty dishes, and a dirty house.

21. Water my flowers.

22. Just send a card to let me know you care.

23. Pray for me and share your faith with me.

24. Tell me how you'd like to help me and when I agree, please do so.

25. Tell me about support groups, so I can share with others.

Reprinted with permission of Seasons Hospice, Inc., Park Ridge, IL, 1998.

Source: Goodman M: Saying good-bye, in Yarbro CH, Frogge MH, Goodman M (eds): *Cancer Symptom Management* (ed 2). Sudbury: Jones and Bartlett, 1999. © Jones and Bartlett Publishers.

Closure Interview

Patient Name: _____ Address: _____

Phone: _____ Appointment date/time: _____

The purpose of this meeting is to identify any possible needs and services you may require in your home and to make referrals for these services. We would also like to talk about your experiences in this healthcare setting and give those present an opportunity to celebrate having known you and your family. We also want to assure you that we are available to assist you and your family at any time if the need arises.

Who would you like to attend?

1. _____
2. _____
3. _____
4. _____
5. _____
6. _____

What services can we establish for you in your home?

Referral: _____ Phone: _____ Done_____ Date: _____

Referral: _____ Phone: _____ Done_____ Date: _____

Referral: _____ Phone: _____ Done_____ Date: _____

Do you currently have hospice care in your home?   No ☐   Yes ☐

Name: _____

Phone: _____

Would you like to have hospice care in your home?   No ☐   Yes ☐

Preferred hospice: _____

Phone: _____

No preference ☐

Medication list:

Drug	Dosage	Schedule	Number of Refills	Comments

Copy sent to referral agency: Yes ☐   No ☐

Comments

Patients's Signature: _____ Date: _____

Nurse's Signature: _____ Date: _____

Source: Goodman M: Saying good-bye, in Yarbro CH, Frogge MH, Goodman M (eds): *Cancer Symptom Management* (ed 2). Sudbury: Jones and Bartlett, 1999. © Jones and Bartlett Publishers.

Index

Note: Page numbers followed by f indicate figures; those followed by t indicate tables.